Cholesterol and Coronary Heart Disease

The Great Debate

Cholesterol and Coronary Heart Disease

The Great Debate

The Proceedings of an International Workshop held at Hilton Head Island, South Carolina, USA

EDITED BY:

Phil Gold M.D.
McGill University, Montreal

Steven Grover M.D.
McGill University, Montreal

Daniel A.K. Roncari M.D.
University of Toronto, Toronto

Published in association with
Kush Medical Communications
(Division of Pharma Com International, Inc.) by

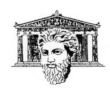

The Parthenon Publishing Group
International Publishers in Medicine, Science & Technology

Casterton Hall, Carnforth,
Lancs, LA6 2LA, UK

120 Mill Road, Park Ridge,
New Jersey 07656, USA

This International Workshop was held under the
auspices of McGill University, Montréal, Sunnybrook
Health Science Centre, Toronto and The University of
Calgary, Calgary and made possible through an educational
grant from the Dairy Bureau of Canada.

Published in the UK by
The Parthenon Publishing Group Limited
Casterton Hall, Carnforth,
Lancs, LA6 2LA, UK

Published in the USA by
The Parthenon Publishing Group Inc.
120 Mill Road,
Park Ridge,
New Jersey 07656, USA

ISBN 1-85070-414-7

Lasertypeset by Martin Lister Publishing Services, Carnforth, Lancs. UK

Contents

Section II. Atherosclerosis and Atherogenesis

Section III. Dietary Cholesterol and Fatty Acids in Health and Disease

Contents

List of Participants

CHAIRMAN:

Phil Gold, CC, MD, PhD, FRCP(C), FACP
Physician-in-Chief
Montreal General Hospital
Director, McGill University Medical Clinic
Douglas G. Cameron Professor
Department of Medicine
Professor, Department of Physiology
Faculty of Medicine
McGill University
Montréal, Québec, Canada

CO-CHAIRMEN:

Steven A. Grover, MD, MPA, FRCP(C)
Director, Centre for Cardiovascular Risk Assessment
Montreal General Hospital
Assistant Professor, Departments of Medicine, Epidemiology and Biostatistics
McGill University
Montréal, Québec, Canada

Daniel A.K. Roncari, MD, PhD, FACP, FRCPC
Physician-in-Chief
Sunnybrook Health Science Centre
Professor of Medicine
University of Toronto
Toronto, Ontario, Canada

PARTICIPANTS:

Paul Bradley Addis, PhD
Professor
Department of Food Science and Nutrition
College of Agriculture and College of Human Ecology
University of Minnesota
St. Paul, Minnesota, USA

Keaven M. Anderson, PhD
Research and Development Division
Centocor, Inc.
Malvern, Pennsylvania, USA

Pierre Budowski, PhD
Professor (Emeritus)
Faculty of Agriculture
The Hebrew University of Jerusalem
Rehovot, Israel

M.T. (Tom) Clandinin, PhD
Professor
Departments of Foods & Nutrition and Medicine
Nutrition and Metabolism Research Group
Faculty of Medicine
University of Alberta
Edmonton, Alberta, Canada

William E. Connor, MD
Professor of Medicine
Head, Section of Clinical Nutrition and Lipid Metabolism
Oregon Health Sciences University
Portland, Oregon, USA

John M. Dietschy, MD
The Jan and Henri Bromberg
Professor and Chief –
Gastroenterology
University of Texas
Southwestern Medical Center
Dallas, Texas, USA

Micheline de Belder
Chief Dietician
Institut de Cardiologie de Montréal
Montréal, Québec, Canada

Ian F. Godsland, BA
Research Director
Wynn Institute for Metabolic
Research
London, United Kingdom

Richard B. Goldbloom, OC, MD
Professor of Paediatrics
Faculty of Medicine
Dalhousie University
Director of Ambulatory Services
IWK Children's Hospital
Halifax, Nova Scotia, Canada

K.C. Hayes
Professor of Biology (Nutrition)
Director, Foster Biomedical
Research Laboratories
Brandeis University
Waltham, MS, USA

Bruce J. Holub, PhD
Professor
Chair, Nutrition Research
Centre for Health Promotion and
Disease Prevention
Department of Nutritional Sciences
University of Guelph
Guelph, Ontario, Canada

Louis Horlick, MD, FRCP(C), FACP
Professor of Medicine (Emeritus)
Department of Medicine
University of Saskatchewan
Royal University Hospital
Saskatoon, Saskatchewan, Canada

Christopher G. Isles
Consulting Physician
Department of Medicine
Dumfries and Galloway Royal
Infirmary
Dumfries, Scotland

Martijn B. Katan, PhD
Professor of Human Nutrition
Department of Human Nutrition
Wageningen Agricultural University
Wageningen, The Netherlands

Stan Kubow, PhD
Assistant Professor
School of Dietetics and Human
Nutrition
Macdonald Campus of McGill
University
Ste. Anne de Bellevue
Québec, Canada

Hélène Laurendeau
Consulting Dietician
Montréal
Québec, Canada

Sheila Murphy
Consulting Dietician
Montréal
Québec, Canada

Cyril R. Nair
Chief, Health Care Statistics
Associate Editor, Health Reports
Canadian Centre for Health
Information Statistics
Ottawa, Ontario, Canada

Mahamed Navab, PhD
Associate Research Cardiologist
Division of Cardiology
UCLA School of Medicine
Los Angeles, California, USA

C. David Naylor, MD, DPhil, FRCP(C)
  Director, Division of
  Clinical Epidemiology Unit and
    Department of Medicine
  Sunnybrook Health Science Centre
  University of Toronto
  Toronto, Ontario, Canada

Howard Parsons, MD, FRCPC
  Associate Professor of Paediatrics
  University of Calgary
  Health Sciences Centre
  Calgary, Alberta, Canada

Emil Skamene, MD, PhD, FRCP(C), FACP
  Professor of Medicine
  McGill University
  Director, McGill Centre for the
    Study of Host Resistance
  Montréal, Québec, Canada

Petr Skrabanek, PhD
  Senior Lecturer
  Department of Community Health
  Trinity College
  University of Dublin
  Dublin, Ireland

William E. Stehbens, MD, D Phil
  Professor of Pathology
  Wellington School of Medicine
  Wellington Hospital
  Newtown, Wellington, New Zealand

Micheline Ste-Marie, MD, FRCP(C)
  Associate Professor
  Department of Paediatrics
  Faculty of Medicine
  Dalhousie University
  Chair, Canadian Paediatric Society
    Nutrition Committee
  IWK Hospital for Children
  Halifax, Nova Scotia, Canada

Hirotsugo Ueshima, MD
  Head and Professor
  Department of Health Science
  Shiga University of Medical Science
  Shiga, Japan

Gloria Lena Vega, PhD
  Associate Professor
  Department of Clinical Nutrition
    and Center for Human Nutrition
  University of Texas
  Southwestern Medical Center
  Dallas, Texas, USA

Kenneth F. Walker, MD, FRCPC
  (alias W. Gifford-Jones)
  Gynecologist and Medical Journalist
  The Toronto Hospital
  Toronto, Ontario, Canada

Randall Wood, PhD
  Professor
  Biochemistry and Nutrition
  Texas A & M University
  College Station, Texas, USA

Katsuhiko Yano, MD
  Senior Investigator
  The Honolulu Heart Program
  Honolulu, Hawaii, USA

Philip L. Yeagle, PhD
  Department of Biochemistry
  University at Buffalo School of
    Medicine
  State University of New York
  Buffalo, New York, USA

Foreword

An International Workshop on Fats and Cholesterol was recently held in Hilton Head, South Carolina, USA, in order to allow experts from around the world in the fields of epidemiology, pathology, cardiology, biochemistry, lipid chemistry and nutrition to discuss the role of dietary cholesterol and animal fat in coronary heart disease.

The opinion that a high cholesterol/fat diet is one of the major environmental agents responsible for the elevation of blood cholesterol, and in turn, for the prevalence of severe atherosclerosis and coronary heart disease, has been promulgated widely in both the lay and scientific press. This notion has been sufficiently forceful to develop cholesterolphobia in the general public. In view of the fact that cholesterol is an essential metabolite and a constituent of every cell in the body, it was felt that a review of the evidence was warranted.

At the end of the conference, the panel concluded that more basic and clinical research is needed in order to both elucidate the pathogenesis of atherosclerosis and thrombogenesis and formulate rational and practical guidelines for coronary heart disease prevention.

Introduction

P. GOLD

It has been said that all progress results from people who, rightly or wrongly, take unpopular positions. This Symposium on Lipids and Coronary Artery Disease offered a unique opportunity, since we drew upon the participation of scientists from a diverse number of places, areas of expertise and opinions concerning the role of cholesterol, and other lipids, in coronary heart disease (CHD). Our goal was not to walk away with a consensus. From a personal perspective, I wanted to learn how a highly intelligent and knowledgeable group of individuals could address the same body of literature and yet hold diametrically opposite opinions concerning cholesterol and CHD. Another of the goals was to determine if we are all saying the same thing but in different ways. On the other hand, if we are, indeed, at odds, then we should attempt to find out why and then design studies that might enable us to resolve our differences of interpretation.

Moreover, if uncertainties were to exist within this group, how could we address the virtually universal impression that has been communicated to the lay population through the media that cholesterol elevation is a 'disease' in itself and not merely a risk factor, and that this 'disease' causes yet another condition called Coronary Heart Disease.

Hopefully, the discussions from this landmark event will have allowed us to determine where there is consensus, where there are differences and how these might be resolved.

Executive Summary

P. Gold, S.A. Grover and D. Roncari

Coronary heart disease (CHD) remains a major cause of death and disability among Canadians despite recent declines in the disease incidence. Given the positive association between serum cholesterol levels and CHD, there is a growing list of expert panels and consensus groups that have recommended low saturated fat diets as part of a community-wide, health promotion strategy. With the apparent unanimous support for a heart-healthy diet, it is difficult to understand why anyone would be interested in an international workshop on fats and cholesterol and their role in the development of CHD.

This workshop was sponsored by the Faculties of Medicine of McGill University, The University of Toronto and The University of Calgary and was supported by an Educational Grant from The Dairy Bureau of Canada and organized by Kush Medical Communications. The interest of the Dairy Bureau in the cholesterol debate is obvious as the consumption of dairy products is declining with the increasing public concerns about saturated animal fats. For the Dairy Bureau to bring together an international group of experts to discuss their research and a broad range of issues surrounding the cholesterol debate would seem unusually altruistic at best or foolhardy at worst if the scientific community has indeed reached a consensus.

The fact that over 30 leading medical scientists with an interest in nutrition science, atherosclerosis, or cardiovascular disease agreed to attend this obviously 'non-consensus' conference is somewhat even more surprising. Given already busy schedules, why would a European expert on the effects of cholesterol lowering diets find the time and interest to discuss coronary risk appraisal with an American biostatistician? Or why would a Canadian molecular biologist who is analyzing the genetic susceptibility of animals to atherosclerosis be interested in the dietary trends in fat and cholesterol intake among the Japanese? Clearly, despite the perceived consensus surrounding the current recommendations for CHD prevention, there remained sufficient topics for discussion to bring researchers from around the world together to Hilton Head, South Carolina.

As one reviews the research papers published in this symposium, it will be clear that there was much excellent science presented at this meeting. While the science was sound, it is interesting to note that many of the results and certainly the conclusions were apparently inconsistent if not conflicting. To summarize these presentations in a few pages would be impossible. We strongly advise anyone interested in diet and CHD to read at least the abstracts of these excellent presentations.

To capture the uncertainty surrounding a number of critical issues in the cholesterol debate, we asked participants to respond to five questions at the start of the conference and at its conclusion. Participants were asked to rate five questions on their degree of importance for the development and/or prevention of coronary heart disease in adults. The degree of importance was rated on a seven-point scale as follows:

(1) Not clinically important at present and *unlikely* to change with additional research;

(2) Not clinically important at present but *could* change with further research;

(3) Not clinically important at present but *will* probably change with further research;

(4) Uncertain;

(5) Presently somewhat important for the prevention of CHD;

(6) Presently very important for the prevention of CHD;

(7) One of the most important factors regarding CHD prevention.

At the conclusion of the conference, participants once again rated the same five questions on their degree of importance. They were also asked to state the most important research questions remaining vis-à-vis the cholesterol debate and to offer any final words of wisdom.

At the onset of the conference, there was wide variation among participants surrounding the degree of importance each placed on the CHD statements (Figures 1–5). After two and a half days of research presentations, the responses to each question still ranged from 1 to 7. These data demonstrate that participants arrived at the conference with a wide spectrum of beliefs and after two and a half days of heated debate they were still very much in disagreement. This reflects the difficulty of reaching a consensus among experienced scientific investigators despite the compelling data at hand.

Although broad variation surrounded the responses to each statement at the end of the conference, there were some trends that were significant (Table 1). The average scores of all participants for each question tended to decline when comparing responses before and after the conference. For instance, on the statement *The role of cholesterol as a risk factor for CHD* the mean response before the conference was 5.4 (± 1.5) compared to 4.9 at the close of the conference ($p < 0.05$). Significant declines were also noted for the statements

Table 1 Responses of participants ($n=31$) before and after the workshop

		Mean response (SD)		
	Questions	Before	After	Difference
1.	The role of cholesterol as a risk factor for CHD	5.4 (1.5)	*4.9 (1.7)	−0.5 (0.2)
2.	The relationship between diet and serum cholesterol	4.8 (1.7)	4.7 (1.6)	−0.1 (0.1)
3.	A diet low in saturated fat and cholesterol to reduce CHD in general public	4.5 (2.0)	4.2 (1.7)	−0.3 (0.3)
4.	Cholesterol screening as part of an annual check-up to identify adults at high risk	4.6 (1.8)	*4.1 (1.9)	−0.5 (0.1)
5.	Cholesterol intervention with diet or drugs for high risk patients	6.0 (1.2)	**5.4 (1.6)	−0.6 (0.2)

*$p<0.05$
**$p<0.01$

Cholesterol screening as part of an annual checkup to identify adults at high risk and *Cholesterol intervention with diet or drugs for high risk patients*. These results suggest that there remains some uncertainty underlying the importance of each of these statements even among experts.

Overall, these data underscore the necessity for further scientific inquiry and public debate surrounding the role of dietary fat and cholesterol in the development of coronary heart disease. The conclusions of consensus conferences must not close the book on additional discussion or further investigation. Rather, consensus conferences should provide the starting point for critical thinking, dissenting opinions and further research.

The questions and opinions of the Hilton Head participants are listed to provide one basis for further thought (Appendices A and B). We trust that the conference proceedings recorded in this publication will stimulate practising health care professionals, public health leaders, patients, and health conscious consumers to ask the necessary questions that must be answered in formulating scientifically sound and practical dietary recommendations for the population at large.

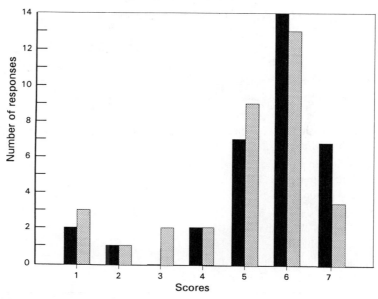

Figure 1 The role of serum cholesterol as a risk factor for CHD

Figures 1–5 The beliefs of participants when surveyed before the conference and at its conclusion. ■ = before conference, ▢ = after conference. Using a seven-point rating scale ('not important' = 1 and 'a great deal of importance' = 7, participants rated the importance of the following statements:

Statement A: The role of serum cholesterol as a risk factor for CHD (Figure 1);

Statement B: The relationship between diet and serum cholesterol levels (Figure 2);

Satement C: A diet low in saturated fats and cholesterol to reduce CHD in the general public (Figure 3);

Statement D: Cholesterol screening as part of an annual checkup to identify adults at high risk of CHD (Figure 4);

Statement E: Cholesterol intervention with diet or drugs for high risk patients (Figure 5).

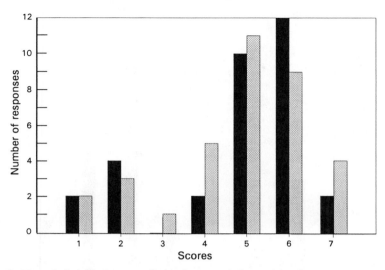

Figure 2 The relationship between diet and serum cholesterol levels

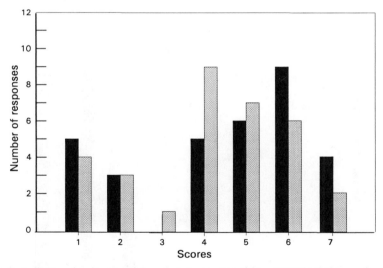

Figure 3 A diet low in saturated fats and cholesterol to reduce CHD in the general public

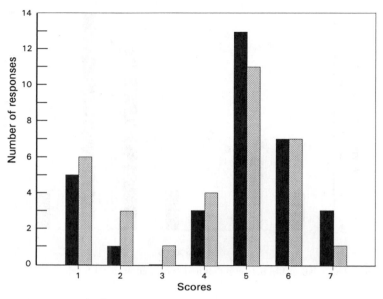

Figure 4 Cholesterol screening as part of an annual checkup to identify adults at high risk of CHD

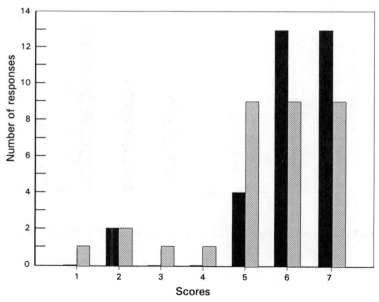

Figure 5 Cholesterol intervention with diet or drugs for high risk patients

Appendix A

'In your opinion, what is the most important research question remaining vis-à-vis the cholesterol debate?'

'Effects on length of life, which the clinical trials have not yet addressed seriously due to the short duration.'

'Need for a better marker for CHD. Need for more research on oxidized lipids in diet and platelet activity.'

'Finding better markers for CHD risk.'

'How does dietary fat affect CHD?'

'What is the early marker in children/youth? What is the mechanism for hyper- and hypo-responders?'

'What remains to be solved scientifically are specific factors that will identify individual risk. My money is on postprandial particles as they affect thrombosis and atherosclerosis.'

'How to apply the scientific information we now have to our populations to prevent coronary disease, especially to the lower socio-economic groups (blacks, poor, unemployed, uneducated).'

'Find a better fraction of the molecule to be able to treat people who are really at risk.'

'Genetic variations that lead to different incidence of atherosclerosis at same LDL-cholesterol level.'

'What are the characteristics of those who do not have high cholesterol but still contract coronary heart disease (or who do not have other identifiable risk factors)?

'The outcome of carefully controlled clinical trials in humans – double blind where ethical – measuring and quantifying morbidity as well as mortality.'

'Need to identify the as yet unidentified genetic factors that increase the risk for atherosclerosis.'

'The effect of diet on CHL/HDL and risk/incidence. The relative benefits of CHL reduction for women, the elderly and children.'

'Continue to identify those dietary variables (and their infraction) that most affect the circulating level of atherogenic lipoproteins (apoB E) relative to HDL.'

'The importance of plasma total CHL/HDL ratio (lowering) combined with plasma triglyceride-lowering by diet needs to be tested on CVD risk.'

'The effect of intervention on all-cause mortality and on CHD mortality in women and the elderly.'

'Why do the French have such low CHD rates in the face of high smoking and high fat intake?'

'Does changing HDL change risk? Does diet affect CHD through platelets? Anti-oxidants? Low cholesterol and stroke?'

'The importance of antioxidant status of individuals with regard to CVD risk.'

'The role of diet in the prevention of CHD in the general population, including children, lower socio-economic groups, women and elderly.'

'The heredity factor.'

'The concern about lowering cholesterol to a level that puts you at risk for other conditions such as cancer, violence, etc. "Treat the whole person".'

'We need a better marker than serum cholesterol for identifying the high risk individuals for CHD.'

'Long-term studies of specific subgroups to show a cost benefit.'

'Basic research to elucidate pathogenesis of atherosclerosis.'

'Research needed towards identification of genetically susceptible (hyper-responders) to diet-induced dyslipidemia.'

'Do we need any more cholesterol research?'

'To determine the underlying molecular changes of acquired vascular fragility seen in atherosclerosis and responsible for its complications.'

'Importance of early intervention.'

'Effectiveness of a community intervention.'

'Identification of genetic factors that may predispose to CHD.'

'Relationship of other risk factors such as high fibrinogen as a cause of CHD.'

'Can dietary fat change mortality? What scientific evidence is there at 10-10-10 (sat-mono-poly) is the best ratio?'

'To determine the optimal levels of serum cholesterol for overall health benefit as well as for prevention of CHD.'

Appendix B

Final word: (Your comments about dietary fat, cholesterol CHD prevention and the conference are invited.)

'The composition of this conference, more so than any other I have attended, appeared driven by strong personal opinions on the subjects under discussion.'

'Widen the scope of research and, therefore, funding of CHD research. There is too much focus on the lipid hypothesis.'

'The question of dietary PUFAs should receive more attention, with respect to their relative and absolute intake, and the efficiency of α-linolenic acid vs. LC-M-3 PUFAs.'

'The conference did not cover: (1) the role of platelets, (2) the developmental aspects of lipoprotein metabolism, (3) lipoprotein phospholipid metabolism, (4) the dynamic measures of cholesterol synthesis, and (5) assessment of the effectiveness of dietary advice, re how will the public use or react to this type of information.'

'The only way to deal with the problem dietary-wise is to affect the food supply generally.'

'I see a growing consensus developing about the importance of nutrition in disease prevention. It is easy to apply and will greatly reduce health care costs.'

'Good to have a meeting that was offering views in an area where the gospel truth tends to prevail.'

'There is need for serious and comprehensive cost assessment of the overall costs and benefits of any proposed intervention, not limited to the target condition.'

'We're on to something important but we should be just as prudent with our public recommendations as with the diets we recommend.'

'Recommendations for cholesterol should be based on multiple risk factors and age. Excellent conference, a real "mind opener".'

'Interesting mix of expertise and bias.'

'Lowering intake of total fat, less saturated fatty acids; less *trans* fatty acids, while eating more complex carbohydrate (fiber) whole grain foods.'

'Lowering dietary fat leads to lower plasma cholesterol which leads to lower CHD is clearly established and is an important basis for prevention and treatment.'

'We still have a long way to go.'

'It seems as if there is enough non-consensus here to keep us all going for the next few decades!'

'I greatly enjoyed this conference, but I do confess a slight feeling of unease about potential commercial exploitation by the sponsor.'

'Much uncertainty still exists although recent dietary pattern changes are likely to be beneficial. We still need further research to identify the relative importance of different diet components to the disease process.'

'Excellent conference! I would have liked to see a presentation made by a dietitian.'

'More importance given to the socio-economic influence on the incidence of CHD and its implication for public health policy.'

'I believe research and education for better prevention and treatment of the major killers CHD, cancer and diabetes must take place within a reasonable space without abuse and creations of hysteria and panic. Cultural characteristics should not be overlooked. Canada should not necessarily follow whatever is recommended for US population.'

'I agree with CCC on cholesterol. Everything in moderation.'

'Should not generalize to public at large, *particularly* to children who are not clearly at risk.'

'There is need to debate the scientific evidence and quality of data in a scientific journal.'

'Superb.'

'Diet is one of the most important risk factors not only for CHD but also for stroke and other diseases.'

'(1) The conference was well organized and stimulating. (2) A significant amount of research is needed to define the nutritional importance of some dietary fats and development of nutritious "designer" foods. (3) Reduce dietary cholesterol; the body can synthesize what it needs. (4) More research is needed in the area of genetics as it relates to CHD prevention.'

'Recommendations for prevention "at large" must be reversed to avoid changing food habits. We don't know the results for future generations. Recommendations must be practical, real fears must be allayed.'

'Too much emphasis on blood cholesterol levels and too little emphasis on lifestyle as a cause of CHD. Why so much talk about cholesterol and so little about how multi-national companies are loading our food with sugar, salt, and directly producing an epidemic of diabetes, atherosclerosis and CHD and other degeneration problems.'

'Let's treat individuals at high risk and not the whole population. Pleased to have the opportunity to attend and would like to participate in the next one which I hope will take place.'

'This conference was very stimulating to me and I have learned a great deal about basic biological mechanisms of diet–cholesterol–CHD connection.'

Section I.
Epidemiological Studies

1

AHA Medical/Scientific Statement
Science Advisory
An updated coronary risk profile –
a statement for health professionals

**K.M. ANDERSON, P.W.F. WILSON, P.M. ODELL and
W.B. KANNEL**

Coronary heart disease (CHD) continues to be the cause of the greatest number of deaths among adult Americans[1]. Although there is a downward trend in cardiovascular mortality rates, morbidity and mortality rates remain high and are of great concern to clinicians and health officials. Using a simple worksheet, a patient's 5- and 10-year CHD risks can be estimated. The components of the profile were selected because they are objective and strongly and independently related to CHD and because they can be measured through simple office procedures and laboratory results.

In the past, investigators with the Framingham Heart Study developed CHD risk equations for use by clinicians in predicting the development of coronary disease in individuals free of disease[2]. Early efforts reflected the experience of study investigators from 1950 to the mid-1960s[3,4]. In addition to age and gender, risk factors included systolic blood pressure (SBP), serum cholesterol, cigarette smoking, glucose intolerance, and left ventricular hypertrophy (LVH). A handbook[5] containing CHD risk tables based on Framingham equations[6] was published in 1973. An even simpler approximation of the equations, by which CHD risk could be estimated by following instructions on a pocket-sized card, soon followed[7]. The equations presented here have several advantages over previous versions. The data base from which they are derived is larger and more recent. In particular, more data for individuals older than 60 years are available. In addition, the influence of high density lipoprotein (HDL) cholesterol, which has been measured in the Framingham Heart Study since 1968, is reflected in these equations. Measurement of the

This article was first published by the American Heart Association, 1991. Reproduced with permission. © American Heart Association.
Requests for reprints should be sent to the Office of Scientific Affairs, American Heart Association, 7320 Greenville Avenue, Dallas, TX 75231.

3

ratio of total cholesterol to HDL cholesterol has been found to be superior to measurement of serum cholesterol as a predictor of CHD[8].

At the baseline examination for this study (1968–1975), all members of the original Framingham cohort were more than 50 years old. To provide current estimates of CHD risk over a large age range, data from the original cohort have been combined with data from the second-generation study population, the Framingham Offspring Cohort, for which 12 years of follow-up have recently been completed. Together, these groups span the ages of 12–82 years; however, only persons 30–74 years old have been included in this study. Those 75 years of age or older were excluded because of possible differences in risk factors in this older group and its potentially large influence in the algorithm determination. Tables 1–4 detail the crude incidence rates of CHD and the distributions of risk factors among the study population by age. From the experience of this group during a 12-year period, estimates of CHD risk have been produced that reflect the approximate combined impacts of total and HDL cholesterol, SBP or diastolic blood pressure (DBP), cigarette smoking, diabetes mellitus, and LVH as measured by electrocardiography (ECG-LVH).

The derivation and uses of the worksheet are detailed in the remainder of this article.

Methods

Population and risk factors

Every member of the original and offspring cohorts who met three basic criteria were included in the study. Requirements for inclusion were 1) age 30–74 years at the time of the baseline examination; 2) measurements available for SBP and DBP, cigarette smoking status, total and HDL cholesterol, and diagnoses (yes or no) of diabetes and ECG-LVH (when information on diabetes or LVH was not available, diagnoses were presumed to be negative); and 3) freedom from cardiovascular disease (stroke, transient ischemia, CHD [includes angina pectoris, coronary insufficiency (unstable angina), myocardial infarction, and sudden death], congestive heart failure, and intermittent claudication) until time of risk factor measurement.

Definitions of risk factors and end points are those considered standard in the Framingham study[9]. In the original cohort, diabetes was diagnosed if a casual whole blood glucose measurement was 150 mg/dl or above or the individual was being treated with insulin or oral hypoglycemics. In the offspring study, a more recent definition, requiring treatment or a fasting glucose level of 140 mg/dl or above from plasma measurement, was used. Measurements of risk factors for the original cohort were taken from the first examination cycle in which HDL cholesterol levels were measured. In most cases (87.7%), this was examination 11 (1968–1971); for some cohort members, it was examination 10 or 12. Follow-up was performed through the 17th examination cycle, a span of approximately 12 years. For the offspring cohort, risk factor measurements were from the first examination cycle (1971–1975), whereas follow-up was performed through the third examination cycle, approximately 12 years later. The study included 5,573 persons (2,983 women and 2,590 men).

Table 1 Prevalence of dichotomous risk factors and crude coronary heart disease incidence by age for men

	Age (yr)					
	30–39	40–49	50–59	60–69	70–74	30–74
CHD incidence (n)(%)*	41 (5)	74 (11)	143 (20)	98 (29)	29 (26)	385 (15)
Cigarette smoking (n)(%)	340 (45)	284 (43)	301 (42)	102 (30)	28 (25)	1,055 (41)
Diabetes (n)(%)	11 (1)	23 (4)	69 (10)	63 (19)	17 (15)	183 (7)
ECG-LVH (n)(%)**	1 (0.1)	4 (0.6)	2 (0.3)	17 (5)	4 (4)	28 (1)
Total (n)	759	655	725	340	111	2,590

*CHD, coronary heart disease; **ECG-LVH, left ventricular hypertrophy by electrocardiography.

Risk factors are age (years), sex (1, woman; 0, man), SBP [average of two office measurements (mm Hg)], DBP [average of two office measurements (mm Hg)], cholesterol [total serum cholesterol measured by the Abell–Kendall method (mg/dl)], HDL cholesterol [determined after heparin–manganese precipitation (mg/dl)], smoking (1, cigarette smoking or quit within past year; 0, otherwise), diabetes [1, diabetes; 0, otherwise (conservative definition is treatment with insulin or oral agents or having a fasting glucose of 140 mg/dl or above[10]], and ECG-LVH (1, definite; 0, otherwise).

Statistical modeling

A parametric regression model was used for risk estimation. Like the logistic model previously used[4,5,11], it provides a simple formula for estimating probabilities of disease given risk factor levels. It has the additional advantage of allowing computation for variable durations of follow-up. The standard accelerated failure time model[12] has been used with two variations, which are described below.

Let T denote the time until CHD from the beginning of follow-up, μ a location parameter, and σ, a scale parameter for $\log(T)$. Throughout, $\log(\ )$

5

denotes the natural logarithm function. Assume that μ and σ depend on risk factors, as will be described, and that:

$$\frac{\log(T) - \mu}{\sigma}$$

follows an extreme value distribution. This implies that T follows the Weibull distribution, which is often used in analyzing studies of times until event.

The location parameter μ is assumed to be a sum of the products of the risk factors multiplied by their corresponding coefficients; for example,

$$\mu = \beta_0 + \beta_1 \times \text{female} + \beta_2 \times \log(\text{age}) + \beta_3 \times \log(\text{SBP})....$$

The exact form taken by this function is presented in "Results". Next, assume that

$$\log(\sigma) = \theta_0 + \theta_1 \times \mu$$

This functional form for σ, as well as others, is discussed in detail elsewhere[13] and provides a highly statistically significant improvement in model fit over the standard model in which σ is held constant. Thus, the unknown parameters to be estimated are $\beta_0, \ldots, \beta_k, \theta_0,$ and θ_1

The models are estimated by the maximum likelihood method, which is implemented with a specialized computer program written by one of the authors. This type of model can also be estimated with PROC NLIN from SAS Institute, Cary, N.C. To reduce the apparently undue influence of the earliest CHD events, those events occurring during the first 4 years of follow-up are coded as such rather than as occurring at the exact time of onset. This methodology is the subject of a separate report[14].

Table 2 Prevalence of dichotomous risk factors and crude coronary heart disease incidence by age for women

	Age (yr)					
	30–39	*40–49*	*50–59*	*60–69*	*70–74*	*30–74*
CHD incidence $(n)(\%)$*	4 (1)	32 (5)	105 (12)	68 (15)	32 (20)	241 (8)
Cigarette smoking $(n)(\%)$	357 (45)	284 (41)	391 (45)	101 (22)	26 (16)	1,159 (39)
Diabetes $(n)(\%)$	4 (0.5)	13 (2)	58 (7)	55 (12)	24 (15)	154 (5)
ECG-LVH $(n)(\%)$**	2 (0.3)	0 (0)	3 (0.4)	3 (0.7)	7 (4)	15 (0.5)
Total (n)	798	693	867	462	163	2,983

*CHD, coronary heart disease; **ECG-LVH, left ventricular hypertrophy by electrocardiography.

Table 3 Distribution of continuous risk factors by age for men

Measurement	Age (yr)					
	30–39	40–49	50–59	60–69	70–74	30–74
Total cholesterol						
5% percentile	144	161	161	160	149	153
Median	197	213	214	216	208	210
95% percentile	264	279	295	292	281	283
HDL cholesterol*						
5% percentile	27	29	28	29	31	28
Median	42	42	44	44	43	43
95% percentile	64	66	68	72	66	67
Total/HDL cholesterol						
5% percentile	2.8	2.9	2.8	3.0	3.0	2.9
Median	4.6	5.0	4.9	4.9	4.8	4.8
95% percentile	7.9	8.1	8.3	7.8	7.6	8.0
SBP (mm Hg)**						
5% percentile	107	109	110	116	112	109
Median	122	125	130	141	142	128
95% percentile	148	157	173	181	181	168
DBP (mm Hg)***						
5% percentile	68	69	70	69	65	69
Median	81	83	84	84	82	82
95% percentile	98	103	105	104	96	102
Total points						
5% percentile	–2	5	11	15	19	1
Median	6	13	18	23	24	15
95% percentile	15	22	26	32	32	27
Total	759	655	725	340	111	2,590

*HDL, high density lipoprotein; **SBP, systolic blood pressure; ***DBP, diastolic blood pressure.

Results

Results are presented in two forms; the first is an updated version of the 1973 report equations[6] that incorporates new data on HDL cholesterol with the present study data described above. Then, an easy-to-calculate point-scoring algorithm that is based on one of the equations is given. It is hoped that the algorithm will be easy to use. Predicted risk may be calculated with SBP or DBP. Because of the high correlation between these two measurements, both cannot be included; the redundancy leads to difficulty in interpretation. Although in general results are similar, separate equations are given for SBP and DBP to accommodate strong user preferences. The equation incorporating

SBP is recommended because SBP is more accurately determined, has a wider range of values, and is a stronger predictor of CHD, particularly in the elderly.

Framingham equations

Computation with the estimated equation is described below. In this section, SBP is used; the equation incorporating DBP is given next. Explanations of some components of the equation are given after the calculations.

Systolic blood pressure equation

There are some differences in equation calculations for men and women, but both calculations begin in the same way. Compute an interim number a that is based on risk factor measurements.

$$a = 11.1122 - 0.9119 \times \log (\text{SBP}) - 0.2767 \times$$
$$\text{smoking} - 0.7181 \times \log (\text{cholesterol/HDL}) - 0.5865 \times \text{ECG-LVH} \quad (1)$$

The next step, computing a second interim value m, is different for men and women. For men, compute

$$m = a - 1.4792 \times \log (\text{age}) - 0.1759 \times \text{diabetes} \quad (2a)$$

For women, compute

$$m = a - 5.8549 + 1.8515 \times [\log (\text{age}/74)]^2 - 0.3758 \times \text{diabetes} \quad (2b)$$

Next, for both sexes, compute
$$\mu = 4.4181 + m \quad (3)$$

$$\sigma = \exp (-0.3155 - 0.2784 \times m) \quad (4)$$

Finally, choose the number of years for which you wish to predict (from 4 to 12) and call it t. Compute

$$u = \frac{\log (t) - \mu}{\sigma} \quad (5)$$

The predicted probability for t is

$$p = 1 - \exp (-e^u) \quad (6)$$

Table 4 Distribution of continuous risk factors by age for women

Measurement	*Age* (yr)					
	30–39	*40–49*	*50–59*	*60–69*	*70–74*	*30–74*
Total cholesterol						
5% percentile	141	152	173	179	183	151
Median	181	200	229	245	246	212
95% percentile	244	268	306	320	305	295
HDL cholesterol*						
5% percentile	36	35	35	36	35	35
Median	55	56	58	56	54	56
95% percentile	81	86	88	87	85	86
Total HDL cholesterol						
5% percentile	2.2	2.3	2.4	2.5	2.7	2.3
Median	3.2	3.5	3.9	4.3	4.5	3.7
95% percentile	5.6	6.2	6.9	7.3	7.2	6.7
SBP (mm Hg)**						
5% percentile	97	100	105	112	118	100
Median	114	119	130	142	150	123
95% percentile	137	153	170	178	186	168
DBP (mm Hg)***						
5% percentile	61	64	65	64	64	63
Median	73	78	81	82	82	79
95% percentile	89	97	100	100	102	98
Total points						
5% percentile	–16	–3	4	8	10	–12
Median	–6	5	12	16	18	8
95% percentile	5	15	22	26	27	22
Total	798	693	867	462	163	2,983

*HDL, high density lipoprotein; **SBP, systolic blood pressure; ***DBP, diastolic blood pressure.

As an example, consider a 55-year-old individual with SBP of 130 mm Hg, total cholesterol of 240 mg/dl, and HDL cholesterol of 45 mg/dl who smokes cigarettes. We assume that neither diabetes nor ECG-LVH has been diagnosed. First, we compute

$$a = 11.1122 - 0.9119 \times \log (130) - 0.2767 - 0.7181 \times \log (240/45) = 5.1947$$

For a man, then compute

$$m = 5.1947 - 1.4792 \times \log (55) = -0.7329$$

$$\mu = -0.7329 + 4.4181 = 3.685$$

$$\sigma = \exp\left[-0.3155 - 0.2784 \times (-0.7329)\right] = 0.894$$

For a woman, compute

$$m = 5.1947 - 5.8549 + 1.8515 \times \left[\log (55/74)\right]^2 = -0.4972$$

$$\mu = -0.4972 + 4.4181 = 3.921$$

$$\sigma = \exp\left[-0.3155 - 0.2784 \times (-0.4972)\right] = 0.8377$$

We let t be 10 years and compute for a man

$$u = \frac{\log (10) - 3.685}{0.894} = -1.546$$

$$p = 1 - \exp\left(-e^{-1.546}\right) = 0.192$$

For a woman, compute

$$u = \frac{\log (10) - 3.921}{0.8377} = -1.932$$

$$p = 1 - \exp\left(-e^{-1.932}\right) = 0.135$$

Diastolic blood pressure equation

The equations incorporating DBP instead of SBP are precisely analogous to those given above.

$$a = 11.0938 - 0.8670 \times \log (DBP) - 0.2789 \times smoking - \\ 0.7142 \times \log (cholesterol/HDL) - 0.7195 \times ECG\text{-}LVH \qquad (7)$$

Again, the next step is different for men and women.
For men, compute

$$m = a - 1.6346 \times \log (age) - 0.2082 \times diabetes \qquad (8a)$$

For women, compute

$$m = a - 6.5306 + 2.1059 \times \left[\log (age/74)\right]^2 - \\ 0.4055 \times diabetes \qquad (8b)$$

Next, compute

$$\mu = 4.4284 + m \tag{9}$$

$$\sigma = \exp(-0.3171 - 0.2825 \times m) \tag{10}$$

Proceed as with the SBP equation to compute predicted probabilities. For example, if DBP is 90 mm Hg, $p = 0.22$ for a man and $p = 0.16$ for a woman.

Model selection

There are several points to consider in the derivations of the models. First, the natural logarithms of continuous covariates were used rather than actual values. Likelihood analysis indicates that such use improves the fit of the model; one reason is that extremely large covariate measurements now receive less emphasis, allowing risk to change more slowly for very large values than for the range of the bulk of the data. This explains the uneven covariate intervals in the risk prediction worksheet.

Second, the addition of a quadratic term for age for women produces a significantly improved model fit. This term accommodates a rapid increase in risk at younger ages and little change at older ages. The maximum age effect in women was arbitrarily forced to occur at the oldest age in the population; otherwise, this would have occurred at a slightly younger age. This change is not statistically significant. Because of the quadratic form of the function, extrapolation to older and younger age groups is particularly questionable.

Third, the ratio of total cholesterol to HDL cholesterol was used because no improved fit was found when the covariates were used separately. Note that the equations do not contain a cholesterol–age interaction term as did some previous prediction models[11]. When serum cholesterol–age and HDL cholesterol–age interaction terms were added to the model, their contributions were negligible. Thus, it appears that including the ratio of total cholesterol to HDL cholesterol in the equations eliminates the need for such interaction terms.

Fourth, except for differences in aging effects, no significantly different effects were found for men and women. A separate coefficient for diabetes was fit for women based on significant differences between men and women in previous studies[15]. Although female smokers were not found to be at increased risk in some previous Framingham reports[2], the offspring cohort provides evidence of such a relation. Thus, no distinction has been made between smoking effects for men and those for women. Using the number of cigarettes rather than a simple yes-or-no code for cigarette smoking did not provide an improvement in model fit. This may be largely due to the fact that

Table 5 Framingham Heart Study coronary heart disease risk prediction chart

1. Find points for each risk factor

Age (if female) (yr)

Age	Points	Age	Points
30	-12	41	1
31	-11	42-43	2
32	-9	44	3
33	-8	45-46	4
34	-6	47-48	5
35	-5	49-50	6
36	-4	51-52	7
37	-3	53-55	8
38	-2	56-60	9
39	-1	61-67	10
40	0	68-74	11

Age (if male) (yr)

Age	Points	Age	Points
30	-2	48-49	9
31	-1	50-51	10
32-33	0	52-54	11
34	1	55-56	12
35-36	2	57-59	13
37-38	3	60-61	14
39	4	62-64	15
40-41	5	65-67	16
42-43	6	68-70	17
44-45	7	71-73	18
46-47	8	74	19

HDL* cholesterol

HDL*	Points	HDL*	Points
25-26	7	67-73	-4
27-29	6	74-80	-5
30-32	5	81-87	-6
33-35	4	88-96	-7
36-38	3		
39-42	2		
43-46	1		
47-50	0		
51-55	-1		
56-60	-2		
61-66	-3		

Total cholesterol (mg/dl)

Chol	Points	Chol	Points
139-151	-3	220-239	2
152-166	-2	240-262	3
167-182	-1	263-288	4
183-199	0	289-315	5
200-219	1	316-330	6

Systolic blood pressure (mm Hg)

SBP**	Points	SBP**	Points
98-104	-2	140-149	3
105-112	-1	150-160	4
113-120	0	161-172	5
121-129	1	173-185	6
130-139	2		

Other factors

Other factors	Points Yes	Points No
Cigarette smoking	4	0
Diabetes		
Male	3	0
Female	6	0
ECG-LVH***	9	0

2. *Add points for all risk factors. Note: Minus points subtract from total.*

$$\overline{\text{(Age)}} + \overline{\text{(Total chol)}} + \overline{\text{(HDL*)}} + \overline{\text{(SBP**)}} + \overline{\text{(Smoking)}} + \overline{\text{(Diabetes)}} + \overline{\text{(ECG-LVH***)}} = \overline{\text{(Total)}}$$

3. *Look up risk corresponding to point total*

Points	Probability (%) 5 yr	Probability (%) 10 yr	Points	Probability (%) 5 yr	Probability (%) 10 yr	Points	Probability (%) 5 yr	Probability (%) 10 yr	Points	Probability (%) 5 yr	Probability (%) 10 yr
≤1	<1	<2	9	2	5	17	6	13	25	14	27
2	1	2	10	2	6	18	7	14	26	16	29
3	1	2	11	3	6	19	8	16	27	17	31
4	1	2	12	3	7	20	8	18	28	19	33
5	1	3	13	3	8	21	9	19	29	20	36
6	1	3	14	4	9	22	11	21	30	22	38
7	1	4	15	5	10	23	12	23	31	24	40
8	2	4	16	5	12	24	13	25	32	25	42

4. *Compare with average 10-year risk*

Age (yr)	Probability (%) Women	Probability (%) Men	Age (yr)	Probability (%) Women	Probability (%) Men	Age (yr)	Probability (%) Women	Probability (%) Men
30–34	<1	3	45–49	5	10	60–64	13	21
35–39	<1	5	50–54	8	14	65–69	9	30
40–44	2	6	55–59	12	16	70–74	12	24

*HDL, high density lipoprotein; **SBP, systolic blood pressure; ***ECG-LVH, left ventricular hypertrophy by electrocardiography.

older smokers in this study reported smoking fewer cigarettes than did younger smokers. Presumably, this confounded possible dose effects with age effects.

Finally, the estimated effect of ECG-LVH is very large but has a large standard error because of the small prevalence of the condition at baseline.

Point score algorithm

Equations 1–6 were used to devise a worksheet that enables users to estimate their CHD risk by assigning a point score to each risk factor (Table 5). Clinicians or patients can insert the appropriate points and add as indicated to obtain a good approximation of CHD risk during a 5- or 10-year period. For comparison, average risk values, by age and sex, for the Framingham population are also given.

If the values used in the sample computations are used in the worksheet, results are as given in Table 6. These results are a close approximation of those obtained with Equations 1–6 (19.2% for a man and 13.5% for a woman).

Discussion

The CHD risk equations and point score prediction probability algorithm attempt to elucidate the multifactorial etiology of CHD and produce possible comparisons and interpretations for clinicians and their patients at risk. The point-scoring technique allows estimation of an individual's 5- and 10-year risks of CHD, whereas the equations may be used for 4- to 12-year estimations. These calculations are based on the Framingham experience for individuals free of cardiovascular disease at baseline, and such calculations are not appropriate for individuals with coronary disease.

Generalization of the Framingham equations to the population at large is always a matter of concern and should be done cautiously. However, it has been demonstrated repeatedly that the Framingham risk model is effective in predicting heart disease in other large population samples in the United States[16–19]. For example, the 1973 equations were used in the Multiple Risk Factor Intervention Trial to predict the number of cases of CHD to be expected during the course of the trial[20]. The trial was administered during the early 1970s, when there was a sharp decrease in CHD mortality rates in the United States and extensive intervention against risk factors was being practiced. Hence, as could be anticipated, the estimates were high for both the usual-care and the special-intervention groups. But they were systematically high, and the relative weightings of risk factors distinguished low- from high-risk individuals.

Table 6 Sample worksheet results

		Points	
Risk factor	*Level*	*Man*	*Woman*
Age	55	12	8
HDL cholesterol*	45	1	1
Total cholesterol	240	3	3
SBP**	130	2	2
Smoking	1	4	4
Diabetes	0	0	0
ECG-LVH***	0	0	0
Total		22	18
10-year risk (%)		21	14

*HDL, high density lipoprotein; **SBP, systolic blood pressure; ***ECG-LVH, left ventricular hypertrophy measured by electrocardiography.

Nonetheless, cautions should be observed when using the equations or worksheet. First, the equations can, of course, be used only with all risk factors measured. These were chosen because they can be measured objectively and because they make independent contributions to the risk equations. Other important risk influences have not been included in the equations, but they should not be underestimated. For example, heredity is a factor of major importance, but information on this subject is difficult to quantify or even obtain accurately. Individuals with family histories of heart disease should view increased risk factors with particular concern and deal with them more vigorously than should persons without such backgrounds. Obesity is another example of a significant risk factor in long-term predictions[21]; however, in shorter-term studies such as this one, its effects tend to be mediated by other risk factors. Hence, it is not included in the equations.

Second, the predictions may not be appropriate for individuals with extremely elevated risk factors such as malignant hypertension and severe diabetes mellitus or extremely high cholesterol and HDL cholesterol levels that place them in the top or bottom few percentiles of the distributions.

Third, the equations may not be directly applicable to populations with very low CHD incidence rates[19]. Although these equations are considered more accurate than earlier versions when incidence rates are low, this has not been tested extensively. Hence, the equations may be inappropriate for use with populations from countries or ethnic groups that have CHD incidence rates that are much lower or higher than the range presented here[18].

When generalization seems reasonable, estimation of CHD risk can be useful in projecting patient progress in clinics at which preventive cardiology is the goal, such as those concentrating on lipid or blood pressure influence. Risk factor scores and calculations can be discussed with patients and provide a framework for intervention. Clinicians can predict possible rewards in the form of improved risk profiles for patients who make the appropriate although often difficult changes in smoking, eating, and exercise habits.

References

1. National Center for Health Statistics (1989). Births, marriages, divorces, and deaths for May 1989. *Monthly Vital Statistics Report*, Vol 38, No. 5. US Dept of Health and Human Services Publication No. (PHS) 89–11200. Hyattsville, Md

2. Kannel, W.B., McGee, D. and Gordon, T. (1976). A general cardiovascular risk profile: The Framingham Study. *Am. J. Cardiol.*, **38**, 46–51

3. Truett, J., Cornfield, J. and Kannel, W. (1967). A multivariate analysis of the risk of coronary heart disease in Framingham. *J. Chronic Dis.*, **20**, 511–24

4. Walker, S.H. and Duncan, D.B. (1967). Estimation of the probability of an event as a function of several independent variables. *Biometrika*, **54**, 167–79

5. American Heart Association (1973). *Coronary Risk Handbook: Estimating the Risk of Coronary Heart Disease in Daily Practice*. Dallas, Tx

6. Gordon, T., Sorlie, P. and Kannel, W.B. (1971). Coronary heart disease, athero-thrombotic brain infarction, intermittent claudication – A multivariate analysis of some factors related to their incidence: Framingham Study, 16-year follow-up. In Kannel, W.B. and Gordon, T. (eds), *The Framingham Study: An Epidemiological Investigation of Cardiovascular Disease*, Section 27. US Government Printing Office No. 426-1301/1345, Washington, DC

7. Brittain, E. (1982). Probability of coronary heart disease developing. *West. J. Med.*, **136**, 86–9

8. Castelli, W.P., Garrison, R.J., Wilson, P.W., Abbott, R.D., Kalousdian, S. and Kannel, W.B. (1986). Incidence of coronary heart disease and lipoprotein cholesterol levels: The Framingham Study. *J. Am. Med. Assoc.*, **256**, 2835–8

9. Shurtleff, D. (1971). Some characteristics related to the incidence of cardiovascular disease and death: Framingham study, 16-year follow-up. In Kannel, W.B. and Gordon, T. (eds), *The Framingham Study: An Epidemiological Investigation of Cardiovascular Disease*, Section 26. US Government Printing Office No. O-414-297, Washington, DC

10. National Diabetes Data Group (1983). Classification and diagnosis of diabetes mellitus and other categories of glucose intolerance. *Diabetes*, **28**, 1039–57

11. Abbott, R.D. and McGee, D. (1987). The probability of developing certain cardiovascular diseases in eight years at specified values of some characteristics: The Framingham Study. In Kannel, W.B., Wolf, P.A. and Garrison, R.J. (eds): *The Framingham Study: An Epidemiological Investigation of Cardiovascular Disease*, Section 37. National Technical Information Service No. PB 87-221644/A5. Springfield, Va

12. Kalbfleisch, J.D. and Prentice, R.L. (1980). *The Statistical Analysis of Failure Time Data*. (New York: John Wiley & Sons, Inc.)

13. Carroll, R.J. and Ruppert, D. (1988). *Transformation and Weighting in Regression.* (New York: Chapman and Hall)
14. Anderson, K.M. (1991). A non-proportional hazards Weibull accelerated failure time model. *Biometrics*, **47**, 281–8
15. Kannel, W.B. and McGee, D.L. (1979). Diabetes and cardiovascular disease: The Framingham study. *J. Am. Med. Assoc.*, **241**, 2035–8
16. Brand, R.J., Rosenman, R.H., Sholtz, R.I. and Friedman, M. (1976). Multivariate prediction of coronary heart disease in the Western Collaborative Group Study compared to the findings of the Framingham Study. *Circulation*, **53**, 348–55
17. Leaverton, P.E., Sorlie, P.D., Kleinman, J.C., Dannenberg, A.L., Ingster-Moore, L., Kannel, W.B. and Cornoni-Huntley, J.C. (1987). Representativeness of the Framingham risk model for coronary heart disease mortality: A comparison with a national cohort study. *J. Chronic Dis.*, **40**, 775–84
18. McGee, D. and Gordon, T. (1976). The results of the Framingham study applied to four other US-based epidemiologic studies of cardiovascular disease. In Kannel, W.B. and Gordon, T. (eds), *The Framingham Study: An Epidemiological Investigation of Cardiovascular Disease*, Section 31. US Dept of Health, Education, and Welfare Publication No. 76-1083. Bethesda, Md, US Government Printing Office
19. Pooling Project Research Group (1978). Relationship of blood pressure, serum cholesterol, smoking habit, relative weight and ECG abnormalities to incidence of major coronary events: Final report of the pooling project. *J. Chronic Dis.*, **31**, 201–306
20. The Multiple Risk Factor Intervention Trial Group (1977). Statistical design considerations in the NHLI Multiple Risk Factor Intervention Trial (MRFIT). *J. Chronic Dis.*, **30**, 261–75
21. Hubert, H.B., Feinleib, M., McNamara, P.M. and Castelli, W.P. (1983). Obesity as an independent risk factor for cardiovascular disease: A 26-year follow-up of participants in the Framingham Heart Study. *Circulation*, **67**, 968–77

Discussion

Dr Skrabanek: I would like to ask Dr Anderson how he reconciles the results he has just presented with another study recently published by the Framingham group in the *International Journal of Epidemiology*. In fact, I refer to this study in my abstract. This group of investigators looked at risk factors and trends in coronary heart disease in a group of middle-aged men and women ranging from 55 to 64, whereas I believe your model was based on men and women aged 30–74. In this narrow segment of what you would call middle-aged men and women aged 55–64, they found that between 1953 and 1983 there was an increased prevalence and mortality of CHD in men. However, during that very same time period of 30 years, all the recognized risk factors such as hypercholesterolaemia, hypertension and smoking significantly decreased. How do you reconcile this – that while all these risk factors were moving in the right direction, CHD was moving in the opposite direction in men?

Dr Anderson: I do not know how much I can say about that. The paper I am familiar with is the Sukowski paper but it does not sound like the one you are referring to.

I will try to comment a little bit about one matter that I am particularly familiar with and that is systolic blood pressure and its changing role as a risk factor. Considering specifically systolic blood pressure, starting in 1950, and our second-generation study in 1970, if you look at the follow-up from the 1970 group in men, systolic blood pressure almost disappears as a risk factor. What appears to have happened is that, when we looked at systolic blood pressure in 1950, we looked at men with very high pressures. Then, they came back 2 years later still with very high pressures. Four years later, they returned in the 1970s treated. So, your point is a good one and it does provide some difficulties for us to know that there is intervention going on, and presumably at this point in time now there would tend to be much more intervention in cholesterol as well. So, you may ask how does this affect our work? Well, it would tend to lessen, at least to some extent, the association between blood pressure and heart disease. So, maybe our estimation of that association is a little bit weak. On the other hand, it is still there and it is reasonably strong. But, I think it is an excellent point – how can you carry out epidemiological studies when intervention is ongoing?

Dr Roncari: When you added HDL to your analysis, what happened to obesity as a potentially independent risk factor?

Dr Anderson: The problem with obesity, whether or not you have HDL or anything else in the model, you really need long term follow-up to find an association. This is because some people who are skinny presumably are skinny because they are sick or in a premorbid condition. So, I do not really have an answer to that since in the follow-up that we had, obesity would not have been a risk factor. We do not have a long enough follow-up after the HDL measurements really to answer that question at this point.

Dr Grover: This is a nice piece of work as it makes some statistical equations, that in the past many people found complicated, somewhat simpler and easier to use. But, the thing that was nice about some of the older Framingham models is that the interaction term between cholesterol and age told us that the association between cholesterol and CHD weakened with age. Other studies have validated this. For instance, if you look at the MRFIT studies across different age groups, again, as you increase in age, the association weakens. How does this model that you have presented here today take that fact into account? No one would suggest that cholesterol does not still remain a risk factor, but clearly it becomes quite a weak factor.

Dr Anderson: There are two things to keep in mind. First of all, the difference in the statistical models allows some lessening of the relative risk with time. Secondly, and more importantly, the message that I am trying to get across is that once you include HDL in the model, this brings back cholesterol to a large extent. For instance, if you do an analysis dividing people by the American cholesterol cutoffs and look below 200 mg/dl, HDL is a strong risk factor in men. There are not enough women with cholesterols under 200 mg/dl for HDL to be a risk factor, but above 240 mg/dl, HDL becomes a strong risk factor in women. Men are pretty much all at high risk and there is not that strong an association up there. But, overall, if you do consider both measures, you can consider them consistently across sex and age groups. If you are considering cholesterol alone without the HDL measurement, I think that could be a mistake, just for the reasons you are pointing out.

Dr Isles: My main concern about some of these risk scores is the effect it might have on a subject's psyche if patients find that they have a high risk and cannot modify it.

Dr Anderson: That is an interesting question. Certainly you cannot alter age and sex and you cannot change the fact that you have diabetes. I do not claim to have the expertise to know whether or not you can reduce left ventricular hypertrophy but I do know that by reducing weight you probably can reduce it to some extent. I also know that you can lower your cholesterol and raise your HDL to some extent, although to small degrees. For the most part, losing weight and improving diet can have moderate effects for most people in most of these risk factors. As well, the combined effect of these factors should have some outcome in relation to risk. I am sure there will be some exceptions, but this is the sort of strategy that we are trying to point out.

Dr Stehbens: I believe that the Framingham study has been one of the prime factors in inhibiting and retarding the elucidation of the cause of atherosclerosis. Your use of coronary heart disease (CHD) as an end-point is totally inappropriate. It is wrong to use it synonymously with coronary atherosclerosis or atherosclerosis in general, and this usage has been acknowledged by publications from the National Institutes of Health. CHD is a very imprecise clinical diagnosis of which only 90% at the most, it has been estimated, are caused by coronary atherosclerosis. So, you are really talking about more than one disease. If you are talking about coronary atherosclerosis, then most people now accept that atherosclerosis commences at least in infancy. I believe it commences *in utero* as small fibromuscular elastic thickenings of the intima. Risk factor is used by epidemiologists as synonymous with cause, but they state that they prefer to use risk factor, rather than cause, because of the lack of precision and lack of confidence in causality. Even Epstein acknowledges that when risk factors are used, causation is merely assumed. This really is an unscientific approach. CHD is an end-stage disease and yet you are correlating risk factors with end-stage disease and assume a causal relationship with atherosclerosis. This completely misrepresents the whole picture to the general public and to other scientists. What you should be looking for as an end-point is the severity of atherosclerosis because atherosclerosis occurs in all of us without any exception. If you cannot measure accurately the severity of atherosclerosis in the individual during life, and I believe you cannot, then such studies are unscientific and the results are worse than suspect.

Dr Anderson: I think you have some legitimate points; on the other hand, Framingham was originated to look for possible causes, not to find the cause itself. It is not an experiment where you are changing things, it is looking for the aetiology. I do not think it can be denied that there is a lot of use that can come out of this study and that experiments have backed up that some risk factors, when altered, can reduce disease incidence.

2
Cardiovascular disease prevention through dietary change

S.A. GROVER

Cardiovascular disease and risk factors

Cardiovascular disease (CVD) remains the most common cause of death among Canadians despite recent advances in its diagnosis and treatment[1]. There are a number of important risk factors associated with the development of cardiovascular disease including cigarette smoking, hypertension, and elevations in total serum cholesterol levels[2-4]. More importantly, there is now irrefutable evidence that modifying these risk factors through life-style changes or medical treatment will delay and possibly prevent the development of cardiovascular diseases such as stroke and coronary heart disease (CHD).

There is no question that cardiovascular disease can be prevented in certain individuals. The question is how much modification is required for how much prevention? We must determine these 'orders of magnitude' to understand the potential efficacy of dietary change for the average Canadian.

The development of CHD is associated with elevations in total serum cholesterol but this relationship weakens with advancing age[2,4]. Accordingly, the potential benefit of lowering total serum cholesterol in an individual is strongly related to the age of that individual and young adults will probably benefit more than the elderly. Men are also more likely to benefit than women.

Serum cholesterol and diet

The benefits of reducing total serum cholesterol have been clearly demonstrated in the Lipid Research Clinic Coronary Primary Prevention trial (LRC-CPPT) and the Helsinki trial using a combination of dietary intervention and drugs[5,6]. However, these trials were restricted to middle-aged men with

---

Some of this material was previously published in *Nutrition Quarterly*, 1990, **14** (3), 51–52 and *J. Am. Med. Assoc.*, 1992; **267**, 816–22.

severely elevated total serum cholesterol levels and it may not be appropriate to extrapolate these encouraging results to women or the elderly.

Regardless of their generalizability, what are the 'orders of magnitude' seen among middle-aged men? Close inspection of the LRC-CPPT data demonstrates that after 7.4 years of treatment, 8.1% of those in the treatment group (using diet and drugs) developed CHD outcomes whereas 9.8% of those in the placebo group (using diet only) did[5]. This represents an absolute reduction of 1.7%. In other words, treating 100 individuals for 7.4 years would prevent 1.7 heart attacks or deaths among high risk individuals (average cholesterol 292 mg/dl or 7.6 mmol/l) vigorously treated with diet and drugs. (The reduction in total serum cholesterol was 13.4% in the diet/drug group vs. 4.9% in the diet only group, a net reduction of 8.5%).

Less aggressive treatment with dietary modification alone would presumably result in less benefit. Among the diet only group of the LRC-CPPT, total serum cholesterol fell only 4.9% even after visiting the clinic every 2 months. Lower risk individuals, such as women, would also presumably benefit less.

The Canadian Consensus Conference on cholesterol recommended that all adult Canadians know their serum cholesterol level[7]. Those with a total serum cholesterol above 200 mg/dl should be encouraged to lower their levels through diet and/or medical management. Unfortunately, while the Consensus Conference weighed the evidence in support of the lipid hypothesis, it did not calculate the number of Canadians who would be affected by these recommendations, the potential benefits that might result, or the total costs to the health care system. In a previous study, we estimated that among adult Canadians without cardiovascular disease, over 53% would be told that their cholesterol level places them at high or moderate risk requiring intervention[8]. The total cost of screening *alone* was calculated to be between $432 and $561 million for the first year only. Clearly, additional information is required before informing over half of adult Canadians that they should become regular consumers of our overburdened health care system.

The Nutrition Recommendations for Canadians were recently revised by the Scientific Review Committee for Health and Welfare Canada[9]. This committee recommended that all Canadians aged 2 years and over should follow a diet low in cholesterol and saturated fat to prevent the development of CHD. Once again, it is assumed that the benefits will more than outweigh the risks as well as the costs. Unfortunately, the current dietary consumption of Canadians and the current CHD risk of Canadians were not estimated, nor were the expected benefits of modifying the Canadian diet.

Predicting the development of CHD – a computer model

To address many of these questions, we have developed a computer model to predict the changes in life-expectancy and morbidity associated with risk factor modification[10]. The CHD primary prevention model calculates the annual probability of dying from CHD or other causes (non-CHD) and the annual risk of specific CHD events for an individual free of CHD at entry into the model (Figure 1).

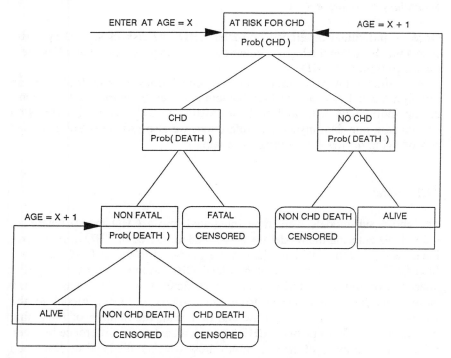

Figure 1 Overview of CHD model. Persons free of CHD enter the model at age x and are at risk of (Prob) CHD events over the following year. Those who develop CHD may suffer a CHD death, or a non-CHD death and are censored. At the end of 1 year, all survivors with CHD age 1 year (x+1) and remain at risk of CHD or non-CHD death. All persons without CHD remain at risk of non-CHD death and the survivors after 1 year re-enter the model at age (x+1). (Reproduced with permission, *J. Am. Med. Assoc.*, 1992, **267**, 816–22. Copyright 1992, American Medical Association)

Non-cardiac events

The risk of all-cause death was based on the 1986 Canadian life tables published by Statistics Canada[11]. These tables present the age-specific annual probability of dying from all causes for men and women in Canada starting at birth and terminating at age 102. These global probabilities were adjusted for specific factors associated with all-cause mortality including cigarette smoking (yes or no), glucose intolerance (yes or no), and the level of diastolic blood pressure (mmHg) based on Framingham results which identified these risk factors to be significantly associated with all-cause mortality[12].

Secondary coronary events

Once an individual developed non-fatal CHD, the risk of secondary CHD events was based on the logistic equations for primary events after adjustment for the presence of CHD.

Accordingly, the previously described probabilities were multiplied by an inflation factor based on the Framingham sex-specific mortality ratios comparing individuals with and without existing CHD[13]. Among those who developed a non-fatal myocardial infarction, we also estimated the increased risk of dying during the ensuing 12 months[13].

CHD model

The above sub-models were then integrated into a CHD model where all individuals entering the model were assumed to be free of CHD at time zero. Each year a number of individuals were predicted to die of CHD, or other (non-CHD) causes. The risk of non-fatal CHD events such as myocardial infarction or angina pectoris/coronary insufficiency was also computed and these individuals then moved from the primary coronary model to the secondary coronary model. At the end of 1 year, the number of remaining individuals at risk for primary CHD was calculated as the difference between those at the beginning of the year minus those who had died and/or developed CHD. The annual cumulative mortality differences among survivors (with and without intervention) over the total life expectancy represented the total years of life saved following intervention. Dividing total years of life saved by the original number of individuals at risk at time zero resulted in the average years of life saved per individual.

Model validation

The accuracy of this computer model was evaluated using data from three CHD primary prevention clinical trials. They included lipid lowering trials such as the Helsinki Heart Study[6] and the LRC-CPPT[5]. The multiple risk factor intervention trial (MRFIT) was also evaluated where the interventions included smoking cessation, cholesterol reduction, and the control of hypertension[14]. The baseline risk profiles of subjects following randomization were obtained from the published reports including summary statistics for age, sex, total serum cholesterol, HDL cholesterol, diastolic blood pressure, and the prevalence of cigarette smokers, left ventricular hypertrophy, and glucose intolerance.

The computer model accurately predicted the results observed in the Helsinki, LRC-CPPT, and MRFIT studies over 5 years, 7.4 years, and 10.5 years respectively. The predicted cumulative event rates closely matched those observed in the clinical trials in terms of CHD events and total mortality (Figures 2–4).

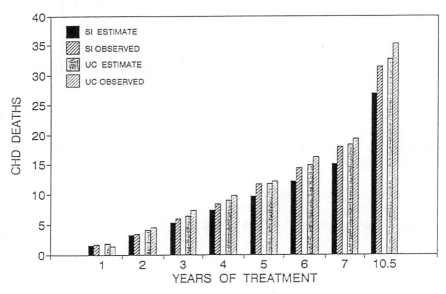

Figure 2 The CHD model and CHD deaths in the MRFIT Study where the estimated results for the special intervention (SI) and the usual care (UC) groups are compared to the observed results. (Reproduced with permission, *J. Am. Med. Assoc.*, 1992, **267**, 816–22. Copyright 1992, American Medical Association)

We also estimated the lifetime benefits of treatment based on the risk factor modification observed over the short-term follow-up of these clinical trials (Figure 5). Among those using cholestyramine in the LRC-CPPT study, the net benefit of treatment would average 1.5 years of life saved for each individual. Among those using gemfibrozil in the Helsinki study, the lifetime benefits of treatment would average 1.3 years of life saved. In the MRFIT

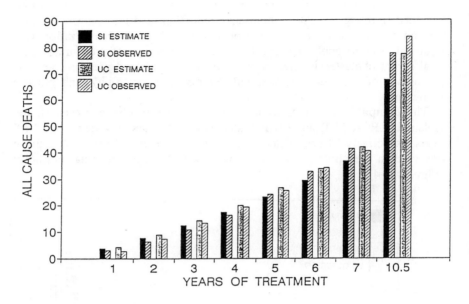

Figure 3 The CHD model and all-cause deaths in the MRFIT Study where the estimated results for the special intervention (SI) and the usual care (UC) groups are compared to the observed results

study, the net benefits for the special intervention group following net reductions in total serum cholesterol, smoking cessation, and blood pressure reduction would average 3.3 years of life saved per individual.

Predicted changes in life expectancy

Using the results of the LRC-CPPT trial where total serum cholesterol fell approximately 5% in the diet only group, we estimated the corresponding change in life expectancy that would occur among Canadians after a similar change in diet. The predicted life-time benefits of cholesterol reduction varied greatly depending upon the baseline level (5.7–7.8 mmol/l or 220–300 mg/dl), the presence or absence of other risk factors, and the age and sex of the individual. For the low risk individuals (no other risk factors, diastolic blood pressure of 80 mmHg), the average increased life expectancy associated with dietary intervention alone was small ranging from 0.03 to 0.32 years for men and 0.04 to 0.19 years for women. Among 'high risk' individuals who smoke and have a diastolic blood pressure of 100 mmHg, the average increased life

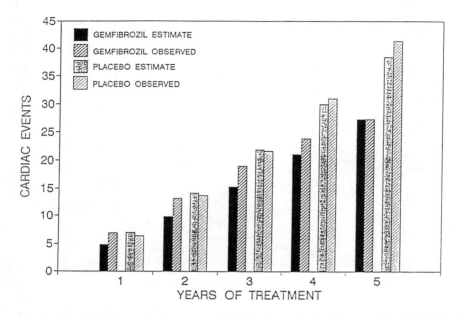

Figure 4 The CHD model and the Helsinki Study where estimated cardiac events (including cardiac death, fatal and non-fatal myocardial infarction) for the gemfibrozil and placebo groups are compared to the observed results. (Reproduced with permission, *J. Am. Med. Assoc.*, 1992, **267**, 816–22. Copyright 1992, American Medical Association)

expectancy would range from 0.05 to 0.60 years for men and 0.05 to 0.24 years for women.

Conclusions

In summary, elevations in total serum cholesterol are associated with an increased risk of CHD. Medical treatment in high risk individuals can prevent CHD. However, we have not demonstrated, either empirically or through critical analyses, that changing the average Canadian diet will substantially change the average life expectancy.

Our computer model suggests that some individuals may benefit from dietary change if they are at 'high risk' due to a high serum cholesterol and/or the presence of other CHD factors. On the other hand, the average change in life expectancy for many groups of Canadians may be less than 1 month as these individuals are already at 'low risk' for CHD.

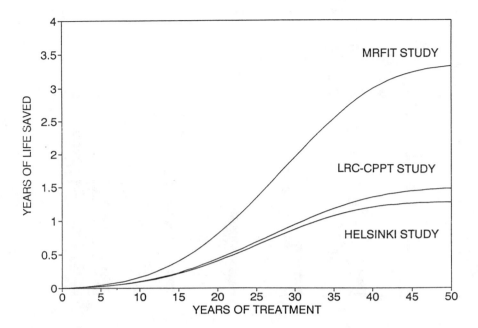

Figure 5 The predicted change in life expectancy (years of life saved) following lifetime risk factor modification observed in three clinical trials including the **MRFIT** Study SI group (+3.3 years), the Helsinki Study Gemfibrozil group (+1.3 years), and the LRC-CPPT cholestyramine group (+1.5 years)

We conclude that the risks, benefits, and costs of dietary modification must be better understood before devising a national strategy. Only then can a scientifically sound and economically feasible program be implemented.

Acknowledgements

This study was supported in part by grants from the National Health Research and Development Program (#6605–3440-H), Health and Welfare Canada; and the Dairy Bureau of Canada (#610015–600).

Dr. Grover is a research scholar supported by Le fonds de la recherche en santé du Québec.

References

1. Nicholls, E., Nair, C., MacWilliam, L. *et al.* (1986). Cardiovascular disease in Canada. *Statistics Canada, Health and Welfare Canada.* 82–544
2. Abbott, R.D. and McGee, D. (1987). The Framingham Study, Section 37. The probability of developing certain cardiovascular disease in eight years at specified values of some characteristics. NIH Publication. no. 87–2284
3. Martin, M.J., Hulley, S.B., Browner, W.S., Kuller, L.H. and Wentworth, D. (1986). Serum cholesterol, blood pressure, and mortality: Implications from a cohort of 361,662 men. *Lancet,* **2**, 933–6
4. Stamler, J., Wentworth, D. and Neaton, J. (1986). Is the relationship between serum cholesterol and risk of death from CHD continuous and graded? *J. Am. Med. Assoc.,* **256**, 2823–8
5. Lipid Research Clinics Program. (1984). The Lipid Research Clinics Coronary Primary Prevention Trial Results: I. Reduction in the incidence of coronary heart disease. *J. Am. Med. Assoc.,* **251**, 351–64
6. Frick, M.H., Elo, O., Haapa, K. *et al.* (1987). Helsinki Heart Study: Primary prevention trial with gemfibrozil in middle-aged men with dyslipidemia. *N. Engl. J. Med.,* **317**, 1237–45
7. The Canadian Consensus Conference on Cholesterol. (1988). Final Report. *Can. Med. Assoc. J.,* **139** (Suppl.), 1–8
8. Grover, S.A., Coupal, L., Fakhry, R. and Suissa, S. (1991). Screening for hypercholesterolemia among Canadians: how much will it cost? *Can. Med. Assoc. J.,* **144**, 161–8
9. The Report of the Scientific Review Committee. Nutrition Recommendations (1990). *Health and Welfare Canada,* no. H49–42/1990E
10. Grover, S.A., Abrahamowicz, M., Joseph, L., Coupal, L., Brewer, C. and Suissa, S. (1992). The benefits of treating hyperlipidemia to prevent coronary heart disease: Predicting changes in life expectancy and morbidity. *J. Am. Med. Assoc.,* **267**, 816–22
11. Statistics Canada. Life Tables, Canada and Provinces, 1985–1987. Ottawa, On: Statistics Canada, 1989. (Health Division. Vital Statistics and Disease Registries Section.) (Formerly catalogue 84–532)
12. Shurtleff, D. (1974). Some characteristics related to the incidence of cardiovascular disease and death: Framingham Study, 18 year follow-up. Section 30. In Kannel, W.B. and Gordon, T. (eds): *The Framingham Study: An Epidemiological Investigation of Cardiovascular Disease.* US Department of Health, Education, and Welfare Publication, NIH 74–599. (Bethesda, Md: US Government Printing Office)
13. Kannel, W.B., Wolf, P.A. and Garrison R.J. (1988). The Framingham Study, section 35, Survival following initial cardiovascular events. Thirty year follow-up. National Heart, Lung, and Blood Institute Publication, NIH 88–2969. (Bethesda, Md: US Government Printing Office)
14. The Multiple Risk Factor Intervention Trial Research Group. (1990). Mortality rates after 10.5 years for participants in the multiple risk factor intervention trial. *J. Am. Med. Assoc.,* **263**, 1795–801

Discussion

Dr Kubow: I wonder if you could reconcile your data showing an age effect with the previous data we saw from Dr Anderson showing no effect of age.

Dr Grover: You have got to remember that where age is in fact concerned, my data are based on Dr Anderson's data. My data are based on publications that Framingham has been putting out for many years. In 1974, I believe it was section 28, Framingham put out a monogram showing that the age–cholesterol interaction was important. In 1987, section 37 of their publication said the same thing and the interaction effect was of the same relative order of magnitude. For years this interaction effect has been there. It is not just Framingham, if you look at the MRFIT study stratified by age, the interaction effect is there as well. Correct me if I am wrong, but Dr Anderson's model is looking at the CHD relationship using total cholesterol to HDL as a ratio. In our particular case I am really not addressing the HDL issue at the moment, I am saying, leave HDL the same but look what happens across total cholesterol. And, remember, our total screening strategies at the moment are largely based on total serum cholesterol, we only do the HDL afterwards. Also remember that our therapies at the moment are largely aimed at lowering total serum cholesterol and it remains to be determined just how efficacious raising HDL cholesterol will be.

Dr Horlick: Although these are extremely interesting data, and very well presented, we are really looking at the whole population here, we are not looking at individuals. As physicians we look at individuals and the figure of a 10% maximum effect from diet is indeed correct if you look at the whole population. But, the data from many nutritional studies have shown that there is a great deal of individual variability in how people respond to diet and that the effect might be quite different from one person to another. Therefore, the physician, when faced with this problem, has to look at the individual characteristics of the person that he is dealing with, rather than with the whole spectrum of the population as a whole. That is my first point.

   My second point is that we are looking at mortality, we are not looking at morbidity. There is a lot of evidence to suggest that alteration of risk factors may have very significant effects on morbidity as well as mortality, and the fact that you may only live an extra couple of days pales into insignificance if you are going to be able to live the last 2 or 3 years of your life without being crippled by an ischaemic event.

Dr Grover: I think both of those points are terribly important. To address your first point, the issue about what an individual can accomplish, I think is true. However, at the present time, our dietary recommendations are for the entire population without any identification of the presence or absence of other risk factors. When you look at the entire population, this is the average reduction you can expect to see, but I quite agree with you. Certainly when I see a patient in my office, before I put him on medication, I give a chance to diet if I believe that person is at significant risk and is going to have significant benefit from lowering that risk through diet or drug intervention.

As far as your second point, I have not had any chance to show you the morbidity numbers and I think they are very important. We have designed our model in such a way that it is capable of determining morbidity as well, because of course, you can censor the individuals at the time they die, or you can censor them at the point where they develop coronary heart disease. So, we can actually look at years free of CHD. In our work in this area it tends to be about twofold greater than years of life saved. So, if you save a year of life, you save 2 years free of coronary heart disease. But again, if you save a day of life, you save 2 days free of CHD, on average.

Dr Katan: I think this is a fascinating set of data and my first question about morbidity was already pre-empted by the previous speaker. The other point I wanted to make was about individuals. When an individual engages in some kind of prudent behaviour he is not thinking about the average impact on the population. For example, when I drive I always use a safety belt. When I was in Naples 2 weeks ago they thought that that was very funny, a little bit ridiculous, and many of the cars do not have them. Indeed, if you calculate the average benefit of wearing a safety belt, I don't know what it is, but I guess it is something in the order of 1 day or 1 hour of gain in life expectancy. But, I am not interested in the population, I am interested in my own risk. If my risk of becoming seriously crippled in an accident is 1% without a belt and 0.3% with a safety belt, I would like a safety belt. You might want to count your data not only in terms of averages, which are very important from a national policy point of view, but also in terms of what is your chance of having a major catastrophe – like having a crippling heart attack in the next 5 years and how much can you do about it. If it then turns out that the chance of having a heart attack is 5% and it is possible to reduce the risk to 3%, people can make their own decision. Some people will say it is too much trouble whereas others will take the 2% gain.

Dr Grover: I agree with you on both of those points. In the Centre of Cardiovascular Assessment at the Montreal General Hospital, we do these simulations with patients showing them what we believe are the outer limits of intervention. Given that information, those who choose to go on to treatment will at least be aware of what they are getting for their treatment. I think it is very motivating. As you know, if you treat these patients, compliance is terrible in many cases. They have nothing to show for what you have done to change their lifestyle. At least in this case you can say, look you have improved your life expectancy and you have lowered your risk and this is what we believe the numbers are. On the other hand, we have people who look at these numbers and say, is that all it is? These are the people who thought they were going to drop dead tomorrow and thought that if they did this they would live forever. When they can realize it is not so black and white, they can make an informed decision.

Dr Holub: I think so many other factors need considering. Last year the Nutrition Recommendations for Canada did not specifically recommend lowering dietary cholesterol from 450 to 300 mg/day. We clearly differ from the American expert committees in this regard. Secondly, there is a very aggressive recommendation that we lower the total fat intake. You eluded to saturated fat as well. Thirdly, there is a very aggressive recommendation that we increase our complex carbohydrate intake including fibre. In 1985 we had an expert committee that recommended that Canadians double their fibre intake to assist the risk of CVD by blood cholesterol-lowering. It can be estimated that there would be approximately a 1–2% drop in blood cholesterol for every 1-gram increase in soluble fibre consumed per day whereas the American Heart and Surgeon General's committees in the United States were not solid on the fibre issue up until 1988. So, I think we need to take the complete package, including the fibre and the total fat, before we regard dietary intervention as having a minimal effect in any age group.

Dr Grover: Your point is well taken but, on the other side of the coin, I would argue that in arriving at those recommendations we also need some hard data about what we believe the benefits would be in some quantitative fashion. To simply say we have got a few studies that say that fibre is good, so let us double fibre, is a bit ridiculous. Similarly, we have studies that show that fat is bad. But, to reduce fat without any real assessment about what the current fibre and fat intake of Canadians is and how much we plan to change it and what we expect the benefits of this change will be, it seems unclear to me how we can arrive at recommendations without this information.

Dr Gold: When recommendations are made from consensus conferences, they are largely based on population studies and are intended to attempt to alter societal patterns of behaviour. However, what I have heard to a large extent this morning is that the same individuals who have made such recommendations but cannot find statistically significant population data to support the recommendations concerning cholesterol and CHD will often mention the potential importance of the recommendations to the well-being of the individual patient. I could not agree more about the concern for the individual patient but I don't think that in the light of the discussions that we are having that one can 'have it both ways'. I think we must decide where and when we are talking about populations and, conversely, when we are talking about the individual patient. I believe that by switching from one to the other without clearly indicating where, when and why is creating a great deal of confusion and that this is one of the points that we must resolve.

3

Coronary risk factors today: a view from Scotland

C.G. ISLES and D.J. HOLE

Introduction

It is accepted that cardiovascular disease is the commonest cause of death in the Western world, and that cardiovascular mortality among those living in Scotland is particularly high[1]. It is also agreed that a large proportion of coronary deaths could be delayed[2,3]. The purpose of this review is to examine the evidence that coronary heart disease (CHD) can be delayed by stopping smoking, lowering cholesterol and reducing blood pressure. Although the development of CHD is also related to psychosocial factors, to obesity and to fibrinogen, there is less agreement here on the benefits of change.

Cigarette smoking

Cigarette smoking appears to be the most important risk factor for CHD in countries where the incidence of CHD is high[4-7]. The rate in smokers has generally been two to three times that of non-smokers and is dose related, with no evidence that non-inhalation or the use of filter cigarettes[4] offers any protection. Recent evidence suggests that passive smokers may also be at risk[8]. Cigarette smoking not only promotes premature coronary atherosclerosis[9] but also has important effects on coagulation[10] and the sympathetic nervous system[11]. All of these may contribute to the increased risk of coronary disease.

There is still some uncertainty, however, concerning the risk associated with pipe smoking and cigar smoking. An apparently paradoxical finding is that pipe and cigar smokers who have never smoked cigarettes may not be at increased risk[4,12], whereas smokers who change from cigarettes to pipes or cigars continue to experience the same risk as current smokers[12]. A recent case control study showed a two-fold excess risk among pipe smokers who had never smoked cigarettes, although the confidence intervals were wide and the estimate of risk did not achieve statistical significance[13]. A likely difficulty, here and in other analyses of pipe and cigar smokers, is that the numbers studied are too small, and the CHD end points too few, for confident predictions of risk.

The best advice to an individual seeking to lower his or her chance of CHD is, of course, not to start smoking, but the problem faced by most doctors in the UK is that many of their patients have smoked for a considerable number of years. Recommendations that patients should stop smoking are based on the widespread belief that CHD rates in ex-smokers approximate those of non-smokers within a year or two of giving up smoking.

Data from the United States[4,14] and the Whitehall Civil Servants Study[6] support this view, but other reports describe an intermediate risk persisting for at least 5 years[15] and a recent analysis from the British Regional Heart Study suggests that this is still evident 20 years after stopping smoking[12]. One explanation for this surprising result is that the British men may only have stopped smoking because they had been advised to do so following the diagnosis of CHD. These findings emphasize the need to persuade individuals never to start smoking, to give up as soon as possible if they are smokers, or as a poor third option to reduce the number of cigarettes smoked if they are unable to stop.

Plasma cholesterol

The importance of plasma cholesterol as a risk factor hardly needs stating[4–7,16] (Figure 1). CHD is rare among populations where plasma cholesterol is below 5.2 mmol/l. Risk appears to increase progressively at levels above this, and a number of lipid lowering drug trials have shown that CHD rates may be lowered by therapy[17–21]. There remain, however, many uncertainties.

Differences between and within countries

Although serum cholesterol and incidence of CHD are strongly correlated between populations[22] and within populations[23], there are differences in CHD rates that cannot readily be explained in this way (Figure 2). Average serum cholesterol is only slightly higher in Scotland than in France and yet CHD mortality is four times more common among Scots men, and six times more common among Scots women[1]. To explain these findings, a number of theories have been proposed that depend on protection against CHD by wine[24], or food such as garlic[25] and olive oil[26]. All of these are consumed in greater quantities in France than in Scotland. This is clearly an area that requires further study.

The possibility exists that at least some of the difference between CHD rates in Scotland and France is artefactual, as a consequence of underdiagnosis

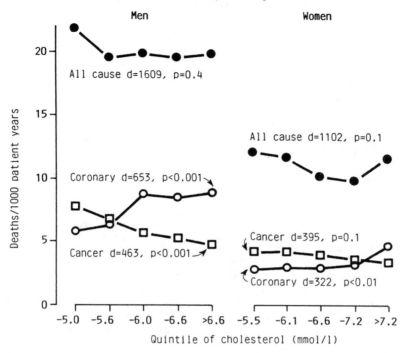

Figure 1 Relation between plasma cholesterol, coronary heart disease, cancer and all-cause mortality in Renfrew and Paisley[16]. Deaths are per 1000 patient years after adjusting for age, body mass index, diastolic pressure, cigarette smoking and social class. The best fit for each of the slopes was shown to be linear by logistic regression analysis, except for all-cause mortality in women which was curvilinear. The *p* values refer to trends across the quintiles of plasma cholesterol

of CHD by the French. Had this been the case, then a higher proportion of less specific cardiac causes of death such as 'cardiac insufficiency' might have been used in France than in Scotland. A recent analysis from the WHO showing that mortality from all cardiovascular diseases in France is considerably lower than in Scotland suggests that this is not so[27].

The geographical variation in CHD rates that exists within Scotland is just as intriguing. The Scottish Heart Health Study recently reported a population survey showing the cardiovascular risk profile and mortality in Edinburgh and north Glasgow[28], and have since extended their findings to cover 10 359 men and women aged 40–59 years across 22 districts in Scotland[29]. The results (Table 1) show that there is a marked variation in coronary mortality both between Glasgow and Edinburgh and within the Glasgow area itself. The authors correctly concluded that serum cholesterol levels in Scotland are high and 'a challenge for action' but it is equally clear that serum cholesterol cannot

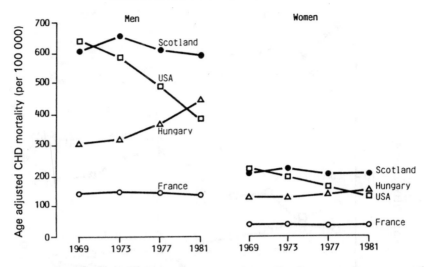

Figure 2 Age adjusted CHD mortality in selected countries for men and women aged 40–69 years[1]. The figure makes no attempt to be fully comprehensive but serves instead to illustrate certain trends. CHD mortality in Scotland was particularly high between 1968 and 1981 at a time when rates in the US were falling. By contrast CHD mortality appeared to be increasing in Hungary and in some other eastern European countries. Rates in France were strikingly low throughout the period of observation, despite the fact that serum cholesterol levels were only slightly lower in France than in Scotland

be responsible for the difference in CHD mortality between the participating centres (Table 1).

Table 1 Serum cholesterol and coronary mortality in Scotland 1984–1986

| | *Men* | | *Women* | |
	Cholesterol (mmol/l)	Coronary SMR	Cholesterol (mmol/l)	Coronary SMR*
Eastwood	6.4	61	6.6	50
Edinburgh	6.4	81	6.7	83
North Glasgow	6.3	117	6.5	121
Monklands	6.4	136	6.7	147

Glasgow and Edinburgh are 50 miles distant; Eastwood is a prosperous suburb of Glasgow and Monklands a poorer area lying to the east of Glasgow; *SMR = standardized mortality rate.

The triglyceride issue

Because triglyceride is positively correlated with total cholesterol, obesity, alcohol intake and diabetes, but negatively correlated with HDL cholesterol, its independent contribution to CHD risk has been difficult to assess[30]. In most univariate analyses serum triglyceride emerges as a positive risk factor, but when other risks are taken into account the significance of triglyceride diminishes[30,31] and this has been taken to mean that high triglyceride is merely a marker for other CHD risk factors[32].

This view is currently being re-examined following analyses from Framingham and Paris. The Framingham group have shown excess CHD risk in men and women with high triglyceride and low HDL irrespective of the total cholesterol level[33]. The French workers, who did not measure HDL, reported excess CHD risk in patients with high triglyceride and normal cholesterol[34]. There is also renewed interest in the possibility that high levels of triglyceride may affect coagulation as well as atherogenesis[35].

For the present, it appears reasonable to conclude that in subjects with high cholesterol the co-existence of high triglyceride adds little in the way of extra risk. However in those with normal cholesterol, triglyceride >3 mmol/l may be associated with increased mortality from CHD, particularly if HDL is <1 mmol/l.

Protective effect of HDL

Of the various lipoprotein fractions studied so far, none has aroused more interest than HDL cholesterol, largely because high levels appear to exert a protective effect against CHD. The evidence comes from several sources notably Framingham[36], the Lipid Clinics Trial[37] and the MRFIT Cohort[38]. A recent paper from the British Regional Heart Study confirms this view[39] reversing a previous report from the same group which suggested that HDL cholesterol might not be protective in British men. The mechanism by which HDL exerts this effect is not known for certain, and the often quoted ability of HDL to carry cholesterol from peripheral cells to the liver for disposal may be too simplistic[40].

For those seeking practical guidelines, patients with high total cholesterol (>6.5 mmol/l) probably do not require treatment if their HDL cholesterol is >2 mmol/l. If, however, HDL cholesterol is <1 mmol/l, the risk of CHD is greatly increased and aggressive therapy is generally indicated.

Cholesterol and cancer

A further area of controversy concerns the inverse relation between serum cholesterol and cancer[41]. An early review dismissed this as a metabolic consequence of cancers already present at the time of screening[42] but findings in other studies suggest that this cannot be the whole explanation[43-46].

In a recent analysis from Renfrew and Paisley in the West of Scotland, a preclinical cancer effect also seems unlikely[16]. An inverse relation between serum cholesterol and cancer was observed in both sexes, although it was significant in men only (Figure 1). It was present for cancer incidence as well as for cancer mortality, and it persisted when new cases or deaths occurring within the first 4 years of follow-up were excluded from the analysis. Cancers with the steepest negative relation were lung cancers in men. It seems unlikely that these cancers could affect cholesterol metabolism many years before the tumours became clinically apparent.

If a preclinical cancer effect is not responsible, what alternative explanations may exist? Two other possibilities deserve consideration: first, that some other factor is lowering cholesterol and independently predisposing to cancer; and second that low levels of serum cholesterol *per se* promote the development of cancer. Both views have their protagonists[47,48], but as yet the issue is unresolved.

So far as drug treatment is concerned, clofibrate was shown to increase cancer mortality[17], but otherwise there has been no significant excess of cancer deaths in the cholesterol lowering drug trials[18-21]. Although reassuring, these results do not entirely exclude a harmful effect. This is because the trials were conducted in men at high risk initially and not among men and women in the general population. The question whether reduction of plasma cholesterol lying initially within the normal range is associated with an increased risk of cancer has not, to our knowledge, been tested.

Hypertension

Hypertension, like plasma cholesterol, is a major risk factor for CHD. The gradient of risk is steep and has been observed in all major prospective observational studies[4-7]. Eventual effects of moderate differences in diastolic pressure on the risks of CHD and stroke have recently been estimated in a meta-analysis of nine studies involving a total of some 420 000 men and women, among whom 5000 CHD events and 8000 strokes were recorded over follow-up intervals of 6 months to 25 years[49]. After adjustment for age, cholesterol and smoking the results indicate that a difference of as little as 6 mmHg in diastolic pressure was associated with 22% fewer fatal and non-fatal myocardial infarctions and 36% fewer strokes. In populations that were free of CHD initially, the relationships were continuous and not J shaped. Moreover, there was no evidence of any threshold pressure below which CHD risk ceased to decline.

In light of these findings the observation that treating mild to moderate hypertension does not appear to reduce the risk of CHD is puzzling. The failure of a number of random controlled trials of treatment to demonstrate a reduction in the incidence of fatal and non-fatal MI indicates that at best the gradient of benefit is small[50-54]. Moreover, a meta-analysis of these and other trials involving a total of 37 000 individuals, 1400 CHD events and 700 strokes confirms this disappointing result. The overall risk of CHD was reduced by only 12% with confidence intervals ranging from 0 to 20%, whereas there was a 43% reduction in the risk of stroke which was highly significant[55].

Several explanations have been proposed to account for these results (Table 2) and the last, that treatment of hypertension may be beneficial in so far as it lowers blood pressure, but harmful in that a new risk or risks may be introduced by therapy, has received most attention. Here, the potential adverse effects of diuretics and beta-blockers on blood lipids have come under great scrutiny, and there is of course the additional concern that diuretics will induce or aggravate hypokalaemia, glucose intolerance and gout.

Table 2 Reasons for failure to reduce risk of CHD in treated hypertensives

1.	Failure to control BP
2.	Slow reversal of risk
3.	Irreversible risk
4.	Association not casual
5.	Other vascular risks, e.g. smoking, cholesterol
6.	Introduction of new risk

So far as the effects on blood lipids are concerned, it is generally agreed that diuretics increase total cholesterol, LDL cholesterol and triglyceride with minimal effects on HDL cholesterol[56]. Beta-blockers are associated with minimal changes in total cholesterol and LDL cholesterol, but reduced HDL cholesterol and increased triglycerides[56]. These alterations are less pronounced with selective beta-blockers and in beta-blockers with ISA[56], but nevertheless it is possible that the changes described both for diuretics and for beta-blockers could augment the risk of CHD. By contrast ACE inhibitors and calcium channel blockers are regarded as lipid neutral[56] and the use of the new highly selective alpha-blocker Doxazosin appears to be associated with a favourable lipid profile, namely reduced levels of total cholesterol, LDL and triglyceride and increased HDL cholesterol[57].

The dilemma for the practising clinician is to decide whether the theoretical advantages of the newer drugs should alter current treatment practices, or whether we should wait for morbidity and mortality studies to prove that ACE inhibitors, calcium channel blockers and alpha-blockers lower the risk of both CHD and stroke, without causing unanticipated harmful effects. The recently published advice of the British Hypertension Society for mild hypertensive patients who require drug therapy is still to use a thiazide diuretic or a beta-blocker first, unless these drugs cause side-effects, are ineffective or are otherwise contra-indicated[58]. An alternative approach in light of earlier comment might be to measure the serum lipids as part of the initial assessment and then tailor the treatment to the patient by taking the results of the lipid profile into consideration.

Multiple risk factors

Increased awareness that CHD is multifactorial in origin has led to a shift of emphasis in both observation studies and intervention trials. Data from Framingham show just how steeply CHD risk rises when combinations of risk factors are present[4], and similar trends can be seen in men and women living in the West of Scotland. Male smokers in Renfrew and Paisley with cholesterol > 6 mmol/l (top 40% of distribution) and diastolic pressure > 97 mmHg (top 20% of distribution) had four-fold higher CHD mortality than men who did not smoke, whose cholesterol was < 6 mmol/l and diastolic pressure < 97 mmHg (Figure 3). The relative risk for women with multiple risk factors was even greater, although this probably reflects the fact that absolute rates for low risk women were lower than for low risk men[16].

Such findings also suggest an explanation for some of the disappointing results of single risk factor intervention trials. Although the authors of the cholesterol lowering trials are entitled to claim significant benefit[17-21] for CHD, it would clearly have been much more satisfying to have shown a reduction in all-cause mortality too. Equally it is a pity that antihypertensive drugs appear to reduce only the risk of stroke in mild to moderate hypertension[50-54], an unexpected result given that CHD is the commonest cause of death in hypertensive patients. The answer may be, of course, that it is unrealistic to expect single risk factor intervention to alter significantly the course of a multifactorial disease.

There is already considerable circumstantial evidence to support a multifactorial approach, and the following three studies serve to illustrate this point. In the Primary Prevention Trial in Gothenberg in Sweden, 686 middle-aged hypertensive men derived from screening a random population sample were followed for up to 12 years[59]. The authors state that individuals at high risk because of their cholesterol levels or smoking habits were offered 'interventive

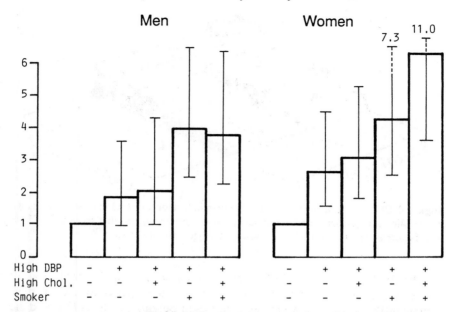

Figure 3 Adjusted relative risk of CHD (with 95% confidence intervals) among men and women in Renfrew and Paisley. For the purposes of this analysis subjects were classified as having high DBP if they were in the top fifth, and high cholesterol in the top two-fifths, of the distribution for each sex

measures' although the nature of these was not specified. Nevertheless the results suggest quite strongly that a combined reduction of blood pressure and cholesterol is necessary in order to achieve a substantial reduction in morbidity (Figure 4). This result is all the more interesting because the drugs used to lower blood pressure in this trial were thiazides and beta-blockers[59].

The North Karelia Study was a comprehensive community programme designed to reduce the incidence of cardiovascular disease in part of Finland where coronary mortality had been particularly high. The neighbouring province of Kuopio, in which there was no special intervention programme, served as a reference area to reflect changes that were taking place elsewhere in Finland. Although the early (5 year) results showed greater reduction in coronary risk factors and coronary mortality in north Karelia than in Kuopio[60], the long term (15 year) change in CHD mortality was similar in both provinces[61]. One interpretation of these findings is that population measures are ineffective in preventing CHD[62], but in our view a more likely explanation is that an increasingly health-conscious population in Kuopio adopted healthier life-styles when they heard of the changes that were being recommended in North Karelia.

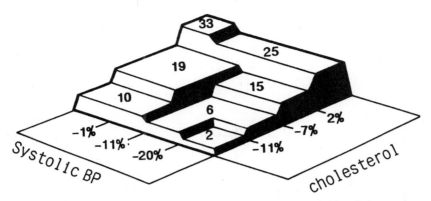

Figure 4 CHD event rates for hypertensive men in Gothenberg trial in relation to change in systolic blood pressure and serum cholesterol. Results suggest that reduction of both risk factors is necessary to achieve a substantial decrease in mortality[59]

The WHO European Collaborative Study was a randomized trial of preventive advice on diet, smoking, obesity, blood pressure and exercise among 60 000 men employed in 80 factories in Belgium, Italy, Poland and the United Kingdom[63]. An important finding was that men in some countries were less inclined to change their life-styles than others. The British seemed most reluctant of all, and hence or otherwise the British CHD mortality showed a small but non-significant increase. However, when risk factors were reduced as in Belgium and Italy, so too was CHD mortality[64]. The best results were seen in Belgium where the reduction in both total CHD (24%) and total mortality (17%) reached statistical significance[65].

Thus, it appears that multiple risk factor intervention is successful in reducing the incidence of CHD, and possibly also of all-cause mortality, in so far as the advice is accepted. The results also suggest that people in different countries may respond very differently to advice about their life-style. To date, the British have been more resistant to the idea of a healthier life-style than have men and women in the rest of Europe and in America.

Acknowledgements

The secretarial assistance of Mrs. Josephine Campbell is gratefully acknowledged. Much of the material used in this paper is drawn from a chapter which will appear in *Preventive Cardiology* edited by Lorimer, A.R. and Shepherd, J. and published by Blackwell Scientific Publications, Oxford, 1991.

References

1. Tunstall-Pedoe, H., Smith, W.C.S and Crombie, I.K. (1986). Levels and trends of coronary heart disease mortality in Scotland compared with other countries. *Hlth Bull.*, **44**, 153–61
2. British Cardiac Society Working Group on Coronary Prevention. (1987). Conclusions and recommendations. *Br. Heart J.*, **57**, 188–9
3. European Atherosclerosis Society Study Group. (1987). Strategies for the prevention of coronary heart disease: a policy statement of the European Atherosclerosis Society. *Eur. Heart J.*, **8**, 77–88
4. Castelli, W.P. (1984). Epidemiology of coronary heart disease: the Framingham study. *Am. J. Med. Symp.*, 4–12
5. Kannel, W.B., Neaton, J.D. and Wentworth, D. (1986). Overall and coronary heart disease mortality rates in relation to major risk factors in 325,348 men screened for the MRFIT. *Am. Heart J.*, **112**, 825–36
6. Reid, D.D., Hamilton, P.J.S., McCartney, P., Rose, G., Jarrett, R. J. and Keen, H. (1976). Smoking and other risk factors for coronary heart disease in British Civil Servants. *Lancet*, **2**, 979–84
7. Shaper, A.G., Pocock, S.J., Walker, M., Phillips, A.M., Whitehead, T.P. and McFarlane, P.W. (1985). Risk factors for ischaemic heart disease: the prospective phase of the British Regional Heart Study. *J. Epidemiol. Commun. Hlth*, **39**, 197–209
8. Hole, D., Gillis, C.R., Chopra, C. and Hawthorne, V. (1989). Passive smoking and cardiorespiratory health in a west of Scotland general population. *Br. Med. J.*, 299, 423–7
9. Strong, J.P. and Richards, M.L. (1976). Cigarette smoking and atherosclerosis in autopsied men. *Atherosclerosis*, **23**, 451–75
10. Kannel, W.B., D'Agostino, R.B. and Belanger, A.J. (1987). Fibrinogen, cigarette smoking and risk of cardiovascular disease: insights from the Framingham Study. *Am. Heart J.*, **113**, 1006–10
11. Winniford, M.D., Wheelan, K.R. and Kramers, M.S. (1986). Smoking induced coronary vasoconstriction in patients with atherosclerosis coronary disease: evidence of adrenergically mediated alterations in coronary artery tone. *Circulation*, **73**, 662–7
12. Cook, D.G., Shaper, A.G., Pocock, S.J. and Kussick, S.J. (1986). Giving up smoking and the risk of heart attacks. *Lancet*, **2**, 1376–80
13. Kaufman, D.W., Palmer, J.R., Rosenberg, L. and Shapiro, S. (1987). Cigar and pipe smoking and myocardial infarction in young men. *Br. Med. J.*, **294**, 1315–16
14. Rosenberg, L., Kaufman, D.W., Helmrich, S.P. and Shapiro, S. (1985). The risk of myocardial infarction after quitting smoking in men under 55 years of age. *N. Engl. J. Med.*, **313**, 1511–14
15. Doll, R. and Peto, R. (1976). Mortality in relation to smoking: 20 years' observation on male British doctors. *Br. Med. J.*, **2**, 1525–36
16. Isles, C.G., Hole, D.J., Gillis, C.R., Hawthorne, V.M. and Lever, A. F. (1989). Plasma cholesterol, coronary heart disease and cancer in the Renfrew and Paisley Survey. *Br. Med. J.*, **298**, 920–4

17. Committee of Principal Investigators. (1978). A cooperative trial in the primary prevention of ischaemic heart disease using Clofibrate. *Br. Heart J.*, **40.**, 1069–118

18. Lipid Research Clinics Program. (1984). The lipids research clinics coronary primary prevention trial results. 1. Reduction in incidence of coronary heart disease. *J. Am. Med. Assoc.*, **251**, 351–64

19. Canner, P.L., Berge, K.G. and Wenger, N.K. (1986). 15 year mortality in coronary drug project patients: longterm benefit with Niacin. *J. Am. Coll. Cardiol.*, **8**, 1245–55

20. Blankenhorn, D.H., Nessim, S.A., Johnson, R.L., Sanmarco, M.E., Azen, S.P. and Cashin-Hemphill, L. (1987). Beneficial effects of combined Colestipol-Niacin therapy on coronary atherosclerosis and coronary venous bypass grafts. *J. Am. Med. Assoc.*, **257**, 3233–40

21. Helsinki Heart Study. (1987). Primary prevention trial with Gemfibrozil in middle aged men with dyslipidaemia. *N. Engl. J. Med.*, **317**, 1237–45

22. Keys, A. (1980). *Seven Countries: A Multivariate Analysis of Death and Coronary Heart Disease.* (Cambridge, Mass: Harvard University Press)

23. Martin, M.J., Hulley, S.B., Browner, W.S., Kuller, L.H. and Wentworth, D. (1986). Serum cholesterol, blood pressure and mortality: implications from a cohort of 361,662 men. *Lancet*, **2**, 933–6

24. St. Leger, A.S., Cochran, A.L. and Moore, F. (1979). Factors associated with cardiac mortality in developed countries with particular reference to the consumption of wine. *Lancet*, **1**, 1017–20

25. Fulder, S. (1989). Garlic and the prevention of cardiovascular disease. *Cardiol. Pract.*, **7**, 30–5

26. Grundy, S.M. (1986). Comparison of monounsaturated fatty acids and carbohydrates for lower plasma cholesterol. *N. Engl. J. Med.*, **314**, 745–8

27. Uemura, K. and Pisa, Z. (1988). Trends in cardiovascular disease mortality in industrialised countries since 1950. *Wrld Hlth Stat. Q.*, **41**, 155–78

28. Smith, W.C.S., Crombie, I.K., Tunstall-Pedoe, H.D., Tavendale, R. and Riemersma, R.A. (1988). Cardiovascular risk factor profile and mortality in two Scottish cities. *Acta Med. Scand. (Suppl.)*, **728**, 113–18

29. Tunstall-Pedoe, H., Smith, W.C.S., Crombie, I.K. and Tavendale, R. (1989). Coronary risk factor and lifestyle variation across Scotland: Results from the Scottish Heart Health Study. *Scot. Med. J.*, **34**, 556–60

30. Hulley, S.B., Rosenman, R.H., Bawol, R.G. and Brand, R.J. (1980). Epidemiology as a guide to clinical decisions: the association between triglyceride and CHD. *N. Engl. J. Med.*, **302**, 1383–9

31. Pocock, S.J., Shaper, A.G. and Phillips, A.N. (1989). Concentration of high density lipoprotein cholesterol, triglycerides and total cholesterol in ischaemic heart disease. *Br. Med. J.*, **298**, 998–1002

32. Concensus Conference. (1984). Treatment of hypertriglyceridaemia. *J. Am. Med. Assoc.*, **251**, 1196–2000

33. Castelli, W.P. (1986). The triglyceride issue: a view from Framingham. *Am. Heart J.*, **11**, 432–7

34. Cambien, F., Jacqueson, A., Richard, J.L., Warnet, J.M., Ducimetiere, P. and Claude, J.R. (1986). Is the level of serum triglyceride a significant predictor of

coronary death in normocholesterolaemic subjects? The Paris prospective study. *Am. J. Epidemiol.*, **124**, 624–32

35. Simpson, H.C.R., Mann, J.I., Meade, T.W., Chakrabarti, R., Stirling, Y. and Woolf, L. (1983). Hypertriglyceridaemia and hypercoagulability. *Lancet*, **1**, 786–90

36. Castelli, W.P., Garrison, R.J., Wilson, P.W.F., Abbott, R.D., Kalousdian, S. and Cannel, W.B. (1986). Incidence of coronary heart disease and lipoprotein cholesterol levels: the Framingham Study. *J. Am. Med. Assoc.*, **256**, 2835–8

37. Gordon, D.J. (For the Lipid Research Clinics coronary primary prevention trial investigators). (1985). Plasma high density lipoprotein cholesterol and coronary heart disease in hypercholesterolaemic men. *Circulation*, **72**, 111–85

38. Watkins, L.O., Neaton, J.D. and Kuller, L.H. (For the MRFIT Research Group). (1985). High density lipoprotein cholesterol incidence in black and white MRFIT usual care men. *Circulation*, **71**, 417A

39. Pocock, S.J., Shaper, A.G., Phillips, A.N., Walker, M. and Whitehead, T.P. (1986). High density lipoprotein is not a major risk factor for ischaemic heart disease in British men. *Br. Med. J.*, 292, 515–19

40. Betteridge, D.J. (1989). High density lipoprotein and coronary heart disease. *Br. Med. J.*, **298**, 974–5

41. McMichael, A.J., Jensen, O.M., Parkin, D.M. and Zaridze, D.G. (1984). Dietary and endogenous cholesterol and human cancer. *Epidemiol. Rev.*, **6**, 192–216

42. International Collaborative Group. (1982). Circulating cholesterol level and risk of death from cancer in men aged 40 to 69 years. *J. Am. Med. Assoc.*, **248**, 2853–9

43. Kark, G.D., Smith, A.H. and Hames, C.G. (1980). The relationship of serum cholesterol to the incidence of cancer in Evans County, Georgia. *J. Chronic Dis.*, **33**, 311–22

44. Beaglehole, R., Foulkes, M.A. and Prior, I.A.M. (1980). Cholesterol and mortality in New Zealand maoris. *Br. Med. J.*, **1**, 285–7

45. Peterson, B. and Trelle, E. (1983). Premature mortality in middle aged men: serum cholesterol as a risk factor. *Klin. Wochenschr.*, **63**, 795–801

46. Schatzkin, A., Hoover, R.N. and Taylor, P.R. (1987). Serum cholesterol and cancer in the NHANES I follow up study. *Lancet*, **2**, 298–301

47. Kark, J.D., Smith, A.H. and Haynes, C.G. (1982). Serum retinol and the relation between serum cholesterol and cancer. *Br. Med. J.*, **284**, 152–4

48. Oliver, M.F. (1988). Reducing cholesterol does not reduce mortality. *J. Am. Coll. Cardiol.*, **12**, 814–17

49. MacMahon, S., Peto, R., Cutler *et al.* (1990). Blood pressure, stroke and coronary disease. Part 1. Prolonged differences in blood pressure. Prospective observational studies corrected for the regression dilution bias. *Lancet*, **335**, 765–74

50. Report by the Management Committee. (1980). The Australian therapeutic trial in mild hypertension. *Lancet*, **1**, 1261–7

51. Amery, A., Brixco, P. and Clement, D. (1985). Mortality and morbidity results from the European Working Party on high blood pressure in the elderly. *Lancet*, **1**, 1349–54

52. Medical Research Council Working Party. (1985). MRC Trial of treatment of mild hypertension: principal results. *Br. Med. J.*, **2**, 97–104

53. IPPPSH Collaborative Group. (1985). Cardiovascular risk and risk factors in a randomised trial of treatment based on the betablocker Oxprenolol: the international prospective primary prevention study in hypertension (IPPPSH). *J. Hypertens.*, **3**, 379–92

54. Wilhelmsen, L., Berglund, G. and Elmfeldt, D. Betablockers versus diuretics in hypertensive men: main results from the HAPPHY trial. *J. Hypertens.*, **5**, 561–72

55. Collins, R., Peto, R. and MacMahon, S. (1990). Blood pressure, stroke and coronary disease. Part 2. Short term reduction in blood pressure. Overview of randomised drug trials in their epidemiological context. *Lancet*, **335**, 827–38

56. Weidmann, P., Euhlinger, D.E. and Gerber, A. (1985). Antihypertensive treatment and serum lipoproteins. *J. Hypertens.*, **3**, 297–306

57. Trost, B.N., Weidmann, P., Riesen, W., Claessens, J., Streulens, Y. and Nelemans, F. (1987). Comparative effects of Doxazosin and Hydrochlorothiazide on serum lipids and blood pressure in essential hypertension. *Am. J. Cardiol.*, **59**, 99G–104G

58. British Hypertension Society Working Party. (1989). Treatment of mild hypertensions. *Br. Med. J.*, **298**, 694–8

59. Samuelsson, O., Wilhelmsen, L., Andersson, O.K., Pennert, K. and Berglund, G. (1987). Cardiovascular morbidity in relation to change in blood pressure and serum cholesterol levels in treated hypertension. Results from the Primary Preventional Trial in Goteborg, Sweden. *J. Am. Med. Assoc.*, **258**, 1768–76

60. Salonen, J.I. , Tuomilehto, J., Puska, P., Nissinen, A. and Kottke, T.E. (1983). Decline in mortality from coronary heart disease in Finland from 1969 to 1979. *Br. Med. J.*, **286**, 1857–60

61. Pyorala, K. (1989). 15 year results of the North Karelia Study. Abstract presented at European Society of Cardiology, Nice

62. McCormick, J. and Skrabanek, P. (1988). Coronary heart disease is not preventable by population interventions. *Lancet*, **2**, 839–41

63. WHO European collaborative Group. (1986). European collaborative trial of multifactorial prevention of coronary heart disease: final report on the 6 year results. *Lancet*, **1**, 869–72

64. WHO European Collaborative Group. (1983). Multifactorial trial in the prevention of coronary heart disease: incidence and mortality results. *Eur. Heart J.*, **4**, 141–7

65. Kornitzer, M., de Backer, G. and Dramix, M. (1983). Belgian Heart Disease Prevention Project: incidence and mortality results. *Lancet*, **1**, 1066–70

Discussion

Dr Roncari: You talked about obesity in your study and I was wondering whether you discriminated between abdominal obesity and diffuse obesity? I ask this question because I believe that on some of the risk factors women become more like men metabolically in terms of risk factors when they develop abdominal obesity. The only other point that I would like to make is that the ratio of oestrogen to androgens may be much more important than the protective effect of oestrogens *per se*.

Dr Isles: Yes, I wish we had looked at the waist hip circumference but in the early 1970s no one had caught on to that yet, so we did not. However, if you extend the curve for body mass index right out and look at those people who have a body mass index of 35 and 40, then there does appear to be an increased risk for coronary heart disease.

Dr Parsons: Your conclusions are based on total cholesterol levels. You have not broken down your cholesterol into HDL and LDL cholesterol. Do you have this information, and if so, when will that information be made available?

Dr Isles: No, in Renfrew and Paisley, in the early 1970s, HDL was not measured routinely. There is, however, a 10% subset, I believe, who had HDL measured, but we do not have enough data on HDL.

Dr Godsland: I am glad to see someone looking at women in detail: they have certainly been disregarded compared to men. There are, however, some discrepancies between findings in your population and in others that have been reported. Firstly, the magnitude of the difference between cholesterol levels in your younger men and women: the Lipid Research Clinics data is probably the largest set of data that has been published in this respect and there does seem to be a cross-over between men and women in cholesterol concentrations as they change with age. But, in the LRC data, up to about 45 years of age men have higher cholesterol levels than women. I was also surprised to see that in your study men had roughly twice the rate of coronary heart disease mortality of women, but the United Kingdom national average is about a sixfold difference. So how representative was your population of men and women in general? Or should we be considering separate populations rather than generalizing?

Dr Isles: First, I would like to address your point about the levels of cholesterol compared to other studies. We only have data from men and women aged 45 onwards and I have thought that they are consistent with the LRC data, in that, from 45 years onwards, the women go up and the men go down slightly. The second point is that I am sure you are right. Our data are representative of men and women living in the west of Scotland who have a very different risk profile from men and women living elsewhere. As well, there are many other factors that we cannot measure under the heading of deprivation that may also be very relevant to the west of Scotland. I do not think that we can generalize from these studies to someone living in California or Japan.

Sheila Murphy: I was interested to see the introduction of social class into the discussion. I was wondering why it was chosen as a risk factor?

Dr Isles: Social class has long been a standard risk factor in the British cardiovascular risk assessments. It probably does define a group of people who have a cluster of other risk factors that adversely affect them in a number of ways. However, it would appear from the results I showed you that the adverse effects of being in a low social class were not accounted for simply by cigarette smoking and the other risk factors because they were all adjusted for.

4

Effect of cholesterol-lowering treatment on coronary heart disease morbidity and mortality: the evidence from trials, and beyond

M.B. KATAN

Sources of information on the role of serum lipoproteins in the development of disease are diverse (Table 1). In the evaluation of drugs, randomized controlled clinical trials are considered indispensable. On the other hand, public health interventions are frequently judged on epidemiologic grounds alone, as was the case regarding the noxious effect of cigarette smoking on the myocardium: the metabolic pathways involved are poorly defined, there are no good animal studies, and, most important, there is no evidence from randomized controlled trials that cessation of smoking is beneficial; yet, its importance is widely accepted. Nor is there persuasive evidence from randomized controlled trials that obesity, lack of exercise, stress, exposure to radioactivity or air pollution, failure to wear a safety belt or helmet, drunk driving or substance abuse will shorten life expectancy.

Table 1 Sources of information on the role of cholesterol in disease

Epidemiology
  Individuals
  Nations
  Trends in time
Hereditary hypercholesterolemia and hypocholesterolemia
Metabolic pathways
Animal experiments
Controlled clinical trials

This article was first published in *Cardiology*, **77** (Suppl. 4), 8–13, and is reproduced by permission of Karger AG, Basel. © 1990, Karger AG Basel.

On several of these points, e.g. exposure to radioactivity or drug abuse, insistence on trial evidence would be pedantic, because epidemiologic and clinical observations plus common sense should persuade anyone that they are unhealthy. In the case of obesity or exercise, setting up and running a properly controlled clinical trial would be a formidable and impossible task. On the other hand, the impact of cholesterol lowering on coronary risk has been studied intensively. Still, calculations have shown that a definitive settling of the diet–heart question would require a trial involving 72,000–145,000 subjects treated for at least 5 years[1]. None of the published trials approach these figures. We will thus have to accept the limitations and look at, but also beyond, trial evidence for the long-term effects of cholesterol reduction on coronary heart disease (CHD) morbidity and mortality.

Effect of cholesterol lowering on CHD

There have been many trials to evaluate the role of cholesterol in the etiology of CHD, and their results have not always been consistent – a common phenomenon in biomedical research. A meta-analysis, in which results of all published trials meeting consistent criteria are entered into a single calculation, then becomes helpful. Such analysis can provide a perspective on the extent to which the outcomes of the various trials agree. Single trials have almost uniformly lacked the statistical power to allow firm conclusions.

Although in most trials, treatment of hypercholesterolemia by diet or by drugs reduced the incidence of CHD, the numbers of patients studied were so small that many of these outcomes could have been due to chance if viewed individually. Statisticians express this by saying that the 95% confidence interval for the reduction in incidence did not exclude a zero effect, or that the effect was not significant. Only combining the data compiled for the 40,000 patients studied in the 20–30 trials published hitherto allows the signal to rise above the noise. Such meta-analyses have shown that reducing total or low-density-lipoprotein (LDL) cholesterol levels consistently reduces the incidence of myocardial infarction and coronary death[2,3]. The effect is graded: the greater the cholesterol reduction, the larger the benefit (Table 2). Benefit has been shown to increase with longer duration of treatment (Table 3) as well. Table 3 also shows that in this respect the trial evidence fits well with epidemiologic observations. It is therefore a logical conclusion that the duration of exposure of the arterial wall to high LDL concentrations determines the chance that an occluding lesion will occur.

Table 2 Relation between cholesterol lowering and reduction in CHD: meta-analysis of randomized, controlled trials

Cholesterol reduction (%)	Reduction in CHD (%)*
5–9	8
10–15	19

Adapted from R. Peto (1988, unpublished analyses)
*In these trials, patients who developed CHD had been receiving treatment for an average of 2 years when symptoms first appeared.

Table 3 Reduction in coronary events associated with a cholesterol reduction of 10% in a meta-analysis of randomized controlled trials

Type of study	Reduction in CHD mean ± SE (%)	Duration of cholesterol reduction until 1st event (years)*
13 short trials	9 ± 5	1–2
8 longer (5–7 years) trials	22 ± 4	3
Comparisons within and between populations	30	~ 50

Adapted from R. Peto (1988, unpublished analyses).
*At the time when CHD symptoms first appeared, patients had on average been receiving treatment or adhering to a specific diet for the number of years indicated.

Value of cholesterol-lowering strategies

Total mortality

If treatment of hypercholesterolemia reduces mortality from CHD and does not cause other diseases, then it should be associated with a reduction in total mortality, i.e. patients should live longer. In practice, this has not been proven to occur[3], perhaps because CHD, like cancer, diabetes, and cerebrovascular accidents, is a disease that mainly affects elderly people, who have a limited life expectancy. The average number of years to be gained by prevention of CHD is small, and the gain is diluted by other competing causes of death. Thus, there is a dilemma involved in cholesterol trials; elderly subjects gain little in life expectancy even if CHD is prevented, and younger subjects experience too few CHD deaths during a trial to allow firm conclusions on the benefit of treatment. (The exceptions are patients with familial hypercholesterolemia, in whom CHD mortality is already high in middle age. With the available pharmaceutical treatment for hypercholesterolemia, a dramatic increase in total life expectancy can be assumed to be discernible in the future among these patients.)

With the majority of CHD deaths occurring in elderly people, is an increased average life span a realistic goal in the primary prevention of CHD? In my opinion, increasing life expectancy among populations of the developed world is a pointless effort. The number of people living to 80 years or more is already growing rapidly, and to many the added years are a mixed blessing. Rather than to further postpone death, a more relevant goal is to reduce the burden of disease that makes the last years or even decades of life miserable. The question then becomes: will cholesterol lowering keep patients free from disease for a longer period rather than simply keep them alive longer? This issue of CHD incidence, as opposed to total mortality, has been largely settled by the trials: reduction of LDL and total cholesterol levels leads to a decreased incidence of CHD[2,3].

Side effects

A second important question is whether treatment of hypercholesterolemia has significant side effects, i.e., whether it actively causes other diseases, especially cancer. Unfortunately, the trials lack the power to give us reliable information on this aspect. Consider cancer deaths in the Helsinki Heart Study (Table 4)[4]. On the face of it, neither this trial nor, for that matter, the Lipid Research Clinics Coronary Primary Prevention Trial[5] showed any evidence

Table 4 Number and causes of deaths in the Helsinki Heart Study

	Number	
Patients	*Placebo* (*n*=2030)	*Gemfibrozil* (*n*=2051)
CHD	19	14
Other causes	24	30
other vascular diseases	4	8
cancer	11	11
other medical causes	3	1
accidents and violence	6	10
Total	43	44

Adapted and corrected from Frick *et al* [4] according to Frick (written communication, 1990), checking of the coding of the patients disclosed some errors in the published[4] mortality data. In the present Table 4, there are therefore 1 death less from other medical causes in both groups, and 2 more deaths from accidents and violence in the placebo group than in the original publication.

that cholesterol lowering promotes cancer. But what if 2 of the 11 patients dying from cancer in the placebo group (Table 4) had succumbed just after the trial had finished instead of during the trial, and 2 more of the drug-treated patients had died of cancer during the trial? Instead of a difference of zero, we would then have had an almost 50% excess of cancer deaths in the group receiving active treatment. The reverse holds for the 'accidents and violence' category: simply transfer 3 cases from the drug to the placebo group, and no one would have worried. In statistical terms, it is said that the difference in violent deaths between the drug and placebo groups was not significant. This means it could have been a coincidence; we simply cannot tell. The numbers are too low to allow a reliable answer; even if all the trials are combined, the numbers are still too low.

Thus, the trials cannot settle the cholesterol-cancer issue. Nor are epidemiologic follow-up studies helpful, because by now it is evident that preexisting but undiagnosed tumors caused reduced serum cholesterol levels[6], so that cancer may cause low cholesterol levels instead of the reverse.

However, much more potent and unequivocal evidence on this issue is available. There are hundreds of millions of people who have had low cholesterol levels all their lives. Such people live in countries where the diet is low in saturated fat and cholesterol. As shown in Figure 1[7,8], there is no evidence that such populations have higher cancer rates than populations with much higher cholesterol levels. If a reduction of cholesterol by 10% should by itself cause cancer[9], then surely the almost twofold difference in cholesterol levels between Finnish and Japanese men should have caused a perceptibly higher death rate from cancer in the Japanese: this was not the case (Figure 1).

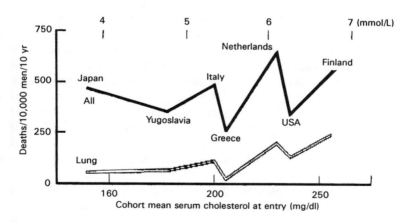

Figure 1 Serum cholesterol levels at entry, and cancer deaths after 6–15 years of follow-up in cohorts of middle-aged men in the Seven Countries Study[7]. Adapted from Katan[8]. Upper curve – total cancer deaths; lower curve – lung cancer deaths

Additional information comes from experiments of nature in the form of genetic disturbances in the regulation of cholesterol levels. That patients with homozygous hyperbetalipoproteinemia (better known as homozygous familial hypercholesterolemia), who have cholesterol levels of 20–30 mmol/l (800–1,200 mg/dl), will often develop myocardial infarctions in the first years of life is well known. It is not always realized that the opposite genetic defect also exists: there are several hundred patients worldwide who suffer from abetalipoproteinemia or homozygous hypobetalipoproteinemia. These patients have an LDL cholesterol level of zero and a total cholesterol level of 0.5–1 mmol/l (20–40 mg/dl). As LDL is the vehicle not only for cholesterol, but also for vitamin E, these patients used to develop massive vitamin E deficiency and its associated neuropathy[10]. Now that this deficiency has been recognized and patients are being treated with mega-doses of vitamin E, they live well into their fifties and sixties. The salient point is that excessive cancer rates are not and have never been a feature of these diseases (P.N. Herbert, MD, PhD, personal communication, 6 October 1987). This observation is hard to reconcile with any theory that moderate LDL cholesterol lowering will deplete cholesterol from some essential tissues or cells and in that way promote the development of malignant tumors. If that were true, patients with zero LDL cholesterol levels would have rampant tumor growth at an early age, which they do not.

Conclusion and perspectives for drug treatment

Evidence from a number of sources, including trials, shows that reducing serum levels of LDL cholesterol will postpone CHD[2,3]. The more extensive the lowering, the larger the gain in CHD-free years. In addition, it appears unlikely that a reduction in the level of LDL cholesterol will by itself promote other diseases, especially cancer. However, this does not exclude the possibility that certain forms of cholesterol-lowering treatment may have specific toxic effects. Epidemiologic and trial evidence suggests that diets low in saturated fat and cholesterol are fairly harmless. However, several of the early cholesterol-lowering drugs, including estrogen, dextrothyroxine, and triparanol, caused serious toxicity, and had to be withdrawn. Clofibrate has also been suspected of carcinogenicity, but trials in humans have yielded contradictory evidence for this adverse effect[11,12].

The new 3-hydroxy-3-methylglutaryl coenzyme A reductase inhibitors have enormous potential for reducing premature CHD and death, and their safety profile to date is satisfactory[13]. However, no drug is completely free from side effects. There is pressure – from patients more than from physicians – to prescribe reductase inhibitors to very large numbers of people who have only minimal serum cholesterol elevations. In this case, the side-effects in the many may outweigh the benefit in the few. This is undesirable not only because of the potential harm to patients not requiring drug therapy, but also because fear of side effects might stop patients with severe hypercholesterolemia from taking these drugs.

Thus, cholesterol lowering as such will probably increase the number of disease-free years for many people in affluent societies. However, the agent used to lower cholesterol should be appropriate to the severity of the hypercholesterolemia, and in the large majority of patients with mild hyper-cholesterolemia diet is a more appropriate form of treatment than drugs.

References

1. Diet-Heart Review Panel: Mass field trials of the diet-heart question – their significance, timeliness, feasibility and applicability. *American Heart Association Monograph*, New York, American Heart Association. 1969, p. 28
2. Peto, R., Yusuf, S. and Collins, R. (1985). Cholesterol-lowering trial results in their epidemiological context. *Circulation, 72*, (Suppl. 3), 451
3. Yusuf, S., Wittes, J. and Friedman, L. (1988). Overview or results of randomized clinical trials in heart disease. II. Unstable angina, heart failure, primary prevention with aspirin, and risk factor modification. *J. Am. Med. Assoc., 260*, 2259–63
4. Frick, M.H., Elo, O., Haapa, K. *et al.* (1987). Helsinki Heart Study: Primary prevention trial with gemfibrozil in middle-aged men with dyslipidemia. Safety of treatment, changes in risk factors, and incidence of coronary heart disease. *N. Engl. J. Med., 317*, 1237–45
5. The Lipid Research Clinics Program. (1984). The Lipid Research Clinics Coronary Primary Prevention Trial results. I. Reduction in incidence of coronary heart disease. *J. Am. Med. Assoc., 251*, 351–64
6. Sherwin, R.W., Wentworth, D.N., Cutler, J.A. *et al.* (1987). Serum cholesterol levels and cancer mortality in 361,662 men screened for the Multiple Risk Factor Intervention Trial. *J. Am. Med. Assoc., 257*, 943–8
7. Keys, A., Aravanis, C., Blackburn, H. *et al.* (1985). Serum cholesterol and cancer mortality in the Seven Countries Study. *Am. J. Epidemiol., 121*, 870–83
8. Katan, M.B. (1986). Effects of cholesterol-lowering diets on the risk for cancer and other non-cardiovascular diseases. In Fidge, N.H. and Nestel, P.J. (eds) *Proceedings of the 7th Atherosclerosis Symposium*, pp. 657–61. (Amsterdam: Elsevier)
9. Feinleib, M. (1983). Review of the epidemiological evidence for a possible relationship between hypercholesterolemia and cancer. *Cancer Res., 43*, 25033–75
10. Herbert, P.N., Assmann, G. and Gotto A.M. Jr. *et al.* (1983). Familial lipoprotein deficiency: Abetalipoproteinemia, hypobetalipoproteinemia, and Tangier disease. In Stanbury, J.B., Wyngaarden, J.B., Fredrickson, D.S. *et al.* (eds), *The Metabolic Basis of Inherited Disease*, 5th edn, pp. 589–621. (New York: McGraw-Hill)

11. Canner, P.L., Berge, K.G., Wenger, N.K. *et al.* (1986). Fifteen-year mortality in coronary drug project patients: Long-term benefit with niacin. *J. Am. Coll. Cardiol.*, **8**, 1245–55
12. Oliver, M.F., Heady, J.A., Morris, J.N. *et al.* (1984). WHO cooperative trial on primary prevention of ischaemic heart disease with clofibrate to lower serum cholesterol: Final mortality follow-up. (Report of the Committee of Principal Investigators.) *Lancet*, **2**, 600–4
13 Bilheimer, D. (1990). Long-term clinical tolerance of lovastatin and simvastatin. *Cardiology*, **77** (Suppl 4), 58–65

Discussion

Dr Skrabanek: I would like to ask Dr Katan about the meta-analysis by Richard Peto because these were unpublished results. There have been few of these meta-analyses published, one in the *British Medical Journal* and I have seen two more of them in the *New England Journal of Medicine*. Your results are showing something quite different from Peto's because they show that total mortality, in either primary or secondary intervention trials, was not changed and heart disease did not change significantly. However, cancer mortality showed a significant increase in the primary prevention trials, as well as other causes including accidents, violence and so on.

Normally meta-analyses are used to change the insignificant to significant, as Richard Peto is doing. But, in this particular instance, your meta-analysis suggests that even when all the insignificant results are pooled together, they are still insignificant in terms of reducing mortality from heart disease. However, they are then significant in increasing cancer mortality. Arguing that cancer and cholesterol are not related because Japanese people do not show increased mortality from violence, or because mean cholesterol levels in populations do not correlate with cancer mortality, is a classical example of an ecological fallacy. One can conclude nothing from this kind of comparison.

In fact, the Ancel Keys study was also an example of an ecological fallacy. As to the genetic defect, we know so little about cancer that I do not think we can conclude anything from the fact that cases of cancer were not described among people with an LDL-C of zero, because of genetic defect. I would tend to conclude that they did not live too long. Secondly, if they have that kind of genetic defect, they may also have a genetic complement which may protect them against cancer. So, I do not see how you can conclude anything about whether cholesterol and cancer are related in an aetiological or pathophysiological way from these two points.

Dr Katan: That is three questions really, one about the various meta-analyses, one about population comparisons and one about the low-cholesterol syndromes.

Different people have now tried to combine the various cholesterol lowering trials and they have used different criteria for which trials to include and which trials not to include. There has been a lot of to-and-fro about what is, and what is not, significant and should it be a one-sided test, a two-sided test and what is the '*p*' value, etc. I am not a statistician and I refuse to let computers make my decisions. What I try to do is to look at the evidence in general and try to decide what is plausible. What I see in these trials is a highly consistent reduction in coronary heart disease morbidity and mortality when cholesterol is reduced. The longer the reduction and the larger the extent of the reduction, the larger the reduction in CHD. Whether a particular analysis of a particular set of trials will show that this is 'significant' or not will not change my conclusion. As far as the comparison of populations is concerned, of course there can be no 100% certainty that lowering cholesterol does not have certain side-effects. That of course is a hallmark of any intervention. We do not know whether in people who smoke, taking away their cigarettes is going to give them some kind of dreadful disease – those studies have not been done. For the very same reason, we do not know whether in people who are obese, if it is safe or even effective, to lose weight; we just try to make do with the data we have. I do not see how you can maintain that eating a cholesterol-lowering diet will increase your risk of cancer, when at the same time you see hundreds of millions of people world-wide in the Mediterranean and Far East who have had these diets all their lives and do not get the cancers. Again, maybe it is my fault in not being a statistician.

As to the low-cholesterol syndrome and the genetic defect involved in it, this is a quite well-defined defect in the apolipoprotein B part of the LDL. In essence, you are postulating that these people do not get cancer because they may have yet another unknown genetic defect or a protecting gene which protects them from a cancer that they should have had because they have low cholesterols. In response, I say that it is a basic rule in science that you should stick with the minimum number of assumptions that will explain the data. The absence of premature cancer in low-cholesterol syndromes fits with the rest of the data. I see no need to assume lots of hypothetical counteracting genes.

Dr Goldbloom: I am sure we would all agree with you that it does not make much sense to attribute violence in society to what we eat. On the other hand, there are well-established relationships between diet and behaviour. I am a little concerned that the tendency to dismiss the differences noted as statistical aberrations may represent a kind of selective treatment of statistically significant differences, in that, if they do not fit with our ideas, we sometimes tend to dismiss them. I recently came across an abstract describing a study related to primates which showed that monkeys on low-fat diets demonstrated significantly more violent behaviour than those on a high-fat intake. I would like to raise the question whether we really know about specific behavioural effects of chronic low-fat intake?

Dr Katan: Let me first correct one point. I am certainly not suggesting that the data prove that there is no problem. What I am saying is, that whether you see a difference in the small numbers, like with the acts of violence, or whether you see no difference, as with cancer, neither of them provides really hard information. This is because the numbers are too small. If the numbers are equal you should not derive comfort from them and say that this proves that there is no problem because the numbers are too small. However, if the numbers are different, you are indeed left with a question that needs to be studied. The only thing I can do is to say that the numbers are too small to give me an answer; I will need to look at other evidence. I find the evidence from populations eating low-fat diets or high-fat, low-saturated-fat diets very comforting; if I weigh this against animal experiments and see that the results are conflicting, then I tend to go with the human evidence. I have seen too many instances where something can be produced in an animal but not in man or, where something occurs in man but not in animals. Again, this is something that needs to be looked at very carefully.

Dr Roncari: If one is trying to determine whether a neoplasm has led to a low total cholesterol level, it is often useful to examine the HDL levels. I thought there was a differentiating point here, in that, in the association between low cholesterol and neoplasia, the HDL-C is also low. This does not pertain in cases where there is a healthy individual with a low total cholesterol level.

Dr Katan: I do not know about those people in the very lowest quintile of the cholesterol distribution where there is no relation between low HDL and low LDL. I certainly have not seen any analyses based on this distribution but maybe Dr Anderson can comment on that.

Dr Anderson: We do not have an awful lot of follow-up on HDL but we did do some measurements using Svedberg fractions many years ago. One thing we are in the process of getting published is a study in men where increased colon cancer rates are observed with lower cholesterols. These rates are even more marked if you look at LDL cholesterol and they are consistent across the age groups. The other curious thing is that it is particularly the low cholesterol, obese men, that have higher rates. This suggests again that maybe it is not the cholesterol-lowering diet, because you might expect that to be associated with lower body weights as well. So, there appear to be some unusual things going on. There are some very real things happening, but I certainly would not attribute any cause to what I know. I would suspect that you are right and I would like to know about the HDLs also.

5

Trends in fat and cholesterol intake, serum cholesterol levels and cardiovascular disease in Japan

H. UESHIMA

Introduction

Japan is now the leading country with the highest longevity in the world. This status was acquired by reducing mortality from stroke and ischaemic heart disease beginning with the period 1965–70[1-3]. On the other hand, fat and cholesterol intake has increased remarkably over the last three decades in accordance with the westernization of lifestyles, and, in particular, dietary habits[1,2].

Many epidemiological follow-up studies on the Japanese have revealed that risk factors for stroke and ischaemic heart disease are no different from those for the US and European countries[4-8]. In Japan, hypertension was also cited as one of the main risk factors for stroke, while hypertension, hypercholesterolaemia and smoking were risk factors for ischaemic heart disease[4-8].

A question that is becoming increasingly raised is why mortality from ischaemic heart disease has declined continuously since 1970 despite increasing trends in fat and cholesterol intake. This paper addresses this question by reviewing trends in mortality from stroke and ischaemic heart disease and changes in dietary habits in Japan.

Materials and methods

The sex and 10-year age-specific mortality rates for stroke and ischaemic heart disease in Japan were obtained from the Vital Statistics reports put out by the Ministry of Health and Welfare in Japan for 1956–88[9]. Since there were no published data on death rates during 1956–67, these were calculated from the number of deaths due to stroke and ischaemic heart disease from the population in each 5-year age group. The population in each 5-year age group was also reported in Vital Statistics reports[9]. The 10-year age-specific mortality rates were then calculated by using the 5-year age-specific mortality rates and standard populations of 5-year age groups in 1960. For the international comparison of stroke and ischaemic heart disease in selected countries in 1960, data reported by Aoki *et al.* was used[10].

Food and nutrient intakes per capita per day during the period 1956–88 were obtained from the National Nutrition Survey[11]. The National Nutrition Survey is carried out annually with family samples selected randomly from the census tract. These family samples are considered to be representative of a given year.

Instead of looking at the serum cholesterol levels, the dietary lipid factors devised by Keys *et al.*, and discussed by Fetcher *et al.*[12], were calculated using data on food intake from the National Nutrition Survey, and from the self-devised data on polyunsaturated and saturated fatty acids and cholesterol content intake by food group[13].

Comparison of plasma cholesterol levels between Japan and the US were made using the data on Japanese males from the National Cardiovascular Survey in Japan in 1980[14], and the data on US white males from the Lipid Research Clinics in 1972–76 in the US[15].

Data from a cross-sectional survey on life insurance company workers aged 20–59 in Tokyo from 1984 to 86 were compared among 10-year age-groups to show recent changes in dietary habits and total cholesterol levels[16,17]. Nutritional intake in this study was based on a 24-h recall study.

Results

Age-specific mortality trends in stroke

Figure 1 shows the sex and age-adjusted stroke mortality for men and women aged 40–69 years in selected countries in 1960. The mortality rate in Japan was the highest amongst these countries and was three-fold that of the US rate. Figure 2 shows trends in age-specific stroke mortality for men. Rates for men aged 50–59 and 60–69 years began to decline around 1965, and the rate of decline for men aged 60–69 years accelerated starting from 1970. For men, aged 40–49 years, the rate initially declined slightly and, then declined more steeply from 1980 onward. The rate for men aged 30–39 years increased up to 1970, but declined subsequently. For women, aged 50–59 and 60–69 years, the declining trends in stroke mortality were almost the same as for men. However, the mortality rate for women in the 40–49 and 30–39 years age groups began to decline before 1965, in contrast to the rates of their male counterparts (Figure 3).

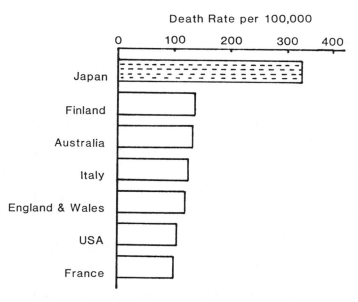

Figure 1 Sex and age-adjusted stroke mortality rate for men and women aged 40–69 years in selected countries in 1960

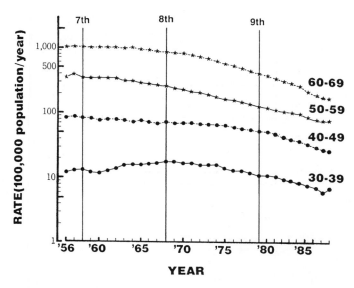

Figure 2 Trends in age-specific mortality from stroke for men in Japan, 1956–1988. The vertical lines labelled '7th', '8th', '9th' represent the revisions of the International Classification of Diseases in Japan

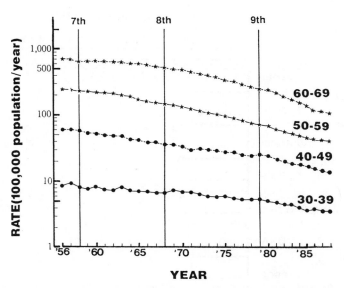

Figure 3 Trends in age-specific mortality from stroke for women in Japan, 1956–1988. The vertical lines labelled '7th', '8th', '9th' represent the revisions of the International Classification of Diseases in Japan

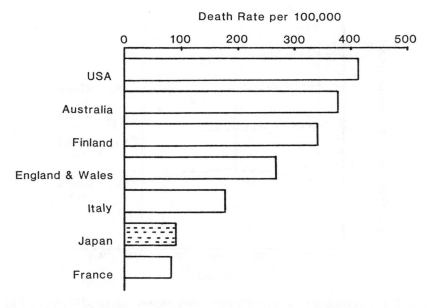

Figure 4 Sex and age-adjusted mortality from ischaemic heart disease for men and women aged 40–69 years in selected countries in 1960

Ischaemic heart disease mortality

Of special interest, in Japan, was the observation that mortality from ischaemic heart disease was the lowest among all industrialized countries (Figure 4). Figure 4 shows that the sex and age-adjusted death rate for ischaemic heart disease in Japan was less than one-fourth of that in the US in 1960. Figure 5 shows age-specific mortality trends in ischaemic heart disease for men. Rates for men aged 50–59 and 60–69 years increased until 1970 but then showed a subsequent decline. Mortality rates for men aged 30–39 and 40–49 years did not increase and did, in fact, decline from 1970. The declining trends for men aged 30–39 and 40–49 were much steeper from 1974 and 1980, respectively. Mortality rates in ischaemic heart disease for women aged 50–59 and 60–69 years increased until 1967, but then decreased from 1970 onwards (Figure 6). Rates for women aged 30–39 years decreased steadily from 1956. Rates for women aged 40–49 years did not change during the 1956–1967 period, but they decreased from 1970 for women in this and other age groups.

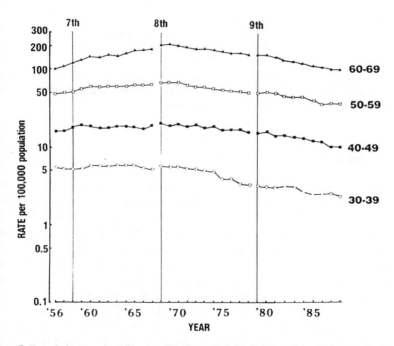

Figure 5 Trends in age-specific mortality from ischaemic heart disease for men in Japan, 1956–1988. The vertical lines labelled '7th','8th','9th' represent the revisions of the International Classification of Diseases in Japan

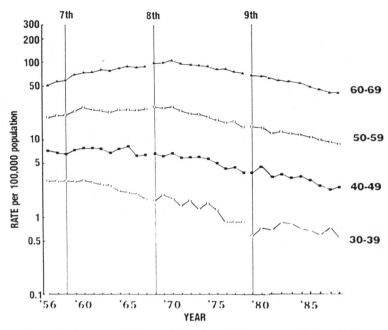

Figure 6 Trends in age-specific mortality from ischaemic heart disease for women in Japan, 1956–1988. The vertical lines labelled '7th', '8th', '9th' represent the revisions of the International Classification of Diseases in Japan

Food and nutrient intake

Meat consumption, as shown in Figure 7, increased remarkably until 1975. The daily consumption of meat per capita, however, was lower than that of fish and shellfish. The consumption of milk and dairy products increased remarkably as well. However, the amount consumed per capita per day in Japan was far lower than the amount consumed in other industrialized countries. Figure 8 shows trends in nutrient intake. It was observed that carbohydrate intake decreased remarkably while fat and animal protein intake increased. However, fat intake was still less than 60 g per capita per day. Therefore, the energy intake from fat was still only 25.5% in 1988.

Figure 9 shows trends in cholesterol and polyunsaturated and saturated fats per capita per day. The intake of lipids increased from 1956, but slowed down after 1972. Cholesterol intake levelled off starting from 1972. The percent changes in cholesterol and polyunsaturated and saturated fatty acids were 107, 50 and 120%, respectively between 1956 and 1972.

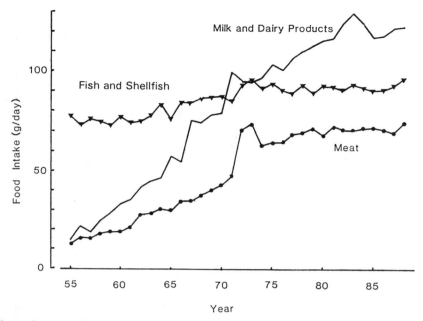

Figure 7 Trends in the food intake of meat, fish and shellfish, milk and dairy products per capita per day in Japan, 1955–1988

Instead of addressing the trends in the serum total cholesterol level, the dietary lipid factor devised by Keys *et al.* was calculated (Figure 10). Keys' lipid factor increased steadily from 1956, in contrast to the decrease in the polyunsaturated/saturated fat (P/S) ratio. The P/S ratio, however, was still over 1.0.

Figure 11 shows the comparison of the plasma total cholesterol levels between Japanese and US white men using the data from the National Survey in Japan in 1980, and Lipid Research Clinics in the US for the period 1972–76. A 20–30 mg/dl difference in the total cholesterol level was found to exist between the two groups in that period. However, recent dietary habits that are characterized by an increase in animal foods in Japan have raised total cholesterol levels both in farmers and white-collar workers (i.e. serum total cholesterol levels around 1985 were 180 and 200 mg/dl for middle-aged male farmers and white-collar workers, respectively).

Nutrient intake and serum total cholesterol level by sex and age group for workers in a life insurance company in Tokyo in 1984–86 are shown in Table 1. Energy intake from fat showed that the younger the age group, the higher the fat energy intake (i.e. in men and women aged 20–29 intake was around 30%). This higher fat intake in the younger rather than in the older generation

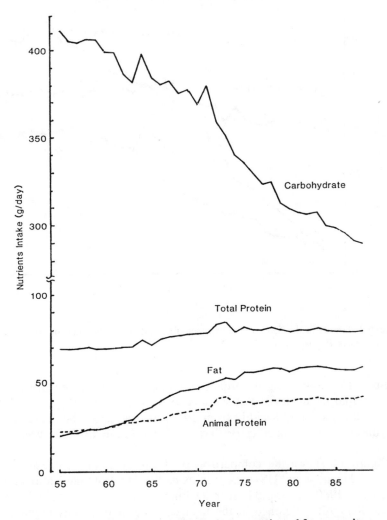

Figure 8 Trends in the nutrient intake of carbohydrate, protein and fat per capita per day in Japan, 1955–1988

was brought about by higher meat and lower fish consumption in the younger generation. This observation also suggested that meat was consumed in greater amounts than fish in the 20–29 and 30–39 age groups compared with the 40–49 and 50–59 age groups (Table 1). However, the polyunsaturated/saturated fatty acid ratio was still over 1.0 for all age groups.

Table 1 Nutrient and fish and shellfish intake and serum total cholesterol level by sex and age group for workers in a life insurance company in Tokyo, 1984–1986. Dietary survey was carried out by a 24-h recall method

	Age group							
	Men				Women			
	20–29 (51)*	30–39 (50)	40–49 (51)	50–59 (49)	20–29 (53)	30–39 (50)	40–49 (49)	50–59 (10)
Energy (cal/day)	2616	2377	2266	2177	1929	1826	1839	1963
Protein (g/day)	91.6	85.5	82.1	81.9	69.8	66.1	74.2	78.5
Fat (g/day)	85.7	74.6	64.6	64.3	72.7	64.2	60.5	67.2
Polyunsaturated fatty acids (g/day)	21.9	19.6	17.1	17.7	17.6	17.2	16.6	15.7
Saturated fatty acids(g/day)	17.4	15.3	13.2	12.8	16.0	13.0	12.4	15.1
P/S ratio	1.4	1.4	1.4	1.5	1.2	1.4	1.5	1.1
Energy from fat (%)	29.5	28.2	25.7	26.6	33.9	31.6	29.6	30.8
Fish and shellfish (g/day)	81.9	92.7	99.4	95.9	62.8	63.5	98.7	118.9
Meat (g/day)	130.2	105.3	86.9	86.5	93.1	77.4	64.1	77.8
Serum total cholesterol (mg/dl)	—	185.3	196.8	206.5	—	180.3	192.9	219.9

* The numerals in parenthesis are the number of subjects.

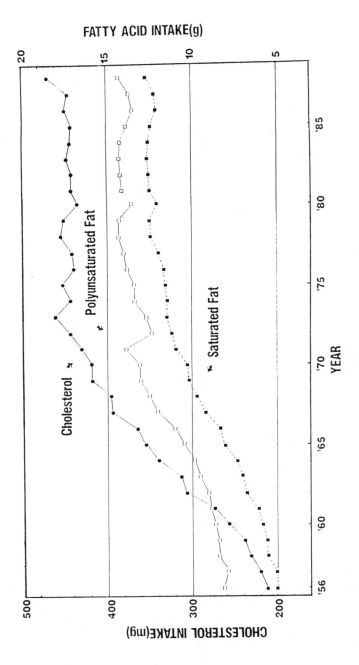

Figure 9 Trends in cholesterol and polyunsaturated and saturated fat intake per capita per day in Japan, 1956–1988

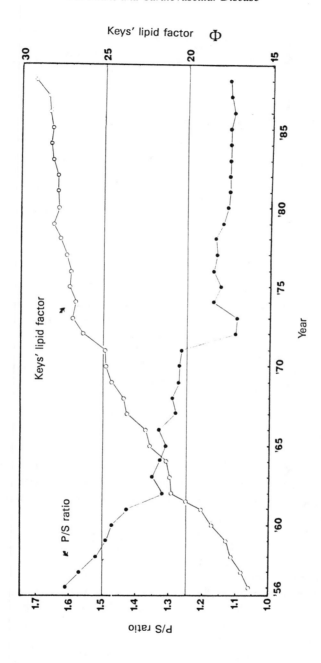

Figure 10 Trends in Keys' lipid factor and in the ratio of polyunsaturated/saturated fat per capita per day in Japan, 1956–1988

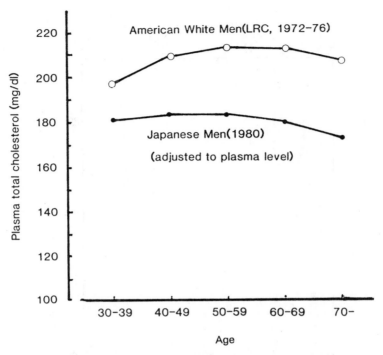

Figure 11 Comparison of the plasma total cholesterol level between Japanese men and US white men. The data on US white men were obtained from Lipid Research Clinics[15], while those on Japanese men came from the Cardiovascular Survey of Japan[14]

Discussion

The principal question of this study was why mortality from stroke and ischaemic heart disease has decreased since the period 1965–70 in Japan, despite remarkable increases in fat and cholesterol intake and in total cholesterol level.

Some clinicians have indicated doubt that the mortality rate from ischaemic heart disease really is declining given that total cholesterol levels in the Japanese are increasing steadily. Moreover, since many doctors have more opportunity to see more patients in clinics in recent years than in the past, they feel they can confidently make this claim regarding increased total cholesterol levels. Further, they believe that since some of the deaths from heart failure can be classified as ischaemic heart disease, the death rate from this disease is underestimated. However, the fact remains that the mortality rate from heart failure and also from heart disease in general has been, and still is decreasing[18]. Therefore, the declining trend in ischaemic heart disease mortality is, in fact, true.

If the declining mortality from ischaemic heart disease is true, then what are its contributing factors? The decline in mortality from ischaemic heart disease in Japan started several years later than the decline in stroke mortality. However, both mortality rates have continued to decline. Therefore, it is expected that common risk factors for ischaemic heart disease and stroke have both contributed to the recent decline. In this sense, the hypothesis that a decrease in blood pressure levels and in the prevalence of hypertension both contribute to the decline in mortality rates is, indeed, quite reasonable[1,2,17,19].

Keys' lipid factor Φ can be used to predict the serum cholesterol levels in a given population[13]. In this regard, we reported that the correlation coefficient between average level of Keys' lipid factor and serum total cholesterol level among several populations was 0.9[13]. According to the change in Keys' lipid factor, a serum cholesterol level of 13 mg/dl was expected for the Japanese between 1956 and 1988. Although there are no data available on exact trends in the serum cholesterol level in Japan, there is no doubt that serum cholesterol levels in the Japanese have increased[1,13,17]. Since a high serum cholesterol level is a risk factor of ischaemic heart disease even for the Japanese[8], the number of people at high risk due to high cholesterol levels has definitely increased[13,16,17]. However, this increased risk was not found to induce an increased trend in the mortality rate from ischaemic heart disease during the period 1970–88 in Japan.

These conflicting results may be partly explained by the decrease in the prevalence of hypertension[17,19] brought about by improvements in lifestyle changes including: less salty foods in daily diets[17,19–21], an increase in the treatment of hypertension[19], and the short exposure time to a relatively higher serum cholesterol level[1,8,13,14,17].

The high P/S ratio of over 1.0 is still prevalent due to higher fish and shellfish consumption and lower fat consumption from meat and dairy products in Japan. High consumption of ω-3 fatty acids, which comes mainly from fish oil may have a favourable effect on the coagulation system and, in turn, aid in the prevention of ischaemic heart disease[22]. The Japanese of today hold the highest per capita consumption ever of fish and shellfish in their history, and also are consuming the highest rate of other animal food sources.

Smoking is a major coronary risk factor. The smoking rate of Japanese men has decreased from over 80% to around 60% over the last two decades[1], although this, even, is very high. This decreasing trend may also have a favourable effect on the reduction of ischaemic heart disease[1].

For stroke, it has been considered in Japan that the increase in animal food source consumption, including meat and dairy products, may prevent stroke occurrence[2–4,6,7,13,17]. Epidemiological follow-up studies have found that people who live in rural areas and who consume few animal food sources with a lower serum total cholesterol level have a higher incidence of and mortality rate from stroke[4,6,7,13,17,23,24]. Kimura *et al.*[4] hypothesized that animal protein may prevent stroke. Previously, we also hypothesized that animal food sources may prevent stroke[6,7,16,17,23,24], that serum cholesterol was not a risk factor for stroke[7,23], and that rather low cholesterol levels are a risk factor for haemorrhagic stroke[7]. With respect to the relationship between serum total cholesterol and stroke, it is not fully understood yet whether or not serum total cholesterol itself directly influences stroke occurrence; it may, in fact, be an indicator of animal food intake and of nutritional status in general[7]. In either case, it may be suggested that recent dietary changes in Japan which are characterized by increases in fat intake, from both animal and vegetable sources, and increased animal protein intake, may partly contribute to the decline in stroke incidence and mortality[2,3,13,17,23,24].

Conclusion

In conclusion, it may be reasoned that recent increases in dietary fat and animal protein intake, which resulted in the increase in serum total cholesterol, reduced the mortality rate from stroke. However, these increases did not increase the mortality from ischaemic heart disease despite a remarkable increase in serum total cholesterol level. There are some possible reasons why the increase in total cholesterol did not adversely affect ischaemic heart disease over the last two decades: firstly, it may have been due to the short exposure period to relatively higher serum cholesterol levels; secondly, it may have been due to the lower levels of cholesterol in Japan compared to the US and European countries; thirdly, favourable changes in other coronary risk factors may have overcome its adverse effect; and finally, the high intake of ω-3 fatty acids which are taken from fish may have contributed to the absence of an adverse effect.

It is important to suggest that careful monitoring and proper education regarding dietary habits be implemented at an early age. Young and old alike should be informed as to the importance of not exceeding the ideal level of serum total cholesterol, because the coronary risk factors for the Japanese are the same as for their US and European counterparts.

References

1. Ueshima, H., Tatara, K. and Asakura, S. (1987). Declining mortality from ischemic heart disease and changes in coronary risk factors in Japan, 1956–1980. *Am. J. Epidemiol.*, **125**, 62–72

2. Ueshima, H. (1990). Changes in dietary habits, cardiovascular risk factors and mortality in Japan. *Acta Cardiol.*, **45**, 311–27

3. Ueshima, H., Tatara, K. and Asakura, S. (1984). Mortality trends in stroke, blood pressure, the treatment rate of hypertension between 1956 and 1980 in Japan. *Jpn J. Public Hlth.*, **31**, 589–99 (in Japanese with English abstract).

4. Kimura, N., Toshima, H., Nakayama, Y. *et al.* (1972). Population survey on cerebrovascular diseases: The ten years experience in the farming village of Tanushimaru and the fishing village of Ushibuka. *Jpn Heart J.*, **13**, 118–27

5. Omae, T., Ueda, K., Kikumura, T., Shikata, T., Fujii, I., Yanai, T. and Hasuo, Y. (1981). Cardiovascular deaths among hypertensive subjects of middle to old age: a long-term follow-up study in a Japanese community. In Onesti, G. and Kim, K.E. (eds). *Hypertension in the Young and Old*, pp. 285–97. (New York: Grune and Stratton)

6. Komachi, Y., Iida, M., Shimamoto, T., Chikayama, Y., Takahashi, H., Konishi, M, Tominaga, S. *et al.* (1971). Geographic and occupational comparisons of risk factors in cardiovascular disease in Japan. *Jpn Circulation J.*, **35**, 189–207

7. Ueshima, H., Iida, M., Shimamoto, T., Konishi, M., Tsujioki, K., Tanigaki, M., Nakanishi, N., Ozawa, H., Kojima, S. and Komachi, Y. (1980). Multivariate analysis of risk factors for stroke: eight-year follow-up study of farming villages in Akita, Japan. *Prev. Med.*, **9**, 722–40

8. Ueshima, H. (1990). Risk factors for ischemic heart disease in the Japanese. *Nichinainaishi*, **79**, 1491–6. (in Japanese)

9. Statistics and Information Department, Ministry's Secretariat, Ministry of Health and Welfare. *Vital Statistics 1956–1988, Japan.* (Tokyo: Kosei Tokei Kyokai), 1958–1990. (in Japanese)

10. Aoki, N., Horibe, H. and Kasagi, F. (1985). *Geographic presentation of mortality from all causes, cerebrovascular diseases, ischemic heart disease, and diabetes mellitus in the world, 1956–1978.* Dept. of Epidemiology, National Cardiovascular Center, 1985

11. Public Health Bureau, Ministry of Health and Welfare. *National Nutrition Survey, 1956–1990.* (Tokyo: Daiichi Shuppan Publishers), 1956–1990. (in Japanese)

12. Fetcher, E.S., Foster, N., Anderson, J.T., Grande, F. and Keys, A. (1967). Quantitative estimation of diet to control serum cholesterol. *Am. J. Clin. Nutr.*, **20**, 475–92

13. Ueshima, H., Iida, M., Shimamoto, T., Konishi, M, Tanigaki, M., Doi, M., Nakanishi, M., Takayama, Y., Ozawa, H. and Komachi, Y. (1982). Dietary intake and serum total cholesterol level: their relationship to different lifestyles in several Japanese populations. *Circulation*, **66**, 519–26

14. Public Health Bureau, Ministry of Health and Welfare. *National Cardiovascular Survey*, 1980. (Tokyo: Japan Heart foundation), 1982. (in Japanese)

15. The Lipid Research Clinics Program Epidemiology Committee. (1979). Plasma lipid distributions in selected north American populations: The Lipid Research Clinics Program Prevalence Study. *Circulation*, **60**, 427–39

16. Ueshima, H., Hirao, Y., Ishikawa, M., Tsukamoto, H., Ozawa, H., Aota, M., Morino, M. and Kagawa, Y. (1987). Dietary habits and serum total cholesterol levels for workers in a life insurance company from a cardiovascular prevention viewpoint. *Jpn Card. Dis. Contr. Assoc.*, **22**, 185–9. (in Japanese)

17. Shimamoto, T., Komachi, Y., Inada, H., Doi, M., Iso, H., Kitamura, A., Iida, M., Konishi, M., Nakanishi, N., Terao, A., Naito, Y. and Kojima, S. (1989). Trends for coronary heart disease and stroke and their risk factors in Japan. *Circulation*, **79**, 503–15

18. Uemura, K. and Pisa, Z. (1988). Trends in cardiovascular disease mortality in industrialized countries since 1950. *Wld. Hlth. Statist. Q.*, **41**, 155–78

19. Ueshima, H., Tatara, K., Asakura, S. and Okamoto, M. (1987). Declining trends in blood pressure level and the prevalence of hypertension, and changes in related factors in Japan, 1956–1980. *J. Chronic Dis.*, **40**, 137–47

20. Intersalt Cooperative Research Group. (1988). Intersalt: an international study of electrolyte excretion and blood pressure. Results for 24 hour urinary sodium and potassium excretion. *Br. Med. J.*, **297**, 319–28

21. Hashimoto, T., Fujita, Y., Ueshima, H., Kagamimori, S., Kasamatsu, T., Morioka, S., Mikawa, K., Naruse, Y., Nakagawa, H., Hara, N., Yanagawa, H. and Elliott, P. (1989). Urinary sodium and potassium excretion, body mass index, alcohol intake and blood pressure in three Japanese populations. *J. Hum. Hypertens.*, **3**, 315–21

22. Dyerberg, J. and Jorgensen, K.A. (1982). Marine oils and thrombogenesis. *Progr. Lipid Res.*, **21**, 255–9

23. Ueshima, H., Iida, M. and Komachi, Y. (1979). Is it desirable to reduce total cholesterol level as low as possible? *Prev. Med.*, **8**, 104–5

24. Tanaka, H., Tanaka, Y., Hayashi, M., Ueda, Y., Date, C., Baba, T., Shoji, H., Horimoto, T. and Owada, K. (1982). Secular trends in mortality from cerebrovascular diseases in Japan, 1960–1979. *Stroke*, **13**, 574–81

Discussion

Dr Skrabanek: You had mentioned that ischaemic heart disease in Japan has been declining because cholesterol has not been changed more recently. However, if cholesterol is supposed to be a risk factor for IHD, and if cholesterol is unchanged, and IHD is declining, the trends obviously do not contribute one way or the other to strengthen the relationship. You showed that between 1955 and 1970, which is a 15-year period, there was quite a dramatic increase in cholesterol and saturated fat intake in Japan. Surely, if you believe that cholesterol is an important risk factor, the 15-year increase would have to be translated into some increase in CHD. If you have cholesterol data from 1955, when do you suppose to see an effect on the disease which is postulated to be related to this? Or, would any kind of time interval do, depending on whether it shows what we want to show? Furthermore, you demonstrated that in Japan and France, in men 40–69 years of age, the death from IHD in 1960 was the same. Obviously you have totally different cultures, totally different diets and totally different levels of cholesterol, smoking, hypertension, everything is different. However, you are telling us that the ischaemic heart disease was the same. If you look in the booklet titled *Cardiovascular Disease In Canada*, which is published by the Canadian Heart and Stroke Foundation, you can see that in 1987 Japan and France had exactly the same CVD rates among females. Why this should happen when Japanese women and French women have nothing in common in their lifestyle is interesting. Yet, when CVD rates are calculated, presumably by summing IHD and stroke together, the sum total is exactly the same. Furthermore, the Heart and Stroke Foundation booklet reveals that there is an inverse relationship between IHD and stroke, the countries who are top for ischaemic heart disease are lowest for stroke. So, I think to link stroke and IHD together, as if they were related to the same risk factors, does not make either epidemiological or clinical sense. What I am really saying is that from the data you have shown, it is impossible to disentangle the effect of anything on anything because there have been so many social and dietary changes. In the Japanese population, smoking is decreasing, blood pressure control is increasing, fish intake is increasing and salt intake is decreasing. Also, you have stroke and ischaemic heart disease at different age groups and sexes and different time periods. How can anyone make sense as to how these things are related?

Dr Ueshima: First, I show the trend in cholesterol intake and other fat intake. If one considers the dietary changes that have occurred in Japan, it can be noted that there has been a general increase in the cholesterol level. However, as I have shown, IHD has not yet increased. I think this is due in part to favourable changes in other risk factors. Also, you must keep in mind that the serum cholesterol levels are still lower than in North America and other European countries. The exposure time is very short, so this may prevent an increase in ischaemic heart disease even with the occurrence of a total serum cholesterol increase.

Secondly, I do not know why the French and Japanese people have the same IHD mortality rates. Currently though, Japanese people have lower mortality rates than the French. I think that one of the factors that may be influential here is the alcohol intake. Alcohol may help prevent IHD, and both the French and the Japanese consume high amounts of alcohol. However, in essence, it is very difficult to determine as there may be many contributing ecological factors. I think that the risk factors are the same. Some epidemiological studies have shown that the risk factors for CHD for Japanese Americans and for Japanese are almost the same as those obtained in other American or European countries. I, however, think that the risk factor distribution is different between America and Japan.

Dr Gold: I don't mean to belabour the point, but there are certainly genetic differences between the populations to which you refer in the East and the West and there are other factors involved both qualitatively and quantitatively to which reference has already been made. If I interpret what you have said correctly, the increased intake in fat and the rise in cholesterol in Japan over the last 30 years, which is a fairly substantive period of time, has led to an increase in longevity due to a decrease in stroke and CHD. Although I fully realize the importance of the lowered blood pressure on the data that you have presented, am I correct in inferring that at the present time your data may also show that an increase in lipid intake, associated with increased serum cholesterol levels, may be protective against stroke and CHD?

Dr Ueshima: Yes, this is possible for stroke, but I do not know the definite rate. Total serum cholesterol may be an indicator of food intake. For example, farmers in the northern part of Japan had low cholesterol levels and rarely ate animal products. However, people who were living in the urban areas of Japan had higher cholesterol levels in comparison. This may be an indicator of food intake. I do not exactly know whether or not cholesterol has a direct effect on stroke prevention.

Dr Gold: I am afraid that I still need a bit of clarification on this matter. If we take stroke out of the picture and consider what you have said here today, is it possible that an increase in lipid intake and an increase in serum cholesterol levels have led, at least in this time period, to a decrease in the incidence of CHD, despite the fact that the study has now been going on for three decades?

Dr Ueshima: Yes, that is correct. It should be noted that the increase in total serum cholesterol was found mostly in the younger generations and not for those over 60 years of age. The older population has not increased their serum cholesterol and in fact the levels are almost steady. However, this group of people has experienced a great decline in blood pressure. This decline in blood pressure may overcome the adverse effects of raising serum cholesterol levels. Also, an increased number of the Japanese people have stopped smoking.

Dr Addis: Have you looked at the changes in antioxidant intake in the diet?

Dr Ueshima: No, we have not.

Dr Stehbens: I understand that at the present time the autopsy rate in Japan is approximately 3%. I also understand that in the Department of Pathology in Tokyo there is a registry of causes of death, as determined by autopsy. I would like to know if you have compared your national mortality rates with the autopsy-derived causes of death?

Dr Ueshima: No.

Dr Stehbens: The other point I would like to raise is that, around the 1950s, when cerebral haemorrhage was regarded as being higher in Japan than anywhere else in the world, this high incidence was really quite spurious. Evidence indicated that this was due to diagnostic fashion and the mortality rates for cerebral haemorrhage, as determined in the Hiroshima autopsy study, revealed that cerebral haemorrhage was not nearly that high. The rates were only a fraction of the national mortality rates for cerebral haemorrhage, and CHD mortality rates were in fact higher than those for cerebral haemorrhage.

Dr Yano: The results of our study and comparative studies of CHD and stroke incidence and mortality among Japanese men living in Hiroshima, Japan, Honolulu, Hawaii and San Francisco, California, indicate that the incidence of CHD is only moderately higher among Japanese men in California and Hawaii compared to those in Japan. On the other hand, the incidence, and also the mortality from stroke, is much higher in Japan compared to Hawaii and California. Comparisons of risk factors indicate that the blood pressure levels are approximately the same between Japan and Hawaii. However, the level of serum cholesterol and also the intake of animal fat and protein are much higher in Hawaii than in Japan. These differences cannot be explained by different diagnostic standards or different methods of risk factor measurement. So, I think that the higher cholesterol levels for Japanese men in Hawaii and California are protective against the stroke incidence and mortality. On the other hand, this much cholesterol difference may not be sufficient to

81

Japanese men in Hawaii and California are protective against the stroke incidence and mortality. On the other hand, this much cholesterol difference may not be sufficient to increase the CHD incidence and mortality in Japanese men in Hawaii and California to the extent of statistically significant level.

Dr Stehbens: I understand that in the 1950s and 1960s, more than 50% of the death certificates in Japan were not signed by medical practitioners. Would you have any idea of that figure at the present time? And, it is not simply Japan, in some parts of France, a high percentage of death certificates are not signed by medical practitioners. This raises another problem with the reliability of national mortality rates.

Dr Ueshima: I am not sure that I follow your comments. The death certificates in Japan were signed by doctors in the 1960s. The diagnosis for stroke was very exact without autopsy because we used the CT scanners and for most of the stroke cases we did CT examinations. As many people have suffered from stroke, we have become better in our ability to diagnose this problem. Unfortunately, we have no autopsy data for IHD so I believe its diagnosis may not be as exact as in other industrialized countries and thus, cases of heart failure may be misclassified. However, even with these misclassifications, heart disease and all cardiovascular disease is declining, hence, I think that the mortality trend is not very different from the true trend.

Hélène Laurendeau: In your conclusion you suggest that older and younger people in your country should be informed about the potential risk of elevated cholesterol. Considering your answer to Dr Gold's question, could you comment on why you made that specific recommendation?

Dr Ueshima: I believe that population strategies are very important. We have discussed the importance of age differences, and sex differences, but, for public health, I believe we should focus on one idea. In Japan we have not seen an increase in mortality from IHD; however, there is the possibility of an increased patient mortality pattern that the younger generation may follow. For example, as people in their early thirties and forties age, they will have higher mean cholesterol levels than their current counterparts in Japan. Dr Yano's studies and other Japanese studies have shown that the risk factors for CVD, especially ischaemic heart disease, are almost the same as in other countries. The difference lies in the distribution of serum cholesterol and other risk factors. So, I think it is very important to educate and inform the public with regard to the harmful effects of excess consumption of fat and cholesterol.

Dr Gold: Would it not strike you equally as well that what you may be doing is reversing a positive trend? What you have said can certainly be interpreted as indicating that after 30 years of increasing lipid intake in Japan, the incidence of CHD has fallen. Taking the decreased blood pressure effect into consideration and with all other factors being equal, you now suggest that because of data gathered in other countries under other circumstances, that you are now prepared to recommend a lowering of fat intake in the Japanese diet. Since we often take periods of time far less than three decades as allowing us to make recommendations concerning population habits, I wonder why you are prepared to ignore your own experience of 30 years and make lipid intake recommendations to your own population based on data accumulated in the West that still appears to be in the process of hot debate?

Dr Ueshima: From my understanding of what you said, I think that the Japanese people have lower cholesterol levels than their counterparts in the West. For example, 30 years ago, men aged 50–60 had very low average cholesterol levels of approximately 160 mg/dl. Presently, even if the Japanese increase their cholesterol a little bit, they would still have lower cholesterol levels than their counterparts in American and European countries. The exposure time is very short in spite of the increase in total serum cholesterol. Also, recent dietary changes have occurred amongst young people and not amongst the elderly. In our elderly population, hypertension and smoking have decreased so the harmful effects of serum cholesterol and increased fat intake, in fact, have been overshadowed by these other favourable risk factor changes.

6
The heart disease crusade – cui bono?

P. SKRABANEK

'We owe almost all our knowledge not to those who have agreed, but to those who have differed' – Charles Caleb Colton

Introduction

In the last decade, mainly under American influence, the cholesterol scare has swept over the Western world. Politicians have declared a war on heart disease, besides a war on cancer, and other wars. Experts talk about the need to change the nation's diet. The screening industry is booming. Drug companies are preparing for the greatest bonanza since the introduction of benzodiazepines. Yet is there any evidence that mass intervention in whole populations is likely to reduce mortality from coronary heart disease (CHD)?

The lipid–heart hypothesis

Despite the fact that cholesterol and fats in diet represent only one out of about 300 risk factors for CHD, cholesterol has been presented by many experts as the arch-villain. In their eagerness to 'do something', these experts have assumed that a risk factor means a causal factor, rather than a marker of the risk. Before whole populations are screened for their cholesterol levels and treated with diet or drugs, basic questions must be answered. These are: Is the measurement of blood cholesterol in screening campaigns reliable? Is there evidence that reduction of cholesterol by recommended diets or by drugs reduces the likelihood of dying from CHD? Is the treatment safe, or, put differently, do the benefits of treatment outweigh, by a reasonable margin, the adverse effects? Are the proposed interventions acceptable to the population?

This article was first presented at the international meeting *Cholestérol et Prévention Primaire*, held in Paris 23–24 February 1990. Reproduced by permission of CIDIL, Paris.

Is the cost of such intervention affordable and justifiable in terms of cost-benefit?

The advocates of mass intervention use evidence in support of their campaign, which is either irrelevant or wrong. What the man in the street wants to know is, would he live any longer if he undergoes screening and subsequent treatment. This question cannot be answered by referring to animal experiments in which herbivores are fed enormous amounts of fat, or to studies comparing rates of CHD in different countries with the fat consumption per capita, as extrapolation of such results to individuals is impermissible (this logical error is known as the ecological fallacy). Of many different levels of evidence used in support of the diet-heart hypothesis (Table 1), only ran-domised controlled trials of intervention are of clinical and practical relevance. As will be shown later, these trials have failed to demonstrate benefit.

Table 1 Levels of evidence for diet–heart hypothesis

A. Animal experimentation		
B. Epidemiology	(1) CHD trends –	dietary correlations
	(2) CHD rates –	inter-country correlations
	(3) CHD rates –	migration studies
C. Human observational studies	(1) Biochemical	Diet effect on blood lipids
	(2) Pathology	Lipids – atherosclerosis
		Atherosclerosis – CHD
	(3) Clinical	Blood lipids – CHD
		Diet – CHD
D. Intervention studies	(1) Single risk factors	– diet trials
		– cholesterol-lowering drugs
	(2) Multiple risk factors	

The lipid–heart hypothesis postulates a series of steps, each of them with ambiguous or conflicting evidence (Figure 1). If the individual links are weak, it is not surprising that the whole chain is also weak.

The relationship between diet and blood cholesterol (Link 1) is at best weak, and generally undemonstrable in observational studies, such as the Framing-ham study and many others. Cholesterol is a crude term, which covers a complex relationship between various fractions and the carrier proteins. It is not surprising, then, that there is no correlation between blood cholesterol and atheromatous changes in the coronary vessels (Link 2). An assumption

86

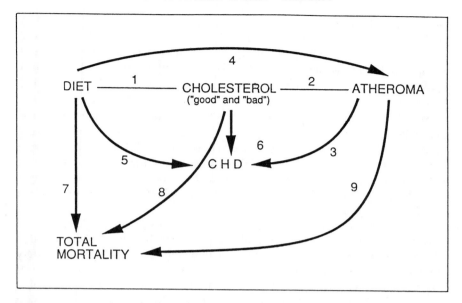

Figure 1 Steps in the lipid–heart hypothesis

that atheroma 'causes' CHD (Link 3) is untenable for two reasons: CHD is not a single pathological entity, and CHD is characterized by acute episodes which are not explained by the presence of atheroma. There is no evidence from human studies for Link 4. Link 5 is of direct clinical relevance, but the relationship has not been supported by numerous trials of dietary modification aiming to prevent CHD. Link 6 has been supported by studies of risk factors for CHD: with increasing levels of blood cholesterol, the risk of CHD increases. The relationship, however, is weak, not linear and does not apply for all ages and all populations. For example, in the Värmland cohort of 93,000 people, age 17–74, in Sweden, the relative risk of death from CHD for men and women was as follows[1]:

Cholesterol (mg/dl)	Men	Women
<224	1.0	1.0
225–249	1.1	0.9
250–275	1.4	0.9
>276	1.8	1.2

Similarly, in Canada, in men, aged 35–64, the relative risk of dying of CHD, with serum cholesterol levels of 240–279 mg/dl versus 200–239 mg/dl was only 0.88[2]. Dietary manipulation aiming at changing cholesterol levels in blood should not be viewed as self-evidently harmless, as in various dietary trials an excess of cancer deaths was observed. This possible adverse effect has been often associated with the use of cholesterol-lowering drugs. For this reason it is essential that Links 7 and 8 are carefully examined before any population intervention is contemplated. After all, ascertainment of the cause of death is often uncertain, particularly in the case of CHD. And what matters, from the point of view of a potential participant in a preventive programme, is not what appears on the death certificate but whether he lives any longer. The possibility that lowering the mean cholesterol in the nation could increase deaths from cancer must be seriously considered.

The introduction of new cholesterol-lowering drugs, which have not yet been properly tested, is fraught with dangers. Geoffrey Rose's warning that 'we cannot accept long-term mass preventive medication... as long-term safety cannot be assured and quite possibly harm may overweigh benefit' was well taken but unlikely to be heeded in the atmosphere of zealous activity and unwarranted optimism. Moreover, without drugs, and with the overwhelming evidence from dietary trials that diet alone is not enough to reduce mortality from CHD, the whole anti-cholesterol crusade founders.

Yet the experts talk about the 'prudent diet' which should be adopted by whole nations. There have been at least 20 different committees which have issued consensus recommendations on what people should eat. The consensus method is, to paraphrase Richard Feynman, like the old Chinese problem of deciding what is the length of the Emperor's nose. As no one was permitted to see the Emperor's face, it was necessary to go around the country, asking all knowledgeable people what they *think* the length of the Emperor's nose was, and averaging it. The result was very accurate because so many estimates were pooled.

High-risk versus low-risk

A sterile debate has been going on now for many years as to whether it would be preferable to concentrate on people with a high risk of dying from CHD, or whether preventive measures should be applied to whole populations with a low average risk. Some participants in this debate, anxious not to make enemies, have opted for recommending both strategies simultaneously. The apparent issue in this debate is the so-called Rose's preventive paradox, which states that in mass prevention each individual has only a small expectation of benefit, while the whole community may accrue a large benefit. On the other hand, while concentrating on high-risk individuals may confer large benefit

Table 2 Primary prevention of CHD

Trial	CHD deaths I	CHD deaths C	Total deaths I	Total deaths C	Lives saved per 1000/yr
MULTIPLE-RISK-FACTOR INTERVENTION					
WHO	428	450[1]	1325	1341[1]	0.1
Göteborg	462	461	1293	1318	0.2
MRFIT[2]	115	124	265	260	excess deaths
Helsinki[2]	4	1	10	5	excess deaths
Oslo[2]	6	13[1]	16	23[1]	2.3
DRUG TRIALS					
Clofibrate[2]	54	48	162	127	excess deaths
Cholestyramine[2]	32	44	68	71	0.2
Gemfibrozil[2]	6	8	45	42	excess deaths

[1]Adjusted for the difference in sample size in the intervention (I) and the control (C) groups.
[2]High risk population.
For references to these trials, see McCormick, J. and Skrabanek, P. (1988). Coronary heart disease is not preventable by population interventions. *Lancet*, **2**, 839–41.

to them, the value to the community is limited. The reason why this debate is irrelevant to the prevention of CHD lies in the negative results of large randomized controlled trials, in which the same negative results were obtained regardless of whether high-risk or low-risk individuals were studied (Table 2).

Randomized controlled trials of primary prevention of CHD

Dietary trials of primary prevention of CHD, carried out in the 1960s, were well reviewed by Borhani, who concluded that these interventions had negative or equivocal results[3].

Table 2 includes all randomised controlled trials in which the lipid–heart hypothesis was tested either in multiple risk factor intervention trials (in which, in addition to cholesterol-lowering diet, smoking reduction, blood pressure control and control of obesity were part of the intervention), or specifically using cholesterol-lowering drugs. All these trials were carried out in middle-aged white men, and their combined results represent about one million man-years data. The amount of time and effort put into the collection of such an enormous database, in face of the monotonous repetition of negative results, is a tribute to the tenacity of belief in the diet–heart hypothesis.

There are several striking features in these results. Firstly, the multiple-risk-factor strategy produced no improvement on the negative results of earlier trials using dietary modification only. That would suggest that none of the so-called risk factors for CHD plays a causal role. Secondly, the drug trials were no improvement on the dietary trials. Whatever could have been theoretically gained in reducing mortality from CHD was annulled or even exceeded by deaths from other causes, possibly induced by the drugs themselves. Thirdly, participants with a high risk of CHD fared no better in these trials than participants with a low risk. In fact, 4 out of the 6 trials with participants selected for their high risk showed an excess of deaths in the intervention group. This important observation has been ignored by the advocates of a high-risk intervention strategy.

It would require a psychologist or a sociologist to unravel why the strikingly negative evidence from these trials has been continuously presented by knowledgeable experts as evidence for the validity of the diet-heart hypothesis, and a vindication of their plans to extend these 'preventive' measures to whole nations. In the largest of these trials, the WHO Collaborative trial, there was no overall benefit, though the authors claimed benefit in the Belgian subgroup of the trial. However, in the UK part of the trial, the intervention group had a somewhat higher rate of fatal CHD (by 8%) and a higher overall mortality (by 11%) than the control group. The authors did not comment why this should be so, when at least one risk factor (smoking) was significantly reduced in the intervention group. Similarly, in the Polish part of the trial, the intervention group had a slight excess in fatal CHD deaths. Overall, with 365,287 man/year observation, there was no difference in CHD mortality between the control and intervention groups ($p=0.8$) and in overall mortality ($p=0.4$). Despite this clear negative result, the authors stated that 'these *benefits* are *large enough* to be of *great* public health importance... but they do not achieve the conventional level of significance, and therefore by themselves constitute only *moderate evidence* that intervention is effective'. It seems that statistics can be pushed aside when they do not support the foregone conclusion. The 'moderate evidence' is then upgraded in their conclusion: 'This trial has yielded *strong* experimental evidence that (intervention) is *effective'*. Even medical students would know that if no difference can be shown in a study involving 60,000 people followed up for 6 years, whatever is being measured has no clinical or practical significance. A better defence of these disappointing results would be to admit that the design of the trial was so bad that no useful information could result from it and that the WHO had wasted some of their resources. Lars Werkö noted that 'the authors and originators of these studies are not prepared to accept inconclusive results. Sophisticated statistical calculations are instead used to create some support for the preconceived ideas behind the trial'[4]. Michael Oliver spoke of 'post-hoc rationalisation of the current negative results by those who are persuaded by the positive effects of life-style changes on risk factors'[5].

The cost

With two exceptions, the costs of trials testing the diet-heart hypothesis have not been made public. We know, however, that one life 'saved' in the Lipid Research Clinics trial cost $50 million. In the MRFIT trial, in which no life was actually saved, the cost would exceed $115 million. Froom estimated, on the basis of the lowest available costs at his university hospital in New York that the initial cost of screening 130 million Americans deemed in need of such screening would be at least $10 billion[6], with an additional $10 billion for cholestyramine prescribed for 5 million patients per year[7]. These costs do not include medical fees and repeat tests (Table 3).

Table 3 Cost of trials, screening and intervention

		Cost of high-risk intervention			
Trial	No. screened	No. treated	Cost ($)	Lives saved	Cost per life saved ($)
MRFIT	361 662	12 866	115 m.	0	>115 m.
LRC	480 000	3 806	150 m.	3	50 m.

Cost of mass lipid screening and intervention	
130 m. persons (one round)	>$10 billion (Froom, 1989)[6]
Cholestyramine for 5 m. persons + medical fees	$10 billion/yr (Moore, 1989)[7]

Conclusions

I would like to conclude with three quotations which neatly summarize the pseudo-science which has been the hallmark of the crusade against CHD:

'Uncertainties and controversy have been swept aside as being obstructive and reactionary, and official recommendations have been sharpened and distorted at each stage of interpretation. The end result is a belief system which is almost totally unrelated to scientific fact'[8].

'Through American evangelism cholesterol campaigns are increasing in other countries. Vast sums are spent and widespread changes are made in the lifestyle of normal people when the accumulated evidence is that total mortality is unchanged or possibly even increased. At all events, the public should be aware that the available facts, as distinct from manipulation and projection of data, are that reduction of elevated plasma cholesterol and modification of related atherogenic lipoproteins does not reduce mortality'[9].

'When one pushes the evangelists into a corner they will admit that there is indeed no evidence but they then turn on to another tack by saying "even if it does no good it can do no harm"... Suppose that a vacuum cleaner salesman called at your house and claimed that his appliance would clean up all known dirt and leave your carpet as good as new. By way of a practical proof he sprinkled your carpet with cigarette ash, food and fluff, switched on his machine and it failed to pick up any of the dust. When this is pointed out to him he said "It didn't fuse the lights, did it?" Would you buy his machine?'[10].

References

1. Törnberg, S.A., Jakobsson, K.F.S. and Eklund, G.A. (1988). Stability and validity of a single serum cholesterol measurement in a prospective cohort study. *Int. J. Epidemiol.*, **17**, 797–803
2. Semenciw, R.M., Morrison, H.I., Mao, Y. *et al.* (1988). Major risk factors for cardiovascular mortality in adults: results from the Nutrition Canada Survey Cohort. *Int. J. Epidemiol.*, **17**, 317–24
3. Borhani, N.O. (1977). Primary prevention of coronary heart disease. A critique. *Am. J. Cardiol.*, **40**, 251–9
4. Werkö, L. (1987). The enigma of coronary heart disease and its prevention. *Acta Med. Scand.*, **221**, 323–33
5. Oliver, M.F. (1986). Prevention of coronary heart disease – propaganda, promises, problems and prospects. *Circulation*, **73**, 1–9
6. Froom, J. (1989). The cholesterol controversy. *Family Practice*, **6**, 232–7
7. Moore, T.J. (1989). The cholesterol myth. *The Atlantic Monthly*, Sept., 37–70
8. Pickard, B. (1986). Dairy products and red meat – villains or victims? In Anderson, D. (ed.), *A Diet of Reason*, pp. 21–39. (London: Social Affair Unit)
9. Oliver, M.F. (1988). Reducing cholesterol does not reduce mortality. *J. Am. Coll. Cardiol.*, **12**, 814–17
10. Mitchell, J.R.A. (1984). What constitutes evidence on the dietary prevention of coronary heart disease, Cosy beliefs or harsh facts? *Int. J. Cardiol.*, **5**, 287–98

Discussion

Dr Katan: I think there are two issues at work in conferences like these. One is the obvious issue on the table which is about figures and data and is this more than that and why would the trend in a country be so and so, and is it because of smoking or what? There is another unspoken and subjective issue which is: What should really be the way we live our lives; which interventions are worth the trouble and discomfort and which are not? One of the reasons why conferences like this sometimes get acrimonious is because the two issues get confused. Often, data are used to mask a sentiment which is really an inborn sentiment and not a matter of data that you can calculate with a computer. I think those inborn convictions need to be put on the table. This brings me, in a roundabout way, to a direct question. Do you feel governments should encourage their populations to quit cigarette smoking?

Dr Skrabanek: I think governments should stay as much out of our private lives as possible. What is happening more recently, is what you could call a tendency towards health fascism. Or you could call it more moderately, health fascism with a human face. The state adopts a nanny state function and tries to instruct you from cradle to grave, from morning to evening, on what you should do. I think that the problem of lifestyle and what it is worth in our life is something which is so philosophical and non-medical that the more doctors stay out of that area the better.

Dr Katan: In other words, you would say no. My point is that the disagreement between you and all those people who do feel that governments should discourage people from smoking is not so much that those people have access to different data, or that they make different calculations, but that they have a different philosophy and outlook on life. As long as we can agree on that perhaps we can avoid useless discussions about whether something increased or decreased because of something else. We have got to realize that there are some basic issues at stake here in prevention, which are based on personal choices, and on subjective matters, that have nothing to do with the data.

Dr Skrabanek: Not everyone would agree that we are meeting here to express our subjective feelings about human happiness. I thought we were here to discuss the nature and the quality of the data. I was trying to show that the data are of such poor quality that it is very difficult to make anything out of it. Perhaps what you are saying is that you can choose, according to your ideology, what you should pick from it. Obviously, we can do it that way, but if we do this, we should also state that it does not follow from the data.

Dr Anderson: In my own personal choice, I think the mortality data are of great interest. However, to confine oneself exclusively to mortality data I think is quite misleading. That is one of the problems I have with what you have talked about.

Dr Skrabanek: You are absolutely right. But, as I was trying to show, even in Framingham, prevalence and incidence of CHD in middle-aged men in the last 30 years actually increased. So, not only was there no effect on mortality, but there are more people involved in Framingham who are diagnosed as having ischaemic heart disease. Hence, it really is not clear whether current concerns with lifestyle are making people any happier or less ill. A few years ago a paper in the *New England Journal of Medicine*, by Barsky, called 'Paradox of Health' showed that when you looked at the indices of well-being in Americans, the sense of well-being or the number of people that actually say that they feel well has decreased while at the same time longevity has increased. I think we have now reached a saturation level and we cannot go any further. We can only retreat to tell people that not everything is in the hands of their doctor.

Dr Godsland: Do you actually have any thoughts about whether CHD can be prevented and if you think that it can, what kind of avenues we might pursue?

Dr Skrabanek: Obviously there is a Nobel prize waiting for the one who can answer this question, I have absolutely no idea.

Dr Isles: I would be interested to know how you interpret the results of the atheroma regression trials.

Dr Skrabanek: There is a problem there because the theory would say that there is no safe threshold for cholesterol. You cannot have it both ways and say that there is no threshold and at the same time say that there is a point at which atheroma starts dissolving, which means that there is a threshold. First of all, the studies are based on surrogate outcomes, you are measuring the diameter of vessels on X-ray or you do something which is basically inaccurate. This still does not answer your question – does the apparent change in the lumen of an artery have any effect in terms of reduced mortality 10, 20 years later? We do not know. I think that this regression theory is possible, but certainly not conclusive evidence, that you could reverse the process.

Dr Isles: I think I sit on this neither being an evangelist on the one side nor a nihilist on the other. But, the atheroma regression trials do appear to show, not only a change in the lumen, but also a reduction in the number of events, as well as a reduction in the number of people going for bypass grafts and having myocardial infarcts. In that group of people who already have established CHD there does seem to me to be reasonable evidence that altering cholesterol, alters their outcome. Would you dispute that?

Dr Skrabanek: No, I do not dispute anything, but a study of this kind was published in *The Lancet* recently from the United States. As you remember, there was quite heated correspondence about it. All I would say is that I would suspend my judgement, I am not saying yes or no.

Dr Grover: I agree with you, I think the secondary regression data looks pretty promising and I think we have to take a good hard look at those studies and ask why it works as well as it does in this group. Firstly, it is clear that this is a carefully chosen group of people. They are a young group of men with premature atherosclerotic disease who have lipid abnormalities. If we look at Greg Brown's study published in the *New England Journal of Medicine* last year, when patients with apolipoprotein abnormalities had their cholesterol lowered, there was not only regression but also a reduction in end-points. I think that this is very promising.

In secondary prevention, if you had a young individual in that same group you would be crazy not to tell them to lower their cholesterol after they have had their first myocardial infarct or their first bypass. I think we run into problems when we let those margins blur and proceed to extrapolate the data on to a 65-year-old women who has never had chest pain in her life and tell her because her cholesterol is 260 mg/dl, she needs to do something as well. I suspect that in the future we are going to see the secondary and the primary prevention studies really take a different path but hopefully this should translate into very different clinical practice guidelines as well.

Dr Walker: Do you believe that studies done during World War II in occupied countries showing a regression of atheromatous lesions are correct?

Dr Skrabanek: If you are referring to those done in Scandinavia, Denmark and Norway, I think you can make very little out of the studies because what you are looking at are diagnostic practices. This kind of evidence is similar to other wartime data for instance, those which claimed that eating bread is a cause of schizophrenia. So, in answer to your question, no credence can be given to that sort of evidence.

Dr Stehbens: In regard to the regression trials, I think you have to really look at those much more carefully than you are suggesting. For a start, many of the trials do include people with a metabolic lipid abnormality and those subjects with lipid abnormalities should be treated completely separately from those who are normolipidaemic.

Secondly, it can be very difficult with the regression trials to determine if the authors are referring to a reduction in the cross-sectional area or a reduction in the transverse diameter of the silhouette in angiography. When you review the papers, they do not in fact say what is significant change, but a number of them indicate that a minimum of 20–25% change either in cross-sectional area or of the diameter of the silhouette is needed to be significant. I think you can get very subtle changes in the wall that cannot be detected. The lumen is not being compared with a normal lumen but with the lumen of an adjacent segment which is also abnormal. Results of this sort are extremely inaccurate. When you have a metabolic lipid abnormality, there is a possibility that a reduction in serum lipids may reduce the space occupied by fat or lipid. Because, after all, it is not necessarily atherosclerosis but a fat storage phenomenon that may be reduced. Starry had a very good paper a few years ago indicating that there is either a change in a thrombus, or organization of a thrombus or lysis, but there is no change in fibrotic lesion.

Dr Grover: I think your comments are well taken, Dr Stehbens, but at the same time one has to remember that if we look at Greg Brown's studies, being the best that have come out to date, these are radiological readings being done blindly. All things being equal, at least radiologically, it appears that something has happened to the lesion. I, like you, have no idea what has happened, but the lumen looks bigger in the group which has had intensive intervention as far as their cholesterol is concerned. Some of the critical end-points of CHD were actually less in this group. I think that this is compelling information and suggests that we should look at these sorts of studies over a much longer term. But, I agree it is a highly selective group of patients and you have to be very cautious about extrapolating that data even to a 75-year-old or 60-year-old who have developed their first myocardial infarct. This is not premature atherosclerosis any more and it is not premature atherosclerosis in someone with an inherited hyperlipidaemia either.

Dr Horlick: The data from the Cholesterol Lowering Atherosclerosis Study (CLAS) would suggest that there was a very wide range of cholesterol levels in this population. The analysis of the data seems to suggest that regression had really not much to do with the cholesterol levels of the individuals at entry. What the important factor was here, was not entirely clear, other than the fact that if you do objective readings of angiograms there is a difference. Clearly, something is going on that is beneficial but we do not know what it is. I do not think anyone would want to extrapolate from this data to a 70-year-old female because I do not think there were any 70-year-old individuals in the CLAS study. I really believe that the CLAS study is still the best study and the one that has the longest follow-up. It is rather interesting that at the 4-year follow-up of the CLAS study the results have been well maintained and have shown some further improvement with the passage of time.

I also wanted to direct some remarks at Dr Skrabanek's paper. In essence, what he has done is to attempt to demolish 50–60 years of the so-called cholesterol hypothesis. I think that this is easy to do if you are careful to select out the bits of information that fit into your preconceived notions. If you want to really look objectively at the whole issue, the best studies done to date, and I am not talking about the ideal studies Katan assured us can never be done, but the best studies that have been done to date indicate that there is a difference in terms not only of total deaths but perhaps more so in terms of morbidity from myocardial infarct, angina, surgical intervention etc., in individuals who have had intervention of one sort or another, either dietary or drug instituted on their part. I do not think that this can be explained away in a facile and humorous fashion as Dr Skrabanek attempted to do. The other point I would like to make, and is in a sense, a defence for the consensus argument, is the fact that there will never be a perfect experiment. And, on the basis of pure reason and science, there will never be agreement on any set of interventions for anything because the final answer will never be in. From a public health point of view, we are dealing with a major killer. It is important that we try and devise methods which can be applied to the population which can reduce death and disability and I think that is what the Consensus Conference attempted to do. They have attempted to do it by judiciously balancing what was known, what was available, and what could be done. I think they can be clearly defended on this basis.

Dr Skrabanek: It seems that the defenders of the consensus are now using the excuse that you can never have a perfect experiment. This is the sort of thing that arises when you have reasonable evidence for something else. It is only when the evidence is not there that people say, of course, you cannot have 1 000 000 monozygotic twins for a given study. But, that really is not the point.

You also mentioned that people who undergo intervention have less morbidity from myocardial infarct, angina and surgical intervention. It seems to me that the more people who are exposed to intervention, the more likely they are to end up in the hands of surgeons because the number of heart operations, coronary bypasses and angioplasty are increasing quite phenomenally. So, your argument is not really true and I think what you are saying in defence of the consensus is that one should be reasonable and take some sort of middle way between half true and half false which will codify something we are to believe in for the next 40 years. ,

There are so many people who have spent 30–40 years working on this. To expect that they proclaim that they have wasted their time is ludicrous, and as a result, they cling to their hypotheses. In fact, some of these hypotheses simply die with their generators. In science, when there is scientific disagreement you go back to the laboratory and do more experiments, research and accumulate more basic knowledge.

When you are trying to learn more about anything you must rely on the falsification method and try to find out the best way to disprove your hypothesis. If you see a discordant result, you should cherish it because that discordant result is hiding some new truth or new observation. What the advocates of consensus do is brush away the discordant results because they do not want to have their peace of mind upset. I agree it is easier, as you say, to be a critic than to produce something constructive. However, if someone produces destructive criticism it is then dismissed as if it were selective data. Criticism is always selective. For example, if one single repeatable phenomenon does not fit into your hypothesis, you have to accommodate that hypothesis with this new piece of information. You cannot stand up and say that it is selective and you did not make a mean of all opinions. This is where the Consensus Conference is misleading because it simply takes the lowest common denominator, rather than selecting the points of disagreement and saying this is where we have to learn more.

Dr Kubow: As a nutritionist, I would like to comment on some of the dietary trials that have been performed to date, in modifying P/S ratio, particularly in the primary and secondary intervention studies. The primary studies in the past have not shown strong effects, or when effects have been shown, I feel that the subject number was either too small or not well controlled. I think the Minnesota Coronary Survey, as one of the more recent studies, was a well-controlled, randomized trial but which showed no differences in cardio-vascular events in subjects fed diets with a high P/S ratio versus subjects who were eating diets with a low P/S ratio. In actual fact, I think the jury is still out in modulating P/S ratios in terms of CHD morbidity or mortality. In terms of secondary intervention trials, there is suggestive evidence of the effect of dietary fat modification on coronary lesion growth that has come out from the Blankenhorn Cholesterol Lowering Atherosclerosis Study. This secondary intervention study showed that there was a positive relationship between total fat consumption and coronary lesion growth in coronary bypass patients. This study did show an effect of quality of fat on lesion growth, but interestingly, a higher dietary P/S ratio was associated with higher coronary lesion growth. So, to make blanket statements in terms of dietary intervention at this point, either in terms of primary or secondary intervention trials, I think is a little premature before we totally investigate this with properly controlled trials.

Section II.
Atherosclerosis and Atherogenesis

7

The role of blood flow in atherogenesis and the dietary cholesterol–fat hypothesis

W.E. STEHBENS

Introduction

It is characteristic of human nature that resentment rather than curiosity is roused when we are advised that evidence dictates long-held beliefs or concepts are false, and though the majority view always attracts supporters and discourages opposition, it is essential that the evidence be assessed logically.

Debate on the role of dietary cholesterol and animal fat in coronary heart disease (CHD) is intensifying, the consensus view maintaining that a high cholesterol/fat diet is the major environmental agent responsible for the elevation of blood cholesterol and low density lipoprotein (LDL) levels and in turn for the prevalence of severe atherosclerosis and CHD. This viewpoint, promulgated widely in both the lay and scientific press with almost religious fervour, has been sufficiently forceful to develop cholesterol phobia in the general public. However it is implausible that cholesterol, an essential metabolite and a constituent of every cell in the body, could possibly be noxious at all blood levels when it is also a precursor of vitamin D, steroid hormones and bile acids and constitutes up to 17% of the dry weight of the brain[1] and when up to 80% is synthesized endogenously and synthesis increases when intestinal absorption decreases and vice versa. On these grounds alone review of the evidence is warranted for it is not possible that cholesterol or LDL could be the principal causal factor of atherosclerosis which is ubiquitous in man and occurs widely in lower animals.

Pathological evidence

Knowledge of atherosclerosis and its underlying mechanisms has been evolving rapidly of late and whilst many clinical investigators may be concerned with CHD, atherosclerosis is implicitly assumed to be the underlying disease process responsible.

Atherosclerosis is a degenerative disease of blood vessels affecting all humans but with individual variation in severity. It also affects many lower species to a lesser degree and despite vegetarian diets such animals as gorillas, chimpanzees and parrots can manifest severe atherosclerosis. The cause of atherosclerosis must be present in all individuals and animals suffering from the disease and it is the variation in severity that requires intense study to provide clues to causation rather than the incidence of a non-pathognomonic complication of the disease.

It is widely acknowledged that atherosclerosis commences with a microscopic zone of fibromusculo-elastic intimal proliferation as a pre-lipid but integral stage of the disease[2]. If examined histologically these intimal thickenings originate at specific anatomical sites about the forks of distributing arteries in the fetus with their localization indicative of haemodynamic influences[3]. They are more pronounced about sites of branching in the aorta and more extensive in the neonate with the same distribution as severe atherosclerosis of later life[2].

In the cerebral arteries these intimal thickenings become thicker, extend and coalesce and progressively merge with overt atherosclerosis without any line of demarcation[4]. Many investigators have maintained they are early manifestations of atherosclerosis, because lipid, when it appears, usually does so deep in the intima indicating that intimal proliferation always precedes the lipid. Indeed the intimal injury hypothesis[5] is a belated acceptance that intimal proliferation about forks is an early manifestation of the disease[6].

These intimal thickenings in the sheep are sites of predilection for spontaneous lipid deposition[7], the same as has been found in human coronary arteries[8]. In the rabbit the pads or cushions are also sites of predilection for dietary-induced lipid deposition[9] but therein lies the only similarity. Ultrastructurally the lipid accumulation in the rabbit differs in pathogenesis from the development of atherosclerosis in man[10]. There are distinct morphological differences, an absence of complications and extravascular lipid storage phenomena that are irreconcilable with atherosclerosis[11,12]. This misrepresentation of the pathology of the cholesterol-fed animal has been instrumental in misleading the scientific community and epidemiologists interested in atherogenesis. Gross over-feeding of animals with cholesterol with or without added fat and ablation of thyroid function produces a fat storage phenomenon. In those animals that develop spontaneously more advanced atherosclerotic lesions than the rabbit the dietary-induced lesions more closely resemble human atherosclerosis. Such lesions can be considered as mixed lesions with fat storage superimposed on atherosclerosis[11,12].

In man atherosclerosis varies in severity from individual to individual and from vascular bed to vascular bed as well as with the anatomical site within the vascular tree (such as forks, unions, curvatures, dilatations). It is most severe in large arteries and in the systemic circulation, less severe in pulmonary arteries and least severe in veins and small blood vessels. The intimal proliferation of the fetus and neonate thicken, extend and coalesce with hypertension accentuating the severity in each vascular bed[2]. The disease slowly and insidiously progresses during a clinically quiescent phase usually lasting for several decades, until the stage of complications sets in. This is associated with intimal tears and ulceration with secondary thromboembolic phenomena and progressive encroachment on the lumen and ischaemic incidents result. Alternatively, progressive ectasia, tortuosity and localized or diffuse aneurysmal dilatation develop with pressure effects and possibly fatal haemorrhage as the result of mural rupture. All these clinical manifestations can be explained on the basis of an acquired pathological fragility or weakness of the vessel wall attributable to a lifetime long haemodynamically-induced engineering failure or fatigue[2]. Aggravation of the disease by hypertension and the complications of atherosclerosis are readily explained by the fatigue hypothesis but not by the lipid hypothesis.

The ultrastructural changes in developing atherosclerosis include dystrophic basement membrane material, cellular fragility with the accumulation of much cell debris (matrix vesicles)[13] with its affinity for lipid and mineralization, loss and fragmentation of elastin, abnormal collagen fibres and separation of endothelial and muscle cells from their basement membranes[14]. These are in all probability manifestations of a loss of cohesion of the vessel wall and of its increasing fragility. Such changes are not induced by cholesterol-feeding[11,12]. The accumulation of lipid and calcium salts is a late or secondary manifestation of atherosclerosis, not the initiator.

Homozygous familial hypercholesterolaemia (FH) is regarded as the strongest evidence in support of hypercholesterolaemia supposedly being the cause of atherosclerosis[15,16]. The homozygous form, the purest form of the disease, is crucial to the lipid/cholesterol controversy. In recent years the vascular changes have been regarded as atherosclerotic but in early literature they were referred to as xanthomatosis or xanthelasma of the aorta, indicating the xanthomatous nature of the lesions and their similarity to the extensive extravascular xanthomatosis that characterizes the disease and also to the foam cell lesions of cholesterol-fed animals. Differences from spontaneous atherosclerosis are quite striking[17,18] and although FH allegedly produces premature accelerated atherosclerosis, in the literature there is not a single case of aortic aneurysm in a subject with homozygous FH. All the evidence indicates that FH, like the excessive administration of cholesterol to susceptible animals, is a fat storage disease.

Pathologically the juxtaposition of advanced atherosclerosis to intima with no demonstrable intimal thickening does not support the causal role of any humoral agent. Moreover surgeons produce accelerated atherosclerosis in venous by-pass grafts[2] in which the vein is subjected to arterial haemodynamics and also in the anastomosed vein of therapeutic arteriovenous shunts for renal dialysis[19]. Yet these veins if left intact like other veins in the subject would remain minimally affected for the remaining years of life. The vessel wall becomes susceptible or receptive to the accumulation of lipids at all blood levels of cholesterol and LDL with the crucial factor being not the presence of a circulating humoral factor such as cholesterol or LDL, but the haemodynamic stresses to which the vessels are subjected.

Coronary heart disease

CHD is an imprecise clinical diagnosis indicating myocardial ischaemia, no matter the underlying cause. It is not a specific disease and in only 90% of subjects with myocardial ischaemia is it considered due to atherosclerosis[20], whilst in up to 20 or even 30% of subjects with clinical CHD the coronary arteries angiographically are normal or nearly so[21,22]. On the other hand, in the Framingham Study up to 30% of cases of severe CHD were symptomless[23] and up to 70% of ischaemic events in subjects continuously monitored had no anginal pain whatsoever[24]. Comparison of discrepancies between clinical diagnoses and autopsy findings reveal a diagnostic error for CHD conservatively at ±30%[25]. Non-specific complications which are common to many diseases such as headache, hypertension, subarachnoid haemorrhage, etc. are not definitive diagnoses in themselves and their clinical management depends on determining the disease responsible for such pathological changes in each instance. Yet in the epidemiology of CHD, no differentiation is made and all subjects are classified together, including metabolic lipid storage diseases[26].

Since it is not possible to measure the severity of atherosclerosis during life, complications of atherosclerosis viz. CHD, stroke or peripheral vascular disease are often used as a clinical marker of severe atherosclerosis. Such a procedure may seem reasonable but in view of the uncertain severity of atherosclerosis in genuine cases of atherosclerotic CHD and the diagnostic error and the non-pathognomonic nature of CHD, it is inappropriate to determine the incidence of CHD instead of the severity of atherosclerosis which is present whether or not the individual has myocardial ischaemia. The inability to measure accurately the severity of ubiquitous atherosclerosis in each individual does not condone the use of incidence of an inappropriate surrogate monitor[27]. In epidemiology and in science generally it is essential that the parameter sought should be measured, not a substitute. An inadequate, inappropriate surrogate provides defective, misleading data. Moreover, when a population or cohort is divided into those with and those without CHD, all have atherosclerosis of some degree of severity. Therefore a risk factor statistically more frequent in the CHD group can only be an aggravating factor – not a cause. The situation is worsened when invalid extrapolations are made from risk factors of CHD which occurs predominantly in late middle age and the elderly to the aetiology of atherosclerosis which commences in infancy if not *in utero* [26].

Myocardial ischaemia can occur in both the cholesterol-fed rabbit and in subjects with homozygous FH but the pathogenesis of the myocardial ischaemia differs from that of conventional coronary atherosclerosis[11,12,17]. Therefore subjects with FH and analogous metabolic storage diseases (Type III hyperlipoproteinaemia) should be excluded from clinical studies of risk factors and from clinical trials. Their inclusion results in selection bias. Such subjects have been preferentially included in some regression studies and results therefrom considered applicable to the whole population[28].

If aortic aneurysm had been used as a surrogate monitor of severe atherosclerosis, lipids would never have received such exclusive attention. Atherosclerosis would not have been regarded as a metabolic disease of lipids, but it would have been essential to exclude hereditary connective tissue disorders from clinical studies.

The majority of investigators in the field of atherosclerosis research are poorly versed in the pathology and natural history of the disease. Unwarranted faith has been placed in the cholesterol-fed animal and FH, the pathology of which has been misrepresented and does not support the cholesterol or lipid hypothesis. Without corroborative pathological and experimental evidence, epidemiological studies lose their significance. The lipid hypothesis is not a theory of the aetiology of atherosclerosis but merely an hypothesis concerned with lipid infiltration of the vascular wall. It does not explain the complications of atherosclerosis such as the intimal tears, ulceration, tortuosity, ectasia and aneurysms which are merely assumed to follow in the wake of lipid deposition in the arterial wall.

It is apparent that some clinicians are more concerned with the incidence of CHD in the belief that elevated blood cholesterol levels result in augmented lipid accumulation in atherosclerotic coronary arteries but this has yet to be demonstrated. Pathological evidence for augmented atherosclerosis in FH and possibly type III hyperlipoproteinaemia is poorly substantiated[17,18] indicating a need for further detailed qualitative and quantitative study of the vascular lesions of normo- and hypercholesterolaemic individuals. Theoretically a lipid dystrophy could affect atherosclerosis by one or more of the following mechanisms (1) fat storage and a space-occupying effect on the intima with encroachment on the lumen thus accentuating the effects of atherosclerosis, (2) similar fat storage superimposed on atherosclerosis providing mixed lesions, (3) interference with general metabolic and reparative functions of endothelial and smooth muscle cells, (4) a secondary haemodynamically-induced degenerative effect on intimal foam cell masses or (5) a totally independent propensity to vascular degeneration and atherosclerosis[18]. On current evidence it is likely that only items 2 and 4 would be applicable.

The epidemiological evidence

The lipid hypothesis is thought to receive strong support from epidemiological studies, which have proven invaluable in acute infectious and occupational diseases. However they are of limited applicability to ubiquitous chronic degenerative diseases that develop insidiously over a lifetime such as atherosclerosis. Results of these epidemiological studies have been widely accepted because the limitations of epidemiological methods are not generally appreciated.

Smith and Pinckney[29] provided a particularly damning survey revealing serious inconsistencies in the data and misrepresentation of the results of clinical studies. This lack of precision in terminology and lack of concern for data accuracy have become major concerns. Logic dictates that even one unexplained inconsistency negates the hypothesis necessitating review of the premises on which the theory rests. However by assuming a multicausal concept of disease processes, atherosclerosis in any individual is said to be a variable mix of risk factors resulting in the same clinical and pathological state without any one factor being essential[30]. An approach like this inhibits testable hypotheses and precludes proof or disproof of a causal role for any one factor and is a reason why the essential cause of atherosclerosis has proven so elusive.

After demonstrating that the vascular pathology of cholesterol-fed animals[11,12] and of FH[17] had been seriously misrepresented, Stehbens reviewed the methodology of the epidemiological approach to CHD. In so doing he identified a number of methodological errors sufficiently serious to invalidate the data and the conclusions derived therefrom. In summary these include the following:

(1) 'Cause' is misused. Rather than being used in its correct lexical sense as the essential prerequisite of atherosclerosis without which the disease does not occur, causation is softened and essentially is non-specific including reasons or conditions why a disease develops. Statistical associations with CHD (endstage atherosclerosis) are used synonymously with cause without proof of causality by non-epidemiological means[27,31].

(2) Misuse of CHD has already been explained[27].

(3) CHD epidemiology relies heavily on national mortality rates which provide defective data and fallacious science[32]. The data pertaining to cerebrovascular disease incorporates even greater error[33].

(4) Dietary data in respect of the primary food constituents is unreliable and extrapolations from such short-term studies, no matter how accurate, cannot seriously be regarded as of consequence in the case of a chronic ubiquitous disease such as atherosclerosis[34,35].

(5)   There is no scientific correlation between dietary fat, serum cholesterol, CHD and atherosclerosis at an individual level within the population even though such correlations can generally but not always be demonstrated between some national and population groups. Most ecological correlations are invalid and in the case of CHD the inapplicability in individuals indicates its lack of validity and biological significance. To claim otherwise is an ecological fallacy. Many ecological correlations with CHD mortality are non-specific characteristics of an affluent society and all that such life styles entail with no evidence of cause and effect[35].

(6)   More than 280 risk factors have been correlated with CHD[36] without evidence of causality and most can have no biological significance. Some of these correlations with end-stage disease may provide reasons why or the conditions under which CHD develops but evidence of causality in respect of atherosclerosis is merely assumed. None of the current risk factors comply with the epidemiological criteria of causation.

(7)   Since the pathogenesis of CHD in FH differs from that in atherosclerosis, subjects with lipid dystrophies such as FH and hyperlipoproteinaemia type III should be excluded from clinical trials. Incorporating such subjects in clinical studies including regression trials is inappropriate, being likely to produce a bias to hypercholesterolaemia[35].

(8)   The young subjects usually studied in CHD epidemiology constitute a young non-representative group and a secondary result is a selection bias to the incorporation of FH subjects[35].

(9)   The age changes in blood cholesterol levels in both sexes do not parallel the CHD mortality rates with increasing age[26].

(10) CHD and atherosclerosis in the age group usually studied are both age dependent and there appears to be a genetic dependence as well. Yet serum cholesterol, hypertension, diabetes mellitus (and glucose intolerance) and body bulk or obesity are not only age and genetically dependent but are interrelated one with another in some as yet inextricable manner and it is acknowledged on pathological grounds that hypertension and diabetes mellitus aggravate the severity of atherosclerosis. In view of the diagnostic inaccuracy associated with CHD, the variable duration and severity of these so-called risk factors, and the above methodological weaknesses, sophisticated statistical analyses are unlikely to determine the true relationship of serum cholesterol levels to the severity of atherosclerosis or even CHD[37].

Progress in medical science results from the pursuit of truth and exactitude and reliability of data in all aspects of clinical studies and trials. Too much faith has been placed on CHD mortality and morbidity rates and angiography in the belief that these can monitor atherosclerosis severity during life. Until it is technologically possible to reliably grade the severity and progression of atherosclerosis, clinical trials will be of limited value and should not be used to support the lipid hypothesis[28]. Nor does the absence of reliable technology condone the use of, or validate, results derived from unscientific methodology.

The role of blood flow

Preoccupation with lipids and the lipid hypothesis has stimulated enormous interest in lipid metabolism. Much of the research has been beneficial but other research avenues have been neglected as a consequence. For example, it has long been recognized that the distribution of atherosclerosis suggests haemodynamics play an important role in lesion localization[2], but in recent years haemodynamics has been considered merely as a localizing factor. Halsted's important observations regarding poststenotic dilatation and aneurysm in aortic coarctation[38] and Holman's subsequent experimental work[39] revealed that dilatation of the aorta and of smaller arteries was a non-specific result caused by vibratory activity of the wall in the post-stenotic area. This dilatation and subsequent mural tearing seemed to be derived from structural failure of the aortic wall, and results of an extensive study of arterial forks and aneurysms led Stehbens[40] to postulate long since that atherosclerosis and berry aneurysms of cerebral arteries were also consequences of engineering fatigue. Atherosclerosis was considered the ultimate manifestation of the degenerative changes caused by fatigue and the proliferative changes which were essentially reparative in nature. Death occurred eventually when degenerative changes predominated and were manifested by serious loss of tensile strength of the wall, the phenomenon which accounted for clinical ischaemic and haemorrhagic events.

Engineering fatigue is the change in mechanical properties of materials caused by repetitive stresses of an intensity less than is normally required to cause single application fracture. The fatigue fracture is due to an ill-understood molecular alteration typified by loss of cohesion and tensile strength, the stressed material failing suddenly under normal operational loading. The vibratory effect is cumulative but the stresses vary in amplitude. Fatigue, an engineering term, affects most solid materials including timber, rubber, bones (stress fractures) and tendons. Stress fractures of bones and tendons in joggers and athletes and march fractures of soldiers are similar in nature. The post-stenotic dilatation of coarctation has also been demonstrated to be due to haemodynamically induced vibrations being thought to be the cause of dissecting aneurysm beyond aortic or pulmonary valvular stenosis[41].

Thoma invoked angiomalacia with medial weakening and dilatation and compensatory intimal thickening to maintain the cross-sectional area of the lumen[42]. This concept is supported by other observations viz.

(1) progressive ectasia of the aorta and cerebral and coronary arteries and concomitant intimal thickening[2],

(2) progressive intimal thickening in lower limb arteries concomitant with medial thinning[43],

(3) medial thinning beneath coronary intimal proliferation in the neonate[44], and

(4) loss of tissue cohesion in the atherosclerotic intima as suggested by many of the degenerative changes seen histologically and ultrastructurally, some being observed in neonates[3,14].

The complications of atherosclerosis occur predominantly in the second clinical phase which arises in the sixth decade and beyond, so to produce atherosclerosis experimentally at an accelerated rate which would validate the fatigue hypothesis, it was necessary to use vascular models of disturbed blood flow in which the vessel wall was subjected to increased frequency or amplitude of the vibrations or both.

Experimental models

(i) Chronic arteriovenous fistulae

Since arteries and veins are both subjected to atherosclerosis and composed of the same cellular and non-cellular connective tissues, though with different architecture, arteriovenous fistulae were fashioned between the common carotid artery and external jugular vein on one side of the neck in a series of sheep without manipulating the diet. Control phlebotomy and arteriotomy were fashioned on the contralateral side. The anastomosed veins exhibited progressive ectasia with tortuosity and irregular aneurysmal dilatation, and their walls assumed features of human atherosclerotic thickening with lipid accumulation, intimal tears, mural thrombosis and calcification. Histologically[45], ultrastructurally[46] and biochemically[47-50] the changes were consistent with those of atherosclerosis. Only the severity was not as great as in advanced atherosclerosis. The pathogenesis of the accelerated lesions was similar to that in man. The human counterpart, seen in therapeutic arteriovenous fistulae for renal dialysis[19], also exhibits similar vascular changes histologically and ultrastructurally consistent with those of atherosclerosis.

(ii) Experimental aneurysms

Berry aneurysms in man develop atherosclerosis at an accelerated rate although the vibrations are of lower amplitude but higher frequency than those associated with arteriovenous fistulae[2,33]. Therefore three types of venous pouch aneurysms were fashioned on the common carotid artery or at the aortic bifurcation in rabbits on a stock diet. Atherosclerosis histologically and ultrastructurally similar to that of man developed at an accelerated rate in the aneurysms and complications included thromboses, calcification and lipid accumulation[51-53].

(iii) The U-shaped bend

Intimal proliferation progressing to atherosclerosis occurs in the carotid siphon of man just beyond the lesser curvature of bends in regions of boundary layer separation. Disturbed flow occurs in such regions in glass models of tortuosities and U-shaped bends[54,55]. In experimental tortuosities lipid-containing intimal proliferation has been reported but not illustrated, so the lipid content was probably minimal[56,57]. Since tortuosities are difficult to control without fixation of the arteries, U-shaped bends were fashioned in rabbits and sheep by transposing a common carotid artery to the opposite side and tying the anastomotic tie-sutures together to fashion a fairly sharp U-bend. The proliferative lesions so formed were similar histologically and in site to those in the human carotid siphon. Lipid was present in the thickenings in sheep but the experiments were terminated before more advanced lesions developed[58].

(iv) Haemodynamic stress and hypercholesterolaemia

Since haemodynamic stress is often considered to be a localizing factor only, experimental arterial aneurysms and arteriovenous fistulae were fashioned by microvascular surgery in hypercholesterolaemic rabbits. The aneurysmal sacs and the anastomosed veins of arteriovenous fistulae were sites of predilection for lipid deposition. Histologically, rather than accentuating the haemodynamically induced changes, the latter were merely honeycombed with lipid-laden macrophages which suggests superimposed lipid storage on haemodynamically induced stress changes in the wall[59,60].

The intimal pads or cushions about arterial forks in the rabbit resemble those in human infants. When hypercholesterolaemia is induced, the progressive changes including lipid deposition are not ultrastructurally those of accelerated atherosclerosis[10]. Lipid storage predominates with separation of the pre-existing constituents rather than the pathogenetic features of the atherosclerotic process appearing which suggests that in these rabbit experiments, dietary fat and cholesterol do not accelerate atherogenesis *per se*.

(v) Atrophic lesions

Atherosclerosis is usually considered to be characterized by proliferation of the intima, although medial thinning and even disappearance of the media may occur in the advanced disease. There may be less intimal proliferation at the flow divider of cerebral arterial forks and at times there is frank atrophy of the media adjacent to the crotch or apex of the fork[33]. These atrophic lesions are the early manifestations of cerebral aneurysm formation and in recent years similar atrophic changes of varying degree have been produced experimentally on the greater curvature of arterial bends[58], at cerebral arterial forks with imbalance of flow in rats[61] and in the afferent artery of arteriovenous fistulae[59]. Their earliest manifestations, observed by scanning electron microscopy, appear to be tears of the internal elastic lamina which are predominantly transversely orientated and visible within a few days postoperatively[62,63]. Similar elastic tears have been observed in human infants on the greater curvature of bends and also in the internal iliac arteries where they are related to haemodynamics and exhibit subsequent calcification and even lipid deposition[64]. Early cerebral aneurysms in man can consist virtually of endothelium and attenuated adventitial remnants and yet subsequently at the sides of the aneurysm severe proliferative atherosclerosis develops[33]. This indicates that the atrophic lesions are manifestations of atherosclerosis and may also exhibit the proliferative disease changes.

Commentary

The lipid hypothesis is based on observations of end-stage atherosclerosis and epidemiological data relevant only to an imprecise clinical diagnosis of one of the complications. It is not a theory of the aetiology of atherosclerosis *per se* but merely of reasons why lipid might accumulate in the arterial wall. It assumes that atherosclerosis and its complications naturally evolve once lipid is present in the vessel wall. The serious and particularly damaging inconsistencies analysed by Smith and Pinckney[29] and the methodological weaknesses in CHD epidemiology[26] indicate that the data provided by such methods are scientifically unacceptable.

In the study of any disease familiarity with the pathology and pathogenesis is essential but unfortunately most investigators are not familiar with the pathology of atherosclerosis. Lack of precision in terminology with CHD commonly used synonymously with atherosclerosis followed by invalid extrapolations from statistical associations with CHD to the aetiology of atherosclerosis. Misrepresentation of the pathology of FH and of the cholesterol-fed animal has contributed to the confusion and controversy over cholesterol but this does not condone the methodological weaknesses and lack of concern for quality of the data in CHD epidemiology. This review does not disprove the lipid hypothesis but it reveals the unscientific basis of the cholesterol–heart disease controversy and is a warning for investigators not to rely unquestioningly on the consensus view.

The mechanical concept of the aetiology and pathogenesis of atherosclerosis here espoused is gaining credence for the vascular system is not immune to the fundamental laws of hydromechanics. Vibrational stress with fatigue failure provides a logical explanation for the acquired fragility and weakness of the vessel wall and the disease complications (ectasia, aneurysms, intimal disruption, dissection and thrombosis)[2]. The variation in susceptibility from vascular bed to vascular bed and the production of accelerated disease in man and even herbivorous animals merely by altering blood flow cast serious doubt on the concept of the disease being caused by some humoral agent in the blood. Vessel wall susceptibility even to lipid and mineralization can be induced haemodynamically and the experimental flow models indicate that haemodynamics can produce lesions similar to atherosclerosis in the absence of an elevated serum lipid or any dietary manipulation. If haemodynamically induced vibrational stress is not the mechanism underlying the development of atherosclerosis in experimental animal models and in venous bypass grafts and arteriovenous shunts associated with renal dialysis in man, then lipid protagonists have to formulate explanations for their nature and pathogenesis and for the inconsistencies and methodological flaws in CHD epidemiology.

Acknowledgements

This research has been supported by the National Heart Foundation of New Zealand, the New Zealand Dairy Board and the New Zealand Meat Research and Development Council.

References

1. McDonald, P., Edwards, R.A. and Greenhalgh, J.F.D. (1987). *Animal Nutrition*, 3rd edn., p. 37. (Harlow: Longman Group Limited)
2. Stehbens, W.E. (1979). *Hemodynamics and the Blood Vessel Wall*. (Springfield, Ill: C.C. Thomas)
3. Stehbens, W.E. (1960). Focal intimal proliferation in the cerebral arteries. *Am. J. Pathol.*, **36**, 289–301
4. Stehbens, W.E. (1963). Histopathology of cerebral aneurysms. *Arch. Neurol.*, **8**, 272–85
5. Ross, R. and Glomset, J.A. (1976). The pathogenesis of atherosclerosis. *N. Engl. J. Med.*, **295**, 369–77, 420–5

6. Stehbens, W.E. (1988). The role of hemodynamics in the proliferative lesions of atherosclerosis. In Yoshida, Y., Yamaguchi, T., Caro, C.G., Glagov, S. and Nerem, R.M. (eds). *Role of Blood Flow in Atherogenesis*, pp. 47–53. (Tokyo: Springer-Verlag)
7. Stehbens, W.E. (1965). Intimal proliferation and spontaneous lipid deposition in the cerebral arteries of sheep and steers. *J. Athero. Res.*, **5**, 556–68
8. Jaffé, D., Hartroft, S., Manning, M. and Eleta, G. (1971). Coronary arteries in newborn children. *Acta Paediatr. Scand.*, **219**, 3–28
9. Stehbens, W.E. (1963). The renal artery in normal and cholesterol-fed rabbits. *Am. J. Pathol.*, **43**, 969–85
10. Stehbens, W.E. and Ludatscher, R.M. (1983).The susceptibility of renal arterial forks in rabbits to dietary-induced lipid deposition. *Pathology*, **15**, 475–85
11. Stehbens, W.E. (1986). An appraisal of cholesterol-feeding in experimental atherogenesis. *Progr. Cardiovasc. Dis.*, **29**, 107–28
12. Stehbens, W.E. (1986). Vascular complications in experimental atherosclerosis. *Progr. Cardiovasc. Dis.*, **29**, 221–37
13. Rogers, K.M. and Stehbens, W.E. (1986). The morphology of matrix vesicles produced in experimental arterial aneurysms of rabbits. *Pathology*, **18**, 64–71
14. Stehbens, W.E. (1975). Cerebral atherosclerosis. Intimal proliferation and atherosclerosis in the cerebral arteries. *Arch. Pathol.*, **99**, 582–91
15. Oliver, M.F. (1981). Serum cholesterol – the knave of hearts and the joker. *Lancet*, **2**, 1090–5
16. Goldstein, J.L. and Brown, M.S. (1983). Familial hypercholesterolemia. In Stanbury, J.B., Wyngaarden, J.B., Fredrickson, D.S., Goldstein, J.L. and Brown, M.S. (eds). *The Metabolic Basis of Inherited Disease*, 5th edn, pp. 672–712. (New York: McGraw Hill)
17. Stehbens, W.E. and Wierzbicki, E. (1988). The relationship of hypercholesterolemia to atherosclerosis with particular emphasis on familial hypercholesterolemia, diabetes mellitus, obstructive jaundice, myxedema and the nephrotic syndrome. *Progr. Cardiovasc. Dis.*, **30**, 289–306
18. Stehbens, W.E. and Martin, M. (1991). The vascular pathology of familial hypercholesterolemia. *Pathology*, **23**, 54–61
19. Stehbens, W.E. and Karmody, A.M. (1975). Venous atherosclerosis associated with arteriovenous fistulas for hemodialysis. *Arch. Surg.*, **110**, 176–80
20. Robbins, S.L., Angell, M. and Kumar, V. (1981). *Basic Pathology*, 3rd edn, pp. 289–99. (Philadelphia: W.B. Saunders)
21. Gazes, P.C. (1988). Angina pectoris: classification and diagnosis, Part 2. *Mod. Concepts Cardiovasc. Dis.*, **57**, 25–7
22. Mukerji, V., Alpert, M.A., Hewett, J.E. and Parker, B.M. (1989). Can patients with chest pain and normal coronary arteries be discriminated from those with coronary artery disease prior to coronary angiography? *Angiology*, **40**, 276–82
23. Kannel, W.B. and Abbott, R.D. (1984). Incidence and prognosis of unrecognized myocardial infarction. *N. Engl. J. Med.*, **311**, 1144–7
24. Cohn, P.F. (1981). Asymptomatic coronary artery disease. Pathophysiology, diagnosis, management. *Mod. Concepts Cardiovasc. Dis.*, **50**, 55–60
25. Stehbens, W.E. (1987). An appraisal of the epidemic rise of coronary heart disease and its decline. *Lancet*, **1**, 606–11

26. Stehbens, W.E. (1990). The lipid hypothesis and the role of hemodynamics in atherogenesis. *Progr. Cardiovasc. Dis.*, **33**, 119–36
27. Stehbens, W.E. (1990). Basic precepts and the lipid hypothesis of atherosclerosis. *Med. Hypotheses*, **31**, 105–13
28. Stehbens, W.E. (1991). Reduction of serum cholesterol levels and regression of atherosclerosis. *Pathology*, **23**, 45–53
29. Smith, R.L. and Pinckney, E.R. (1988). *Diet, Blood Cholesterol and Coronary Heart Disease: A Relationship in Search of Evidence.* (Santa Monica: Vector Enterprises Inc.).
30. Evans, A.S. (1978). Causation and disease: a chronological journal. *Am. J. Epidemiol.*, **108**, 249–58
31. Stehbens, W.E. (1985). The concept of cause in disease. *J. Chronic Dis.*, **38**, 947–50
32. Stehbens, W.E. (1990). Review of the validity of national coronary heart disease mortality rates. *Angiology*, **41**, 85–94
33. Stehbens, W.E. (1972). *Pathology of the Cerebral Blood Vessels.* (St. Louis: C.V. Mosby)
34. Stehbens, W.E. (1989). Diet and atherogenesis. *Nutr. Rev.*, **47**, 1–12
35. Stehbens, W.E. (1989). The controversial role of dietary cholesterol and hyper-cholesterolemia in the etiology of atherosclerosis. *Pathology*, **21**, 213–21
36. Hopkins, P.N. and Williams, R.R. (1986). Identification and relative weight of cardiovascular risk factors. *Cardiol. Clin.*, **4**, 3–31
37. Stehbens, W.E. (1990). The epidemiological relationship of hypercholesterolemia, hypertension, diabetes mellitus and obesity to coronary heart disease and atherogenesis. *J. Clin. Epidemiol.*, **43**, 733–41
38. Halsted, W.S. (1916). An experimental study of circumscribed dilation of an artery immediately distal to a partially occluding band, and its bearing on the dilation of the subclavian artery observed in certain cases of cervical rib. *J. Exp. Med.*, **24**, 271–86
39. Holman, E. (1954). On circumscribed dilatation of an artery immediately distal to a partially occluding band: Poststenotic dilatation. *Surgery*, **36**, 3–24
40. Stehbens, W.E. (1958). *Intracranial Arterial Aneurysms and Atherosclerosis.* (University of Sydney: Thesis)
41. Heath, D., Edwards, J.E. and Smith, L.A. (1958). The rheologic significance of medial necrosis and dissecting aneurysm of the ascending aorta in association with calcific aortic stenosis. *Proc. Mayo Clin.*, **33**, 228–34
42. Thoma, R. (1921). Über die Intima der Arterien. *Virchows Arch.*, **230**, 1–45
43. Dible, J.H. (1964). The ageing and collateral peripheral artery. *Lancet*, **1**, 520
44. Levene, C.I. (1956). The pathogenesis of atheroma of the coronary arteries. *J. Pathol. Bacteriol.*, **72**, 83–6
45. Stehbens, W.E. (1974). Haemodynamic production of lipid deposition, intimal tears, mural dissection and thrombosis in the blood vessel wall. *Proc. R. Soc. Lond.*, Series B, **185**, 357–73
46. Stehbens, W.E. (1974). The ultrastructure of the anastomosed vein of experimental arteriovenous fistulae in sheep. *Am. J. Pathol.*, **76**, 377–400

47. Davis, P.F. and Stehbens, W.E. (1985). The biochemical composition of haemo-dynamically stressed vascular tissue. I. The lipid, calcium and DNA concentration in experimental arteriovenous fistulae. *Atherosclerosis*, **56**, 27–37

48. Rogers, K.M., Fraser, J.K., Yong, R.Y.Y., McIntosh, C.J. and Stehbens, W.E. (1985). Elevated lysosomal enzymes in experimental aneurysms in sheep. *IRCS Med. Sci.*, **13**, 224

49. Rogers, K.M., Merrilees, M.J. and Stehbens, W.E. (1985). The effect of haemo-dynamic stress on the glycosaminoglycan content of blood vessel walls of experimental aneurysms and arteriovenous fistulae. *Atherosclerosis*, **58**, 139–48

50. Davis, P.F. and Stehbens, W.E. (1986). The biochemical composition of haemo-dynamically stressed vascular tissue. II. The concentration of protein and connective tissue components in the salt extracts of experimental arteriovenous fistulae. *Atherosclerosis*, **60**, 55–9

51. Stehbens, W.E. (1981). Chronic vascular changes in the walls of experimental berry aneurysms of the aortic bifurcation in rabbits. *Stroke*, **12**, 643–7

52. Stehbens, W.E. (1981). Chronic changes in experimental saccular and fusiform aneurysms in rabbits. *Arch. Pathol. Lab. Med.*, **105**, 603–7

53. Stehbens, W.E. (1985). The ultrastructure of experimental aneurysms in rabbits. *Pathology*, **17**, 87–95

54. Stehbens, W.E. and Fee, C.J. (1985). Hydrodynamic flow in U-shaped and coiled glass loops simulating arterial configurations. *Angiology*, **36**, 442–51

55. Stehbens, W.E., Fee, C.J. and Stehbens, G.R. (1987). Flow in glass models simulating arterial tortuosities under steady flow conditions. *Q. J. Exp. Physiol.*, **72**, 201–14

56. Imparato, A.M., Lord, J.W., Texon, M. *et al.* (1961). Experimental atherosclerosis produced by alteration of blood vessel configuration. *Surg. Forum*, **12**, 245–7

57. Texon, M., Imparato, A.M. and Lord, J.W. (1960). The hemodynamic concept of atherosclerosis. *Arch. Surg.*, **80**, 47–53

58. Stehbens, W.E. (1986). Experimental arterial loops and arterial atrophy. *Exp. Mol. Pathol.*, **44**, 177–89

59. Stehbens, W.E. (1973). Experimental arteriovenous fistulae in normal and cholesterol-fed rabbits. *Pathology*, **5**, 311–24

60. Stehbens, W.E. (1981). Predilection of experimental arterial aneurysms for dietary-induced lipid deposition. *Pathology*, **13**, 735–48

61. Hazama, F. and Hashimoto, N. (1987). An animal model of cerebral aneurysms. *Neuropathol. Appl. Neurobiol.*, **13**, 77–90

62. Greenhill, N.S. and Stehbens, W.E. (1983). Scanning electron-microscopic study of experimentally-induced intimal tears in rabbit arteries. *Atherosclerosis*, **49**, 119–26

63. Martin, B.J., Stehbens, W.E., Davis, P.F. and Ryan, P.A. (1989). Scanning electron microscopic study of haemodynamically-induced tears in the internal elastic lamina of rabbit arteries. *Pathology*, **21**, 207–12

64. Meyer, W.W., Walsh, S.Z. and Lind, J. (1980). Functional morphology of arteries during fetal and post-natal development. In Schwartz, C.J., Werthessen, N.J. and Wolf, S. (eds). *Structure and Function of the Circulation*, Vol. 1, pp. 95–379. (New York: Plenum Press)

Discussion

Dr Godsland: I think you have brought up a very important point, which is the structural aspects of atherosclerosis, which may have been pushed into the background somewhat by the emphasis given to the rather more accessible metabolic variables. There are two points. Firstly, you seem to be implying that atherosclerosis in familial hypercholesterolaemia differs from other kinds of CHD. Is that apparent in the structural characteristics of the lesions?

Dr Stehbens: Yes, it has a different distribution as well.

Dr Godsland: The other point was that you make a nice case for cholesterol deposition in the artery being secondary to mechanical fatigue damage. That makes sense for LDL and total cholesterol, but how can you accommodate that with the independent association seen with HDL?

Dr Stehbens: I think there, again, is another epidemiological error. Usually HDL has an inverse relationship to the LDL level. It has never been shown that a high level of HDL is protective against atherosclerosis. It has only been deduced by variation with the LDL level that HDL could possibly be protective. That is what Dr Yerushalmy referred to as the substitution game. After all, I have already explained why using CHD as your end-point is invalid.

Dr Grover: Do you think that lipids play absolutely no role in the genesis of the atherosclerotic lesion in CHD? Is there no role for them?

Dr Stehbens: I did not say that. It plays a role in the pathogenesis the same as calcium does, because it is there, so does muscle, and so forth, but it certainly is not causative.
  However, if you have a lipid abnormality, such as familial hypercholesterolaemia, there is the possibility that it may not only have an effect on storage or on a space-occupying lesion in the blood vessel wall, but it may interfere with the normal metabolism of the cell. By no means am I saying that lipids do not have a role to play, but their role certainly is not causative. My prime interest is in the cause of atherosclerosis and not the various reasons why coronary heart disease develops clinically.

Dr Grover: Is it not conceivable, though, that the genesis of atherosclerosis, given that it may be multifactorial, could be different in different individuals?

Dr Stehbens: No, I do not believe that and I do not like the term multicausal. There is no specific disease that I know of that has more than one cause.

116

Again, you are relying on the epidemiological misuse of cause. I think that this is the result of epidemiologists using cause as they see fit and their inclusion of contributory factors, conditional factors and aggravating factors, and even one has suggested that the vermiform appendix is one of the causes of acute appendicitis! This loose usage of terms reveals the essence of their approach and the majority of people do not understand the limitations of epidemiological methods.

8
Cellular and lipoprotein interactions in early atherogenesis

M. NAVAB, S.Y. HAMA and A.M. FOGELMAN

In the early stages of atherogenesis, retention of low density lipoprotein (LDL) in the subendothelial space is increased in the lesion prone areas[1,2]. Monocyte adhesion to endothelium increases followed by monocyte transmigration into the artery wall. LDL in the subendothelial space can be modified and exert several biological effects[3-6] or can accumulate in the differentiated monocyte-macrophage and lead to foam cell formation[7]. Medial smooth muscle cells (SMC) are then attracted to the intima where they proliferate, take up the modified LDL and produce additional foam cells. This may be followed by fatty streak formation, and by infiltration of lymphocytes and their interactions with other intimal cells[8]. With continued lipid accumulation and foam cell formation inflammatory mediators are further released leading to more complex cellular interactions and eventual formation of atheromatous plaque[8]. Functional and anatomical alterations in the endothelial lining of the affected sites can lead to the denudation of the vessel wall and exposure of the subendothelium resulting in the adhesion and aggregation of platelets and the activation of the coagulation cascade[8]. This can result in the production of fibrin which eventually may lead to arterial lesions due to formation of fibrin clot. In the following sections a brief review of some aspects of lipoprotein–cell and cell–cell interactions that may play a role in atherogenesis is presented.

Lipoprotein–cell interaction

Accumulating evidence suggests that oxidized lipoproteins may play a critical role in the development of atherosclerosis. These lipoproteins have been observed in atherosclerotic plaques in human[9,10] and in experimental animals[11-13]. Additionally, the development of lesions in cholesterol-fed or Watanabe rabbits can be diminished by treatment with antioxidants such as probucol or butylated hydroxytoluene[14,15]. In early stages of atherogenesis, however, the subendothelial space is basically acellular and LDL modification must occur in the presence of some plasma antioxidants and thus it is unlikely that highly oxidized LDL is produced.

Berliner and colleagues[3] have reported that LDL preparations obtained by storage or by mild iron oxidation were indistinguishable from native LDL to the LDL receptor and were not recognized by scavenger receptor. Treatment of endothelial cells (EC) with $0.1\ \mu g/ml$ of this minimally modified LDL (MM-LDL) caused a significant increase in the production of a chemotactic factor for monocytes (MCP-1) and increased monocyte binding. In contrast neutrophil binding was not increased after such exposure. Activity in the MM-LDL was found primarily in the polar lipid fraction. MM-LDL was toxic for EC from one rabbit but not toxic for the cells from another rabbit. The resistant cells became sensitive when incubated with lipoprotein in the presence of cyclohexamide, whereas the sensitive strain became resistant when preincubated with sublethal concentrations of MM-LDL[3]. Additionally, Rajavashisth *et al.*[4] demonstrated that treatment of human aortic endothelial cells (HAEC), with MM-LDL resulted in a rapid and large induction of the expression of granulocyte-macrophage colony-stimulating factor (GM-CSF), macrophage CSF (M-CSF) and granulocyte CSF (G-CSF). These growth factors are known to affect differentiation, survival, proliferation, migration and metabolism of macrophage/ granulocytes, and G-CSF and GM-CSF also affect the migration and proliferation of EC. The authors suggested that since macrophages are important in the development of atherosclerosis, the expression of the CSFs by the artery wall cells due to interaction with modified LDL may contribute to this disease[4]. Cushing and colleagues[5] have demonstrated that incubation of HAEC or HASMC with microgram levels of MM-LDL produced a dramatic increase in the induction of mRNA for MCP-1. This increase was time and dose dependent. The increase in mRNA levels for MCP-1 seen for HAEC appeared to remain high for at least 24 h whereas the increase in the mRNA observed in HASMC reached a maximum 8 h after the treatment with MM-LDL. Liao *et al.*[6] examined the biological activity of MM-LDL *in vivo*. After the injection of $50-100\ \mu g$ of MM-LDL into the mice, M-CSF activity in sera increased by up to 26-fold while injection of native LDL did not produce such an effect. Injection of MM-LDL into a mouse strain (C3H/HeJ) that is resistant to bacterial endotoxin gave similar results. This indicated that LPS and MM-LDL trigger cytokine production through distinct pathways. Additionally, MM-LDL induced, in various tissues, a dramatic increase in mRNA for JE, the mouse homologue of MCP-1. Native LDL or highly modified LDL did not produce these effects[6].

LDL has been demonstrated to undergo modification by EC[16,17], SMC[16,18], and monocyte-macrophages[19] in culture in the absence of serum. In previous studies the inclusion of even small amounts of serum in the incubation media prevented the modification of LDL[7]. Although the mechanism of modification of LDL in the vessel wall is not well understood, it must occur in the presence of plasma components with antioxidant properties such as α-tocopherol, ceruloplasmin, or transferrin. We have used a co-culture of HAEC, HASMC and studied the modification of native LDL in the presence of serum. We have observed that incubation of LDL with artery wall cells results in the oxidative modification of LDL with certain biological activities. Incubation of co-cultures of HAEC and HASMC with LDL in the presence of 5–10% human serum resulted in a 7.2-fold induction of mRNA for MCP-1, a 2.5-fold increase in the levels of MCP-1 protein in the co-culture super-natants, and a 7.1-fold increase in the transmigration of monocytes into the subendothelial space of the co-cultures. Monocyte migration was inhibited by 91% by antibody to MCP-1. Media collected from the co-cultures that had been incubated with LDL induced target EC to bind monocyte but not neutrophil-like cells. Media collected from co-cultures that had been incubated with LDL induced monocyte migration into the subendothelial space of other co-cultures that had not been exposed to LDL. In contrast, media from separate cultures of EC or SMC and incubated with the same LDL did not induce monocyte migration when incubated with the target co-cultures. High density lipoprotein (HDL), when presented to co-cultures together with LDL, reduced the increased monocyte transmigration by 91%. Virtually all of the HDL mediated inhibition was accounted for by the HDL_2 subfraction. HDL_3 was essentially without effect. Apolipoprotein AI was also ineffective in preventing monocyte transmigration while phosphatidylcholine liposomes were as effective as HDL_2 suggesting that lipid components of HDL_2 may have been responsible for its action. Preincubating LDL with β-carotene or with α-tocopherol did not reduce monocyte migration. However, pretreatment of LDL with probucol or pretreatment of the co-cultures with probucol, β-carotene or α-tocopherol prior to the addition of LDL prevented the LDL induced monocyte transmigration. Addition of HDL or probucol to LDL *after* the exposure to co-cultures did not prevent the modified LDL from inducing monocyte transmigration in fresh co-cultures. We, therefore, have concluded that co-cultures of human aortic cells can modify native LDL even in the presence of serum or plasma, resulting in the induction of MCP-1, and that HDL and antioxidants prevent the LDL induced monocyte transmigration.

Cell–cell interaction

Under normal conditions there are only a limited number of SMC and monocytes present in the subendothelial space[20]. However, in the course of development of an atherosclerotic lesion there is a marked migration of monocytes and SMC into the subendothelial space. The presence of EC, SMC, and monocytes in such a confined space might be predicted to favour cellular interactions. In tissue culture, the interaction of EC and SMC has been shown to lead to increased LDL receptor activity[21], increased lysosomal cholesteryl esterase activity[22] and reduced rates of SMC proliferation[23]. The co-culture of SMC and EC has also been shown to alter the amount and the composition of the extracellular matrix[24]. Recently two laboratories[25,26] have shown that bovine EC and pericytes or SMC, when cultured together, produced active transforming growth factor β in the culture medium. Both EC[27] and SMC[28] have been shown to express message for connexin 43, a member of the family of related gap junction proteins. The induction of connexin 43 as a result of the interaction of EC, SMC, and monocytes in co-culture has not been previously reported. We have demonstrated that the co-culture of adult HAEC with HASMC taken from the same donor resulted in increased levels of several biologically important molecules when the cells were cultured under conditions permitting direct cell–cell contact. Moreover, we have shown that the addition of human monocytes to the co-culture markedly enhanced the levels of these matrix components. We have also presented evidence indicating that cell–cell interaction results in increased induction of mRNA for connexin 43 and that interleukins 1 and 6 are involved in increased levels of matrix proteins. As stated above, in normal arteries very few SMC are found in the subendo-thelial space[20]. Higher numbers of SMC in association with EC have been observed in experimental atherosclerosis and in atherosclerotic human ar-teries[29]. Accumulating evidence indicates that substantial direct physical contact and interaction occurs between EC and SMC *in vitro*[21-26,30,31] and *in vivo*[32-35]. In our *in vitro* studies, the interaction between HAEC and HASMC produced a 2- to 4-fold increase in M-CSF and GM-CSF levels in the culture media. M-CSF can support the growth and survival of monocyte-macrophages *in vitro* even in the absence of serum growth factors[36]. From the study of autopsy specimens of human coronary arteries, Stary[29] speculated that many of the monocyte-macrophages in the subendothelial space would have died unless their survival had been supported by growth factors[29]. M-CSF produced by the interaction of EC and SMC could potentially act as one such factor. GM-CSF could be another one. GM-CSF has been shown to prolong the survival, differentiation, proliferation and development of responsive cells *in vitro*[36]. Lang *et al.*[37] demonstrated that the expression of GM-CSF gene in transgenic mice led to the accumulation of monocyte-macrophages in tissues such as eyes, striated muscle, and in peritoneal cells expressing this gene and resulted in substantial tissue damage[37].

The increased induction of the gap junction protein connexin 43 in co-cultures of EC and SMC indicates the possibility of increased junctional communication and interaction between the EC and SMC in these co-cul-tures[38]. In our studies, addition of human monocytes from nine different donors (but not from three others) to the co-cultures amplified the production of the extracellular matrix molecules. Addition of monocytes to co-cultures also produced a marked induction of connexin 43 raising the possibility of increased direct heterotypic cellular communications.

Upon activation, monocytes demonstrate markedly increased activities for numerous factors including for IL-1[39]. We have observed that during the process of monocyte transmigration into the subendothelial space of the co-cultures the cells acquire the typical appearance of spread monocytes suggesting the activation of these cells[40]. Leukocyte interleukins have also been reported to induce cultured EC to produce a highly organized pericellular matrix[41]. Injection of IL-1 into rats has been reported to produce elevated serum levels of fibronectin[42]. IL-1 induces IL-6 in certain cell types[43]. Hagiwara and co-workers[44] demonstrated that hepatocytes stimulated by IL-1 produced increased levels of IL-6 and that in turn resulted in elevated levels of fibronectin in cultured hepatocytes. Lanser and Brown[45] have shown that increased fibronectin production by rat hepatocytes exposed to conditioned medium from stimulated monocytes is due to IL-6. In our studies, the significant inhibition of monocyte-induced increase in fibronectin levels in co-cultures of artery wall cells by neutralizing antibodies to IL-1 and to IL-6 strongly suggests the involvement of these cytokines in the monocyte–artery wall cell interactions.

Both collagen type I and fibronectin have been implicated in atherogenesis[46]. Increases in collagen have been shown in several experimental models of atherosclerosis[47]. Additionally atherosclerotic lesions of human intima are known to have an increased collagen content[48] and collagen type I was reported to be the prominent form in the diseased vessels[49]. Increased levels of fibronectin were seen in rabbit aorta 4 weeks after cholesterol feeding[50]. Moreover, substantial levels of fibronectin have been observed in the extracellular matrix of fatty streaks and in some areas of fibrous plaque containing large numbers of subendothelial cells in human arteries[51].

The results of the studies reported here suggest that the migration of SMC and monocytes into the subendothelial space of the early atherosclerotic lesion may lead to cell–cell interactions that result in production of several biologically important molecules that may amplify lesion development. Consistent with this notion are the reported findings that high levels of M-CSF mRNA are present in the atherosclerotic lesions of both Watanabe Heritable Hyperlipidaemic and cholesterol-fed rabbits[4].

Based on the findings presented in this and in previous reports[3–8,11,52] we propose the following scheme for the sequence of events in the development of foam cells in the artery wall: LDL becomes trapped in microenvironments in the extracellular matrix of the subendothelial space secluded from plasma antioxidants. Reactive oxygen species and/or oxidized cellular lipids may be transferred to LDL and initiate the propagation of LDL lipid peroxidation. Since at the early stages of atherogenesis the subendothelial space is largely acellular and does not contain a significant number of monocyte-macrophages

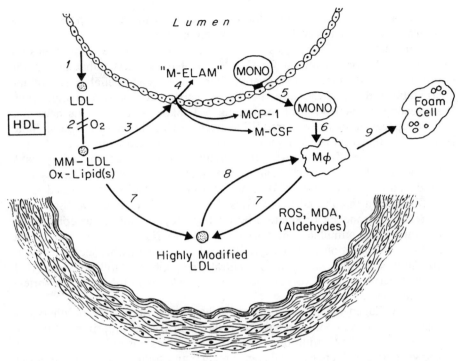

Figure 1 A proposed model for foam cell formation in the artery wall. Plasma LDL enters the largely acellular subendothelial space [1] where it is trapped in microenvironments secluded from plasma antioxidants [2]. LDL lipid is oxidatively modified giving rise to a mildly oxidized LDL, MM-LDL. Once formed MM-LDL stimulates the overlaying endothelium [3] to produce an adhesion molecule(s) for blood monocytes, 'M-ELAM' [4] and to secrete MCP-1 and M-CSF. These molecular events lead to the following cellular events: monocyte attachment to the EC; MCP-1 induced monocyte migration into the subendothelial space of the artery wall [5] and M-CSF induced differentiation into monocyte-macrophages [6]. Macrophage products such as reactive oxygen species (ROS), and malondialdehyde (MDA) can then further modify MM-LDL to a highly modified (oxidized) form [7] which is then recognized by the macrophage scavenger receptor [8] leading to cholesterol ester accumulation and foam cell formation [9]. If HDL is present in sufficient concentrations the formation of biologically active MM-LDL is prevented

releasing high levels of pro-oxidants, the resulting LDL is only minimally oxidized. This minimally modified LDL (MM-LDL) then can induce the overlaying endothelium to express an adhesion molecule(s) for monocytes[3], secrete MCP-1[3,5] and macrophage-colony stimulating factor[4]. These molecular events in turn induce monocyte binding, migration into subendothelial space, and monocyte differentiation into macrophages[36]. The macrophages could subsequently release reactive oxygen species[7], and aldehydes, further modifying the MM-LDL into a highly modified form which is then recognized and taken up by the macrophage scavenger and/or oxidized LDL receptor[53], resulting in foam cell formation[54]. Additionally we hypothesize that if HDL (presumably HDL_2) is present in sufficient concentrations the formation of biologically active MM-LDL is prevented and the inflammatory reaction may be blocked.

Acknowledgements

We thank Drs. Margarete Mehrabian and Richard Bork for providing us with the cDNA for MCP-1; Drs. George Popjak, Guy Chisolm, Judith Berliner and Sampath Parthasarathy for valuable discussions, Greg Hough and Cynthia Harper for their excellent technical assistance; and the members of the UCLA Heart Transplant Team for collecting the aortic specimens.

This work was supported in part by the US Public Health Services grants HL 30568, IT 32 HL 07412, and RR 865; by the Laubisch, Rachel Israel Berro; and M.K. Grey Funds.

References

1. Schwenke, D.C. and Carew, T.E. (1989). Initiation of atherosclerotic lesions in cholesterol-fed rabbits: I. Focal increases in arterial LDL concentration precede development of fatty streak lesions. *Arteriosclerosis*, **9**, 895–907
2. Schwenke, D.C. and Carew, T.E. (1989). Initiation of atherosclerotic lesions in cholesterol-fed rabbits: II. Selective retention of LDL vs. selective increase in LDL permeability in susceptible sites of arteries. *Arteriosclerosis*, **9**, 908–18
3. Berliner, J.A., Territo, M.C., Sevanian, A., Ramin, S., Kim, J.A., Bamshad, B., Esterson, M. and Fogelman, A.M. (1990). Minimally modified low density lipoprotein stimulates monocyte endothelial interactions. *J. Clin. Invest.*, **85**, 1260–6
4. Rajavashisth, T.B., Andalibi, A., Territo, M.C., Berliner, J.A., Navab, M., Fogelman, A.M. and Lusis, A.J. (1990). Modified low density lipoproteins induce endothelial cell expression of granulocyte and macrophage colony stimulating factors. *Nature*, **344**, 254–7
5. Cushing, S.D., Berliner, J.A., Valente, A.J., Territo, M.C., Navab, M., Parhamai, F., Gerrity, R., Schwartz, C.J. and Fogelman, A.M. (1990). Minimally modified low density lipoprotein induces monocyte chemotactic protein 1 in human endothelial cells and smooth muscle cells. *Proc. Natl Acad. Sci.*, **87**, 5134–8
6. Liao, F., Berliner, J.A., Mehrabian, M., Navab, M., Demer, L.L., Lusis, A.J. and Fogelman, A.M. (1991). Minimally modified low density lipoprotein is biologically active *in vivo* in mice. *J. Clin. Invest.*, **87**, 2253–7

7. Steinberg, D., Parthasarathy, S., Carew, T.E., Khoo, J.C. and Witztum, J.L. (1989). Beyond Cholesterol. Modifications of low-density lipoprotein that increase its atherogenicity. *N. Engl. J. Med.*, **320**, 915–24

8. Ross, R. (1986). The pathogenesis of atherosclerosis. An update. *N. Engl. J. Med.*, **314**, 488–500

9. Morton, R.E., West, G.A. and Hoff, H.F. (1986). A low density lipoprotein sized particle isolated from human atherosclerotic lesions is internalized by macrophages via a non-scavenger mechanism. *J. Lipid Res.*, **27**, 1124–34

10. Hoff, H.F. and Gaubatz, J.W. (1982). Isolation, purification and characterization of a lipoprotein containing Apo B from the human aorta. *Arteriosclerosis*, **42**, 273–97

11. Haberland, M.E., Fong, D. and Cheng, L. (1988). Malondialdehyde altered protein occurs in atheroma of WHHL rabbits. *Science (Wash.)*, **241**, 215–18

12. Palinski, W., Rosenfeld, M.E., Yla-Herttuala, S., Gurtner, G.C., Socher, S.S., Butler, S.W., Parthasarathy, S.,Carew, T.E., Steinberg, D. and Witztum, J.L. (1989). LDL undergoes oxidative modification *in vivo. Proc. Natl Acad. Sci.*, **86**, 1372–80

13. Chisolm, G.M. and Morel, D.W. (1988). Lipoprotein oxidation and cytotoxicity: effect of probucol on streptozotocin-treated rats. *Am. J. Cardiol.*, **62**, 20B–26B

14. Carew, T.E., Schwenke, D.C. and Steinberg, D. (1987). Antiatherogenic effect of probucol unrelated to the hypocholesterolemic effect: evidence that antioxidants *in vivo* can selectively inhibit LDL degradation in macrophage rich fatty streaks and slow progression of atherosclerosis in the WHHL rabbit. *Proc Natl Acad. Sci.*, **84**, 7725–9

15. Bjorkhem, I., Henriksson-Freyschuss, A., Breuer, O., Diczfalusy, U., Berglund, L. and Henriksson, P. (1991). The antioxidant butylated hydroxytoluene protects against atherosclerosis. *Arterioscl. Thromb.*, **11**, 15–22

16. Morel, D.W., DiCorleto, P.E. and Chisolm, G.M. (1984). Endothelial and smooth muscle cells alter low density lipoprotein *in vitro* by free radical oxidation. *Arteriosclerosis*, **4**, 357–64

17. Steinbrecher, U., Parthasarathy, S., Leake, D.S., Witztum, J.L. and Steinberg, D. (1984). Modification of low density lipoprotein by endothelial cells involves lipid peroxidation and degradation of low density lipoprotein phospholipids. *Proc. Natl Acad. Sci.*, **83**, 3883–7

18. Heinecke, J.W., Rosen, H. and Chait, A. (1984). Iron and copper promote modification of LDL by human arterial smooth muscle cells. *J. Clin. Invest.*, **74**, 1890–4

19. Cathcart, M.K., Morel, D.W. and Chisolm, G.M. (1985). Monocytes and neutrophils oxidize low density lipoprotein making it cytotoxic. *J. Leukocyte Biol.*, **38**, 341–50

20. Rhodin, J.A.G. (1980). Architecture of the vessel wall. In Bohr, D.F., Somlyo, A.P. and Sparks, Jr., H.V. (eds), *Handbook of Physiology, The Cardiovascular System II*, Ch. 1, pp. 1–31. (Bethesda, Md: American Physiological Society)

21. Davies, P.F., Truskey, G.A., Warren, H.B., O'Connor, S.E. and Eisenhare, B.H. (1985). Metabolic cooperation between vascular endothelial cells and smooth muscle cells in co-culture: Changes in low density lipoprotein metabolism. *J. Cell Biol.*, **101**, 871–9

22. Hajjar, D.P., Marcus, A.J. and Hajjar, K.A. (1987). Interactions of arterial cells. Studies on the mechanisms of endothelial cell modulation of cholesterol metabolism in co-cultured smooth muscle cells. *J. Biol. Chem.*, **262**, 6976–81

23. Hajjar, D.P., Falcone, D.J., Amberson, J.B. and Heffon, J.M. (1985). Interaction of arterial cells. I. Endothelial cells alter cholesterol metabolism in co-cultured smooth muscle cells. *J. Lipid Res.*, **26**, 1212–23

24. Merrilees, M. J. and Scott, L. (1981). Interaction of aortic endothelial and smooth muscle cells in culture. Effect on glycosaminoglycan levels. *Atherosclerosis*, **39**, 147–61

25. Antonelli-Orlidge, A., Sunders, K.B., Smith, S.R. and D'Amore, P.A. (1989). An activated form of transforming growth factor beta is produced by cocultures of endothelial cells and pericytes. *Proc. Natl Acad. Sci.*, **86**, 4544–8

26. Sato, Y. and Rifkin, D.B. (1989). Inhibition of endothelial cell movement by pericytes and smooth muscle cells: Activation of a latent transforming growth factor beta 1-like molecule by plasmin during coculture. *J. Cell Biol.*, **109**, 309–15

27. Larson, M., Haudenschild, C.C. and Beyer, E.C. (1990). Gap junction messenger RNA expression by vascular wall cells. *Circ. Res.*, **66**, 1074–80

28. Lash, J.A., Critser, E.S. and Pressler, M.L. (1990). Cloning of a gap junctional protein from vascular smooth muscle and expression in two cell mouse embryos. *J. Biol. Chem.*, **265**, 13113–17

29. Stary, H. (1989). Evolution and progression of atherosclerotic lesions in coronary arteries of children and young adults. *Arteriosclerosis*, **9** (Suppl. I), 19–32

30. Jones, P. (1979). Construction of an artificial blood vessel wall from cultured endothelial and smooth muscle cells. *Proc. Natl Acad. Sci.*, **76**, 1882–6

31. Davies, P.F., Olesen, S.P., Clapham, D.E., Morrel, C.M. and Shoen, D.J. (1988). Endothelial communication. State of the art lecture. *Hypertension*, **11**, 583–582

32. Thoma, R. (1921). Uber Die Intima der Arterien. *Virchows Arch. Path. Anat. Physiol.*, **230**, 1–45

33. Bruns, R.R. and Palade, G.E. (1968). Studies on blood capillaries. I. General organization of blood capillaries in muscle. *J. Cell Biol.*, **37**, 244–76

34. Huttner, I., Boutet, M. and More, R.H. (1973). Gap junctions in arterial endothelium. *J. Cell Biol.*, **57**, 247–52

35. Spagnoli, L.G., Villaschi, S., Neri, L. and Palmieri, G. (1982). Gap junctions in myo-endothelial bridges of rabbit carotid arteries. *Experientia*, **38**, 124–5

36. Metcalf, D. (1989). The molecular control of cell division, differentiation commitment and maturation in haemopoietic cells. *Nature*, **339**, 27–30

37. Lang, R.A., Metcalf, D., Cuthbertson, R.A., Lyons, I., Stanley, E., Kelso, A., Kannourakis, C., Williamson, D.J., Klinthworth, C.K. and Konda, T.J. (1987). Transgenic mice expressing a hematopoietic growth factor gene (GM-CSF) develop accumulation of macrophages, blindness, and a fatal syndrome of tissue damage. *Cell*, **51**, 875–86

38. Eghbali, B., Kessler, J.A. and Spray, D.C. (1990). Expression of gap junction channels in communication-incompetent cells after stable transfection with cDNA encoding connexin 32. *Proc. Natl Acad. Sci.*, **87**, 1328–31

39. Dayer, J. M., de Rochemonteix, B., Burrus, B., Demczuk, S. and Dinarello, C.A. (1986). Human recombinant interleukin 1 stimulates collagenase and prostaglandin E2 production by human synovial cells. *J. Clin. Invest.*, **77**, 645–8

40. Adams, D.O. and Hamilton, T.A. (1984). The cell biology of macrophage activation. *Ann. Rev. Immunol.*, **2**, 283–98

41. Montesano, R., Mossaz, A., Ryser, J.-E., Orci, L. and Vassalli, P. (1984). Leukocyte interleukins induce cultured endothelial cells to produce a highly organized glycosaminoglycan rich pericellular matrix. *J. Cell Biol.*, **99**, 1706–15

42. Hagiwara, T., Kono,I., Nemoto, K., Kashiwagi, H. and Onozaki, K. (1989). Recombinant interleukin-1 triggers the increase of circulating fibronectin levels in rats. *Int. Arch. Allergy Appl. Immunol.*, **89**, 376–80

43. Elias, J.A. and Lentz, V. (1990). IL-1 and tumor necrosis factor synergistically stimulate fibroblast IL-6 production and stabilize IL-6 messenger RNA. *J. Immunol.*, **145**, 161–6

44. Hagiwara, T., Suzuki, H., Kono, I., Kashiwagi, H., Akiyama, Y. and Onozaki, K. (1990). Regulation of fibronectin synthesis by interleukin-1 and interleukin-6 in rat hepatocytes. *Am. J. Pathol.*, **136**, 39–47

45. Lanser, M. E. and Brown, G.E. (1989). Stimulation of rat hepatocyte fibronectin production by monocyte condition medium is due to interleukin 6. *J. Exp. Med.*, **170**, 1781–6

46. Mecham, R.P., Whitehouse, L.A., Wrenn, D.S., Parks, W.C., Griffin, G.C., Senior, R.M., Crouch, E.C., Sternmark, K.R. and Voelkel, N.F. (1987). Smooth-muscle mediated connective tissue remodeling in pulmonary hypertension. *Science. (Wash.)*, **237**, 423–6

47. Mayne, R. (1986). Collagenous proteins of blood vessels. *Arteriosclerosis*, **6**, 585–93

48. Levene, C.I. and Poole, J.C.F. (1962). The collagen content of the normal and atherosclerotic human aortic intima. *Br. J. Exp. Pathol.*, **43**, 469–71

49. Smith, E.B. (1965). The influence of age and atherosclerosis on the chemistry of aortic intima. *J. Atheroscl. Res.*, **5**, 241–8

50. Uematsu, M., Tanouchi, J., Ishihara, K., Fujii, K., Toshida, Y., Doi, Y. and Kamada, T. (1989). Hypercholesterolemia without mechanical interventions induces early accumulation of fibronectin during fatty streak formation. *Arteriosclerosis*, **9**, 769a (Abstr.)

51. Shekhonin, B.V., Domogatsky, S.P., Idelson, G.L., Koteliansky, V.E. and Rukosuev, V.S. (1987). Relative distribution of fibronectin and type I, III, IV, V collagens in normal and atherosclerotic intima of human arteries. *Atherosclerosis*, **67**, 9–16

52. Navab, M., Liao, F., Hough, G.P., Rossi, L.A., Van Lenten, B.J., Rajavashisth, T.B., Lusis, A.J., Laks, H., Drinkwater, D.C. and Fogelman, A.M. (1991). Interaction of monocytes with coculture of human aortic wall cells involves interleukins 1 and 6 with marked increases in connexin 43 message. *J. Clin. Invest.*, **87**, 1763–72

53. Sparrow, C. P., Parthasarathy, S. and Steinberg, D. (1989). A macrophage receptor that recognizes oxidized low density lipoprotein but not acetylated low density lipoprotein. *J. Biol. Chem.*, **264**, 2599–604

54. Brown, M.S. and Goldstein, J.L. (1990). Scavenging for receptors. *Nature*, **343**, 508–9

Discussion

Dr Vega: I wonder, have you characterized the Apo-B protein in the minimally modified LDL, and is it degraded?

Dr Navab: It may be modified but it is not degraded. That is an interesting question. In highly modified LDL, the modified LDL that was reported during the 1980s, depending on the type of modification, you could have a high degree of modification on the Apo-B or fragmentation which was observed in SDS-PAGE. But, in our preparations so far we have not been able to show any changes in the Apo-B. We are very anxious to see what the principal lipid components are in this lipoprotein which makes it active both *in vitro* and *in vivo*.

Dr Vega: Would you know, or have you looked for, release of TNF from macrophages during incubation of this minimally modified LDL with the macrophages?

Dr Navab: A paper has been submitted by Dr Ana Jewett for publication which shows that incubation of human peripheral blood monocytes, with small doses of minimally modified LDL, e.g., 5–10 μg, induces TNF-α and IL-1β to the degree that γ-interferon does and the effect of a combination of minimally modified LDL and γ-interferon is synergistic.

Dr Hayes: Your model would imply that the plasma tocopherol status of the host, particularly in the LDL, would be very important to the circumstances. Have you measured, or better yet, attempted to modify the tocopherol concentration in your model?

Dr Navab: We are very interested in this question. Although we found that LDL, incubated with α-tocopherol, did not become resistant to modification, Dr Esterbauer has reported that it is possible to get increased incorporation. If you incubate the LDL with α-tocopherol, in the presence of high levels of plasma or serum, you do get increased incorporation.

Several studies on the effect antioxidants on LDL modification are in progress both in animals and in humans in Finland and in Austria. But the issue is complicated because there is a large variation among different individuals. We have seen this in our experiments too. We have used 40 or 50 different preparations of LDL in the past 2 years and there is a large difference in their resistance (or sensitivity) to modification. This is partly due to the antioxidant content of LDL. There is a large variability in the α-tocopherol content of LDL particles. Some of the LDL particles do not contain β-carotene, also the licopene levels are different. The other point is the fatty acid content of LDL.

As Dr Parthasarathy has shown, when you feed rabbits with Trison, the safflower oil which has more oleic acid, you make the LDL highly resistant to oxidation. So, the composition of fatty acids in the LDL molecule also affects its degree of resistance to modification.

The issue of antioxidant intake by the public is going to be another controversial one which we will be hearing about soon. We must be cautious about recommending anything before the issue is well studied. Just because a compound is not harmful, it does not mean that one has to recommend it. We must wait for the results of studies investigating in more detail the role of antioxidants in the LDL modification and atherosclerosis.

Dr Walker: From a clinical standpoint, do you recommend that your patients use mega doses of Vitamin C or E?

Dr Navab: No, we need more information on this subject. It has been reported that a daily intake of 200 IU of Vitamin E will have the same effect as would four times as much vitamin E on the serum levels, the LDL content of α-tocopherol or its resistance to oxidation. You would have to go to very high levels to see further increase in resistance of LDL to oxidation and that may not have physiological implications or relevance. No, nobody knows what the recommendations should be at this stage. We need more studies.

Dr Skamene: You have shown a variety of macrophage-related phenomena which all make sense in piecing together this hypothesis. Do you know which of these are cause and effect phenomena, which of them are unrelated to the cause, which of them are epiphenomena? In other words, did you do any correlation of this *in vitro* analysis with the states of resistance or susceptibility, for example the activity of macrophage growth factors, which you showed to be elevated?

Dr Navab: That is an important question. No, these were the results of recent experiments we have been involved with and we do not intend to extrapolate to the *in vivo* situations. As I mentioned, at this time this is a hypothesis, trying to dissect out some of the early events in atherogenesis, and obviously the studies you mentioned have to be done.

9
Animal models for studying the pathogenesis of atherosclerosis

J.L. STEWART-PHILLIPS, J. LOUGH and E. SKAMENE

Introduction

Atherosclerosis is a progressive disease characterized by both cellular prolifer-ation and necrosis and the accumulation of lipid and connective tissue elements to form fibro-fatty plaques in the intima of large elastic and medium-sized muscular arteries. Initial atherosclerotic lesions, or fatty streaks, appear in the aorta in the first year of life[1]. Gradually other vessels of the arterial tree are affected by such lesions which may vary in their composition, but always contain intra- and extracellular lipid. By 10 years of age, fatty streaks are seen to include clusters of lipid-containing macrophages and smooth muscle cells, known as foam cells. Within another 5 years, foci of necrosis become apparent and by 30 years of age fibrous plaques have developed. These progressively increase in size and extent and may undergo calcification, thrombosis, ulceration or haemorrhage. The composition of such atheromatous plaques is comparable to those observed in humans and those which either appear spontaneously or are induced by diet in many species of animals.

Current theories regarding the pathogenesis of atherosclerosis focus on two main elements – smooth muscle cell proliferation in response to endothelial injury and the excessive accumulation of arterial lipids due to abnormal lipoprotein metabolism and/or infiltration. In reality there is probably no single common event which initiates the atherogenic process. According to Schwartz et al.[2] atherogenesis involves 'complex cascades of interactions among environmental factors, components of blood, including platelets, monocytes and lipoproteins, the cells of the arterial wall, namely endothelial and smooth muscle cells, patterns of blood flow and arterial connective tissue elements. It is likely that the expression of these interacting cascades is at least in part under significant genetic control'. This last concept has been the subject of intense investigation in recent years. The most common consequence of atherosclerosis is coronary heart disease (CHD) and of the major risk factors for CHD which clearly have genetic components, hyperlipidaemia is the

131

strongest, most consistent and most closely associated with the progression of atherosclerosis in humans and experimental animals[3].

A considerable number of genes control the levels of circulating lipids including genes for apolipoproteins, lipoprotein receptors, lipid transfer proteins and enzymes involved in lipid synthesis, absorption and metabolism and bile metabolism[4]. Undoubtedly, variation among these genes contributes to the hereditary component of atherosclerosis. For example, patients with familial hypercholesterolaemia, a disease shown by Goldstein and Brown[5] to have a single gene transmission, lack, or who are deficient in functional low density lipoprotein (LDL) receptors in their tissues, have very high plasma LDL concentrations and develop precocious atherosclerosis. However, this is a relatively rare disorder and it is generally accepted that the more common type of progressive atherosclerosis described at the beginning of this paper would be polygenic with the genes responsible acting at a number of steps in the atherogenic process.

Because of the multifactorial, polygenic basis of atherosclerosis and its long natural progress in man, most genetic studies have been conducted in animal models. This paper, which is by no means intended to be a comprehensive review of the subject, will briefly examine some common animal models for studying the genetic basis of the disease and then describe in detail the use of inbred and recombinant inbred (RI) mouse strains for investigating the genetic determinants of susceptibility and resistance to diet-induced atherosclerosis.

Animal models used in genetic studies of atherosclerosis

Animal models have been used to study atherosclerosis since cholesterol-fed rabbits were first observed to develop aortic lesions over 80 years ago (see Ref. 6 for short review). The use of such models has made an immeasurable contribution to our understanding of the pathogenesis of atherosclerosis. However, the choice of experimental animal is usually based on accessibility, familiarity, affordability, availability of metabolic data and ease of handling, rather than on the relevance or suitability of the animal to the pathogenic mechanism being investigated[6]. Therefore, it is essential to recognize the limitations of each model when extrapolating experimental findings to the human situation. This is particularly true of genetic experiments. Different strains of animals of the same species often show different susceptibilities to atherosclerosis which correlate with variations in serum lipids and lipoproteins. This may facilitate the identification of the phenotypic traits which are linked to susceptibility/resistance to the development of the disease but it gives no information on the genetic mechanisms, such as organization and regulation of the genes, involved. For this, elaborate breeding experiments are necessary which have their own set of criteria for suitability of an animal model.

Various species of birds, which are relatively hypercholesterolaemic and prone to develop atherosclerotic lesions, have been used as models to study the pathogenesis of atherosclerosis. They include chickens, turkeys, ducks and geese, none of which are extensively used today, particularly in genetic experiments. Pigeons, which exhibit strain differences in the development of atherosclerotic lesions, however, provide a popular model for studying the aetiology of atherosclerosis, including the identification of phenotypes associated with resistance and susceptibility to the disease. Quail, which can be bred to give atherosclerosis-susceptible and resistant strains, may also prove useful as a model for studying the genetic basis of atherosclerosis.

Almost every mammalian species appears to have been used in atherosclerosis experiments at some time. However, the three which have most relevance for genetics studies and which will be described in this paper are non-human primates, the rabbit and the mouse.

1. Pigeons

In 1959, Clarkson et al.[7] reported that aortic atherosclerosis occurs spontaneously in White Carneau pigeons. A difference in susceptibility to atherosclerosis between White Carneau and Show Racer pigeons was then reported by Prichard[8] who suggested that a polygenic mode of inheritance is involved. The heritability of cholesterol levels was subsequently studied in different strains of pigeons by Patton et al.[9] who concluded that this was also polygenic. Using high and low serum cholesterol-differentiated lines of White Carneau and Racing Homer pigeons, Patton et al.[10] then studied diet-induced atherosclerosis, concluding that differences between the strains were indicative of genetic variation and that independent mechanisms may control susceptibility to aortic and coronary disease.

When comparing the effects of diet on atherogenesis in White Carneau and randomly bred pigeons, Wagner[11] observed a significantly higher incidence of atheromata in the former but similar cholesterol, triglyceride, glucose, uric acid, calcium and phosphorus levels, blood pressures and adrenal and thyroid weights. He concluded that genetic factors affecting susceptibility to atherosclerosis in these pigeons must function at the arterial wall level. Further investigation by Rowe and Wagner[12] suggested that a difference in post-translational processing of arterial wall proteoglycans may reflect distinct functional properties mediating resistance or susceptibility to atherosclerosis. Compared with randomly bred pigeons, White Carneau pigeons have structurally distinct proteoglycan monomers which may have increased binding affinity for LDL. This in turn may accelerate atheroma formation. These findings indicate that pigeons may have a particular role as a model for studying the genetic determinants of susceptibility/resistance to atherosclerosis which act at the level of the arterial wall.

2. Quail

Japanese quail have been genetically selected for high susceptibility or resistance to diet-induced atherosclerosis[13]. Susceptibility may possibly involve Marek's disease herpes virus[14]. Viral DNA has been found in the aortas of susceptible quail and it increases with the severity of the aortic lesion. Indeed, the integrated viral gene(s) are co-selected with atherosclerosis susceptibility. Interestingly, Herpes simplex virions[15] and genomic mRNA[16] and cytomegalovirus antigens[17] have been found in human arterial cells from atherosclerosis patients. This observation coupled with the fact that atherosclerotic lesions in quail resemble those observed in humans indicate that these birds may provide a very useful model for studying the aetiology of atherosclerosis as well as for investigating the genetic determinants of susceptibility and resistance to the disease.

3. Non-human primates

As with other types of study, the animals of choice for investigating the genetic basis of atherosclerosis would be non-human primates. Physiologically, they are closest to man and they may be bred to give hypo- and hyperresponders to an atherogenic diet. However, they are also expensive, less easy to handle than other species, not available in the large numbers required for genetic experiments and difficult to breed, having long gestation and maturation times. The induction of atherosclerotic lesions is also a relatively lengthy process compared with rabbits or mice. However, non-human primates have been invaluable in identifying some of the basic, genetically-determined defects in lipoprotein metabolism which promote atherogenesis and in studying lesion promotion and the components of atherosclerotic plaques.

Clarkson *et al.*[18,19] used squirrel monkeys to investigate the possible link between variation in circulating cholesterol levels and aortic and coronary atherosclerosis. They concluded that hyperresponders (i.e. those animals developing severe hypercholesterolaemia) were more prone to develop atherosclerosis, xanthelasma and xanthomatosis. The results of breeding experiments suggested that there is a high degree of genetic control of plasma cholesterol levels, possibly by a single dominant gene. Although the data on genetic control related only to cholesterol level and not to atherogenesis, a strong correlation between the two was suggested. More recent studies of these non-human primates fed cholesterol showed that 65% of the variability in serum total cholesterol concentration was due to genetic factors[20]. Hyporesponders demonstrated a greater and faster increase in the faecal excretion of bile salts. Hoover and Hayes[21] postulated that the difference between atherosclerosis-susceptible squirrel monkeys and resistant celus monkeys lies in a difference in their response to endothelial injury. However, the results of their experiments indicate that the acute response to intimal injury does not mediate vulnerability to atherosclerosis in monkeys.

Selective breeding of baboons also yields hypo- and hyperresponders to a cholesterol and saturated fat-enriched diet. Differences in the rate of cholesterol biosynthesis, plasma high density lipoprotein (HDL) concentrations and their effect on cholesterol movement in and out of the body pool have all been observed[20]. Genetic analyses have been performed using progeny of these 'positive assortative matings'. The examination of lipoprotein profiles revealed several phenotypes that clustered in families. A major gene appears to affect HDL cholesterol levels when animals consume either a chow or a high fat and cholesterol diet[22].

The different responses of hyper- and hyporesponder rhesus monkeys to dietary cholesterol appears to be due to differences in intestinal absorption of cholesterol while hyperresponder macaques appear to demonstrate 'mesenchymal susceptibility', i.e. at the level of the artery wall, independent of serum cholesterol levels[20].

One of the disadvantages of using any species, including non-human primates, in genetic studies is the necessity of feeding them diets containing high concentrations of saturated fat and/or cholesterol in order to induce atherosclerotic lesion formation within a reasonable time. The question has arisen of whether lesions produced under such circumstances are truly representative of human atheroma. However, Pigtail monkeys have recently been used to investigate atherogenesis during low level hypercholesterolaemia and studies of both fatty streak formation[23] and conversion of the fatty streak to a fibrous plaque[24] indicate that the cellular events which take place during these processes are practically identical to those which occur during very high levels of hypercholesterolaemia in non-human primates and in other species. This suggests that employing higher levels of hypercholesterolaemia for shorter periods of time is quite valid for studying the pathogenesis of atherosclerosis in animal models.

4. Rabbits

Although the rabbit is the classic animal model for atherosclerosis research, it too has major limitations in genetic experiments. Breeding, housing and handling are all less easy compared with the mouse. More importantly, it is much less well-defined genetically as strains are not so highly inbred and RI strains are not available. Even so, the rabbit has contributed valuable information on putative determinants of susceptibility and resistance to atherosclerosis.

New Zealand White (NZW) and Dutch Belt strains of rabbit differ significantly in their susceptibility to atherosclerosis[25], the development of which is related to dietary cholesterol and consequent plasma levels of cholesterol. Shore and Shore[26] observed different alterations in plasma lipoproteins of the two strains in response to a cholesterol-enriched diet. Susceptible NZW rabbits exhibit higher levels of very low density lipoprotein (VLDL), intermediate density lipoprotein (IDL) and LDL and lower levels of HDL, particularly HDL_3, than resistant Dutch Belt rabbits. On both cholesterol-rich and normal diets, Dutch Belt rabbits exhibit higher HDL_3/HDL_2 ratios than do NZW rabbits. It was suggested that, by directing synthesis of lipoproteins, genetic factors influence cellular flux and metabolism of cholesterol in rabbits.

Other rabbit strains also exhibit different responsiveness to dietary cholesterol. For example, concentrations as low as 0.08% cholesterol in the diet will discriminate between the two inbred strains – AX/JU (hyperresponders) and 111VO/JU (hyporesponders)[27]. This is in contrast to rats and mice where much higher amounts of cholesterol have to be used. Furthermore, hypo- and hyperresponsiveness to dietary cholesterol and to the type of fatty acids in the diet coincides in these rabbit strains as it does in man. Differences in cholesterol metabolism between the hypo- and hyperresponsive rabbits also parallel the human situation. Therefore these strains could be used to study those aspects of cholesterol metabolism which are experimentally inaccessible in man as well as to investigate the genetic basis of hypo- and hyperresponsiveness.

Hereditary hyperlipidaemic New Zealand White rabbits[28] which were bred from a male observed to be severely hypercholesterolaemic when fed normal chow have been proposed as models for studying the pathogenesis of atherosclerosis. They are apparently distinct from Watanabe heritable hyperlipidaemic (WHHL) rabbits in that the underlying mechanism of hypercholesterolaemia appears to be over-production of VLDL and LDL, comparable to familial combined hyperlipidaemia in humans. Arterial lesions in these rabbits are characterized by lipid accumulation.

The genetic basis of the susceptibility to atherosclerosis of the homozygous WHHL rabbit is a lack of functional LDL receptors[29-31]. This animal therefore serves as a model for the study of human familial hypercholesterolaemia. The cholesterol-fed heterozygous WHHL rabbit has also been proposed as a model for studying the pathogenesis of atherosclerosis[32]. Atherosclerotic lesions observed after 24 weeks of cholesterol treatment are characterized by necrosis, cholesterol clefts, fibrous caps and calcification and resemble those found in humans. In contrast, aortic lesions seen in NZW rabbits after 24 weeks of cholesterol feeding are more fibrous, contain foam cells and do not resemble human plaques.

5. Mice

Thompson[33] reported in 1969 that mice of an inbred strain – C57BL/6J – make a good model in which to study the production of dietary atheroma. Not only are they small, cheap and easy to handle but they survive well on an atherogenic diet and develop lesions relatively quickly, at approximately the same time and in the same easily identifiable region of the aortic valve. A number of other inbred mouse strains were surveyed and found to have variable susceptibility to diet-induced atherosclerosis[34]. Experiments with crossbred and backcrossed mice of the most and least susceptible strains (C57Br/cdJ and CBA/J, respectively) indicated a polygenic system of inheritance of susceptibility or resistance to atherosclerosis[35]. A significant positive relationship between high fat, high cholesterol feeding, serum total cholesterol levels and size and extent of arterial lesions was also revealed. It was concluded that this relationship depends on a multifactorial type of inheritance, more complicated than a simple additive dominance model, and with no special maternal or paternal influence.

The findings of Roberts and Thompson prompted the use of C57BR/cdJ and CBA/J mice in a number of studies of the pathogenesis of atherosclerosis. A correlation between the resistance of CBA/J mice to the development of diet-induced atherosclerosis and their capacity to prevent large increases in serum cholesterol, to suppress abnormal α- and pre-β-migrating lipoproteins and to maintain elevated serum apo E/total apoprotein ratios was observed[36]. Conversely, mice of the susceptible C57Br/cdJ strain were found to have significantly higher free cholesterol, esterified cholesterol and total lipid values and a markedly lower mean phosphatidylcholine/free cholesterol ratio than mice of the resistant strain[37]. The results of Breckenridge *et al.*[38] suggest that the development of atherosclerosis in C57BR/cdJ mice on an atherogenic diet results from a greatly increased accumulation of cholesterol rich VLDL and IDL and a depletion of HDL, all of which are characterized by decreased phosphatidylcholine/free cholesterol ratios.

The mouse is the classical mammal for genetic studies. Each inbred strain represents a unique gene pool in which naturally occurring polymorphisms have become fixed. This has resulted in it having by far the most extensive gene-linkage map of any mammal. As mentioned previously, a number of highly inbred strains are either susceptible or resistant to diet-induced atherosclerosis, making them ideal models for studying the genetics of the disease. Indeed, Lusis *et al.*[39,40] employed 40 inbred strains to investigate the genetic factors controlling the structure of HDL in mice. They discovered structural variations of the two major apolipoproteins of mouse HDL, apo A-1 and apo A-11 and concluded that these are inherited as single Mendelian genes exhibiting co-dominant expression[40].

In order to locate these genes, Apoal and Apoa2, their strain distribution patterns (SDPs) were compared with previously typed genetic markers segregating among recombinant inbred (RI) strains derived from atherosclerosis susceptible C57BL/6J (B) and atherosclerosis resistant BALB/cBy (C) or C3H/HeJ (H) mice[40]. RI strains are produced by crossing two inbred strains, selecting pairs at random from the F_2 generation and propagating them by brother–sister mating for at least 20 generations. This establishes a set of new inbred strains, each of which is a mixture of the two progenitor strain genomes where the alleles from either one have become fixed in a homozygous form at each locus. The strains can be phenotyped to obtain a strain distribution pattern (SDP) which is characteristic of any given locus. As linked loci have similar SDPs, comparing the SDP of a trait under investigation with established SDPs can be used to map the gene expressing that particular trait to its chromosome. The replicable genotype of RI strains also permits the linkage analysis of genes determining traits measured as incidence. In this way Apoa2 was located on mouse chromosome 1 and results suggested a location for Apoal on chromosome 9 [40].

Lusis *et al.* then investigated the inheritance of the variation in structure of HDL in two sets of RI strains as described above and concluded that the variation is probably controlled by a single major gene, Hdl-l, that is either tightly linked to or identical with the Apoa2 gene on chromosome 1 [40]. This finding was further investigated using the congenic strain, B6.C-*H-25ᶜ*, which carries the minor histocompatibility allele *H-25ᶜ* transferred from BALB/cBy onto the genetic background of C57BL/6By by 14 successive backcrosses. Apoa2 maps very near the *H-25ᶜ* locus. Both Apoa2 and Hdl-l were found to be transferred along with *H-25ᶜ* in these congenic mice, confirming the tight linkage of Apoa2 and Hdl-l on chromosome 1.

Using both B×H RI strains and RI mice derived from the SJL/Bm and SWL/Bm strains, Lusis *et al.*[41] have mapped a gene for apo E (Apoe) to chromosome 7. A further five RI sets, including C×B and B×H, have been used to map a gene for apo B (Apob) to chromosome 12.

The work of Lusis *et al.* was the first demonstration of the advantages of using RI mice to investigate the genetic basis of variations in lipoproteins which may determine atherosclerosis resistance and susceptibility. Paigen *et al.*[42] consequently used female RI mice derived from B and H or B and C progenitors to identify a gene, Ath-1, which appears to determine both susceptibility to atherosclerosis induced by feeding a diet enriched with cocoa butter and cholesterol and serum HDL levels. This gene was mapped to a location in close proximity to Apoa2 on chromosome 1. Phenotypic characterization of Ath-1 indicates that it is responsible for a rapid decrease in both

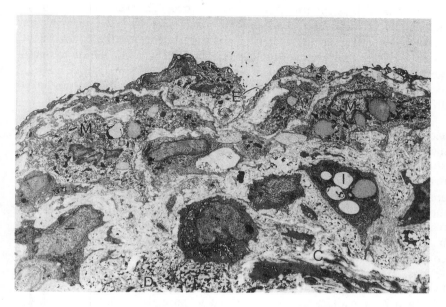

Figure 1 Electron micrograph showing an early atheromatous plaque in the ascending aorta of a C57BL/6J mouse fed an atherogenic diet for 20 weeks. The endothelium (E) appears to be attenuated but intact. Both lipid-filled macrophages (M) and myointimal (I) cells are present surmounting areas of connective tissue deposition (C) and residual cell debris (D). Magnification ×3780

HDL lipid and HDL apolipoprotein levels in susceptible B mice fed an atherogenic diet. This is primarily mediated at the level of HDL catabolism[43]. Using various RI mouse strains, Jiao et al.[44] showed that HDL-cholesterol concentrations are significantly correlated with HDL particle size and are strongly linked to Apoa2. A similar relationship between LDL-cholesterol, LDL particle size and Apob, the gene which codes for apo B, the major apoprotein carried by LDL could not be established, although the results of the genetic analysis do suggest that a major gene is responsible for determining LDL particle size.

Paigen et al.[45] have used female RI mice derived from susceptible strain B and resistant strain A/J (A), to identify a second gene, Ath-2, which determines atherosclerosis susceptibility and HDL levels in response to a diet rich in cocoa butter and cholesterol. However, they have been unable to map Ath-2 to its chromosome or to identify its gene product.

We are also using mice derived from A and B strains to study the genetic determinants of susceptibility and resistance to diet-induced atherosclerosis.

The diet used is a modification of the Hartroft–Thomas diet, employing coconut oil in place of cocoa butter[46], mixed with 10–50% normal chow powder, depending on the design of the experiment. Unlike cocoa butter, coconut oil has a hypercholesterolaemic effect which is in addition to that of the free cholesterol included in the diet. Both male and female mice are used because in our experience there is no consistent, significant sex-linked difference in response to this diet.

B mice show fatty streak-like lesions in the valve sinus region of the ascending aorta within 5 weeks of starting the atherogenic diet. By 10 weeks the lesions are clearly discernible and can be scored according to size and the number of foam cells they contain. By 20 weeks, foam cell penetration into the media, cellular necrosis and bulging of the lesion into the aortic lumen are observed (Figure 1). These lesions progress until at 35 weeks after starting the atherogenic diet they can be described as truly resembling the fibro-fatty plaques of human atherosclerosis[47]. At this time early fatty streak-like lesions may be observed in the aortas of some A mice. Control mice fed rodent chow containing 4% unsaturated fat and 0.022% cholesterol do not develop such lesions. However, 18 month-old B mice which have been maintained on breeder mouse chow, which contains 12% (mostly saturated) fat and approximately 0.25% cholesterol, are observed to have developed aortic lesions similar to those induced by 10 weeks of atherogenic diet feeding.

Analysis of the inheritance of resistance and susceptibility to diet-induced atherosclerosis in mice derived from the A and B strains[48] indicates that:

1. These mice carry a major gene with alleles for susceptibility (S) and resistance (R). All $F_1(A \times B)$ hybrids develop lesions, which are as severe as those observed in B mice, indicating that the S allele is dominant.

2. $F_1(A \times B)$ hybrid mice backcrossed to A segregate into three groups – totally resistant, moderately susceptible and fully susceptible with a ratio of 2:1:1, which would indicate that a second gene is modifying the degree of susceptibility to diet-induced atherosclerosis in these mice.

3. Other minor genes probably modify the expression of the susceptibility alleles in mice which develop diet-induced atherosclerosis as suggested by the observation that some of the offspring of $(A \times B)$ mice backcrossed to B develop more severe atherosclerosis than mice of the parent B strain. Furthermore, although $A \times B / B \times A$ RI mice segregate into totally resistant and susceptible on the basis of aortic lesion score, there is a continuum of lesion scores among the susceptible strains which is consistent with this trait being determined by a number of different genes. Indeed, as mentioned previously, atherosclerosis is a polygenic disease so any trait under investigation such as atheroma formation

would be expected to show a quantitative variation amongst RI strains of mice. In particular, the observation that mice of several RI strains have higher lesion scores than B mice suggests that A mice may carry gene(s) for susceptibility which are not phenotypically expressed in that parent strain but whose effects can be unmasked by genetic recombination with the major susceptibility gene derived from the B progenitor. Such a gene could be Ath-1 or Ath-2.

A linkage analysis of susceptibility and resistance to diet-induced atherosclerosis with known allelic markers in A×B/B×A RI mice has been undertaken by comparing the SDP of susceptibility and resistance with the SDPs of 155 allotypic markers identified so far in the genome of these strains (Table 1). This gives a tentative location for the major gene, which we have designated Ath-3, close to the coat colour gene c on chromosome 7.

By analysing the phenotypic expression of flanking genes of Ath-3 in backcross mice, we hope to establish a more precise location for that gene. A physical map of the region surrounding the gene can then be constructed by saturating the relevant chromosomal segment with RFLP markers. A locus less than 1 centimorgan from a marker gene will give an entry point for future cloning of the new gene. Alternatively, identification of the gene product will enable specific cDNA probes to be constructed and used both to confirm the location of the gene in the mouse genome and to locate its human homologue.

Although there is quite a strong correlation between serum HDL-cholesterol levels and resistance/susceptibility to diet-induced atherosclerosis in mice derived from the A and B strains, concordance between the SDPs of the two traits is not complete. However, our evidence indicates that Ath-3 does code for some aspect of HDL structure or function but that the influence of other genes modifies its expression in A×B mice.

One of the reasons for our choice of A and B mice as a model to study the genetics of diet-induced atherosclerosis is that they offer us a set of RI mouse strains derived from progenitors which exhibit inherited variations in their spectrum of macrophage functions as well as genetic differences in susceptibility to atherosclerosis. It has been established by several investigators that this cell is central to the atherogenic process. B and A mice exhibit marked variations in a number of different macrophage functions which result in the expression of either the susceptible or resistant phenotype in a variety of diseased states[49,50]. In general, macrophage inflammatory responses are poor in mice of the A strain which is partly due to the presence of the Hc⁰ allele on chromosome 2, leading to a lack of C5a complement component[51]. Both the chemotactic responses of A macrophages and their adherence to substratum are depressed when compared with those of B[52]. Furthermore, the macrophages of A mice produce less IL-1[53] in response to microbial lipopolysaccharide and their ability to be activated into microbicidal and tumouricidal

Table 1 Strain distribution of atherosclerosis susceptibility and resistance and linked loci in A×B/B×A RI mice

Locus	1	2	4	5	6	7	8	9	10	13	14	15	17	18	19	21	22	24	25
									A×B										
Gpi-1	b	a	b	a	a	a	b	a	b	b	a	a	a	b	b	a	b	b	b
		x				x								x		x			
Tam-1	b	b	b	a	a	b	b	a	b	b	a	a	a	a	b	a	a	b	b
		x				x						x	x	x		x			
Ath-3	b	a	b	b	a	b	b	a	b	a	a	b	b	b	b	b	a	b	b
c		b	a	b	b	a	b	b	a	b	a	a	b	b	b	b	b	a	b	b
					x															
Hbb	b	a	b	a	a	b	b	a	b	a	a	b	b	b	b	b	a	b	b

Locus	2	4	8	9	10	11	13	14	16	19	22
					B×A						
Gpi-1	a	b	b	a	a	a	a	b	b	b	b
		x						x			x
Tam-1	a	a	b	a	o	a	a	a	b	b	a
					x				x	x	
Ath-3	a	a	b	a	a	b	a	a	a	a	a
c	a	a	b	a	a	b	a	a	a	a	a
		x				x			x		
Hbb	b	a	b	a	a	a	a	a	b	a	a

A×B = strain derived from A/J mother and C57BL/6J father; B×A = strain derived from C57BL/6J mother and A/J father; a = allele inherited from A parent; b = allele inherited from B parent; o = strain not typed; x = crossover.

cells is impaired[54]. There appears to be a genetically determined deficiency in signal transduction of the plasma membrane of macrophages in A mice[55] which may account for their various deficiencies.

It is not unreasonable to suggest that part of the strain difference in susceptibility to atherosclerosis observed between A and B mice is also due to differences in macrophage activity. For example, the recruitment of macrophages to lesion sites and their adhesion to vascular endothelium, two areas where atherosclerosis-resistant A mice are deficient, are recognized steps in the atherogenic process. Therefore, a number of macrophage functions in both normal and atherogenic diet-fed A and B mice[56] are being analysed for concordance with the distribution pattern of atheroma formation (Table 2).

Table 2 The effects of dietary* and exogenous[†] lipids on various traits of macrophage activity which show genetically-determined differences in A/J and C57BL/6J mice

Trait	A/J	C57BL/6J	Effect of lipid
Inflammatory response	Deficient	Efficient	Decrease*
Chemotaxis	Deficient	Efficient	Decrease*[†]
Phagocytosis	Deficient	Efficient	No effect[†B]
Respiratory burst	Efficient	Efficient	Decrease[†B]
			No effect[†A]
Cytotoxic activity	Deficient	Efficient	Decrease*
IFN-γ production	Low	High	Increase*[B]
Adhesion to endothelium	Deficient	Efficient	Increase*[B]

[A]The effect of lipid in A mice only; [B]the effect of lipid in B mice only.

This approach will identify any linkage between macrophage dysfunction and the development of atherosclerosis, i.e. it will determine which traits have cause-and-effect relationships as opposed to association by chance gene assortment.

As genetic linkages are invariably conserved in evolution, the mapping of a gene for susceptibility or resistance to atherosclerosis in the mouse will facilitate the search for its correlate in humans. The loci for a number of genes involved in lipid metabolism have already been shown to be homologous in mice and humans as judged by the conservation of flanking markers[4]. For example, the human homologue of Apoe, APOE, is located on the long arm of chromosome 19, closely linked to APOC1 and APOC2 which code for apo C-1 and the lipoprotein lipase activator apo C-11, respectively. Proximal to APOE is the LDL receptor gene, LDLR. The murine homologue of LDLR, however, has been mapped to chromosome 9. Also on chromosome 9 are Apoal and Apoa4, the human homologues of which, Apo A-1 and Apo A-lV map to chromosome 11.

Conclusions

No animal model can hope to perfectly emulate the pathogenesis of human atherosclerosis. However, different species can contribute different insights into the mechanisms underlying the development of the disease as long as they are carefully selected for their suitability to the type of study proposed. Thus, the mouse would appear to be the best model for studying the genetic determinants of resistance and susceptibility to diet-induced atherosclerosis. Susceptibility is associated with low serum HDL-cholesterol levels and high

LDL/VLDL levels as it is in humans and the atherosclerotic lesions induced have many of the characteristics of human atheroma. Furthermore, in genetic terms, the mouse is the best-defined of all mammals and affords a wide spectrum of the inbred, RI and congenic strains needed for comprehensive genetic studies.

References

1. McGill, H.C. (1984). Persistent problems in the pathogenesis of atherosclerosis. *Arteriosclerosis*, **4**, 443–51
2. Schwartz, C.J., Valente, A.J., Sprague, E.A., Kelley, J.L, Suenram, C.A., Graves, D.T., Rozek, M.M., Edwards, E.H. and Delgado, R. (1986). Monocyte-macrophage participation in atherogenesis: Inflammatory components of atherogenesis. *Semin. Thromb. Hemostas.*, **12**, 79–86
3. Wilson, M.A. (1986). An approach to the hyperlipoproteinemias. *Cardiology*, 52–60
4. Lusis, A.J. (1988). Genetic factors affecting blood lipoproteins: the candidate gene approach. *J. Lipid Res.*, **29**, 397–429
5. Goldstein, J.L. and Brown, M.S. (1979). The LDL receptor locus and the genetics of familial hypercholesterolemia. *Annu. Rev. Genet.*, **13**, 259–89
6. Armstrong, M.L. and Heistad, D.D. (1990). Animal models of atherosclerosis. *Atherosclerosis*, **85**, 15–23
7. Clarkson, T.B., Prichard, R.W., Netsky, M.G. and Loflund, H.B. (1959). Atherosclerosis in pigeons: its spontaneous occurrence and resemblance to human atherosclerosis. *Arch. Pathol.*, **68**, 143–7
8. Prichard, R.W., Clarkson, T., Loflund, H.B. and Goodman, H.O. (1964). Pigeon atherosclerosis. *Am. Heart J.*, **67**, 715–7
9. Patton, N.M., Brown, R.V. and Middleton, C.C. (1974). Familial cholesterolemia in pigeons. *Atherosclerosis*, **19**, 307–14
10. Patton, N.M., Brown, R.V. and Middleton, C.C. (1974). Atherosclerosis in familial lines of pigeons fed exogenous cholesterol. *Atherosclerosis*, **21**, 147–54
11. Wagner, W.D. (1978). Risk factors in pigeons genetically selected for increased atherosclerosis susceptibility. *Atherosclerosis*, **31**, 453–63
12. Rowe, H.A. and Wagner, W.D. (1985). Arterial dermatan sulfate proteoglycan structure in pigeons susceptible to atherosclerosis. *Arteriosclerosis*, **5**, 101–9
13. Shih, J.C.H., Pullman, E.P. and Kao, K.J. (1983). Genetic selection, general characterization and histology of atherosclerosis-susceptible and resistant Japanese quail. *Atherosclerosis*, **49**, 41–53
14. Pyrzak, R. and Shih, J.C.H. (1987). Detection of specific DNA segments of Marek's disease herpes virus in Japanese quail susceptible to atherosclerosis. *Atherosclerosis*, **68**, 77–85
15. Gyorkey, F., Melnick, J.L., Guinn, G.A., Gyorkey, P. and DaBakey, M.E. (1984). Herpesviridae in the endothelial and smooth muscle cells of the proximal aorta in atherosclerotic patients. *Exp. Mol. Pathol.*, **40**, 328–39

16. Benditt, E.P., Barrett, T. and McDougall, K.J. (1983). Viruses in the etiology of atherosclerosis. *Proc. Natl. Acad. Sci. USA*, **80**, 6386–9

17. Melnick, J.L., Dreesman, G.R., McCollum, C.H., Petrie, B.L., Burek, J. and DeBakey, M.E. (1983). Cytomegalovirus antigen within human arterial smooth muscle cells. *Lancet*, **2**, 644–7

18. Clarkson, T.B., Loflund, H.B., Bullock, B.C. and Goodman, H.O. (1971). Genetic control of plasma cholesterol levels: studies on squirrel monkeys. *Arch. Pathol.*, **92**, 37–45

19. Loflund, H.B., Clarkson, T.B., St. Clair, W. and Lehner, N.D.M. (1972). Studies on the regulation of plasma cholesterol levels in squirrel monkeys of two genotypes. *J. Lipid Res.*, **13**, 39–47

20. Clarkson, T.B., Jayo, J.M. and Anthony, M.S. (1989). Individual differences in the susceptibility of nonhuman primates to diet-induced atherosclerosis. In Crepaldi, G., Gotto, A.M., Manzato, E. and Baggio, G. (eds). *Atherosclerosis VIII*, pp. 145–8. (Amsterdam: Elsevier)

21. Hoover, G.A. and Hayes, K.C. (1984). Aortic intimal response to endothelial removal in cebus and squirrel monkeys. *Arteriosclerosis*, **4**, 165–75

22. McGill, H.C. and Kushwaha, R. Development and utilization of genetic dislipoproteinemias in baboons. In Crepaldi, G., Gotto, A.M., Manzato, E. and Baggio, G. (eds). *Atherosclerosis VIII*, pp. 149–52. (Amsterdam: Elsevier)

23. Masuda, J. and Ross, R. (1990). Atherogenesis during low level hypercholesterolemia in the non-human primate. I. Fatty streak formation. *Arteriosclerosis*, **10**, 164–77

24. Masuda, J. and Ross, R. (1990). Atherogenesis during low level hypercholesterolemia in the non-human primate. II. Fatty streak conversion to fibrous plaque. *Arteriosclerosis*, **10**, 178–87

25. Adams, W.C., Gaman, E.M. and Feigenbaum, A.S. (1972). Breed differences in the responses of rabbits to atherogenic diets. *Atherosclerosis*, **16**, 405–11

26. Shore, B. and Shore, V. (1976). Rabbits as a model for the study of hyperlipoproteinemia and atherosclerosis. In Day, C.E. (ed.) *Atherosclerosis Drug Discovery*, pp. 123–41. (New York: Plenum)

27. Katan, M.B., Meijer, G.W. and Beynen, A.C. (1989). Inbred rabbit strains as models for human hypo- and hyperresponders to dietary cholesterol. In Crepaldi, G., Gotto, A.M., Manzato, E. and Baggio, G. (eds). *Atherosclerosis VIII*, pp. 119–23. (Amsterdam: Elsevier)

28. La Ville, A., Turner, P.R., Pittilo, M., Martini, S., Marenah, C.B., Rowles, P.M., Morris, G., Thomson, G.A., Woolf, N. and Lewis, B. (1987). Hereditary hyperlipidemia in the rabbit due to overproduction of lipoproteins. 1. Biochemical studies. *Arteriosclerosis*, **7**, 105–12

29. Kita, T., Brown, M.S., Watanabe, Y. and Goldstein, J.L. (1981). Deficiency of low density lipoprotein receptors in liver and adrenal gland of the WHHL rabbit. An animal model of familial hypercholesterolemia. *Proc. Natl. Acad. Sci. USA*, **78**, 2268–72

30. Bilheimer, D.W., Watanabe, Y. and Kita, T. (1982). Impaired receptor-mediated catabolism of low density lipoprotein in the WHHL rabbit. An animal model of familial hypercholesterolemia. *Proc. Natl. Acad. Sci. USA*, **79**, 3305–9

31. Buja, L.M., Kita, T., Goldstein, J.L., Watanabe, Y. and Brown, M.S. (1983). Cellular pathology of progressive atherosclerosis in the WHHL rabbit. An animal model of familial hypercholesterolemia. *Arteriosclerosis*, **3**, 87–101

32. Atkinson, J.B., Hoover, R.L., Berry, K.K. and Swift, L.L. (1989). Cholesterol-fed heterozygous Watanabe heritable hyperlipidemic rabbits: a new model for atherosclerosis. *Atherosclerosis*, **78**, 123–36

33. Thompson, J.S. (1969). Atheromata in an inbred strain of mice. *J. Atheroscler. Res.*, **10**, 113–22

34. Roberts, A. and Thompson, J.S. (1976). Inbred mice and their hybrids as an animal model for atherosclerosis research. In Day, C.E. (ed.) *Atherosclerosis Drug Discovery*, pp. 313–17 (New York: Plenum)

35. Roberts, A. and Thompson, J.S. (1977). Genetic factors in the development of atheroma and on serum total cholesterol levels in inbred mice and their hybrids. *Prog. Biochem. Pharmacol.*, **13**, 298–305

36. Morrisett, J.D., Kim, H.-S., Patsch, J.R., Datta, S.K. and Trentin, J.J. (1982). Genetic susceptibility and resistance to diet-induced atherosclerosis and hyperlipoproteinemia. *Arteriosclerosis*, **2**, 312–24

37. Kuksis, A., Roberts, A., Thompson, J.S., Myher, J.J. and Geher, K. (1983). Plasma phosphatidylcholine/free cholesterol ratio as an indicator for atherosclerosis. *Arteriosclerosis*, **3**, 389–97

38. Breckenridge, W.C., Roberts, A. and Kuksis, A. (1985). Lipoprotein levels in genetically selected mice with increased susceptibility to atherosclerosis. *Arteriosclerosis*, **5**, 256–64

39. LeBoeuf, R.C., Puppione, D.L., Schumaker, V.N. and Lusis, A.J. (1983). Genetic control of lipid transport in mice. I. Structural properties and polymorphisms of plasma lipoproteins. *J. Biol. Chem.*, **258**, 5063–70

40. Lusis, A.J., Taylor, B.A., Wangenstein, R.W. and LeBoeuf, R.C. (1983). Genetic control of lipid transport in mice. II. Genes controlling structure of high density lipoproteins. *J. Biol. Chem.*, **258**, 5071–8

41. Lusis, A.J., Taylor, B.A., Quon, D., Zollman, S. and LeBoeuf, R.C. (1987). Genetic factors controlling structure and expression of apolipoproteins B and E in mice. *J. Biol. Chem.*, **262**, 7594–604

42. Paigen, B., Mitchell, D., Reue, K., Morrow, A., Lusis, A.J. and LeBoeuf, R.C. (1987). Ath-1, a gene determining atherosclerosis susceptibility and high density lipoprotein levels in mice. *Proc. Natl. Acad. Sci. USA*, **84**, 3763–7

43. LeBoeuf, R.C., Doolittle, M.H., Montcalm, A. and Martin, D.C. (1990). Phenotypic characterization of the Ath-1 gene controlling high density lipoprotein levels and susceptibility to atherosclerosis. *J. Lipid Res.*, **31**, 91–101

44. Jiao, S., Cole, T.G., Kitchens, R.T., Pfleger, B. and Schonfeld, G. (1990). Genetic heterogeneity of plasma lipoproteins in the mouse: control of low density lipoprotein particle sizes by genetic factors. *J. Lipid Res.*, **31**, 467–77

45. Paigen, B., Nesbitt, M.N., Mitchell, D., Albee, D. and LeBoeuf, R.C. (1989). Ath-2, a second gene determining atherosclerosis susceptibility and high density lipoprotein levels in mice. *Genetics*, **122**, 163–8

46. Stewart-Phillips, J.L., Lough, J. and Skamene, E. (1988). Genetically determined susceptibility and resistance to diet-induced atherosclerosis in inbred strains of mice. *J. Lab. Clin. Med.*, **112**, 36–42

47. Stewart-Phillips, J.L. and Lough, J. (1991). Characteristics of the atherosclerotic lesions induced by a high fat diet in C57BL/6J mice. *Atherosclerosis* (In press)

48. Stewart-Phillips, J.L., Lough, J. and Skamene, E. (1989). Ath-3, a new gene for atherosclerosis in the mouse. *Clin. Invest. Med.*, **12**, 121–6

49. Stevenson, M.M., Kongshaven, P.A.L. and Skamene, E. (1981). Genetic linkage of resistance to Listeria monocytogenes with macrophage inflammatory responses. *J. Immunol.*, **127**, 402–7

50. Skamene, E. and Stevenson, M.M. (1985). Genetic control of macrophage response to infection. In Furth, R. Van (ed.) *Mononuclear Phagocytes – Characteristics, Physiology and Function*, pp. 647–53. (Dordrecht: Martinus Nijhoff)

51. Gervais, F., Stevenson, M.M. and Skamene, E. (1984). Genetic control of resistance to Listeria monocytogenes: Regulation of leukocyte inflammatory responses by the Hc locus. *J. Immunol.*, **132**, 2078–83

52. Thomson, D.M.P., Stevenson, M.M. and Skamene, E. (1985). Correlation between chemoattractant-induced leukocyte adherence inhibition, macrophage chemotaxis and macrophage inflammatory responses in vivo. *Cell. Immunol.*, **94**, 547–57

53. Brandwein, S.R., Skamene, E., Aubut, J.A., Gervais, F. and Nesbitt, M.N. (1987). Genetic regulation of lipopolysaccharide-induced interleukin-1 production by murine peritoneal macrophages. *J. Immunol.*, **138**, 4263–9

54. Skamene, E., James, S.L., Meltzer, M.S. and Nesbitt, M.N. (1984). Genetic control of macrophage activation for killing of extracellular targets. *J. Leuk. Biol.*, **35**, 65–9

55. Hamilton, T.A., Somers, S.A., Becton, D.L., Celada, A., Schreiber, R.D. and Adams, D.O. (1986). Analysis of deficiencies in IFN-mediated priming for tumor cytotoxicity in peritoneal macrophages from A/J mice. *J. Immunol.*, **137**, 3367–71

56. Stewart-Phillips, J.L. and Phillips, N.C. (1991). The effect of a high fat diet on murine macrophage activity. *Int. J. Immunopharm.*, **13**, 325

Discussion

Dr Hayes: I am interested in the cluster of proteins apparently on chromosome 7. Do you have any indication that it is, in fact, several genes that are being expressed or could it be one cytokine that accounts for the entire set of reactions?

Dr Skamene: No, there are quite clearly recombinations between the several genes in that area. That portion of mouse chromosome 7 is synthetic to human chromosome 11. There are several genes there which cause variation in the different facets of macrophage function. These have been, for whatever reason, conserved in evolution in close linkage.

Dr Dietschy: Did you give us the other lipid levels, that is, the animals which do not develop atherosclerosis? Do they have the same LDL and VLDL cholesterol levels as animals who do not develop the disease?

Dr Skamene: The animals which are fully resistant are those which have low cholesterol and low LDL and high HDL. What I was talking about were the animals which fall into the susceptible category.

Dr Dietschy: The animals that do not develop atherosclerosis have lower levels, so why would you jump immediately to the vessel wall and not conclude that the gene is actually regulating lipid levels? I am not entirely clear because there are many genes that alter lipid levels.

Dr Skamene: I guess I was not clear. The single gene, which divides the mice into fully resistant and into the range of susceptible, controls the lipid level as a single factor. We found differences in the degree of susceptibility to be polygenic, but one gene, designated Ath-3, apparently determines serum HDL levels and may exert a major effect. We have tentatively mapped this gene to mouse chromosome 7.

Dr Dietschy: So, given a similar level of lipids, there is a set of genes that controls the severity of the atherosclerotic lesion?

Dr Skameme: Yes.

Dr Dietschy: But there must be many more than one gene regulating lipid levels. We know of dozens already that control different steps of lipid levels. Is this unique to this mouse model?

Dr Skamene: What this model shows are the genes which were fixed in different allelic distribution in the two parental strains. It is quite likely that a number of other genes have been fixed in an identical allelic fashion in the two progenitors and, therefore, we do not see their effect. What we see is the manner in which the two strains differ. We do not see the genes which are important in controlling other traits in which those two kinds of strains are identical.

Dr Katan: I would like to comment on two points. Firstly, the diet that you give is rather extreme, 5% cholesterol by weight in a human diet would be equivalent to 100 eggs a day or one egg every 5 minutes, 7 days a week. In addition, you give large amounts of cholic acid which is a strong detergent. Dr Beynen in our laboratory has experimented with similar diets, diets containing a lot less cholesterol and a lot less cholic acid than with your rats. He observed severe liver damage on these diets – hepatomegaly, major elevation of transaminases, and enormous accumulation of cholesterol in the liver. So, I would be somewhat worried whether you are not measuring some kind of resistance to toxicity, or for instance, cholic acid rather than a gene normally involved in lipid metabolism.

Secondly, your findings seem to be related to those of René Leboeuf who has also studied these genes in mice and actually named her sites Ath1 and Ath2. Could you comment on the relation between her findings and yours and, are they on the same chromosome?

Dr Skamene: To answer your first question, yes, it is an extreme diet and it is basically used to produce the lesion quickly. As I said, we can show the same differences if we keep the two mouse strains on a normal diet for 3 years. We have not seen pathologically any changes which would suggest liver damage. The fact that we see lesions in the aorta which resemble plaques and that we measure morphological lesions, not death, should alleviate any concerns that we are looking at some toxic phenomenon.

René Leboeuf used other inbred mouse strains on a very similar diet. The two genes which you refer to both control lipoprotein metabolism and they are not linked to the gene referred to here.

Dr Goldbloom: Do the genetically susceptible mice die prematurely?

Dr Skamene: This is a difficult question to answer. In fact, we have stumbled on this observation in our experiments dealing with the genetic determination of longevity. The A/J mice, which are the resistant mice, have a life span of 2 years, which is an equivalent of 66 human years. The B6 mice, which are the susceptible mice, live 3 years and we find the lesion only toward the end of their life span. So, in fact, you might say that if you could devise a way to prolong the life of the resistant mouse, somehow we could perhaps see the lesions as well. But, the experimental set up is such that it precludes us from answering that.

Dr Clandinin: Is the A/J mouse the one that develops the rapidly developing changes in auto-immunity and the lymphomas in later life?

Dr Skamene: No. The A/J mouse develops many other things, but not lymphomas, but it is very resistant to mouse AIDS.

10
Obesity and associated apolipoprotein abnormalities: relation to coronary heart disease

D.A.K. RONCARI

Obesity, defined by a body weight greater than 120% of reference or a body mass index greater than $27\,kg/m^2$, is associated with a high degree of cardiovascular morbidity and mortality, including of course coronary heart disease[1]. Indeed, obesity is generally associated with one or more of the following risk factors: hypertension, non-insulin dependent diabetes, and dyslipoproteinaemias (dysapolipoproteinaemias), and is the subject of this paper. The obese state itself is an independent atherogenic risk factor[1-3].

Obesity both triggers the development of a variety of lipoprotein-apolipoprotein abnormalities and aggravates them[1,4-6]. Individuals with specific genetic susceptibility to dyslipoproteinaemia are generally most affected by the development of obesity, manifesting the more pronounced abnormalities.

Hepatic production of very low density lipoproteins (VLDL) is augmented in obesity, particularly when the body weight is increasing or when the corpulence is maintained[1]. The accelerated flux of free fatty acids from adipose tissue is considered to be an important factor in VLDL overproduction[1]. Apolipoprotein B (apo B-100) is an indispensable constituent of the developing VLDL particles, which eventually are converted, via intermediate density lipoproteins (IDL), to low density lipoproteins (LDL)[7,8]. Sniderman and associates have postulated, and have adduced supportive evidence, for a critical role of specific cholesterol esters in controlling the production of apo B in hepatocytes[9]. According to this proposed mechanism, the apo B-cholesterol ester complex would then move from the rough endoplasmic reticulum to the smooth endoplasmic reticulum where they incorporate newly formed triglycerides and other constituents[9]. Depending on the rate of production of apo B, as well as the quantity of available triglycerides, the ratio of apo B to cholesterol esters varies, accounting in great part for the heterogeneity of VLDL particles[9,10]. The denser particles, i.e. those with higher apo B/cholesterol ester ratios, are more atherogenic. Another significant influence on the production of VLDL is the insulin level, accounting for the accentuation of VLDL-triglyceride secretion in obesity[1].

VLDL are converted to the more highly atherogenic IDL and LDL, through progressive hydrolytic stripping of their triglycerides by hepatic triglyceride lipase and lipoprotein lipase[7,8]. Thus, the lipoproteins become increasingly enriched in cholesterol esters.

Intermediate density lipoproteins containing apolipoprotein isoforms E-2 and E-4 are associated with dyslipidaemias[4,8,11]. These isoforms impart genetic propensity to dyslipidaemia, which is further unmasked and aggravated by obesity, especially abdominal obesity. The E-4 isoform has the highest affinity for both the hepatic LDL receptor (apo B-100/apo E receptor) and the hepatic apolipoprotein E receptor (recent findings suggest that this is the low density lipoprotein receptor-related protein, which is identical to the receptor for α_2-macroglobulin)[8,12]. The increased affinity of isoform E-4 for both receptors leads to more efficient hepatic uptake of both dietary and endogenous cholesterol, resulting in suppression of apo B-100/apo E receptor activity, and thus increased plasma LDL-cholesterol levels. Apolipoprotein E-4 apparently also augments intestinal cholesterol absorption[12]. In subjects with the E-4 isoform, a positive correlation exists between total abdominal fat accumulation, as well as intra-abdominal fat deposition (as determined by computed tomography) and LDL-apo B levels[11]. Those with the E-4 isoform, moreover, reveal a more general positive correlation with VLDL, LDL, and apo B. On the other hand, subjects with the apo E-2 isoform have a particular association with VLDL, as well as a negative correlation with high density lipoprotein (HDL)-cholesterol[4,11].

Upon conversion of IDL to LDL, apo B-100 becomes the exclusive apolipoprotein and these highly atherogenic particles are particularly enriched in cholesterol ester[7,8]. In obesity, there is augmented flux of the atherogenic VLDL, IDL and LDL [1]. Thus, even in the absence of elevated plasma levels, their excessive turnover imposes a substantial risk for coronary heart disease. Specific fatty acids have differing influences on plasma LDL-cholesterol levels. Myristic (14:0) and palmitic acid (16:0) raise their levels, as does probably lauric acid (12:0), stearic acid (18:0) is neutral, while oleic acid (18:1) and linoleic acid (18:2) decrease plasma LDL-cholesterol[12–14]. In addition, n-3 fatty acids, i.e. eicosapentaenoic (20:5) and docosahexaenoic (22:6) acids, decrease both LDL-cholesterol and VLDL-triglyceride levels, particularly in subjects with elevated VLDL-triglycerides[15]. *Trans*-mono-unsaturated acids (mainly elaidic acid – *trans* 18:1) which are formed by hydrogenating vegetable oils to provide a solid texture to margarines and shortenings, also raise plasma LDL-cholesterol (while decreasing HDL-cholesterol)[13]. While much more research is required, it appears that obesity may accentuate the effect of the cholesterol-raising fatty acids.

152

While some of the best characterized conditions associated with elevated LDL-cholesterol levels are based on defects of clearance of these particles, much more common is the situation of augmented production of LDL, and more specifically, LDL-apo B[8]. As mentioned, there is only one molecule of apo B in each LDL particle, while the content of cholesterol and its esters varies appreciably. Sniderman and associates described the syndrome of hyperapobetalipoproteinaemia, which represents the extreme situation with highest apo B/cholesterol ester ratios[10,16]. This is a highly atherogenic state, despite the frequently normal plasma cholesterol and triglyceride concentration. To make the diagnosis, it is essential to measure apo B levels, which reflect the important feature, namely, the number of LDL particles[10]. Parenthetically, while the beneficial effects of n-3 fatty acids have already been mentioned for some circumstances, these actually augment the production of apo B in hyperapobetalipoproteinaemia[17]. Denser VLDL and LDL particles, as found in hyperapobetalipoproteinaemia, occur frequently in the setting of familial combined hyperlipidaemia, which has variable expression in different family members[8]. The obese state probably has an aggravating effect in both this form of hyperlipidaemia and in pure hyperapobetalipoproteinaemia.

In both abdominal and diffuse obesity (particularly massive obesity, which is most commonly childhood-onset, in which the adiposity includes the limbs), the HDL species containing apolipoprotein A-1 (e.g. HDL2) are decreased, partly because of increased binding and disposal in the expanded adipose tissue[1,18]. Moreover, in abdominal obesity, increased hepatic triglyceride lipase activity is augmented, contributing to the decrease in HDL2-cholesterol[19].

Some obese children reveal a similar profile of lipoprotein-apolipoprotein abnormalities as described[6,20,21]. Other obese children do not manifest them until reaching puberty or early adult life. In both children and adults, effective dietary and exercise measures generally result in decreased hepatic apolipoprotein B and VLDL production, lowering of plasma VLDL-triglycerides and LDL-cholesterol, and frequently elevation of apo A-1 containing HDL species, notably HDL2[21-23]. The specific dietary composition influences HDL2 levels, i.e. diets enriched in oleic acid raise them, those containing *trans*-fatty acids decrease them, while enrichment with linoleic acid decrease or increase HDL2, depending upon other factors[13,14]. Appropriate weight loss, moreover, has lasting ameliorative effects on lipoprotein-apolipoprotein abnormalities, reflecting long-term changes in adipose tissue metabolism[21,23]. The ultimate degree of benefit brought about by effective dietary and exercise measures is dictated by genetic factors.

While much remains to be learned about lipoprotein(a), including the possible effects of obesity on its metabolism and its levels, it is gaining increasing interest because it is both atherogenic and thrombogenic[24]. Lipoprotein(a) represents a family of lipoprotein particles containing a single copy of apo B-100, generally linked to a single copy of apolipoprotein(a) of variable mass. The apo B allows binding to cholesterol esters, triglycerides, and other lipids. Heterogeneity results from the variable number of kringles of apolipoprotein(a) which is genetically dictated[24]. The thrombotic influence is derived from the structural similarity between apolipoprotein(a) and plasminogen, implicating lipoprotein(a) in interference with the fibrinolytic system. The LDL receptors are involved in clearing lipoprotein(a) from the circulation through interaction with the apo B moiety. Indeed, subjects with familial hypercholesterolaemia plus high levels of lipoprotein(a), have a significantly greater risk for coronary heart disease. Lipoprotein(a) levels are relatively elevated in obese subjects and decrease upon weight loss[25].

It is interesting that while the liver is the major site of lipoprotein, apolipoprotein, and lipid production (the small intestine is also a significant site, but mainly in relation to lipid absorption), adipose tissue metabolism modulates these hepatic functions, and contributes appreciably to their pathophysiology in obesity[1]. A major site of VLDL-triglyceride clearance is adipose tissue, where adipose cell-derived lipoprotein lipase, affixed onto the capillary endothelium, cleaves the triglycerides[1,7,8]. Apolipoprotein C-2 is the essential activator of lipoprotein lipase. Pertinent to the pathogenesis of obesity, lipoprotein lipase activity is increased in this state, and its activity rises even further upon weight loss[26]. This apparently paradoxical response contrasts with most other metabolic abnormalities associated with obesity, which improve with weight reduction[1]. Thus, lipoprotein lipase would facilitate weight regain in susceptible subjects.

Using cultured pre-adipocytes from persons with massive obesity (defined by body weight higher than 170% of reference, or by body mass index higher than $37 kg/m^2$), we have found several cellular and molecular abnormalities, as recently reviewed[27]. Pre-adipocytes from the massively obese replicate excessively, as a result of the inordinate production of specific mitogenic growth factors which act through paracrine/autocrine mechanisms[27,28]. Adipose tissue of massively obese subjects also has a much greater number of pre-adipocyte clones with a particular susceptibility to differentiation[29]. *In vivo*, important factors for differentiation in the obese include accelerated turnover of glucocorticoids and the hyperinsulinaemia characteristic of massive obesity[1]. We have also found that mature fat cells can dedifferentiate in culture and then regain the ability to replicate[27]. We have thus proposed that under conditions of prolonged adherence to diet and exercise, the complement of supernumerary fat cells can decrease; however, as indicated by our studies in culture, the reverted cells, which are depleted of triglycerides, have the genetic susceptibility to replicate and then differentiate excessively. Thus, with each cycle of adherence and then relapse (overeating and physical inactivity), there would be an ever increasing production of new mature fat cells, leading to progression of the corpulence[27]. In turn, at each stage of adiposity, there would be an influence of adipose tissue on hepatic lipoprotein–apolipoprotein metabolism, as well as metabolism of lipoproteins and their products in the fat tissue itself. Similarly, the cellular and biochemical abnormalities localized to abdominal and intra-abdominal depots in abdominal obesity, would influence both hepatic metabolism and clearance of lipoproteins and their products in the fat tissue itself.

References

1. Roncari, D.A.K. (1986). Obesity and lipid metabolism. In Spittell, J.A. and Volpé, R. (eds.) *Clinical Medicine*, 2nd edn, pp. 1–57. (Philadelphia: Harper and Row)
2. Hubert, H.B., Feinleib, M., McNamara, P.M. and Castelli, W.P. (1983). Obesity as an independent risk factor for cardiovascular disease: a 26-year follow-up of participants in the Framingham Heart Study. *Circulation*, **67**, 968–77
3. VanItallie, T.B. (1990). The perils of obesity in middle-aged women. *N. Engl. J. Med.*, **29**, 928–9
4. Eto, M., Watanabe, K. and Ishii, K. (1989). Apolipoprotein E polymorphism and hyperlipoproteinemia in obesity. *Int. J. Obes.*, **13**, 433–40
5. Laakso, M. and Pyorala, K. (1990). Adverse effects of obesity on lipid and lipoprotein levels in insulin-dependent and non-insulin-dependent diabetes. *Metabolism*, **39**, 117–22
6. Zwiauer, K., Widhalm, K. and Kerbl, B. (1990). Relationship between body fat distribution and blood lipids in obese adolescents. *Int. J. Obes.*, **14**, 271–7
7. Havel, R.J. and Kane, J.P. (1989). Structure and metabolism of plasma lipoproteins. In Scriver, C.R., Beaudet, A.L., Sly, W.S. and Valle, D. (eds). *The Metabolic Basis of Inherited Disease*, 6th edn, pp. 1129–38. (New York: McGraw-Hill)
8. *Ibid*: Disorders of the biogenesis and secretion of lipoproteins containing the B apolipoproteins. pp. 1139–64
9. Cianflone, K., Yasruel, Z., Rodriguez, M.A., Vas, D. and Sniderman, A.D. (1990). Regulation of apoB secretion from HepG2 cells: Evidence for a critical role for cholesterol synthesis in the response to a fatty acid challenge. *J. Lipid Res.*, **31**, 2045–55
10. Teng, B., Thompson, G.R., Sniderman, A.D., Forte, T.M., Krauss, R.M. and Kwiterovich, P.O., Jr. (1983). Composition and distribution of low density lipoprotein fractions in hyperapobetalipoproteinemia, normolipidemia and familial hypercholesterolemia. *Proc. Natl. Acad. Sci. USA*, **80**, 6662–6
11. Pouliot, M.C., Despres, J.P., Moorjani, S., Lupien, P.J., Tremblay, A. and Bouchard, C. (1990). Apolipoprotein E polymorphism alters the association between body fatness and plasma lipoproteins in women. *J. Lipid Res.*, **31**, 1023–9
12. Gotto, A.M. (1991). Cholesterol intake and serum cholesterol level. *N. Engl. J. Med.*, **324**, 912–13
13. Grundy, S.M. (1990). Trans monounsaturated fatty acids and serum cholesterol levels. *N. Engl. J. Med.*, **323**, 480–1

14. Garg, A., Bonanome, A., Grundy, S.M., Zhang, Z. and Unger, R.H. (1988). Comparison of a high-carbohydrate diet with a high-monounsaturated-fat diet in patients with non-insulin-dependent diabetes mellitus. *N. Engl. J. Med.*, **319**, 829–34

15. Leaf, A. and Weber, P.C. (1988). Cardiovascular effects of n-3 fatty acids. *N. Engl. J. Med.*, **318**, 549–57

16. Teng., B., Sniderman, A.D., Soutar, A.K. and Thompson, G.R. (1986). Metabolic basis of hyperapobetalipoproteinemia: Turnover of apolipoprotein B in low-density lipoprotein and its precursors and subfractions compared with normal and familial hypercholesterolemia. *J. Clin. Invest.*, **77**, 663–72

17. Sullivan, D.R., Sanders, T.A., Trayner, I.M. and Thompson, G.R. (1986). Paradoxical elevation of LDL apoprotein B levels in hypertriglyceridemic patients and normal subjects ingesting fish oil. *Atherosclerosis*, **61**, 129–34

18. Despres, J.P., Moorjani, S., Ferland, M., Tremblay, A., Lupien, P.J., Nadeau, A., Pinault, S., Theriault, G. and Bouchard, C. (1989). Adipose tissue distribution and plasma lipoprotein levels in obese women. Importance of intra-abdominal fat. *Arteriosclerosis*, **9**, 203–10

19. Despres, J.P., Ferland, M., Moorjani, S., Nadeau, A., Tremblay, A., Lupien, P.J., Theriault, G. and Bouchard, C. (1989). Role of hepatic-triglyceride lipase activity in the association between intra-abdominal fat and plasma HDL cholesterol in obese women. *Arteriosclerosis*, **9**, 485–92

20. Burns, T.L., Moll, P.P. and Lauer, R.M. (1989). The relation between ponderosity and coronary risk factors in children and their relatives. The Muscatine Ponderosity Family Study. *Am. J. Epidemiol.*, **129**, 973–87

21. Zwiauer, K., Kerbl, B. and Widhalm, K. (1989). No reduction of high density lipoprotein2 during weight reduction in obese children and adolescents. *Eur. J. Pediatr.*, **149**, 192–3

22. Epstein, L.H., Kuller, L.H., Wing, R.R., Valoski, A. and McCurley, J. (1989). The effect of weight control on lipid changes in obese children. *Am. J. Dis. Child.*, **143**, 454–7

23. Eckel, R.H. and Yost, T.J. (1989). HDL subfractions and adipose tissue metabolism in the reduced-obese state. *Am. J. Physiol.*, **256**, E740–6

24. Scanu, A.M. and Fless, G.M. (1990). Lipoprotein(a). Heterogeneity and biological relevance. *J. Clin. Invest.*, **85**, 1709–15

25. Sonnichsen, A.C., Richter, W.O. and Schwandt, P. (1990). Reduction of lipoprotein(a) by weight loss. *Int. J. Obes.*, **14**, 487–94

26. Schwartz, R.S. and Brunzell, J.D. (1981). Increase of adipose tissue lipoprotein lipase activity with weight loss. *J. Clin. Invest.*, **67**, 1425–30

27. Roncari, D.A.K. (1990). Abnormalities of adipose cells in massive obesity. *Int. J. Obes.*, **14**, 187–92

28. Cooper, S.C. and Roncari, D.A.K. (1989). 17-Beta-estradiol increases mitogenic activity of medium from cultured preadipocytes of massively obese persons. *J. Clin. Invest.*, **83**, 1925–9

29. LeBlanc, P.E., Roncari, D.A.K., Hoar, D.I. and Adachi, A.M. (1988).Exaggerated triglyceride accretion in human preadipocyte-murine renal line hybrids composed of cells from massively obese subjects. *J. Clin. Invest.*, **81**, 1639–45

Discussion

Dr Stehbens: I believe you said that adiposity causes certain lipid abnormalities and I cannot quite understand how adiposity *per se* can cause a lipid abnormality. If, on the other hand, you had said that adiposity is associated with some lipid abnormalities, which suggest that the lipid abnormalities led quite frequently to adiposity, then I could understand it. But, I cannot understand how adiposity, *per se*, produces a lipid abnormality.

Secondly, you said that Apo-a is thrombogenic. Now, thrombosis in man, and I think experimentally, is a secondary phenomenon and is associated with a loss of endothelium. There is also usually a very severe lesion of the intima and I cannot quite see how Apo-a would induce that sort of change in the vessel wall leading to a loss of endothelium and disruption of connective tissues underneath. I would also like to know how you harvested your pre-adipose cells from the omentum and whether or not you excluded the possibility that they might be mesothelial cells. How did you identify them as pre-adipose cells?

Dr Roncari: Well, to take the second part first, both lipoproteins-a and apolipoproteins-a have actually been found in arteries and in vein grafts. I do not know what the problem is. I can visualize quite readily how this lipoprotein, because of interference with plasminogen function, would aggravate the tendency to thrombosis. But, of course, I realize there has to be an underlying lesion for this thrombotic event. It has been found directly localized in arteries and vein grafts.

In regard to the second part of your question, there is abundant evidence indicating that adipose tissue does influence lipoprotein production and metabolism through the various interconversions and through the effects of free fatty acids. In obesity, as I mentioned, there is increased flux of free fatty acids to the liver and that leads to increased VLDL synthesis. There is, as I mentioned, lipoprotein lipase, which modifies and converts lipoproteins from one to the other so, it is directly involved.

Dr Stehbens: But you inferred that adiposity was the cause and now you have just said it is associated with it, but which comes first?

Dr Roncari: Normally, there is modulation and regulation. In obesity, this is exaggerated. For example, in obesity there is increased lipoprotein lipase activity and increased flux of free fatty acids. So, what happens normally is exaggerated in the obese state. As far as our pre-adipocytes, I have several articles from the *Journal of Clinical Investigation* where we characterize these cells. We have cloned them. They have all the characteristics of mesenchymal cells. We have done extensive biochemical and molecular biology studies and for example, they uniquely show adipose differentiation and specific gene expression. For example, lipoprotein lipase, adipsin, glycerophosphodehydrogenase go up a 1000-fold and these are all features that are practically exclusive to pre-adipocytes. They have been very well characterized.

Dr Goldbloom: You mentioned that lipid abnormalities are primarily associated with abdominal obesity. As a paediatrician, one of the problems I have sometimes in reading the literature on clinical studies of obesity is the failure to distinguish between obesity of childhood onset, which is now recognized to be overwhelmingly genetically determined, and obesity of adult onset. I am wondering, are there differences here between these two types of obesity, abdominal or otherwise?

Dr Roncari: Yes, that is a good question. As I mentioned, HDL depression occurs in all forms of obesity, although it may be worse in abdominal obesity. As you know, childhood onset obesity, and most of these massively obese individuals we studied had childhood onset obesity and it is a diffuse obesity.

11
Modulation of membrane function by cholesterol

P.L. YEAGLE

Cholesterol has long been known to be an essential component of mammalian cells. Yet despite much study, the role cholesterol plays in mammalian cell biology has remained a mystery. Without cholesterol, mammalian cells cannot experience normal growth. As a consequence, most mammalian cells are capable of making their own cholesterol.

Many steps are involved in cholesterol biosynthesis. Even after the synthesis of lanosterol, 18 enzymatically catalysed steps remain to produce cholesterol[1]. Much valuable cellular energy is therefore utilized in the complex biosynthetic pathway for cholesterol. Why this occurs is not fully understood. Bloch has suggested that evolutionary pressure for a more biologically competent sterol led to the development of the pathway from lanosterol to cholesterol[2]. However the molecular details describing why the cholesterol structure is required have not yet been fully described.

Some studies are available on specificity for sterol structure by sterol-requiring cells. *In vitro* experiments have shown that lanosterol cannot fully substitute for cholesterol as the essential sterol for cell function[3]. For example, *Mycoplasma mycoides* can be adapted to grow on low cholesterol media. However, they cannot grow in the total absence of cholesterol. Lanosterol will not support cell growth in the absence of cholesterol. However, growth will occur at nearly the same rate in cells fed low cholesterol levels supplemented with high (relatively) lanosterol, as in cells fed high (relatively) cholesterol levels[4]. This sterol synergism has pointed to a special role for cholesterol in supporting cell growth in which the particular chemical structure of cholesterol is required.

The requirement of cholesterol for normal function of mycoplasma is mirrored in yeast by an analogous requirement for ergosterol. Yet one sterol cannot substitute for the other; cholesterol cannot fully substitute for ergosterol in yeast, and ergosterol cannot support normal mammalian cellular function. Anaerobic growth of *Saccharomyces cerevisiae* requires ergosterol supplement to the culture medium. Supplementation only with cholesterol will not support normal growth[5]. Yet cholesterol is more effective at modifying the properties of lipid bilayers than is ergosterol (see below). These data point to a specific sterol recognition interaction, crucial to normal cellular function, that is different in yeast than it is in mycoplasma.

The requirement for cholesterol in mammalian cells is not well understood due to the paucity of available mammalian sterol auxotrophes. Therefore other methods have been used to explore the role of cholesterol. In mammalian cells, inhibition of cellular cholesterol biosynthesis inhibits cell growth[6]. In addition to the role of metabolic products from mevalonate other than cholesterol in cell growth, cholesterol itself played a role since the addition of cholesterol in the culture medium would restore cell growth[7].

Data such as these suggest that a unique sterol structure leads to biological competence in each sterol-requiring organism. What defines that biological competence is central to the discussion in this article. From this analysis emerges an hypothesis for the essential role of cholesterol in mammalian (and other cholesterol-requiring) cells.

Cholesterol has been the subject of extensive investigation for many years. Cholesterol is predominantly found in the membranes of cells, due to its largely hydrophobic structure. Much effort has been expended exploring the fascinating effects cholesterol has on the bulk properties of lipid bilayers, including cholesterol effects on permeability[8] and molecular ordering[9,10], lateral phase separations[11], reduction of the enthalpy of phospholipid phase transitions from the gel to the liquid crystalline state[12], to name just a few. As will be seen in the following, this line of study has provided information about some of the effects of cholesterol on biological membrane function (for a review, see Ref. 13). However, these effects are not as highly specific for sterol structure as are some of the biological effects. Therefore, the search for the role of cholesterol in mammalian cells has broadened to encompass more specific effects that may be due to the interaction between cholesterol and membrane proteins.

Since the primary location of cholesterol in cells is in the membranes of the cells, the ability of cholesterol to modify membrane function has been the focus of much interest. In particular, the modulation by cholesterol of the function of membrane proteins has been examined, both by modifying the cholesterol content of the native membranes in which the protein is found, and by reconstituting the membrane proteins into membranes of defined lipid content. Studies of this sort have led to three different classes of observations.

(1) An increase in the level of cholesterol in the membrane leads to a proportionate decrease in membrane protein function. An example can be seen in Figure 1. In this example, the equilibrium constant for the Meta I–Meta II transition of rhodopsin was measured as a function of the cholesterol content of reconstituted membranes[14]. The data show an

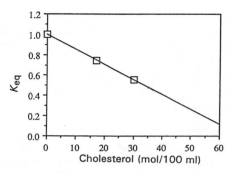

Figure 1 Effect of membrane cholesterol on the equilibrium constant for the Meta I–Meta II transition of bovine rhodopsin in reconstituted systems at 37 °C as a function of cholesterol content of the membranes (mol/ 100 ml with respect to the total lipid content of the membranes). Data replotted from ref. 14

inverse relationship between the function of the membrane protein and the cholesterol content of the membrane. For rhodopsin, cholesterol apparently acts as a negative modulator, or an inhibitor, at high cholesterol levels. Similar inhibitory effects of cholesterol have been observed on rhodopsin activation of the cyclic GMP cascade[15], alkaline phosphatase[16], UDP-glucuronosyltransferase[17], thymidine transport[18], and anion transport[19].

(2) An increase in the level of cholesterol in the membrane leads to a proportionate increase in membrane protein function. This can be seen at low membrane cholesterol levels for the Na^+-K^+-ATPase in Figure 2. From a cholesterol/phospholipid mole ratio of 0 to about 0.35, an

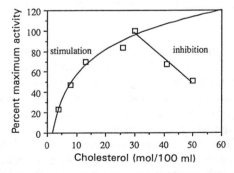

Figure 2 Effect of membrane cholesterol on the ATPase activity of the bovine kidney Na^+-K^+-ATPase. Cholesterol content was modified by incubation of the native membranes with lipid vesicles, with or without cholesterol, which resulted in intermembrane cholesterol transfer and alterations in the cholesterol level in the native membrane. Data replotted from ref. 37

increase in cholesterol in the membrane leads to an increase in the ATP hydrolysing activity of this enzyme in the modified native membrane. Stimulation of other membrane functions by cholesterol has been observed, including Na^+-Ca^{2+} exchange[20], ATP–ADP exchange[21], carrier mediated lactate transport[22] and the acetyl choline receptor[23,24]. (At high membrane cholesterol levels, inhibition is observed as described in the examples in (1)).

(3)   Some membrane functions appear to be insensitive to cholesterol levels in the membrane. Figure 3 shows data for the ATPase activity of the rabbit sarcoplasmic reticulum. As membrane cholesterol content was varied over a wide range, no alteration in ATPase activity was observed. Other membrane functions such as sucrase, lactase and maltase activities of the rat intestinal microvillus are apparently unaffected by alterations in the membrane cholesterol level[16].

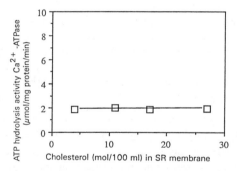

Figure 3 Effect of membrane cholesterol on the ATPase activity of the rabbit muscle sarcoplasmic reticulum Ca^{2+}-ATPase[44]. Membrane cholesterol levels were modified as described in Figure 2

The challenge is to find an explanation for these varied observations. The approach to be taken here is to identify the known effects of cholesterol on membrane structure and to use these properties to explain the observed effects of cholesterol on membrane function. A review of the available literature indicates that there are at least two general classes of interactions in which cholesterol can engage while in a membrane.

The most studied is the class of bulk effects on the lipid bilayer of the membrane. An example of this can be seen in the reduction of passive permeability of a membrane to neutral solutes upon the addition of cholesterol[8]. In phosphatidylcholine bilayers, cholesterol is the most effective sterol at reducing passive permeability. Cholesterol reduces permeability in direct proportion to the level of cholesterol in the membrane. Cholesterol, at a level of 50 mol/100 ml with respect to the membrane phospholipid, virtually eliminates passive glucose permeability in phosphatidylcholine bilayers.

Passive permeability has been modelled in terms of packing defects in the lipid bilayer (for a more detailed description see Ref. 25). These packing defects result because of non-cooperative isomerizations of carbon–carbon single bonds such that adjacent chains do not exactly mimic each other in conformation[26]. This leads to transient packing defects into which small molecules can fit. By moving from defect to defect, small molecules can transit the lipid bilayer. The smaller the molecule the more rapidly the transmembrane movement. Hence the relatively free permeability of membranes to water.

The presence of cholesterol in the membrane, in particular the fused ring system of the sterol, reduces the conformational flexibility of the hydrocarbon chains of the membrane lipids, causing them to adopt an average conformation in which most carbon–carbon single bonds are in the *trans* configuration[9]. This leads to more effective packing and a reduction in the packing defects. Permeability of the membrane to small, uncharged molecules is consequently reduced (see Figure 4).

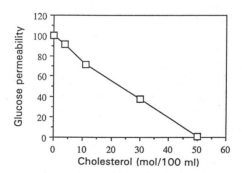

Figure 4 Reduction in passive glucose permeability of egg phosphatidylcholine bilayers by cholesterol. Data replotted from ref. 8

Litman and co-workers have approached this issue from a different perspective, using the properties of a fluorescent probe to calculate the effective 'free volume' in a membrane[27]. The concept of free volume is related to the defects in packing just discussed. The addition of cholesterol reduces the 'free volume' in the membrane. Figure 5 shows an example of the influence of cholesterol on this 'free volume' parameter.

Also shown in Figure 5 is the influence on the 'free volume' parameter of the incorporation of an integral membrane protein in the membrane bilayer[28]. The example shown is the reconstitution of rhodopsin into a phosphatidylcholine bilayer. Clearly, a membrane protein, upon incorporation into a lipid bilayer, reduces the available 'free volume', analogous to the incorpora-

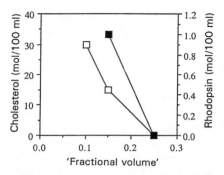

Figure 5 'Free volume' parameter (fractional volume) as determined from diphenylhexatriene fluorescence in egg phosphatidylcholine bilayers as a function of added cholesterol and rhodopsin. Data replotted from refs. 27 and 28

tion of cholesterol into the membrane. Apparently, to accommodate a membrane protein in a membrane requires some flexibility in the volume occupied by the protein. This flexibility can be achieved by scavenging free volume from packing defects in the lipids.

One would already anticipate that the influence of cholesterol on the properties of the lipid bilayer may be antagonistic to the need for 'free volume' by the integral membrane protein. In such a case, cholesterol might be expected to inhibit the function of such a membrane protein.

The other interaction between cholesterol and membrane components that could be important to membrane function is a direct interaction between the sterol and the membrane protein. Studies have shown an apparent binding of cholesterol to some integral membrane proteins, including glycophorin[29] and band 3 [30,31] from the human erythrocyte membrane. In the case of the latter protein, cholesterol has been shown to be an inhibitor of function[19]. Time-resolved fluorescence studies of a fluorescent derivative of cholesterol have also suggested cholesterol–protein interactions in the human erythrocyte membrane[32]. Furthermore, cholesterol binding to the fusion protein of Sendai virus has been reported[33].

The possibility that cholesterol can bind directly to membrane proteins suggests a mechanism of sterol modulation of membrane proteins in a manner analogous to effectors of water-soluble proteins. One would predict that such a mechanism would also give rise to a structural specificity in the sterol modulation of membrane proteins. The degree of such specificity would be governed by nature of the sterol–protein interactions.

Interestingly, cholesterol has been suggested to not interact directly with the Ca^{2+}-ATPase of rabbit sarcoplasmic reticulum[34,35]. For the same protein, cholesterol has been shown to be ineffective at modulating activity[36].

This discussion has led to the hypothesis that cholesterol likely modulates the function of biological membranes by more than one mechanism.

(1)   Cholesterol alters the bulk biophysical properties of membranes. Cholesterol increases the orientational order of the lipid hydrocarbon chains of membranes and reduces the 'free volume' available to membrane proteins for conformation changes that may be required for membrane protein function. In this role, cholesterol likely inhibits membrane function.

(2)   Cholesterol may bind directly to membrane proteins and regulate their function. In this role cholesterol may stimulate or may inhibit membrane function.

The discussion can now return to the specific cases provided above for cholesterol modulation of membrane proteins. The first case was that of bovine rhodopsin reconstituted into membranes containing varying levels of cholesterol[14]. Increasing cholesterol levels inhibited the Meta I to Meta II transition. Increasing cholesterol levels also inhibited the ability of this photoreceptor to activate the cGMP cascade[15].

Comparison of Figure 1 and Figure 4 shows that the relationships described for cholesterol effects on 'free volume' and cholesterol inhibition of the Meta I to Meta II transition are remarkably similar. These data suggest that: (1) 'free volume' may be required by the protein for function; (2) cholesterol reduces the 'free volume' available to the protein in the bilayer; (3) cholesterol thereby inhibits the function of rhodopsin in the membrane.

The second case provided above for cholesterol modulation of membrane function was that of the Na^+–K^+-ATPase. Cholesterol stimulates the Na^+–K^+-ATPase at low to moderate membrane cholesterol levels (see Figure 2). Lanosterol and ergosterol were shown to be unable to fully substitute for cholesterol in this stimulation of the enzyme[37].

Figure 6 regraphs the data for several different enzymes describing the dependence of these enzymes on cholesterol level in the membrane. Each of these examples reveals a stimulation of enzyme activity at low membrane cholesterol content and an inhibition of enzyme activity at high membrane cholesterol content. Each enzyme exhibits maximal activity at somewhat different cholesterol levels in the membrane, although all of these enzymes operate near maximum activity at the level of cholesterol in the plasma membrane in which these enzymes reside. Furthermore the data predict that these enzymes exhibit little, or no activity in the absence of cholesterol. These results suggest that cholesterol is required for these enzymes to express normal activity.

More recently, an extensive study of the influence of several sterols on the activity of the Na^+–K^+-ATPase provided greater insight into the specificity

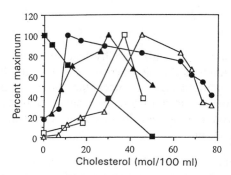

Figure 6 Replot of data on the effects of cholesterol on membrane enzymes. Open squares, Na, Ca exchange[20]; solid triangles, Na$^+$–K$^+$-ATPase[37]; solid circles, glutamate transport[17]; open triangles, GABA transport[17]; solid squares, glucose permeability[8]

of the stimulation for sterol structure[20]. For each of these sterols, previous measurements have provided a measure of the ability of these sterols to reduce the packing defects and favour an all-*trans* conformation of the carbon–carbon single bonds in the lipid hydrocarbon chains[38]. One such parameter is the reduction in the area per headgroup for the phospholipids in monolayers. This is a measure of the so-called 'condensing effect' of sterols.

Figure 7 shows a plot of the extent of the 'condensing effect' of the sterols (reduction in area per lipid headgroup at a fixed sterol level in the monolayer of phospholipid) as a function of the ability of each of these sterols to support ATP hydrolysing activity of the Na$^+$–K$^+$-ATPase. Each point represents a

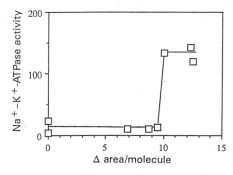

Figure 7 Relationship between the Na$^+$–K$^+$-ATPase activity in the presence of various sterols[20] and the condensing effect of cholesterol on phosphatidylcholine bilayers, represented as the additional reduction in area per headgroup due to the presence of the sterol in the membrane at 50 mol/100 ml[38]. The sterols represented in this graph are androstanol, epicholesterol, ergosterol, stigmasterol, 7-dehydrocholesterol, cholesterol, and cholestanol

166

different sterol. What is evident from this graph is that no simple direct proportionality exists between the ability of the sterol to 'condense' the phospholipids in a monolayer and the ability of the sterols to support activity of the enzyme under otherwise constant conditions in a reconstituted system. A similar lack of a simple relationship is observed between the reduction by sterol in passive permeability of the membrane to small solutes and the activity of Na^+–Ca^{2+} exchange. (It should be noted that the details of these relationships can depend upon the phospholipid composition of the membrane[20]. This may be due to organization of cholesterol-rich regions in the plane of the membrane that is dependent upon phospholipid composition[39].)

These data indicate that the activation of the Na^+–K^+-ATPase by sterol is not a process that is modulated by the condensing or ordering of the membrane lipids by cholesterol. Not only is there no correlation in Figure 7 with enzyme activity, but the small amounts of cholesterol that are required to activate some of the enzymes (see Figure 6) do not have an equivalently dramatic effect on the ordering of the hydrocarbon chains of the membrane lipids at those same low cholesterol levels. At the membrane cholesterol levels that do significantly affect the bulk properties of the lipid bilayer, one observes inhibition of enzyme activity (see below).

What is suggested by the graph in Figure 7 is that activation of the Na^+–K^+-ATPase by sterol at low to moderate sterol levels in the membrane is highly structurally specific. Such structural specificity can be best explained by a direct interaction of sterol with membrane protein. The shape of the activation curve of the Na^+–K^+-ATPase is similar to a binding isotherm. Although such direct interactions between sterol and protein have not yet been studied in these enzyme systems, the data reviewed previously in this article indicated that direct sterol–protein interactions involving membrane proteins were possible.

With this model, the data on cholesterol modulation of the Na^+–K^+-ATPase can be explained by the competition of two effects. One is stimulation of the enzyme by cholesterol at low to moderate cholesterol levels. Stimulation in this model would result from a direct interaction of the sterol with the protein. The other is inhibition of the enzyme by cholesterol at high membrane cholesterol levels. Inhibition in this model would result from a restriction of conformational changes by the enzyme required for function due to a reduction in free volume available within the lipid bilayer by the presence of the cholesterol. Figure 2 schematically shows this division between the two effects of cholesterol on the Na^+–K^+-ATPase.

These two effects of cholesterol on the Na^+–K^+-ATPase compete so as to produce a region of membrane cholesterol levels that support maximal activity. Interestingly for the kidney Na^+–K^+-ATPase, maximal activity is observed at the cholesterol level of the native membrane[37]. This is appropriate for an organ in which the Na^+–K^+-ATPase is very important to the function of that organ. Thus cholesterol homeostasis may be important to ion transport in the kidney. In contrast in the human erythrocyte, where high fluxes of sodium and potassium are not as crucial to cellular function, the membrane cholesterol level determines operation of the erythrocyte Na^+-K^+-ATPase at sub-maximal activity.

In summary at this point, cholesterol regulates the activity of the Na^+-K^+-ATPase in two ways. At low membrane cholesterol levels, cholesterol stimulates the enzyme. At high membrane cholesterol levels, cholesterol inhibits the Na^+-K^+-ATPase. The stimulation of the Na^+-K^+-ATPase is likely due to binding of cholesterol to the enzyme, analogous to modulators of water soluble enzymes. The stimulation is specific for the structure of the sterol. The inhibition is likely due to inhibition of the ability of the enzyme to undergo the conformational changes required for function through the effects of high membrane cholesterol on the bulk properties of the membrane.

For those enzymes in which only inhibition by cholesterol is observed, one could postulate that there are no sites for effective interaction between sterol and protein. In this case, the only effect would be the influence of cholesterol on the bulk properties of the bilayer, thereby indirectly affecting the ability of membrane proteins to undergo conformational changes. Of course, the other possibility of cholesterol acting as a negative effector by binding to the enzyme is possible and may be important to regulation of the HMGCoA reductase[40,41].

One other case should be considered; that is the case of the membrane protein whose activity is not affected by the presence of cholesterol in the membrane. The Ca^{2+}-ATPase of rabbit muscle sarcoplasmic reticulum provides an example (see above). In this case there would presumably be no sites on the protein at which cholesterol could bind. Available data suggest that is the case. Furthermore, the portion of the protein in the membrane may not have to undergo significant conformational changes that absorb 'free volume' from the lipid bilayer during its functional cycle. That may be reasonable for this protein in which the ATPase active site is on the portion of the protein that is outside of the lipid bilayer[42].

Based on the above analysis, it is possible to formulate an hypothesis for the essential role of cholesterol in cholesterol-requiring cells: that the essential role of cholesterol in cell function is to activate membrane enzymes that are necessary for cellular function and growth. A mechanism for such structurally specific sterol stimulation of membrane function would be interactions between cholesterol and membrane proteins that are structurally specific.

Studies on the sterol requirement of a human macrophage-like cell line support this hypothesis *in vivo*. A highly specific sterol requirement was found for growth of this cell line in sterol-depleted media[43]. Examining this sterol requirement for evidence of bulk effects on membrane properties yields the same conclusion as found above for the Na^+-K^+-ATPase. Figure 8 shows a plot of the ability of sterols to promote cell growth versus the condensing effect

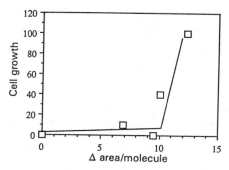

Figure 8 Relationship between the influence of sterols on cell growth of a human macrophage-like cell line[43] and the condensing effect of the sterols (see Figure 7)

of the sterols. As in the case of the Na^+-K^+-ATPase, no simple relationship is observed. Rather, it again appears that structurally specific interactions involving cholesterol and cellular components capable of specific recognition of the chemical structure of cholesterol, such as membrane proteins, are crucial to the growth of the cell.

References

1. Faust, J.R., Trzaskos, J.M. and Gaylor, J.L. (1988). In Yeagle, P.L. (ed.) *Biology of Cholesterol*, pp. 19–38. (Boca Raton: CRC Press)
2. Bloch, K. (1976). In Kornberg, A., Horecker, B.L., Cornudella, Z. and Oro, J. (eds.) *Reflections in Biochemistry*, p. 143. (Oxford: Pergamon Press)
3. Dahl, C. and Dahl, J. (1988). In Yeagle, P.L. (ed.) *Biology of Cholesterol*, pp. 147–72. (Boca Raton: CRC Press)
4. Dahl, J.S., Dahl, C.E. and Bloch, K. (1980). Sterol in membranes: Growth characteristics and membrane properties of *Mycoplasma capricolum* cultured on cholesterol and lanosterol. *Biochemistry*, **19**, 1467–72
5. Andreason, A.A. and Stier, T.J.B. (1953). Anaerobic nutrition of *Saccharomyces cerevisiae*. Ergosterol requirements for growth in a defined medium. *J. Cell. Comp. Physiol.*, **41**, 23
6. Chen, H.W., Kandutsch, A.A. and Waymouth, C. (1974). Inhibition of cell growth by oxygenated derivatives of cholesterol. *Nature*, **251**, 419
7. Brown, M.S. and Goldstein, J.L. (1974). Suppression of 3-hydroxy-3-methyl-glytaryl-coenzyme A reductase activity and inhibition of growth of human fibroblasts of 7-ketocholesterol. *J. Biol. Chem.*, **249**, 7306
8. Demel, R.A., Bruckdorfer, K.R. and Deenen, L.L.M.v. (1972). The effect of sterol structure on the permeability of liposomes to glucose, glycerol and Rb+. *Biochim. Biophys. Acta*, **255**, 321–30

9. Gally, H.U., Seelig, A. and Seelig, J. (1976). Cholesterol-induced rod-like motion of fatty acyl chains in lipid bilayers, a deuterium magnetic resonance study. *Hoppe-Seyler's Z. Physiol. Chem.*, **357**, 1447–50

10. Stockton, B.W. and Smith, I.C.P. (1976). A deuterium NMR study of the condensing effect of cholesterol on egg phosphatidylcholine bilayer membranes. *Chem. Phys. Lipids*, **17**, 251

11. Smutzer, G. and Yeagle, P.L. (1985). Phase behavior of DMPC-cholesterol mixtures; a fluorescence anisotrophy study. *Biochim. Biophys. Acta*, **814**, 274–80

12. Estep, T.N., Mountcastle, D.B., Biltonen, R.L. and Thompson, T.E. (1978). Studies on the anomalous thermotropic behavior of aqueous dispersions of dipalmitoylphosphatidylcholine-cholesterol mixtures. *Biochemistry*, **17**, 1984–9

13. Yeagle, P.L. (1985). Cholesterol and the cell membrane. *Biochim. Biophys. Acta Biomembrane Rev.*, **822**, 267–87

14. Mitchell, D.C., Straume, M., Miller, J.L. and Litman, B.J. (1990). Modulation of metarhodopsin formation by cholesterol-induced ordering of bilayer lipids. *Biochemistry*, **29**, 9143

15. Boesze-Battaglia, K. and Albert, A. (1990). Cholesterol modulation of photoreceptor function in bovine rod outer segments. *J. Biol. Chem.*, **265**, 20727–30

16. Brasitus, T.A., Dahiya, R., Dudeja, P.K. and Bissonnette, B.M. (1988). Cholesterol modulates alkaline phosphatase activity of rat intestinal microvillus membranes. *J. Biol. Chem.*, **263**, 8592–7

17. Rotenberg, M. and Zakim, D. (1991). Effects of cholesterol on the function and thermotropic properties of pure UDP-glucuronosyltransferase. *J. Biol. Chem.*, **266**, 4159–61

18. Saito, Y. and Silbert, D.F. (1979). Selective effects of membrane sterol depletion on surface function thymidine and 3-O-methyl-D-glucose transport in a sterol auxotroph. *J. Biol. Chem.*, **255**, 1102–7

19. Gregg, V.A. and Reithmeier, R.A.F. (1983). Effect of cholesterol on phosphate uptake by human red blood cells. *FEBS Lett.*, **157**, 159–64

20. Vemuri, R. and Philipson, K.D. (1989). Influence of sterols and phospholipids on sarcolemmal and sarcoplasmic reticular cation transporters. *J. Biol. Chem.*, **264**, 8680–5

21. Kramer, R. (1982). Cholesterol as activator of ADP-ATP exchange in reconstituted liposomes and in mitochondria. *Biochim. Biophys. Acta*, **693**, 296–304

22. Grunze, M., Forst, B. and Deuticke, B. (1980). Dual effect of membrane cholesterol on simple and mediated transport process in human erythrocytes. *Biochim. Biophys. Acta*, **600**, 860–8

23. Craido, M., Eibl, H. and Barrantes, F.J. (1982). Effects of lipids on acetylcholine receptor. Essential need of cholesterol for maintenance of agonist-induced state transitions in lipid vesicles. *Biochemistry*, **21**, 3622–7

24. Fong, T.M. and McNamee, M.G. (1986). Correlation between acetylcholine receptor function and structural properties of membranes. *Biochemistry*, **25**, 830–40

25. Yeagle, P.L. (1987). *The Membranes of Cells*, pp. 1–292. (Orlando: Academic Press)

26. Seelig, A. and Seelig, J. (1974). The dynamic structure of fatty acyl chains in a phospholipid bilayer measured by deuterium magnetic resonance. *Biochemistry*, **13**, 4839–45

27. Straume, M. and Litman, B.J. (1987). Equilibrium and dynamic structure of large, unilamellar, unsaturated acyl chain phosphatidylcholine vesicles. Higher order analysis of 1,6-diphenyl-1,3,5-hexatriene and 1-[4-trimethylammonio]-6-phenyl-1,3,5-hexatriene anisotropy decay. *Biochemistry*, **26**, 5113–20

28. Straume, M. and Litman, B.J. (1988). Equilibrium and dynamic bilayer structural properties of unsaturated acyl chain phosphatidylcholine-cholesterol-rhodopsin recombinant vesicles and rod outer segment disk membranes as determined from higher order analysis of fluorescence anisotropy decay. *Biochemistry*, **27**, 7723–33

29. Yeagle, P.L. (1984). Incorporation of the human erythrocyte sialoglycoprotein into recombined membranes containing cholesterol. *J. Membrane Biol.*, **78**, 201–10

30. Klappauf, E. and Schubert, D. (1977). Band 3 from human erythrocyte membranes strongly interacts with cholesterol. *FEBS Lett.*, **80**, 423–5

31. Schubert, D. and Boss, K. (1982). Band 3 protein-cholesterol interactions in erythrocyte membranes. *FEBS Lett.*, **150**, 4–8

32. Yeagle, P.L., Albert, A.D., Boesze-Battaglia, K., Young, J. and Frye, J. (1990). Cholesterol dynamics in membranes. *Biophys. J.*, **57** (in press)

33. Asano, K. and Asano, A. (1988). Binding of cholesterol and inhibitory peptide derivatives with the fusogenic hydrophobic sequence of F-glycoprotein of Sendai virus: possible implication in the fusion reaction. *Biochemistry*, **27**, 1321–9

34. Warren, G.B., Houslay, M.D., Metcalfe, J.C. and Birdsall, N.J.M. (1975). Cholesterol is excluded from the phospholipid annulus surrounding an active calcium transport protein. *Nature*, **255**, 684–7

35. London, E. and Feigenson, G.W. (1978). Fluorescence quenching of Ca^{2+}-ATPase in bilayer vesicles by a spin-labeled phospholipid. *FEBS Lett.*, **96**, 51–4

36. Johannsson, A., Keightley, C.A., Smith, G.A. and Metcalfe, J.C. (1981). Cholesterol in sarcoplasmic reticulum and the physiological significance of membrane fluidity. *Biochem. J.*, **196**, 505–11

37. Yeagle, P.L., Rice, D. and Young, J. (1988). Cholesterol effects on bovine kidney Na^+ K^+ATPase hydrolyzing activity. *Biochemistry*, **27**, 6449–52

38. Demel, R.A., Bruckdorfer, K.R. and Deenen, L.L.M.v. (1972). *Biochim. Biophys. Acta*, **255**, 311–20

39. Hui, S.W. (1988). In Yeagle, P.L. (ed.) *Biology of Cholesterol*, pp. 213–33. (Boca Raton: CRC Press)

40. Heusden, G.H.P.v. and Wirtz, K.W.A. (1984). Hydroxylmethylglutaryl CoA reductase and the modulation of microsomal cholesterol content by the nonspecific lipid transfer protein. *J. Lipid Res.*, **25**, 27–31

41. Bjorkhem, I., Buchmann, M.S. and Skrede, S. (1985). On the structural specificity in the regulation of the hydroxymethylglutaryl-CoA reductase and the cholesterol-7α-hydroxylase in rats. Effects of cholestanol feeding. *Biochim. Biophys. Acta*, **835**, 18–22

42. MacLennan, D.H., Brandl, C.J., Korczak, B. and Green, N.M. (1985). Amino-acid sequence of a Ca^{2+} Mg^{2+}-dependent ATPase from rabbit muscle sarcoplasmic reticulum, deduced from its complementary DNA sequence. *Nature*, **316**, 696–700

43. Esfahani, M., Scerbo, L. and Devlin, T.M. (1984). A requirement for cholesterol and its structural features for a human macrophage-like cell line. *J. Cell. Biochem.*, **25**, 87–97

Discussion

Dr Parsons: I enjoyed your talk. My question has to do with control of the amount of the cholesterol that one finds in the membrane. What is controlling it, is it not the physical properties, like for example, the membrane fluidity?

Dr Yeagle: Membrane fluidity is a very complicated topic. What one is seeing in the stimulation of membrane function by cholesterol is a lack of correlation of the enzyme activity with the effect that the cholesterol has on the properties of the lipid bilayer. Furthermore, there is a strong structural specificity for stimulation at membrane enzymes by sterol. So, it is on the basis of that, that I look to some other kinds of mechanisms for the regulation or for the modulation of these enzymes. This is really what drives me to this concept of a protein involvement since in biology, interactions between these kinds of molecules lead to a much greater specificity.

Dr Parsons: I will readdress my question. Not that I am in disagreement with what you are saying, but intracellular membranes have a much lower cholesterol content than the plasma membrane. They all have enzymes and they are all going to be modulated. What I am asking is what determines the level of cholesterol that you will find in the mitochondria versus the plasma membrane?

Dr Yeagle: We actually attempted to answer that question several years ago, in terms of what controls the level of cholesterol in the membranes. There is a tremendous cholesterol gradient between plasma membranes and intracellular membranes. It has been shown that, while not necessarily always effective, it is possible to get cholesterol transfer even through the aqueous phase, from one membrane to another. Also, there is a tremendous shuttling of membraneous material between plasma membrane and intracellular membranes. So, the question arises, how on earth do you keep that tremendous cholesterol gradient between plasma membranes and intracellular membranes? We examined the issue to see if lipid content, in particular, phospholipid content, might in and of itself, through thermodynamic means, create this cholesterol gradient. We found that there are roles for various phospholipids in controlling the cholesterol content which are not overwhelmingly satisfactory for a typical situation, such as between endoplasmic reticulum and plasma membrane. It turns out that it is extremely satisfactory for a specialized system such as the outer segment of rod cells between the disc and the plasma membrane. We know that there is an important role of phosphotyletholamine in that regard. It is true that Silbert also did some experiments a number of years ago simply incubating mitochondria with plasma membrane or endoplasmic reticulum, and found that the gradient would break down, but it would not break down entirely. So, there is a thermodynamic component and the rest of it must be kinetic, which is not adequately described at this point. But, it is ironic that the site of cholesterol synthesis is in fact a site that is very poor in cholesterol content. Obviously, membrane enzymes at the ER are either examples, such as our calcium pump protein, which are not affected by cholesterol or such as with HMG CoA reductase, which may be affected by low levels of cholesterol and the threshold for modulation is simply that much lower than it is in the plasma membrane. I also do not mean to imply that plasma membrane levels are fluctuating all over the place, and thereby modulating the enzyme activities, I mean something very different. I mean that cholesterol homeostasis is required for proper plasma membrane function.

Dr Holub: I too enjoyed your talk. I have two questions that I would like you to help me with please. Firstly, a comparison of individuals with serum cholesterol levels of 400 mg/dl vs. 200 shows only about a 12–14% higher level of platelet cholesterol in the former group. I am interested in the strategies for the cell, in this case the platelet, resisting a greater increase in cholesterol in the membrane. Secondly, would you comment on *in vitro* vs. *in vivo* studies? In particular, when looking at cholesterol-enriched membranes derived via *in vivo* studies, with cholesterol accretion, there is a concomitant change in the fatty acid composition of the membrane phospholipid which could have important effects. The latter (fatty acid changes) would not occur in an *in vitro* enrichment system.

Dr Yeagle: With respect to the first question, if the system is allowed to come to some sort of thermodynamic equilibrium before cholesterol starts to segregate out and become pure cholesterol patches in the membrane, the typical plasma membrane is high in cholesterol relative to whatever lipid matrix it can tolerate. So, I think the issue that it is difficult to get the plasma membrane to consist of higher amounts of cholesterol has a lot to do with the capacity for that membrane to contain cholesterol without having the so-called phase separations. Phase separations produce membranes that do not have the properties that biological membranes need to have.

Your second question has to do with fatty acid content and the roles the various phospholipid and fatty acid contents have. There is a tremendous amount of literature with respect to both biological membranes and modelling of membrane type studies. At this point all I can say is that the cholesterol interactions with lipids do change and it is very complex. The issues surrounding this, with respect to that compared to the biology of the membrane, are a long way from being adequately described or being bridged from the model studies to the biological studies at this point. I would still tend to think that those effects would tend to be less important than some of the ones that we have just discussed. To be fair, the data are not yet adequate and so we do not really know.

Dr Yano: I wonder if your hypothesis could explain an epidemiological finding that there is an indirect association of low serum cholesterol with a high risk of haemorrhagic stroke. If so, is there any, as you suggest, threshold of low serum cholesterol on the adverse effect?

Dr Yeagle: I believe you can see from the data that I have presented that one does have to go to pretty low-cholesterol levels in those plasma membranes before you start to lose significant activity from important enzymes. And, they are very important enzymes. They do not come much more important than the plasma membrane sodium–potassium pump, for example. You would need a state that would produce a rather large change in plasma membrane cholesterol to inhibit that enzyme, however. Frankly, within the cell, that is probably the last membrane that would allow its cholesterol content to be changed. All of this points back to the essential nature of the activation by cholesterol for cell survival. Quite simply, we have elegant control mechanisms to keep ourselves reasonably far from that threshold below which disaster strikes. So, I think the elegant control mechanisms which are in place to maintain the plasma cholesterol levels are very potent. It is very difficult to manipulate a situation to the point where it is going to cause disaster. I would not worry, therefore, about not having enough cholesterol in the diet.

Section III.
Dietary Cholesterol and Fatty Acids in Health and Disease

12
Hyporesponders and hyperresponders to changes in diet

M.B. KATAN and A.C. BEYNEN

Introduction

The level of serum cholesterol in man is sensitive to the type of fat and the amount of cholesterol in the diet. The quantitative effects of these dietary components can be predicted using empirical formulas[1-3]. However, such predictions of serum cholesterol changes only hold good for group means and not for individual subjects. It has often been suggested that in certain individuals (hyporesponders) the level of serum cholesterol is relatively insensitive to dietary challenge whereas in others (hyperresponders) the effect of diet is much more pronounced.

The subject of hyporesponsiveness and hyperresponsiveness is of practical interest. Patients with hypercholesterolaemia generally receive dietary advice from clinicians to lower their serum cholesterol levels. Frequently, such advice turns out to be ineffective. Although lack of compliance may be involved, it is possible that certain patients are insensitive to cholesterol-lowering diets and need a different form of therapy.

Hyporesponders and hyperresponders to dietary cholesterol

The existence of human hyporesponders and hyperresponders to dietary cholesterol has been frequently assumed[4,5], but has proved very difficult to substantiate experimentally. Table 1 illustrates this. Six volunteers first abstained from cholesterol-rich products for 10 days, and then took six egg yolks per day for another 10 days. The study was repeated with the same subjects 1 year later. The average response for the group was fairly similar from one experiment to another, but the 'hyperresponders' in the first experiment were not necessarily hyperresponders in the second experiment, and neither were those initially classified as hyporesponders consistently unresponsive the second time. Similar experiments were performed in 1942

Table 1 Changes in serum cholesterol levels in six human volunteers after daily consumption of six egg yolks for 10 days

| | *Change in serum cholesterol (%)* | | | | | |
	A	B	C	D	E	F
Expt 1	+5	−3	+17	+17	+27	+5
Expt 2	+16	+12	+26	+25	+4	+3

Twelve months elapsed between Expt 1 and Expt 2; the design was otherwise identical. The pre-experimental and experimental serum cholesterol values were both based on two blood samples obtained on successive days. After Katan and Beynen[6].

by Messinger and co-workers[7]. They fed patients a dietary supplement of 150 g of egg-yolk powder per day emulsified in milk, providing 3750 mg cholesterol. The experiment was repeated in four of these patients and the response was reproducible in only two of them. The patient who displayed the highest cholesterolaemic response in the first experiment showed the lowest response in the second experiment. These two studies illustrate that the variability in the response to dietary cholesterol observed in single short-term experiments by itself does not prove the existence of human hyperresponders and hyporesponders.

We carried out three controlled dietary trials with the same subjects to study the question whether individuals do exist with a consistently high or low serum cholesterol response to dietary cholesterol[8]. In each trial the volunteers successively consumed a low-cholesterol and a high-cholesterol diet, the cholesterol component of the diets (provided by egg yolk) being the only variable. Subgroups of putative hyporesponders and hyperresponding subjects, with mean serum cholesterol increases of 0 and 19%, respectively, were selected from a larger population in a first trial and then underwent a second and a third experiment. Although the response in each subject was only partly reproducible, the selected hyperresponders showed significantly higher serum cholesterol responses in the second and third trial than the hyporesponders (Table 2). Standardized regression coefficients for individual responses in two experiments ranged from 0.34 to 0.53 ($n=32$).

Under less controlled conditions we found similar results. In 1976 Bronsgeest-Schoute *et al.*[9] studied the serum cholesterol response to discontinuation of egg consumption in subjects who habitually consumed at least one egg/day. When eggs were eliminated from the diet, daily cholesterol intake decreased from about 800 mg to 300 mg. Mean serum cholesterol fell only slightly (by 3%), but the individual responses varied from −20% to +8%. In 1982, 34 of these subjects were re-investigated[10], and at our request they again eliminated eggs and egg-containing products from their diet. The differences in serum cholesterol response between individuals were partly reproducible; the

Table 2 Effect of egg-yolk cholesterol on serum cholesterol in three controlled trials with the same subjects

	Change in serum cholesterol (mmol/l)	
	Hyporesponders (n=15)	*Hyperresponders* (n=17)
Selection trial	−0.01±0.21	+0.96±0.27
First reproducibility trial	+0.06±0.35	+0.28±0.38*
Second reproducibility trial	+0.47±0.26	+0.82±0.35**

Results are expressed as means±SD. Change significantly different from that in the hyporesponders (one-tailed Student's *t*-test); *, $p < 0.05$; **, $p < 0.005$. Based on Katan *et al.*[8].

individual responses in 1976 and 1982 were positively correlated ($r=0.32$, $n=34$, $p < 0.05$).

Thus it appears that at least part of the cholesterolaemic response to dietary cholesterol in man is individually determined. It is also clear that one will always find subjects who appear hyperresponsive in one experiment and hyporesponsive in another. This is caused by the diet-independent within-person variability of serum cholesterol. Serum cholesterol fluctuates within subjects on a constant diet with a periodicity of two to three days and an amplitude of up to 1.5 mmol/l[11,12]. Thus, the timing of the actual pre- and post-diet change blood samples can be such that the observed response to diet change appears much larger than the actual mean response, and the subject will be falsely labelled as hyperresponder. The reverse can also be the case, and the subject will be mislabelled as hyporesponder.

In our controlled studies[8] we calculated that the within-person error variance was still responsible for about 25% of the apparent variance in response between subjects even if we used 12 independent blood samples to determine each person's response to dietary cholesterol. Thus it is probably fallacious to characterize a patient as hyperresponsive or hyporesponsive to diet therapy if this is based on the results of a few blood samples only. A large number of serum cholesterol measurements is needed before and after the dietary challenge, and even then the observed response should be interpreted with caution.

Characteristics of hyporesponders and hyperresponders to dietary cholesterol

The characteristics of hyporesponders and hyperresponders to dietary cholesterol are of interest. Knowledge of the hyperresponder profile may help in identifying beforehand which patients will benefit most from dietary therapy. In our controlled studies with low-cholesterol and high-cholesterol diets[8], we found no relation of responsiveness with age, sex, intestinal transit time, ratio of primary to secondary steroids in the faeces and within-subject variability of serum cholesterol while on a constant diet[13]. Both serum total and HDL_2 cholesterol on the low- and high-cholesterol diets were positively associated with responsiveness to dietary cholesterol. It should be stressed that the values for serum total cholesterol and those for calculating the responsiveness variable were based on independent sets of measurements. Thus hyperresponders tended to have higher levels of serum total, but also of HDL_2 cholesterol concentrations than hyporesponders.

Body mass index, total body cholesterol synthesis (based on sterol balance data) and the habitual intake of cholesterol were negatively associated with the cholesterolaemic response to dietary cholesterol. Multivariate analysis was performed to take into account the correlations among the variables with predictive value. It then appeared that body mass index and body cholesterol synthesis did not contribute significantly to the explanation of variance in responsiveness[13].

In conclusion, our repeated controlled studies suggest that a low habitual cholesterol intake, a high serum HDL_2 cholesterol level, or a low body weight do not make one less susceptible to dietary-cholesterol-induced hypercholesterolaemia. The negative association of the response of serum cholesterol with body mass index and the positive association with HDL cholesterol were also seen in the other cohort discussed above, where the effect of cessation of egg consumption on serum cholesterol was studied in subjects who habitually consumed at least one egg/day[10]. Similar associations were reported by Oh and Miller[14].

Metabolic basis for hypo- and hyperresponsiveness to dietary cholesterol

We feel that individual differences in the efficiency of absorption of intestinal luminal cholesterol could be the primary determinants of the phenomenon of hypo- and hyperresponsiveness. This idea is based on animal studies with different species of monkeys. In three studies hyperresponsive monkeys absorbed a significantly higher percentage of dietary cholesterol than did hyporesponders (Table 3).

In an unusual patient, an 88-year-old man who for psychological reasons had eaten about 25 eggs per day for many years, a normal serum cholesterol level, i.e. hyporesponsiveness, was associated with a great reduction in the efficiency of cholesterol absorption from the intestine[18]. If human

Table 3 Mean serum cholesterol concentrations and cholesterol absorption in monkeys on low- and high-cholesterol diets

	Low-cholesterol diet		*High-cholesterol diet*	
	Serum cholesterol (mmol/l)	*Cholesterol absorption (%)*	*Serum cholesterol (mmol/l)*	*Cholesterol absorption (%)*
Squirrel monkeys				
Hypo (*n*=3)	4.5		4.9	55
Hyper (*n*=4)	6.1		8.3	62
Rhesus monkeys				
Hypo (*n*=5)	2.4	46	6.6	45
Hyper (*n*=5)	3.5	60	18.1	53
African green monkeys				
Hypo (*n*=3)	3.6		3.9	37
Hyper (*n*=9)	3.6		7.3	56

Based on data taken from Lofland *et al.*[15], Eggen[16] and St. Clair *et al.*[17].

hyperresponders indeed have a higher efficiency of cholesterol absorption than hyporesponders, then the rate of endogenous cholesterol synthesis must be higher in hypo- than hyperresponders because less cholesterol will reach the tissues from the gut, and synthesis will be less repressed[19]. Indeed, we have shown that whole-body cholesterol synthesis, when calculated from sterol balance data, is negatively associated with the increase in serum cholesterol when going from the low- to the high-cholesterol diet. This negative association was found irrespective of whether cholesterol synthesis was measured on the low- or high-cholesterol diet ($r=-0.43$; $n=32$). However, the relation did not persist on multivariate analysis[13].

Hypo- and hyperresponsiveness to saturated fatty acids

In man the nature of the fat in the diet is more important as a determinant of the serum cholesterol concentration than the amount of cholesterol. Thus it is relevant to know whether hypo- and hyperresponders to dietary fatty acid composition also exist, and whether hyperresponders to dietary cholesterol are also hyperresponsive to saturated fatty acids and other dietary components that affect serum cholesterol levels.

Jacobs *et al.*[20] recently re-analysed data from some of the classical dietary trials performed between 1963 and 1966 by Keys, Grande and Anderson in

Minnesota, USA. In these experiments the amount of cholesterol and the type of fat in the diet varied, and at least two serum cholesterol values per dietary period were known. Analysis of data for 48 subjects who had participated in two or more diet experiments showed that individual diet responsiveness was consistent from experiment to experiment in most men. Quantitative statistical data on the consistency of differences in responsiveness between individuals were not given. However, it was stressed that these differences were small. Most of the men showed a responsiveness within 30% of the value predicted by the formula of Keys[20], and only 2 out of 58 men could reliably be labelled 'non-responder'. Thus it appears that subjects with a consistently high or low response of serum cholesterol to the nature of dietary fatty acids do exist. However, total insensitivity of serum cholesterol to a fat-modified diet is rare, and what is taken to be lack of responsiveness is usually due to random fluctuations and does not constitute a permanent characteristic of the subject in question.

We have addressed the question whether human subjects hypo- or hyper-responsive to dietary cholesterol are also hypo- or hyperresponsive, respectively, to saturated fatty acids in the diet. Twenty-three subjects who participated in the three controlled trials on the effect of dietary cholesterol[8] were also tested for their response to saturated versus polyunsaturated fatty acids. In this experiment cholesterol intake was kept constant at an average of 41 mg/MJ (almost 500 mg/day), but the energy percentage of dietary polyunsaturated fatty acids was kept at 21% for the first 3 and then changed to 5% for the next 3 weeks; the polyunsaturated:saturated fatty acids ratios were 1.91 and 0.22, respectively. The response of serum cholesterol to the change in dietary fatty acid composition in this experiment was positively correlated with the mean response to dietary cholesterol in the three preceding experiments ($r=0.50; n=23; p<0.05$). This indicates that in humans hyperresponsiveness to dietary cholesterol is associated with hyperresponsiveness to saturated fat[21].

References

1. Keys, A., Anderson, J.T. and Grande, F. (1965). Serum cholesterol response to changes in the diet. I. Iodine value of dietary fat versus 2S-P. *Metabolism*, **14**, 747
2. Keys, A., Anderson, J.T. and Grande, F. (1965). Serum cholesterol response to changes in the diet. II. The effect of cholesterol in the diet. *Metabolism*, **14**, 759
3. Keys, A., Anderson, J.T. and Grande, F. (1965). Serum cholesterol response to changes in the diet. IV. Particular saturated fatty acids in the diet. *Metabolism*, **14**, 776
4. Connor, W.L. and Connor, S.L. (1972). The key role of nutritional factors in the prevention of coronary heart disease. *Prev. Med.*, **1**, 49

5. Reiser, R. (1978). Oversimplification of diet: coronary heart disease relationships and exaggerated diet recommendations. *Am. J. Clin. Nutr.*, **31**, 865

6. Katan, M.B. and Beynen, A.C. (1983). Hyper-response to dietary cholesterol in man. *Lancet*, **1**, 1213

7. Messinger, W.J., Porosowska, Y. and Steele, J.M. (1950). Effect of feeding egg yolk and cholesterol on serum cholesterol levels. *Arch. Intern. Med.*, **86**, 189

8. Katan, M.B., Beynen, A.C., de Vries, J.H.M and Nobels, A. (1986). Existence of consistent hypo- and hyperresponders to dietary cholesterol in man. *Am. J. Epidemiol.*, **123**, 221

9. Bronsgeest-Schoute, D.C., Hermus, R.J.J., Dallinga-Thie, G.M. and Hautvast, J.G.A.J. (1979). Dependence of the effects of dietary cholesterol and experimental conditions on serum lipids in man. Part 3. The effect on serum cholesterol of removal of eggs from the diet of freeliving habitually egg-eating people. *Am. J. Clin. Nutr.*, **32**, 2193

10. Beynen, A.C. and Katan, M.B. (1985). Reproducibility of the variations between humans in the response of serum cholesterol to cessation of egg consumption. *Atherosclerosis*, **57**, 19

11. Keys, A. (1967). Blood lipids in man. A brief review. *J. Am. Diet. Assoc.*, **51**, 508

12. Demacker, P.N.M., Schade, R.W.B., Jansen, R.T.P and Laar, A. van 't (1985). Intra-individual variation of serum cholesterol, triglycerides and high density lipoprotein cholesterol in normal humans. *Atherosclerosis*, **45**, 259

13. Katan, M.B. and Beynen, A.C. (1987). Characteristics of human hypo- and hyperresponders to dietary cholesterol. *Am. J. Epidemiol.*, **125**, 387

14. Oh, S.Y. and Miller, L.T. (1985). Effect of dietary egg on variability of plasma cholesterol levels and lipoprotein cholesterol. *Am. J. Clin. Nutr.*, **42**, 421

15. Lofland, H.B., Clarkson, T.B., St. Clair, R.W. and Lehner, N.D.M (1972). Studies on the regulation of plasma cholesterol in squirrel monkeys of two genotypes. *J. Lipid Res.*, **13**, 39

16. Eggen, D.A. (1976). Cholesterol metabolism in groups of rhesus monkeys with high or low response of serum cholesterol to an atherogenic diet. *J. Lipid Res.*, **17**, 663

17. St. Clair, R.W., Wood, L.L. and Clarkson, T.B. (1981). Effect of sucrose polyester on plasma lipids and cholesterol absorption in African green monkeys with variable hypercholesterolaemic response to dietary cholesterol. *Metabolism*, **30**, 176

18. Kern Jr., F. (1991). Normal plasma cholesterol in an 88-year-old man who eats 25 eggs a day. Mechanisms of adaptation. *N. Engl. J. Med.*, **324**, 896

19. Dietschy, J.M. and Wilson, J.D. (1970). Regulation of cholesterol metabolism. Third of three parts. *N. Engl. J. Med.*, **282**, 1241

20. Jacobs, D.R., Anderson, J.T., Hannan, P., Keys, A. and Blackburn, H. (1983). Variability in individual serum cholesterol response to change in diet. *Arteriosclerosis*, **3**, 349

21. Katan, M.B., Berns, M.A.M., Glatz, J.F.C., Knuiman, J.T., Nobels, A. and de Vries, J.H.M (1988). Congruence of individual responsiveness to dietary cholesterol and to saturated fats in humans. *J. Lipid Res.*, **29**, 883

Discussion

Dr Kubow: I was wondering how long you fed subjects in your initial cholesterol trials? I am thinking in particular about Dr Eddington's work in the *American Journal of Nutrition* who, after approximately 6–8 weeks' feeding, found that subjects who were initial hyperresponders to dietary cholesterol, whether they were hypercholesterolaemic or normocholesterolaemic, did not respond in a hyper fashion after such a time length of feeding.

Dr Katan: The duration of each diet in our studies ranged for 2 to 4 weeks. It has been our experience that most of the response to dietary cholesterol, and to saturated fats, is expressed within the first week. You can see a little change in the next couple of weeks, but I wonder if Dr Connor would care to comment since he has done so many trials on dietary cholesterol.

Dr Connor: With regard to the duration, we have a study published in the *Journal of Lipid Research**** in one hypercholesterolaemic lady and one hypocholesterolaemic man. We carried out these studies for 22 weeks. Each individual responded well and continued to have the same baseline. These were metabolic ward studies. Dietary cholesterol was increased for 11 weeks after a cholesterol-free diet established a stable baseline value. Dietary cholesterol increased the plasma cholesterol level greatly. The change occurred by 2–3 weeks and was maintained for the 11 weeks of the high cholesterol diet.

We have done other studies in prison volunteers and likewise found the degree of consistency maintained throughout the period of high dietary cholesterol feeding. I would suggest, however, that the consistency depends upon the change that one makes in the amount of dietary cholesterol. In other words, we used almost cholesterol-free diets and then added increments of dietary cholesterol up to 600–1000 mg per day. This was, in fact, the cholesterol consumption in our country many many years ago and it is, of course, a good deal lower now. So, the difference in serum cholesterol levels is dependent upon the difference in amounts of dietary cholesterol. I think that this prevails in the animal experiments as well. I wanted to ask Dr Katan if he has any data with a lower baseline amount of dietary cholesterol than the baseline presented of around about 110 mg of cholesterol per day? Our baseline dietary cholesterol intakes were close to zero.

---

* Lin, D.S. and Connor, W.E. The long-term effects of dietary cholesterol upon the plasma lipids, lipoproteins, cholesterol absorption and the sterol balance in man: the demonstration of feedback of inhibition of cholesterol biosynthesis and increased bile acid excretion. *J. Lipid Res.*, 1980; **21**, 1042–52

Dr Katan: No, we really cannot feed them a diet that is palatable and consists of natural attractive foods that has less than 100 mg per day.

Dr Connor: But, if you had your baseline at 300 mg per day and then compared it with 600 or 900, what do you think your result would be?

Dr Katan: Much less because, as you have shown and as Ancel Keys has shown, most of the response is in the lower region. You get much more of a response from very low to moderate than from moderate to high.

Dr Grover: The low and high response is an interesting idea. However, I think it would be interesting if we extrapolate from your data to what we see in the community today. For example, if you take someone from a 900 mg cholesterol to a 100 mg cholesterol diet, on average we are looking at a 22 mg/dl change in their serum cholesterol. If we extrapolate from that, an 800 mg change in cholesterol consumption results in a 22 mg/dl change in serum cholesterol. If we then look at the diets that Canadians and Americans consume today, you could propose that taking them from a 450 mg cholesterol diet to a 300 mg cholesterol diet, or 100 or 150 mg change, we can presumably expect one-eighth of that change at best, which is about 2 or 3 mg/dl. Does this not support the idea that dietary intervention, certainly looking only at the cholesterol consumption, has only a very modest result in terms of serum cholesterol in the average individual?

Dr Katan: I cannot calculate that quickly by heart what the expected effect of going from 450 mg to 300 mg is going to be* but certainly the effect of dietary cholesterol in man is quite a bit less than the effect of saturated fatty acids. So, just changing cholesterol intake and leaving the saturated fatty acids where they are, is not going to do a lot for your serum cholesterol.

The one benefit of lowering cholesterol and saturated fatty acids simultaneously is that you also have an interaction term. So, if you eat a food that contains both a lot of cholesterol and a lot of saturated fatty acids, there will be a larger cholesterol-raising effect than with the sum of two foods with the same composition eaten separately. But, there has been a misconception surrounding dietary cholesterol, as opposed to saturated fatty acids; this stemmed from animal experiments because some animals are very sensitive to cholesterol, especially rabbits, while man is not.

Dr Gold: In terms of what has been said, and perhaps Dr Connor could comment on this, is there a breakthrough level? That is, is there a relationship

---

* Note added in proof: The predicted effect is 4 mg/dl.

between increasing the intake of cholesterol and the level of serum cholesterol or does the serum cholesterol remain rather stable and then break through when one gets to a certain high level of cholesterol intake; or is it the other way around?

Dr Katan: No, it is the other way around. It is a saturation phenomenon. If you are someone who is eating three eggs per day and you cut out two of them, you get some decrease in serum cholesterol, but not spectacularly. However, if you then cut out that last egg, then you get a much larger effect. It works the other way around too. If you are on a totally vegetable diet and you add a little bit of cholesterol, the way Dr Connor has done, you get a large effect. If you then add another two eggs, you get less and less of an effect, it keeps going up, but there is a saturation effect. Ancel Keys has described it as a square root function, so it keeps going up, but most of the effect is in the low regions of intake.

Dr Gold: With blood pressure we have now described the so-called 'white coat' effect in terms of walking into a doctor's office and so on. Has anyone ever looked at the effect of knowing you are going to have your cholesterol checked? Is there a mind-set that may raise cholesterol, or lower it, when you go to see your doctor?

Dr Katan: There have been a number of studies on the effect of various mental stresses on the serum lipids. I do not know if seeing a doctor was one of them, but filling in tax returns was certainly studied. These studies have, in general, shown effects on serum triglycerides and serum free fatty acids. But, insofar as I have seen the literature, I think there has been little effect on serum LDL cholesterol or total cholesterol. How do you feel about this, Dr Connor?

Dr Connor: I am a little uncertain about the effects of stress. Stuart Wolfe did some stress studies in medical students before and after exams and showed some increase in the plasma cholesterol levels after stress. I think those studies have never been fully confirmed so I would leave a question mark about the acute effects of stress.

To refer back to what Dr Katan said about the amounts of dietary cholesterol, I certainly agree with what he has proposed. We have suggested that there is a threshold amount of dietary cholesterol below which there will be no effect on the plasma cholesterol and LDL level and above which one would see a somewhat linear response. This would continue until you get to a level of about 300–400 mg per day and then after this, if you continued to increase dietary cholesterol, there would be no further effect on the plasma cholesterol level. There will be compensatory mechanisms that will be set into play, one of them being a profound increase in the synthesis of bile acids, that does not seem to take place at lower levels of dietary cholesterol. So, I think that we have to think of a threshold.

The other concept that I would like to introduce is the concept of a ceiling beyond which further increments of dietary cholesterol will not change the plasma level. I think that this accounts for some of the paradoxes in different experimental studies and results in the literature. One needs to keep the threshold and ceiling concepts in mind.

Dr Parsons: Size, gender and age are clinical variables that correlate with plasma cholesterol levels with the population size. I assume that your population ranged from 30 to 100 kg and you gave them all one egg. When you take the variability out on the basis of per kg, do you see your data coming closer together? Is there a dose response on that basis?

Dr Katan: Actually, we did not give them all one egg. We gave them cholesterol relative to their energy intake. Those with a high energy intake, for instance, a big athlete training for a rowing match, may have received four eggs and a tiny girl with few activities may have had half an egg per day. We saw the same response in both. So that confirmed the concept of Ancel Keys that cholesterol should be expressed relative to calories and that if you have a larger caloric turnover you can handle more dietary cholesterol, as you can handle more of every dietary nutrient. We saw no differences between young or old people or between men and women in response.

13

Re-examination of the dietary fatty acid–plasma cholesterol issue: is palmitic acid (16:0) neutral?

K.C. HAYES, P. KHOSLA, A. PRONCZUK and S. LINDSEY

Introduction

For almost 40 years we have realized that dietary fat alters the plasma cholesterol concentration, but the degree to which various fats or their composite fatty acids modulate these effects and the mechanism(s) involved are not well understood[1]. The situation has been complicated recently because the original findings of Keys[2] and Hegsted[3], with particular regard to the effects of specific fatty acids, have been brought into question[4,5]. Whereas the dietary P/S ratio and intake of total saturated fats were thought to constitute the main impact, attention is now focused increasingly on the contribution from monounsaturated fats[1,4,6].

The point of this discussion is *not* to dismiss dietary saturated fat as a key variable in the cholesterol response, but rather to point out often over-looked subtleties in the metabolism of the specific fatty acids incorporated in the fats we eat. This oversight has come to light now that research has focused on specific lipoproteins and their metabolism, as opposed to assessment of the total plasma cholesterol and triglycerides in previous years.

Fat and energy as stressors

The point to be emphasized is that fatty acids are metabolized in a highly dynamic pattern of metabolic interrelationships such that the impact on plasma cholesterol of any given fatty acid, e.g. myristic acid (14:0), can be ameliorated or exacerbated by the mix of accompanying nutrients (especially other fatty acids and cholesterol) that are consumed and metabolized along with it[5,7]. This translates into the notion that 'high-stress metabolism', such as trying to cope with the dietary burden of excess calories accompanied by an excessive cholesterol intake (>500 mg per day) and a low-fibre, highly-refined carbohydrate diet (which increases hepatic VLDL triglyceride secretion) exerts a negative impact on hepatic lipoprotein secretion and turnover. This imbalance enhances the chances of an LDL build-up and HDL depletion. On the other hand, the severe restriction of calories, inclusion of dietary complex carbohydrate and fibre, increased polyunsaturated fatty acids (PUFA) and a reduced level of cholesterol, can greatly minimize the 14:0 effect.

The apparent reason for this disparate effect is simple enough, namely that lipoprotein metabolism is greatly altered (opposite almost) under the two situations outlined above. Unfortunately the mechanisms involved are more complicated than simply documenting the observed response. In the first instance, energy and cholesterol are being pumped into the lipoprotein transport system in excess, straining the normal metabolic ability to keep pace, in part, because all the necessary ingredients (e.g. PUFA or fibre) are not present in sufficient amounts to facilitate removal. By contrast, in the second scenario, not only are the components of the diet in better balance (PUFA, fibre, low fat, etc.), but more importantly a low energy and low cholesterol intake are, in effect, causing the body to reverse energy flow with a net *output* of these components from body reserves. In the latter case the balance between metabolic hormones and body metabolic processes are at their highest efficiency and better prepared to cope with the energy flux.

The point is that the problem of hypercholesterolaemia and atherogenesis only occurs (typically for the average person) in response to sustained periods (years) of energy excess and adipose tissue expansion[8,9]. This, in turn, is affiliated with decreased low-density lipoprotein receptor (LDLr) activity and polygenic hypercholesterolaemia[10]. An increased body mass index is also associated with decreased HDL-cholesterol[8,9]. During periods of reduced caloric intake and decreased cholesterol production, evidence now exists that cholesterol and fat are actually removed from the arteries[11].

Dietary fat and lipoproteins

How does the above atherogenic scenario translate into plasma lipoprotein profiles? To address this problem, we have conducted a series of experiments over the last few years utilizing purified diets of defined fatty acid composition (Table 1).

As just mentioned, obesity is associated with expanded VLDL and LDL pools and decreased HDL[8-10]. Specific aspects of the dietary fatty acid relationship impact lipoproteins and are modulated by an influential genetic component governing lipoprotein metabolism. These interactions were demonstrated in our recent comparative study of several fats in three species of monkeys[12]. In that experiment only coconut oil (diet 2) and butter (diet 4)

Table 1 Fatty acid composition of purified monkey and hamster diets

Diet [a]	12:0	14:0	16:0	18:0	20:0	16:1	18:1	18:2	18:3	Others[c]
			Dietary [b] fatty acids (% of total)							
1	—	0.2	11.9	2.2	—	0.2	25.1	59.9	0.6	—
2	47.5	22.2	12.9	4.1	—	—	10.8	2.5	—	—
3	—	1.1	23.1	13.5	—	2.8	46.7	11.9	0.9	—
4	7.2	9.9	32.9	15.1	—	2.2	28.9	3.0	0.8	—
5	—	4.7	15.1	3.7	—	6.7	19.2	22.6	0.3	27.7
6	15.8	12.0	15.4	4.4	—	6.6	14.5	3.4	0.2	27.7
7	—	2.2	24.6	18.8	—	3.7	46.4	4.3	—	—
8/13/19	18.8	18.8	10.7	3.3	—	—	9.4	8.5	0.9	—
9/20	23.8	9.6	8.6	3.0	0.2	0.2	37.0	16.0	1.2	—
10/21	13.4	5.8	25.1	3.6	0.2	—	37.2	13.3	0.8	—
11/14/22	0.2	1.0	40.3	4.1	0.3	—	37.0	15.4	1.0	—
12/15/23	0.4	0.7	23.4	3.9	0.3	—	41.1	27.2	2.7	—
16	1.5	1.3	6.3	2.5	—	0.1	13.7	72.8	0.2	—
17	2.3	1.4	40.7	4.8	—	—	39.1	9.8	0.4	—
18	1.6	1.3	5.2	0.3	—	0.1	74.1	14.4	0.4	—
24	2.3	7.5	21.9	6.5	0.4	0.9	35.8	20.4	4.3	—

	Total SFA[d]	Total MUFA[e]	Total PUFA[f]	P/S [g]
1	14.3	25.3	60.4	4.22
2	86.7	10.8	2.5	0.03
3	37.7	49.5	12.8	0.34
4	65.1	31.1	3.8	0.06
5	23.5	25.9	50.6	2.15
6	47.6	21.1	31.3	0.66
7	45.6	50.1	4.3	0.09
8/13/19	80.6	9.4	9.4	0.12
9/20	45.2	37.2	17.2	0.38
10/21	48.1	37.2	14.1	0.29
11/14/22	45.9	37.0	16.4	0.36
12/15/23	28.7	41.1	29.9	1.04
16	11.6	13.8	73.0	6.29
17	49.2	39.1	10.2	0.21
18	8.4	74.2	14.8	1.76
24	38.6	36.7	24.7	0.64

[a]*Dietary fats:* **1**, corn oil; **2**, coconut oil; **3**, lard; **4**, butter; **5**, 2/3 fish oil, 1/3 corn oil; **6**, 2/3 fish oil, 1/3 coconut oil; **7**, tallow; **8, 13 and 19**, 90% coconut oil/ 10% soybean oil; **9 and 20**, 45% coconut oil/40% high-oleic safflower oil/ 15% soybean oil; **10 and 21**, 45% palm oil/ 22% coconut oil/ 20% high-oleic safflower oil/ 13% soybean oil; **11, 14 and 22**, 90% palm oil/ 10% soybean oil; **12, 15 and 23**, 45% palm oil/ 40% soybean oil/ 15% high-oleic safflower oil; **16**, high-oleic safflower oil; **17**, palm oil; **18**, high-linoleic safflower oil; **24**, 52% butter/ 32% canola oil/ 16% corn oil.

[b]Diets 1–18 fed to monkeys, diets 19–24 fed to hamsters. The composition of the purified diets has been described elsewhere [5,11,12,16]. Monkey diets were fed with fat contributing 31% energy except for Nos. 13–18, in which 40% energy was derived from fat. Hamster diets were fed with fat contributing 13% energy. Diets 8–24 were cholesterol-free. Diets 1–7 had cholesterol added to them in order to equalize for the cholesterol present in fish oil (MAXEPA®), which was used to formulate diets 5 and 6. For all formulated diets, the fatty acid composition was determined by GLC.

[c]20:4n-6, 20:5n-3, 22:5n-3 and 22:6n-3 fatty acids.

[d]Total saturated fatty acids (12:0, 14:0, 16:0, 18:0, 20:0).

[e]Total monounsaturated fatty acids (16:1, 18:1).

[f]Total polyunsaturated fatty acids (18:2, 18:3, 20:4n-6, 20:5n-3, 22:5n-3 and 22:6n-3).

[g]Ratio of PUFA/SFA.

were uniformly hypercholesterolaemic in all three species, whereas relatively saturated beef tallow (diet 7) and lard (diet 3) were scarcely different from corn oil (diet 1) in their ability to raise cholesterol (Tables 1 and 2). On the other hand, replacing two-thirds of the corn oil or coconut oil with fish oil (diets 5 and 6, respectively) induced an equally marked decline in cholesterol levels, even though the fatty acid composition of the fish oil blends contained more saturates and less polyenes than corn oil (Tables 1 and 2). The inference was that neither all saturates (12:0, 14:0, 16:0) nor all polyenes (n-6, n-3) were equally effective in modulating the plasma cholesterol response. Furthermore, the strong genetic influence was apparent in the relative non-responsiveness of the plasma cholesterol in rhesus monkeys (30% shift between corn oil and coconut oil) compared with the sensitivity of cebus monkeys (85% shift between these dietary fats) (Table 2).

To examine the implication of these results we undertook two further sets of studies, one in hamsters, the other continuing with monkeys. The monkey study[5] was designed to explore two aspects of the problem. The first examined

Table 2 Effect of short-term feeding of dietary fats on plasma lipids in monkeys[a]

	Dietary fat blend				
	1, 2[b]	3	4	5, 6[c]	7
Monkeys raised on corn oil					
Plasma cholesterol[d]	174 ± 9^{el}	181 ± 12^{f}	193 ± 11^{g}	138 ± 10^{efgh}	189 ± 14^{h}
LDL-cholesterol[d]	86 ± 7^{el}	93 ± 11^{f}	103 ± 7^{eg}	71 ± 9^{fgh}	94 ± 10^{h}
HDL-cholesterol	77 ± 5^{e}	75 ± 5^{f}	74 ± 7^{g}	59 ± 4^{efgh}	76 ± 6^{h}
LDL-C/HDL-C[d]	1.15 ± 0.11^{el}	1.28 ± 0.15	1.50 ± 0.12^{e}	1.27 ± 0.15	1.27 ± 0.11
Monkeys raised on coconut oil					
Plasma cholesterol[d]	256 ± 20^{efgh}	199 ± 20^{ei}	199 ± 18^{fj}	157 ± 16^{gijk}	204 ± 16^{hk}
LDL-cholesterol[d]	153 ± 17^{efgh}	104 ± 15^{e}	111 ± 13^{fi}	90 ± 12^{gi}	106 ± 11^{e}
HDL-cholesterol	86 ± 7^{ef}	78 ± 8^{g}	71 ± 6^{eh}	56 ± 3^{fghi}	82 ± 7^{i}
LDL-C/HDL-C[d]	1.88 ± 0.24^{ef}	1.33 ± 0.18^{e}	1.59 ± 0.17	1.57 ± 0.16	1.33 ± 0.13^{f}

24 monkeys (8 cebus, 8 rhesus and 8 squirrel) had been raised from birth for 8–12 years on cholesterol-free purified diets containing either corn oil (12 monkeys, 4 per species) or coconut oil. They were then fed either their basal diet or the test diet for 8 week periods.

[a]Adapted from[12]. Values are mean $\pm$ SEM; $n = 12$.

[b]For the short term study (8 weeks), both the basal (corn oil or coconut oil) and test diets were supplemented with the indicated amounts of cholesterol (mg/kcal): corn oil or coconut oil , 0.11, butter 0.10, tallow, 0.06, lard 0.05.

[c]Monkeys raised on corn oil were fed 2/3 fish oil, 1/3 corn oil, (diet 5) whilst those raised on coconut oil were fed 2/3 fish oil, 1/3 coconut oil (diet 6). Both diets contained 0.11 mg/kcal cholesterol.

[d]Two-factor repeated-measures analysis of variance revealed significant interaction between original diet and short-term response to fats.

[efghijk]Means in rows sharing a common superscript significantly different by repeated-measures ANOVA and Fisher's protected LSD paired analysis ($p < 0.05$).

[l]Indicates significant difference between basal corn oil and coconut oil diets by Student t-test ($t < 0.05$).

the general response in plasma cholesterol level during a progressive shift in the dietary P/S ratio, and the second assessed specific comparisons between individual saturated fatty acids when the P/S ratio was held constant, specifically comparing the effect of 12:0 + 14:0 vs. 16:0. Again it was apparent that monkey species differed in the magnitude of their response, but more importantly 16:0 (diets 10 and 11) was less cholesterolaemic than 12:0 + 14:0 (diets 8 and 9) in any of the three species of monkeys (Table 3).

In fact, no difference was noted in the exchange of 5% energy as 16:0 for an equal amount of 18:2 (between 5% and 10% kcal as 18:2, diet 11 vs. 12, Table 1) in rhesus monkeys, and only a modest effect of this exchange was evident in the more responsive cebus monkey (Table 3). On the other hand, when dietary 18:2 represented only 2.7% of the total energy (diet 8, Table 1) the impact of 12:0 + 14:0 was clearly evident in rhesus plasma cholesterol and had a major impact on cebus (Table 3). These dietary fatty acid exchanges

Table 3 Plasma lipids of three species of monkeys fed diets with five different fat blends[a]

Species	N	8	9	10	11	12
			Dietary fat blend[b]			
			Total cholesterol (mg/dl)			
Rhesus	8	212 ± 15^{cd}	197 ± 10	201 ± 11^{ef}	184 ± 11^{cf}	183 ± 10^{de}
Cebus	8	246 ± 17^{cdef}	191 ± 8^{dgi}	186 ± 13^{ehj}	161 ± 11^{cgh}	151 ± 9^{fij}
Squirrel	5	245 ± 20^{c}	239 ± 38	233 ± 33	216 ± 22	193 ± 25^{c}
Combined sp.	21	232 ± 10^{cdef}	205 ± 11^{ehj}	203 ± 10^{dgi}	183 ± 9^{cgh}	173 ± 9^{fij}
			LDL-cholesterol (mg/dl)			
Rhesus	8	113 ± 13^{cde}	88 ± 9^{d}	88 ± 5	82 ± 8^{c}	81 ± 6^{e}
Cebus	8	111 ± 16^{cdef}	82 ± 10^{eg}	70 ± 10	62 ± 5^{cd}	55 ± 5^{fg}
Squirrel	5	113 ± 11^{c}	116 ± 27^{d}	112 ± 21	100 ± 19	69 ± 18^{cd}
Combined sp.	21	112 ± 8^{cdef}	92 ± 8^{egi}	87 ± 7^{dh}	79 ± 6^{cg}	68 ± 5^{fhi}
			HDL-cholesterol (mg/dl)			
Rhesus	8	84 ± 5	92 ± 6	81 ± 4	86 ± 5	88 ± 5
Cebus	8	121 ± 10^{cde}	101 ± 6^{df}	103 ± 16	79 ± 13^{c}	85 ± 9^{ef}
Squirrel	5	101 ± 11	106 ± 12	106 ± 13	97 ± 8	98 ± 9
Combined sp.	21	102 ± 6^{cd}	99 ± 4^{ef}	96 ± 6	86 ± 6^{ce}	89 ± 4^{df}
			LDL-C/HDL-C			
Rhesus	8	1.38 ± 0.20	1.00 ± 0.12	1.10 ± 0.08	0.98 ± 0.12	0.92 ± 0.06
Cebus	8	1.15 ± 0.22^{c}	0.85 ± 0.14	0.80 ± 0.18	0.69 ± 0.05^{c}	0.68 ± 0.07
Squirrel	5	1.13 ± 0.04	1.05 ± 0.14	1.07 ± 0.12	1.04 ± 0.14	0.67 ± 0.11
Combined sp.	21	1.23 ± 0.11^{cde}	0.95 ± 0.08^{df}	0.98 ± 0.09^{g}	0.89 ± 0.07^{c}	0.77 ± 0.05^{efg}

[a]Adapted from[5]. Values are mean ± SEM.
[b]See legend to Table 1 for description of fat blend and the fatty acid composition.
[cdefghij]Means sharing a common superscript in a given row are significantly different ($p < 0.05$).

and the different responses emphasize two aspects of the issue, namely (1) the highly diverse genetic contribution was evident between the diverse sensitivity of rhesus and cebus monkeys, and (2) the potential to elicit different responses depending upon the relative amount or 'threshold' level of key fatty acids, especially 18:2 and 14:0 (expressed as percent dietary energy).

Mechanism of fatty acid effect: lipoprotein kinetics

To explore the mechanism underlying the metabolic differences induced by specific fatty acids, we re-fed two of the diets (diets 8 and 11, Table 1) to rhesus monkeys in a second study[13], in order to compare the effects of 12:0 + 14:0 vs. 16:0 + 18:1. Apo B kinetics were evaluated following the simultaneous injection of ^{125}I-VLDL and ^{131}I-LDL. Since the rhesus plasma cholesterol was only moderately responsive to changes in fat saturation, we were surprised to find a major difference in the metabolism of apo B lipoproteins under these dietary circumstances. Specifically, 16:0 + 18:1 in-duced a three-fold higher VLDL apo B transport rate, whereas 12:0 + 14:0 induced an increase (five-fold greater than 16:0 + 18:1) in the transport rate of LDL apo B derived from VLDL-independent sources (i.e. increased 'direct' production of LDL apo B) resulting in a two-fold increase in the circulating

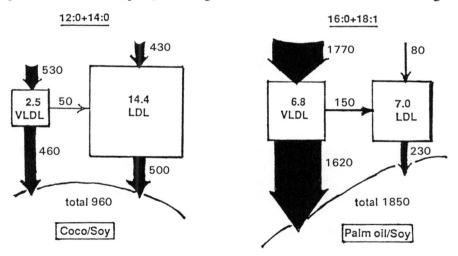

Figure 1 Apo B kinetics were determined in rhesus monkeys fed a coconut oil–soybean oil (12:0 + 14:0) diet or the same diet with palm oil–soybean oil (16:0 + 18:1). Vector arrows depict relative rates (μg/kg/h) of secretion and clearance by the liver into and from the VLDL and LDL apo B pools. Pool sizes are in mg/kg (see text and reference 13 for detailed description)

LDL pool and slight decrease in HDL relative to $16:0 + 18:1$. These changes, in turn, had a significant, negative impact on the LDL/HDL ratio. This detrimental shift towards LDL expansion, typical of 14:0-rich diets (see Tables 2 and 3), took place even though $16:0 + 18:1$ caused a two-fold greater flux of apo B through the lipoprotein pool. These relationships are summarized in Figure 1.

As Figure 1 suggests, $16:0 + 18:1$ enhanced triglyceride synthesis and VLDL production, whereas $12:0 + 14:0$ reduced VLDL output but increased 'direct LDL' production. In the process of VLDL catabolism HDL is generated[14], and VLDL remnants return to the liver via the LDL receptor[15] (Figure 2). Thus clearance of the increased VLDL produced by $16:0 + 18:1$ depends on adequate LDLr activity[1,16]. The direct production of LDL generally has been considered to be a minor component of hepatic lipoprotein secretion on other occasions[1,15], but these studies provide the first evidence that direct LDL production may be a major factor in the expansion of the LDL pool by specific saturated fatty acids, notably $12:0 + 14:0$. As discussed elsewhere[5,13], it is likely that 14:0 was responsible for most of the effect.

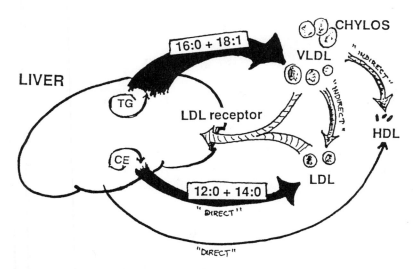

Figure 2 Using the diet comparison described by Figure 1, the relative impact of dietary $12:0 + 14:0$ vs. an equal caloric exchange with $16:0 + 18:1$ on lipoprotein metabolism is depicted. While $16:0 + 18:1$ enhance VLDL production, $12:0 + 14:0$ favour the 'direct' production of LDL and down-regulation of the LDL receptor. Under normal circumstances increased VLDL production and catabolism would increase the indirect generation of HDL with rapid clearance of VLDL remnants via the LDL receptor. Any circumstance that down-regulates the LDL receptor would potentially slow VLDL remnant clearance, resulting in increased LDL and decreased indirect generation of HDL

Hepatic mRNA abundance

To further investigate this metabolic scenario at the molecular level, similar dietary fat blends (although representing only 13% energy from fat) were fed to Syrian hamsters, and certain hepatic mRNAs associated with cholesterol metabolism were measured. In the first study[16] we found that 18:1 greatly increased apo A1 mRNA and LDLr mRNA abundance compared to oils containing 20:5n3, and to a lesser extent, 18:2n6 (Figure 3). A subsequent study[17] also revealed that the highest apo A1 (HDL) and LDLr mRNA abundance was associated with the 16:0+18:1-rich diets compared to several others, including 12:0+14:0 and an American Fat Blend rich in 14:0 (Table 4).

Collectively, these observations in monkeys and hamsters point to a major metabolic disparity resulting from consumption of 14:0 vs. 16:0-rich fats. Not only is the cholesterolaemia greater with 14:0, but the distribution of cholesterol among lipoproteins appeared to differ such that dietary 14:0 tended to increase LDL (in both monkeys and hamsters) more than HDL, i.e. the opposite of the 16:0+18:1 effect. It is not entirely clear at this point whether 16:0 or 18:1 are equal, or whether one is selectively more important than the other in the HDL response. Although the second monkey study[5] (where 12:0+14:0 and 16:0 were exchanged) implied that 16:0 alone might induce these positive changes (Table 3) the mRNA data in hamsters suggested that 18:1 provided the greatest mRNA abundance for the LDLr and apo A1[16,17]

Table 4 Relative abundance of mRNA in hamsters fed different fat blends[a]

Criterion	Dietary fat blend[b]					
	19	20	21	22	23	24
Apo A1 mRNA (% of control)						
Liver	$91\pm7^{e\text{-}h}$	$112\pm5^{d,g}$	115 ± 6^{e}	$118\pm4^{c,f}$	115 ± 6^{h}	$100\pm4^{c,d}$
Gut	$90\pm10^{c\text{-}e}$	119 ± 12^{c}	119 ± 11^{d}	113 ± 12	131 ± 10^{e}	100 ± 11
Apo E mRNA (% of control)						
Liver	104 ± 5	111 ± 5	121 ± 7^{c}	$123\pm7^{d,e}$	110 ± 7^{e}	$100\pm8^{c,d}$
Gut	108 ± 3	108 ± 3	102 ± 5	105 ± 6	113 ± 7	100 ± 12
Apo B mRNA (% of control)						
Liver	95 ± 8^{d}	$125\pm10^{c,d}$	109 ± 6	112 ± 6	112 ± 6	$100\pm9c$
Gut	118 ± 5	125 ± 14	130 ± 8	125 ± 8	120 ± 12	100 ± 12
LDLr mRNA (% of control)						
Liver	$137\pm16^{c,h,i}$	$141\pm23^{d,j}$	$158\pm20^{e,h,j,k}$	$154\pm19^{f,i}$	$142\pm14^{g,k}$	$100\pm11^{c\text{-}g}$
Gut	103 ± 15	127 ± 14	119 ± 7	117 ± 11	128 ± 17	100 ± 16

[a] Adapted from[17]. Values are mean $\pm$ SD ($n=10$ per diet).
[b] See legend to Table 1 for description of fat blend and the fatty acid composition.
[c,d,e,f,g,h,i,j,k]Mean values sharing a common superscript in a given row are significantly different by a one-factor ANOVA ($p<0.05$).

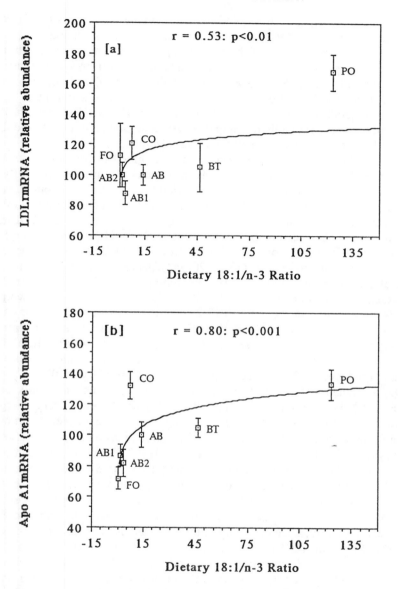

Figure 3 Regression analysis (log) of the hepatic mRNA abundance for the LDL receptor and apo A1 against independent dietary fatty acid variables, revealed the depressing effect of n3 fatty acids and stimulating effect of 18:1 on both LDL receptor (top) and apo A1 (below). The dietary fats represented are AB1 (5% American Fat Blend: fish oil, 4:1), AB2 (5% American Fat Blend: fish oil 3:2), BT (5% beef tallow); PO (5% palm oil), CO (5% canola oil). Fish oil was MAXEPA®

(Figure 3, Table 4), the latter reflecting HDL synthesis. Work is in progress to separate these potential differences in animal models and humans.

It is noteworthy that one of the most complete descriptions of the plasma cholesterol response to individual dietary fatty acids covering a wide range in fat saturation in humans[3] (2 years, 36 diets) also distinguished between 14:0 and 16:0, identifying 14:0 as four times more cholesterolaemic than 16:0. But a subsequent study by these same investigators using semisynthetic fats[18], led them to conclude that their original observations were incomplete and that 12:0, 14:0, and 16:0 were equally cholesterolaemic.

Having obtained these monkey data, which agreed in principle with the Hegsted and Keys regression equations in humans (Figure 4), especially if 16:0 was considered neutral, we were puzzled by the inference from current reports[4,6,19] that 18:1 was as effective as 18:2 in human diets in terms of its cholesterol-lowering ability. At the same time 18:1 did not exert the HDL-depressing effect often seen with high levels of 18:2. An HDL-enhancing effect would be consistent with our data, i.e. 18:1 drives apo A1 mRNA abundance whereas increasing polyenes (18:2, 20:5n3) decrease apo A1 (Figure 3). Several reports demonstrate that the circulating HDL shows a modest but persistent decline between 3% and 30% dietary kcals as 18:2, with a significant decline detectable when 18:2 reaches approximately 20% or more dietary energy[20]. However, the Keys and Hegsted regressions and our data in monkeys and hamsters would suggest that 18:1 is rather neutral in its ability to lower plasma cholesterol, at least when counteracting the cholesterol elevation induced by dietary saturated fatty acids (especially 14:0).

Our explanation for this discrepancy involves the concept of fatty acid 'thresholds', i.e. the amount of any fatty acid (as a percent dietary energy) above or below which its presence either begins or ceases to exert an impact on cholesterol metabolism[27] (Figure 5). Evaluation of the discrepancy between the Keys and Hegsted data and more recent studies[4,6,19] concerning the impact of 18:1 suggest that the latter studies exchanged 18:1 for 18:2 above the critical 'threshold' for 18:2. This threshold relationship is readily discerned in the regression of the plasma cholesterol response against the dietary 18:2% en for human or monkey data (Figure 6). In other words, in recent human studies a relatively high percentage of dietary energy was fed as 18:2 (above it's 6% en 'threshold') in the relative absence of 14:0 in the saturated fat pool. By contrast, Keys and Hegsted typically examined the 18:1 for 18:2 exchange between 1 and 6% energy with normal to exaggerated levels of 14:0 often present in the diet, 14:0 tending to raise the total cholesterol substantially as discussed above. Since 14:0 reportedly decreases the LDLr activity[21,22] in addition to causing 'direct' LDL production[13], its absence in the diet would mean that minimal dietary 18:2 is needed to assure maximal LDLr activity, allowing a neutral fatty acid such as 18:1 to appear to be as efficient as 18:2 when the saturated fat load is insignificant (Figure 5). Specifically, when the

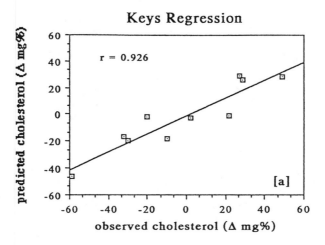

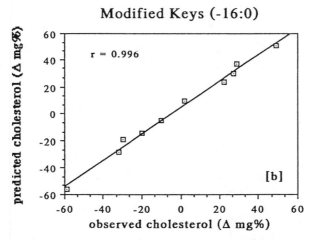

Figure 4 Correlations between the predicted vs. the observed plasma cholesterol values are depicted. Predicted values were generated using the regular Keys regression equation (a) or a modified version (b) in which palmitic acid (16:0) was considered neutral. The data points (taken from Table 3) represent the mean changes for three species of monkeys with comparisons between all possible combinations for the five dietary fat blends examined

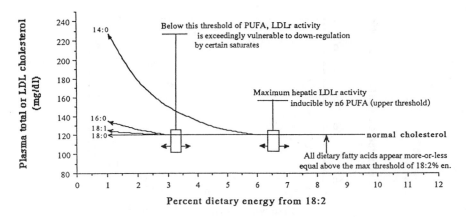

Figure 5 In the above scenario the fatty acid 'threshold' refers to the concentration of a dietary fatty acid (as percent dietary energy) above or below which its presence or absence in the diet will modulate cholesterol metabolism as reflected in the total plasma cholesterol or LDL/HDL ratio. According to the above scheme the threshold for linoleic acid (18:2) would vary depending on the relative concentration of other fatty acids in the diet, particularly the amount and chain length of dietary saturates (14:0, 16:0, 18:0). Although generated on the basis of data from normocholesterolaemic monkeys fed a common diet in which only the dietary fat composition varied, it is conceivable (probable) that any threshold will vary depending on other related factors impacting LDL receptor activity, such as the type of dietary protein, level of fat, type of carbohydrate, fibre content, dietary cholesterol load and the inherent LDL receptor status of the host

exchange is made above the 6% energy 'threshold' for 18:2, this residual 6% en as 18:2 is more than enough to exert a maximal cholesterol lowering effect no matter what other fatty acids (except 14:0) are present. Thus substituting 18:1 'seems equivalent' to 18:2 because the plasma cholesterol (i.e. LDL) will not decline further based on the mix of saturates and unsaturates present in the diet. According to this reasoning, at least two factors need to be considered in future studies of dietary fat saturation: 1) the nature of the 'challenge' contributed by each saturated fatty acid, with the percent energy from 14:0 being most critical and 2) the counterbalance or 'threshold' percent energy contributed by polyenes, primarily 18:2 in the typical diet.

If one examines this relationship carefully in the study best designed to expose it[3], 14:0 appears to have 3–4× the cholesterol-elevating power that 18:2 has for reducing it. Hegsted[3] used percent energy contributed by each fatty acid to express this relationship, which is probably the best procedure when dietary fat represents 30–40% of total energy. This relationship between key fatty acids is consistent with the analysis of our cebus data collected for 13 cholesterol-free diets (Hayes and Khosla, unpublished observations). When

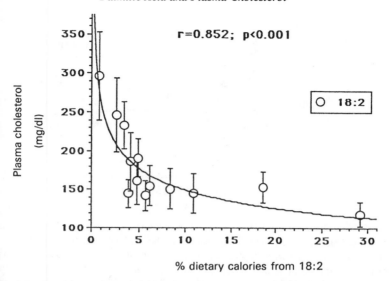

Figure 6 The correlation of the percent dietary energy from linoleic acid (18:2) plotted against the observed plasma cholesterol concentration in cebus monkeys reveals a threshold for 18:2 at 5–6% en. Values shown are the mean±SD. The data were obtained from a total of 16 monkeys with 4–10 monkeys rotated through 13 different cholesterol-free purified diets (diets 1, 2, and 8–18, Table 1) for 6–12 week periods. For each diet, the 18:2 content (as a percentage of total fatty acids, Table 1) was multiplied by the percent energy contributed by the dietary fat (31% or 40% energy) to calculate the percent energy contributed by 18:2

the dietary 18:2/14:0 ratio was examined (Figure 7), these two dietary fatty acids explained 78% of the variation in total plasma cholesterol and 88% of the LDL/HDL ratio response, relationships that were scarcely improved by adding several other fatty acids into the regression. This relationship presumably reflects the impact on LDLr activity, i.e. the receptors would be 'maximally up-regulated' during high intake of 18:2 and minimal intake of 14:0 or 'maximally shut down' during high intake of 14:0 and minimal consumption of 18:2. Because of the disparate power of these two fatty acids, presumably on LDLr activity and 'direct' production of LDL, minimal 14:0 requires considerable 18:2 to balance it. Thus 0.5% en as 14:0 may require as much as 3–4% en as 18:2, whereas 1–2% 14:0 may require 6–8% of 18:2 to counter its impact. In a practical sense 14:0 seldom represents more than 2.5% energy in the human diet, so the upper 18:2 'threshold' should never exceed about 12% energy in the worst-case scenario. This is conjecture at this point since a direct test across sufficient ratios has never been examined in any species, and other dietary factors, such as cholesterol, fibre, protein, etc., and the inherent host LDLr status, presumably affect the relationship.

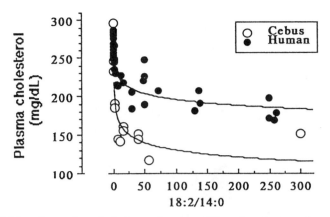

Figure 7 The observed total cholesterol concentrations in cebus monkeys and humans are regressed against the percent dietary energy as the 18:2/14:0 ratio. This ratio provided the simplest, most predictive expression of the relationship and suggests that maximum lowering of cholesterol is achieved when the ratio is 10 or more. The monkey data represent 13 cholesterol-free diets (see legend to Figure 6). The human data (representing 36 diets) are taken from Hegsted *et al.*[3]. In the latter study, diets also contributed 110–686 mg cholesterol per day

We examined the 18:1 vs. 18:2 relationship along with 16:0 in monkeys[26], feeding the atypical fatty acid profiles (diets 16–18, Table 1) present in the Mattson–Grundy diets[4]. The results were both revealing and supportive of the above hypothesis, exposing the importance of the host status (LDLr activity) as another potential variable in such studies (Figure 8). As implied by our previous data[5] and the Hegsted regression equation[3], 18:1 and 16:0 were essentially neutral and similar, whereas the 18:2-rich safflower oil diet (32% energy as 18:2) induced a significantly lower cholesterol level (due to a decrease in HDL) in the more sensitive cebus monkey, but not in rhesus. In essence, *without* 14:0 or cholesterol in the diet and with adequate 18:2 present (at or above its critical threshold) the plasma cholesterol does not increase in normocholesterolaemic individuals fed 16:0. Nor does 18:1 lower the cholesterol more than 16:0 or 18:0 under such circumstances. Furthermore, if one examines the literature carefully, in no case does 18:1 lower an elevated plasma cholesterol level as effectively as 18:2 if the exchange with 18:1 takes place below the critical 'threshold' of 18:2 needed for the mix of saturates in the diet.

Puzzled by the discrepancy between the monkey data[26] and the Mattson–Grundy human data[4], we re-examined the latter with the idea that the host status may have influenced the plasma lipid response, especially since the human population studied was hypercholesterolaemic. When the plasma cholesterol response was separated into high, medium, or low responders to the 'saturated fat' (i.e. palm oil), the low responders (cholesterol values less

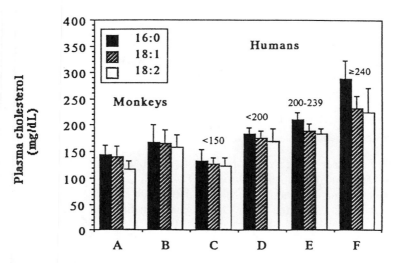

Figure 8 Comparison of the effects of dietary 16:0, 18:1 and 18:2 on plasma cholesterol concentrations in primates. A and B represent data from cebus and rhesus monkeys, respectively[26]. C to F represent human data obtained from the literature: C, reference 25; D to F, reference 4. The human data represent both normocholesterolaemic subjects[25] and hypercholesterolaemic subjects[4]. The mean plasma cholesterol of the normocholesterolaemic subjects at the time of study was 166 ± 29 mg/dl ($n=12$) and for the hypercholesterolaemic subjects this value was 263 ± 50 mg/dl ($n=20$). In plotting D to F, the 20 hypercholesterolaemic subjects were grouped into the indicated categories (<200 mg/dl, $n=7$; 200–239 mg/dl, $n=7$; ≥ 240 mg/dl, $n=6$) based on the plasma cholesterol concentrations measured after consumption of the 16:0-rich diet. Values are means $\pm$ SD. Only in subjects with total cholesterol above 200 mg/dl does 16:0 appear more cholesterolaemic than 18:1 or 18:2.

than 200 mg/dl during palm oil) also revealed similar total cholesterol responses during 18:1 and 18:2 consumption (Figure 8). Only as the total plasma cholesterol increased above 200 mg/dl did 16:0 appear more cholesterolaemic than 18:1 or 18:2. The point we would make, referring again to Figure 2 and the role that the LDLr plays in controlling the size of the LDL pool and, ultimately, the total cholesterol pool, is that down-regulation of the LDL receptor associated with polygenic hypercholesterolaemia[10] would deter clearance of the VLDL remnant by the liver. This would increase VLDL conversion to LDL and further expand the LDL pool. The above scenario also suggests that the influence of fat saturation on cholesterol metabolism would be biased by the presence of cholesterol in the diet because absorbed cholesterol would tend to down-regulate the LDL receptor, thereby affecting the extent to which a given saturated fatty acid would appear cholesterolaemic. For example, under these conditions the increased VLDL production[13] associated with $16:0 + 18:1$ would lead to cholesterolaemia. Numerous examples of this dietary cholesterol effect are reported, including recent examples in hamsters[23] and monkeys[24].

The implication of these various studies suggests the need to focus our attention on individual dietary fatty acid relationships rather than dietary fats or aggregates of saturates and polyenes.

Acknowledgements

The studies described herein were supported in part by Best Foods (Union, NJ), Mead Johnson Nutrition Division (Evansville, IN), National Livestock and Meat Board (Chicago, IL), National Institute of Health – DK #35375 (Bethesda, MD), and the Palm Oil Research Institute of Malaysia (Kuala Lumpur, Malaysia). We are grateful to Drs. Zouhair Stephan, Deborah Diersen-Schade and George Patton for their contribution to these studies.

References

1. Grundy, S.M. and Denke, M.A. (1990). Dietary influences on serum lipids and lipoproteins. *J. Lipid Res.*, **31**, 1149–72
2. Keys, A., Anderson, J.T. and Grande, F. (1957). Prediction of serum cholesterol responses of man to changes in fats in the diet. *Lancet*, **2**, 959–66
3. Hegsted, D.M., McGandy, R.B., Myers, M.L. and Stare, F.J. (1965). Quantitative effects of dietary fat on serum cholesterol in man. *Am. J. Clin. Nutr.*, **17**, 281–95
4. Mattson, F.H. and Grundy, S.M. (1985). Comparison of effects of dietary saturated, monounsaturated, and polyunsaturated fatty acids on plasma lipids and lipoproteins in man. *J. Lipid Res.*, **26**, 194–202
5. Hayes, K.C., Pronczuk, A., Lindsey, S. and Diersen-Schade, D. (1991). Dietary saturated fatty acids (12:0, 14:0, 16:0) differ in their impact on plasma cholesterol and lipoproteins in nonhuman primates. *Am. J. Clin. Nutr.*, **53**, 491–8
6. Mensink, R.P. and Katan, M.B. (1989). Effect of a diet enriched with monounsaturated or polyunsaturated fatty acids on levels of low-density and high-density lipoprotein cholesterol in healthy women and men. *N. Engl. J. Med.*, **321**, 436–41
7. Hayes, K.C. (1989). Dietary saturated fatty acids and low density or high density lipoprotein cholesterol (letter to the editor). *N. Engl. J. Med.*, **322**, 402–4
8. Berns, M.A.M., de Vries, J.H.M. and Katan, M.B. (1989). Increases in body fatness as a major determinant of changes in serum total cholesterol and HDL in young men over a ten year period. *Am. J. Epidemiol.*, **130**, 1109–22
9. Denke, M.A., Sampos, C.T. and Grundy, S.M. (1990). Excess body weight: an unrecognized cause of high blood cholesterol. *Circulation*, **82**, (Suppl. III), Abstract 228
10. Grundy, S.M. and Vega, G.L. (1985). Influence of mevinolin on metabolism of low density lipoproteins in primary moderate hypercholesterolemia. *J. Lipid Res.*, **26**, 1464–75
11. Blankenhorn, D.H., Nessim, S.A., Johnson, R.L., Sanmarco, M.E., Azen, S.P. and Cashin-Hemphill, L. (1987). Beneficial effects of combined cholestipol–niacin

therapy on coronary atherosclerosis and coronary venous bypass grafts. *J. Am. Med. Assoc.*, **257**, 3233–40

12. Pronczuk, A., Stephan, Z.F., Patton, G. and Hayes, K.C. (1991). Species variation in the atherogenic profile of monkeys: Relationship between dietary fats, lipoproteins, and platelet aggregation. *Lipids*, **26**, 213–22

13. Khosla, P. and Hayes, K.C. (1991). Dietary fat saturation in rhesus monkeys affects LDL concentrations by modulating the independent production of LDL apolipoprotein B. *Biochim. Biophys. Acta*, **1083**, 46–56

14. Tall, A.R. (1990). Plasma high density lipoproteins. Metabolism and relation to atherogenesis. *J. Clin. Invest.*, **86**, 379–84

15. Havel, R.J. (1984). The formation of LDL: mechanisms and regulation. *J. Lipid Res.*, **25**, 1570–6

16. Hayes, K.C., Lindsey, S., Pronczuk, A. and Dobbs, S. (1988). Dietary 18:1/18:2 ratio correlates highly with hepatic FC and mRNAs for apo A1, apo E and the LDL receptor. *Circulation*, **78**, (Suppl. 14), Abstract 0383, pII–96

17. Lindsey, S., Benattar, J., Pronczuk, A. and Hayes, K.C. (1990). Dietary palmitic acid (16:0) enhances HDL cholesterol and LDL receptor mRNA abundance in hamsters. *Proc. Soc. Exp. Biol. Med.*, **195**, 261–9

18. McGandy, R.B., Hegsted, D.M. and Meyers, M.L. (1970). Use of semisynthetic fats in determining the effects of specific dietary fatty acids on serum lipids in man. *Am. J. Clin. Nutr.*, **23**, 1288–98

19. Chan, J.K., Bruce, V.M. and McDonald, B.E. (1991). Dietary α-linolenic acid is as effective as oleic and linoleic acid in lowering blood cholesterol in normolipidemic men. *Am. J. Clin. Nutr.*, **53**, 1230–4

20. Shepherd, J., Packard, C.J., Patsch, J.R., Gotto, A.M. Jr. and Taunton, O.D. (1978). Effects of dietary polyunsaturated and saturated fat on the properties of high density lipoproteins and the metabolism of apolipoprotein A–1. *J. Clin. Invest.*, **61**, 1582–92

21. Spady, D.K. and Dietschy, J.M. (1988). Interaction of dietary cholesterol and triglycerides in the regulation of hepatic low density lipoprotein transport in the hamster. *J. Clin. Invest.*, **81**, 300–9

22. Nicolosi, R.J., Stucchi, A.F., Kowala, M.C., Hennessy, L.K., Hegsted, D.M. and Schaefer, E.J. (1990). Effect of dietary fat saturation and cholesterol on LDL composition and metabolism. In vivo studies of receptor and nonreceptor-mediated catabolism of LDL in cebus monkeys. *Arteriosclerosis*, **10**, 119–28

23. Ohtani, H., Hayashi, K., Hirata, Y., Dojo, S., Nakashima, K., Nishio, E., Kurushima, H., Saeki, M. and Kajiyama, G. (1990). Effects of dietary cholesterol and fatty acids on plasma cholesterol level and hepatic lipoprotein metabolism. *J. Lipid Res.*, **31**, 1413–22

24. Rudel, L.L., Haines, J.L. and Sawyer, J.K. (1990). Effects on plasma lipoproteins of monounsaturated, saturated, and polyunsaturated fatty acids in the diet of African green monkeys. *J. Lipid Res.*, **31**, 1873–82

25. Becker, N., Illingworth, D.R., Alaupovic, P., Connor, W.E. and Sunberg, E.E. (1983). Effects of saturated, monounsaturated, and ω-6 polyunsaturated fatty acids on plasma lipids, lipoproteins, and apoproteins in humans. *Am. J. Clin. Nutr.*, **37**, 355–60

26. Khosla, P. and Hayes, K.C. (1992). Comparison between the effects of dietary saturated (16:0), monounsaturated (18:1), and polyunsaturated (18:2) fatty acids on plasma lipoprotein metabolism in cebus and rhesus monkeys fed cholesterol-free diets. *Am. J. Clin. Nutr.*, **55**, in press

Discussion

Dr Vega: In your studies of the comparison of the effects of the 16 and 18 fatty acids vs. the 14 and 12 there was a marked rise in the triglyceride levels in the monkeys. I wonder if you have measured the activity of lipoprotein lipase and hepatic lipase in the $16:0 + 18:1$ vs. the $14:0 + 12:0$ groups. A change in enzyme activity would account for an apparent increase in the production of VLDL and rechannelling of apo B from the LDL pathway to the VLDL pathway.

Dr Hayes: No, we have not measured the lipases. We have noted that increase in plasma triglycerides characteristically when we feed the 16:0-rich diets. We suspect, on the basis of the data I presented, that the triglyceridaemia is due primarily to a production increase. Previous data exist in humans and animals that show lipase activity is decreased with saturated fat (*Metabolism*, 1970, **19**, 1020). That study measured lipoprotein lipase, not hepatic lipase.

Dr Connor: I think your data are very interesting and perhaps illustrate that saturated fats act differently upon the plasma cholesterol level, as you indicated, depending on the species of animals. We found that saturated fat feeding to rabbits, a species which is very sensitive to dietary cholesterol, had a negligible effect in the rabbit. The exception was coconut oil. Cocoa butter, the fat of chocolate, had no effect. I wonder if you fed a small amount of dietary cholesterol as Dr Dietschy did in his studies if there would be harmony between your data and his data?

Dr Hayes: That is a good point. We think the response to fatty acids depends not only upon species, but more critically on the LDL receptor 'setpoint' in the individual (or species) which depends on genetics as well as environmental factors. For example, Rudel (*J. Lipid Res.*, 1990, **31**, 1873) fed the Mattson–Grundy dietary fats to his African green monkeys with a high level of cholesterol, approximately five times the intake of what you and I would eat. In this situation he was able to show, depending on when he measured the levels of lipoproteins, that 16:0 was cholesterolaemic relative to 18:1, which was higher than 18:2. This makes the point that if you alter the LDL receptor activity, either by feeding cholesterol to African green monkeys or due to genetic differences such as those attributable to the genetic makeup of rats or rabbits, the dietary fatty acids can exert a different impact depending on the LDL receptor set-point at the time. Furthermore, the fatty acids are probably interacting with each other to influence cholesterol metabolism. In everyday physiology, the body deals with these interactions. I suspect we have a lot to learn about these interrelationships because we do not eat tripalmitin or tristearin or trilaurin, we eat mixtures of fats and oils.

14
The potential health aspects of lipid oxidation products in food

P.B. ADDIS and G.J. WARNER

Introduction

The idea that some of the products of *in vivo* lipid oxidation are deleterious to human health is not new. However, the concept that *dietary* lipid oxidation products and thermally altered lipids are injurious has attracted much interest recently and is the subject of this review. Regulatory activity by government agencies in the EEC has already occurred with rather tight controls placed on the degree of oil and shortening deterioration permitted during deep-frying. The US Food and Drug Administration (FDA) has been researching 'process-induced' toxic products such as the cholesterol oxidation products and also has an interest in determining any potentially deleterious effects on consumers of consumption of French-fried foods, especially if fried in heavily used, deteriorated oils, shortenings and tallows.

On balance, and in spite of the interest of regulatory agencies, the possible health aspects of lipid oxidation products remain highly controversial. Two excellent examples of the controversial nature of dietary lipid oxides are the areas of research dealing with possible toxic effects of heated fats and, a related area, the possible role of dietary cholesterol oxides and fatty acid oxidation products in coronary heart disease (CHD). On the heated-fat issue, numerous publications, in some cases published as early as the 1930s, reported toxic effects in rats consuming heated fats. Other studies showed no effects or no serious effects if reduced levels of heated fats were fed. Although it is difficult to know whether a consensus may have been reached by researchers on the heated-fat issue, a number of authors have opined that, where deleterious effects were seen, the studies did not reflect the practical situation of a restaurant for two reasons:

This article was first published in *Free Radicals and Food Additives*, Aruoma, O.I. and Halliwell, B. (eds.), Ch. 5, pp. 77–119, reproduced by permission of Taylor and Francis Ltd.

(1)   levels of heated fats fed were unrealistically high; and

(2)   fats were heated far more severely than would be the case in a restaurant.

However, recent studies will be cited to challenge the conclusion concerning the benign nature of abused oils on two accounts.

In the first place, it must be recognised that in the earlier studies the pathological end-points used were crude. In no work that the authors are aware of was arterial injury, atherosclerosis, or other phenomena related to CHD included. Yet, in recent years much evidence has accumulated on a lipid oxidation product – CHD connection. Secondly, research has also demonstrated that the levels of most atherogenic chemicals found in heated fats may in fact be reduced (when extremely abusive heat treatments are employed), by being replaced by dimers, trimers and polymers of fatty acids and triglycerides. The possible atherogenicity of the latter group of lipids has not been assessed. Clearly, it is time to re-examine the abused- or heated-fat issue using more precise and realistic heat treatments, relevant levels of intake, and appropriate pathological end-points.

A second but closely related area of intense debate and controversy deals with the relative atherogenicity of lipids vs. oxidation products of lipids, *viz.* cholesterol vs. cholesterol oxides and fatty acids vs. fatty acid hydroperoxides and/or secondary oxidation products. Of course, superimposed upon the foregoing questions are the sometimes acrimonious debates about the degree to which diet influences serum cholesterol and the degree to which serum cholesterol is related to CHD. The viewpoint that hypercholesterolaemia is an epidemic in most Western countries and is the primary cause of CHD (the lipid hypothesis) is promoted by the National Heart, Lung and Blood Institute (NHLBI) and the American Heart Association (AHA). In the face of severe criticism the NHLBI and AHA have steadfastly supported the 'lipid hypothesis' and have, in terms of funding, studiously ignored other promising areas of research such as dietary lipid oxidation products.

A very large number of research publications support the idea that oxidized lipids are far more deleterious to arterial health than the native lipids themselves. Therefore, cholesterol is viewed as harmless unless it is converted to one or more of a number of autoxidation products. However, here again unanimity is not to be found and one of our objectives is to explore both sides of this important issue.

Many more deleterious effects, and some potentially beneficial effects of oxidized lipids have been reported. Cancer, membrane effects, enzyme effects, mutagenicity, and cytoxicity are suggested. In many cases, the foregoing effects are interrelated: atherogenicity may be based on cytotoxicity which, in turn, is possibly caused by a combination of membrane and enzyme disturbances. In addition, numerous other related phenomena complicate these issues. As is true for most food chemical toxicological issues, the nutritional status of the subjects being studied is important – especially with regard to antioxidant nutrients. Therefore, yet another complicating issue (nutrition) is superimposed on the question of lipid oxidation products and health. Other factors which complicate the determination of the health effect of lipid oxidation products include:

(1)   the complex multifactorial nature of many diseases;

(2)   the exponential increase in research publications related to the subject;

(3)   extensive advances in the knowledge of food chemistry and food analysis;

(4)   rapid advances in food processing;

(5)   the development of convenience foods;

(6)   the extended shelf-life expected of some foods; and

(7)   the alterations of some foods (ironically) to conform to a 'healthy' concept.

An example of (7) is the substitution of a more polyunsaturated fat for a saturated fat in a food. Such an alteration may lessen the hypercholesterolaemic properties of the food but at the same time increase its potential to form lipid oxidation products.

It is difficult to visualize all the possible ramifications of the research area represented in this chapter. It would also be easy to underestimate the importance of lipid oxidation product research to the health of the consumer, to long-term developments in food technology, and to future directions that research takes in medicine and nutrition.

Because of the great interest in health aspects of lipid oxidation products, several extensive reviews, some fairly recent, have been published and the authors have attempted to avoid simple reiteration of what has been published earlier. Rather, we have attempted to, in addition to reviewing the literature, emphasize the most recent studies, making some new connections between what might appear to be unrelated research. Reviews recommended to the serious student of health aspects of lipid oxidation products include Simic and Karel (1980); Smith (1981), Dhopeshwarkar (1981), Ross (1981), Addis *et al.* (1983), Alexander (1983), Finocchiaro and Richardson (1983), Addis (1986), Ross (1986), Smith (1987), Morin *et al.* (1987), Yagi (1987, 1988), Addis and Park (1989), Smith and Johnson (1989), and Steinberg *et al.* (1989).

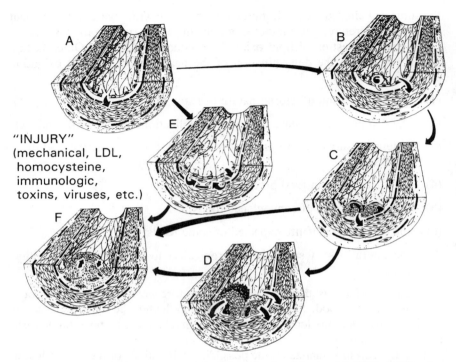

"INJURY"
(mechanical, LDL,
 homocysteine,
 immunologic,
 toxins, viruses, etc.)

Figure 1 The revised response-to-injury hypothesis. Advanced intimal proliferative lesions of atherosclerosis may occur by at least two pathways. The pathway demonstrated by the clockwise (long) arrows to the right has been observed in experimentally induced hypercholesterolaemia. Injury to the endothelium (A) may induce growth factor secretion (short arrow). Monocytes attach to endothelium (B), which may continue to secrete growth factors (short arrow). Subendothelial migration of monocytes (C) may lead to fatty-streak formation and release of growth factors such as PDGF (short arrow). Fatty streaks may become directly converted to fibrous plaques (long arrow from C to F) through release of growth factors from macrophages or endothelial cells or both. Macrophages may also stimulate or injure the overlying endothelium. In some cases macrophages may lose their endothelial cover and platelet attachment may occur (D), providing three possible sources of growth factors – platelets, macrophages, and endothelium (short arrows). Some of the smooth-muscle cells in the proliferative lesion itself (F) may form and secrete growth factors such as PDGF (short arrows). An alternative pathway for development of advanced lesions of atherosclerosis is shown by the arrows from A to E to F. In this case, the endothelium may be injured but remain intact. Increased endothelial turnover may result in growth-factor formation by endothelial cells (A). This may stimulate migration of smooth-muscle cells from the media into the intima, accompanied by endogenous production of PDGF by smooth muscle as well as growth factor secretion from the 'injured' endothelial cells (E). These interactions could then lead to fibrous-plaque formation and further lesion progression (F). From Ross (1986). Reproduced courtesy of *The New England Journal of Medicine*.

Coronary heart disease

Introduction

Coronary heart disease (CHD) is highly complex and its aetiology remains highly controversial. However, attempting to introduce newer concepts, for example, that lipids are less important than the corresponding lipid oxidation products, will further complicate the issue. Therefore, it is useful to cover CHD initially without including lipid oxidation products in the discussion.

The prevailing opinion, that atherosclerosis is simply an accumulation of cholesterol on arteries, has been clearly shown to be erroneous. Therefore, the 'lipid hypothesis' has become less well accepted by serious researchers and has been replaced by a competing hypothesis, i.e. 'response-to-injury' (see Figure 1). As will be seen, elements of both hypotheses are needed to explain CHD in sufficient detail for conducting adequate research, but the 'injury' hypothesis generally displays excellent concordance with the concept that dietary lipid oxides are a factor in CHD (Addis and Park, 1989).

There are two key hypotheses concerning the relationship of diet to CHD:

(1) dietary lipids are key factors in causing hypercholesterolaemia; and

(2) elevated serum cholesterol is a key risk factor in CHD.

Although the AHA and NHLBI have instituted extensive education programmes to convince Americans (on the one hand) that diet is a major cause of elevated blood cholesterol level in coronary heart disease, one major conclusion emanating from a review by Smith (1988) suggested that, diet, at best, is only negligibly related to CHD when considering a particular population. Most major blood epidemiological studies reveal an extremely weak relationship between blood cholesterol and CHD, often showing an increase in annual CHD rate of less than 1% across most, or all, of the blood cholesterol range. This suggests that diet cannot possibly have more than a very minor influence on CHD. It is worth noting that Smith's minimization of the role of diet refers only to dietary influence on CHD via the diet serum cholesterol connection. Diet may still have an important influence on CHD, but the specific factor(s) of importance need further clarification. For example, assume for the moment that dietary lipid oxides are a significant factor in CHD. The vast majority of research publications would indicate that the deleterious effects of lipid oxides are exerted via effects which are unrelated to an elevation of blood cholesterol.

In spite of the shortcomings of the diet–CHD hypothesis (Smith, 1988), traditional recommendations have included reducing dietary cholesterol and saturated fat, increasing consumption of vegetable oils and perhaps including some fish and fibre. Interestingly, many revisions have been necessary over the years. Hence, deep-fat-fried (low-fat) fish like the cod have given way to oily fish such as the salmon, trout and mackerel, prepared by poaching, broiling or baking. Also, it is now realized that vegetable shortening (primarily containing omega-6 (ω-6) fatty acids and a considerable amount of saturated fat) may not be an ideal lipid for prevention of CHD. Some of the newer concepts related to diet and hyperlipidaemia have been reviewed by Addis and Park (1989).

Certain animal products have been targeted as being contributors to CHD by the AHA and NHLBI, especially eggs, beef, lamb and pork. It is clearly difficult to justify the limitation placed on eggs based on the cholesterol content of *c.* 250 mg per yolk (Addis and Park, 1989). Likewise, an objective assessment of animal fats, which are very high in oleic and stearic acids, indicates that most of the fat present is hypocholesterolaemic, not hypercholesterolaemic (Smith, 1988; Addis and Park, 1989).

Nevertheless, in spite of all its shortcomings, the 'lipid-hypothesis' view of the diet–CHD relationship may have had some beneficial effects. The food and animal industries are actively developing numerous low-calorie, low-fat, low-cholesterol, high-fibre and fat-substituted foods which, on the whole, may be useful to the consumer. It is difficult to argue against reducing the fat and calorie content of foods and of diets, irrespective of one's view of the 'lipid hypothesis'. In most cases, lowering dietary lipid content will also result in reducing exposure of humans to lipid oxidation products.

To promote a clear understanding of CHD, as well as oxidation products as possible aetiogenic factors, Addis and Park (1989) divided CHD into three arbitrary phases: arterial injury, atherosclerosis and myocardial infarction, the latter phase induced by thrombosis and/or arterial spasm. The roles of lipids, lipid oxidation products, and other factors in each of the foregoing phases will be discussed. It is interesting to note that adverse effects of oxidation products have been reported for all three phases of CHD. Inquiry into other important biological effects will follow, but it must be emphasized that these effects may be closely related to the potential adverse influence on CHD of lipid oxidation products.

Arterial injury

The 'response-to-injury' hypothesis (Figure 1) is not new, being originally proposed by Virchow in 1856 (Ross, 1981) and, as it is currently viewed, begins with endothelial injury and includes a strong proliferative response from medial smooth-muscle cells (Ross, 1986). Intimal smooth-muscle cell hyperplasia appears to be a key mechanism of the intimal thickening which is the cause of the arterial wall thickening seen in atherosclerosis (Thomas and Kim, 1983). Table 1 summarizes, in an abbreviated manner, the incredibly

Table 1 Abbreviated and modified summary of temporal arterial changes in male pigtail monkeys (*Macaca nemestrina*) fed an atherogenic diet

Time (days)	Microanatomical site	Nature of alteration (atherogenesis)[1]
12	Luminal surface	Adherence of monocytes
30	Subendothelium; lumen	Protrusions, foam cells, covered by endothelium
60	Subendothelium	Increased foam cells; fatty streaks macroscopically visible
90	Subendothelium; endothelium	Increased number and diameter of foam cells; fatty streaks cause endothelial separation and release of foam cells into the circulation
120	Luminal surface; subendothelium	Continuation of all foregoing processes. Monocytes and platelets may begin recruitment of smooth-muscle cells out of the intima
150	Luminal surface; subendothelium	Fatty streaks throughout aortal tree; elastic fibres and collagen exposed; fibrous plaque; platelet thrombi; mural thrombi. Platelets secrete platelet-derived growth factor (PDGF), stimulating hyperplasia of smooth-muscle cells.
180–395	Intima and media and luminal surface	Increased involvement of smooth-muscle cells in foam cell and fatty streak formation. Fibrous plaque formation continues

[1]Control monkeys, fed a nonatherogenic diet, displayed some subendothelial macrophages, apparently functioning normally as scavengers. At day 90 of the experiment, plasma cholesterol was 124.1 ± 6.2 (mg dl^{-1}) for controls and 604.7 ± 15.1 for monkeys on atherogenic diet. Adapted from Faggiotto *et al.* (1984) and Faggiotto and Rose (1984).

complex series of pathological changes which culminate in a mature plaque, as revealed by the research of Faggiotto *et al.* (1984) and Faggiotto and Ross (1984). Briefly summarized, the endothelial injury evokes a response from circulating monocytes which attach to the endothelium, exhibit subendothelial migration, convert to macrophages and accumulate lipid, convert to foam cells, and form fatty streaks of sufficient thickness to disturb more of the overlying endothelium; recruitment of more monocytes and also platelets follows, then subendothelial migration, recruitment of smooth-muscle cells from the medial to the intimal layer, secretion of platelet-derived growth factor (PDGF), smooth-muscle-cell multiplication, and smooth-muscle-cell and macrophage conversion into foam cells. By this stage, plaque is well on its way to maturation and atherosclerosis, the sequel to arterial injury, is now the predominant phase of interest. Again, the arbitrary nature of the dividing line between the first two phases of CHD is apparent (Addis and Park, 1989).

However, the traditional thinking has low-density lipoprotein (LDL) playing a pivotal role by transporting lipid (chiefly cholesterol esters) into the arterial wall, facilitating foam cell formation, and it is for this reason that the primary strategy for reducing the risk of CHD has been to lower blood lipids, especially LDL.

Atherosclerosis

Lowering blood lipids through dietary modification will ostensibly lower LDL, reduce the amount of cholesterol available for foam cell formation and slow or perhaps even reverse some aspects of atherosclerosis so as to lessen the chances of clinical manifestation. Evidence favouring the foregoing hypothesis includes the studies involving feeding cholesterol to rabbits, human clinical trials including dietary modification and life-style changes, and epidemiological data. As is discussed later in this chapter, all three studies have serious shortcomings, but a fairly safe and moderate view, as it pertains to humans, probably would consider a prudent diet to be high in soluble fibre, low in total fat (30% of kcal) and low in saturated fat (<10% of kcal). A recent review of the role of dietary lipids in atherosclerosis has been published (Addis and Park, 1989).

Myocardial infarction

Either thrombosis or arterial spasm (or a combination) may cause a myocardial infarction. Without either thrombosis or spasm, arterial injury and atherosclerosis are rendered far less threatening from the clinical standpoint. Recent research has been centred, therefore, on the prevention of thrombosis and spasm by adjusting the fatty acid ω-6/ω-3 of the diet. The hypothesis that fish oils (ω-3) are beneficial in preventing CHD is based on the observations that ω-3 fatty acids alter eicosanoid metabolism so as to inhibit platelet aggregation and arterial spasm. Inhibition of platelet thrombosis and arterial spasm may well prevent atherosclerotic arteries from incurring myocardial infarction (Leaf and Weber, 1987, 1988; Addis and Park, 1989). Furthermore, considering the important role of platelets (PDGF) and monocytes in early stages of the disease, an interrupting or slowing of the atherosclerotic process may also be possible by increasing dietary ω-3 and/or decreasing ω-6 fatty acids (Leaf and Weber, 1987, 1988).

Modified LDL

In the foregoing brief coverage of the traditional views on CHD, the possible role of lipid oxidation products was omitted. This was done to maintain a coverage of CHD which is relevant to the views of both the NHLBI and AHA. However, there is a growing amount of evidence that dietary lipid oxidation products are a significant factor in CHD.

Recent reviews of modified LDL (mLDL) include those by Jurgens *et al.* (1987), Heinecke (1987) and Steinberg *et al.* (1989). Interest in mLDL (and dietary lipid oxidation products) has been stimulated in part by the fact that the relationship between serum cholesterol and CHD risk is far from perfect. Many exceptions occur over the entire range of serum cholesterol values (Addis and Park, 1989; Steinberg *et al.*, 1989). In recent years, interest has been focused on possible post-secretory modifications of LDL which might amplify its atherogenicity because of strong evidence that the LDL receptor (Brown and Goldstein, 1976) is not a factor in LDL uptake by diseased arteries. In familial hypercholesterolaemic (FH) patients, fatty streaks form in spite of a deficiency of LDL receptors. Also, macrophages and monocytes cannot be converted to foam cells incubated in culture with LDL. Relatively few LDL receptors occur and those that do occur are down-regulated, making it difficult to load sufficient cholesterol ester so as to convert macrophages into foam cells.

The first mLDL created *in vitro* was by Goldstein *et al.* (1979) who acetylated LDL to form a mLDL and noted greatly accelerated uptake by macrophages of mLDL over LDL. Later work demonstrated that cultured endothelial cells, smooth-muscle cells, monocytes and macrophages can modify LDL by oxidative mechanisms to form a variety of derivative LDLs, all of which have properties similar to the acetylated mLDL (for details see Steinberg *et al.*, 1989). Interestingly, the oxidative modification of LDL to form a mLDL can be inhibited by butylated hydroxytoluene (BHT) and vitamin E and may be inhibited by superoxide dismutase (for details see Addis and Park, 1989 and Steinberg *et al.*, 1989). At this point it must be suggested that the use of common food components and additives which are antioxidants (see also Chapter 6) could have a dual benefit: i.e. retardation of lipid oxidation in foods, reducing exposure to humans, and reducing *in vivo* formation of mLDL. Research is urgently needed on these possibilities and their potential practical significance.

The nature of the modification of LDL involves far more than lipid oxidation; indeed, the critical step involves covalent attachment of secondary lipid oxidation products of ε-amino groups of lysine residues of apolipoprotein B$_{100}$, a requirement for recognition by the scavenger receptor (Steinberg *et al.*, 1989). The scavenger receptor is not down-regulated, is specific for mLDL and is the primary mechanism of foam-cell production. Compounds

Table 2 Cholesterol oxidation products in oxidatively modified low-density lipoproteins

Sterol[1]	Control LDL[2]	OxLDL[3]
Cholesterol	687	358
7α-Hydroxycholesterol	—	56
Cholesterol-β-epoxide	—	48
Cholesterol-α-epoxide	—	21
7β-Hydroxycholesterol	—	60
Cholestanetriol	—	—
7-Ketocholesterol	—	181
25-Hydroxycholesterol	—	—

[1]Sterols expressed as μg sterol/mg LDL protein.
[2]Control LDL (200 μg) was incubated for 20 h at 37°C in phosphate-buffered saline pH=7.4) with 200 μM EDTA
[3]Oxidatively modified LDL (200 μg) was incubated for 20 h at 37°C in phosphate-buffered saline (pH = 7.4) with 5 μM CuSO$_4$.

commonly seen in lipid oxidation of foods, including malonaldehyde and 4-hydroxy-nonenal, are among those known to react with the ε-amino groups of lysine residues (Hoff *et al.*, 1989). Steinberg *et al.* (1989) state that cholesterol is oxidized during oxidative formation of mLDL, 'which could enhance its cytotoxicity and atherogenicity', and cites Peng and Taylor (1983). However, nowhere in the published scientific literature that the authors are aware of, is there a direct report of cholesterol oxidation products in oxidatively modified LDL. Representative data given in Table 2 show extensive oxidation of cholesterol in oxidatively modified LDL formed by *in vitro* incubation with copper. The work of Peng and Taylor (1983) has clearly demonstrated the cytotoxicity and atherogenicity of cholesterol oxidation products (but not their existence in mLDL). Clearly, the cytotoxicity of oxidatively modified LDL, an important factor in atherogenesis, involves the lipid oxidation products contained in it.

Steinberg *et al.* (1989) have reviewed the compelling evidence which favours the existence of mLDL *in vivo* and hypothesized several mechanisms whereby mLDL may accelerate atherosclerosis. Some of these mechanisms are incorporated in a modified manner in our own postulate outlined in Figure 2, the details of which are discussed later in this chapter. However, one of the mechanisms hypothesized by Steinberg *et al.* (1989) is important to consider in detail because it may provide a linkage to the possible role of dietary lipid oxidation products in LDL modification. Steinbrecher *et al.* (1984) and Palinksi *et al.* (1989) have provided excellent evidence that the plasma of rabbits and humans contain antibodies which react with mLDLs. Therefore, mLDL could be atherogenic by 'uptake' of immune complexes by macro-

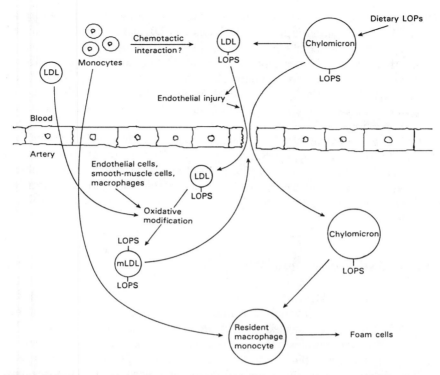

Figure 2 Scheme to illustrate postulated and hypothesized mechanisms whereby dietary lipid oxidation products (LOPS) could cause arterial injury and also accelerate foam cell production. This figure is modified from Steinberg *et al.* (1989) and uses concepts provided by them and by Taylor *et al.* (1979), Naruszewicz *et al.* (1987) and Yagi (1988)

phages through the Fc receptor. Lesser degrees of lysine conjugation with aldehydes are required to stimulate antibody formation than to generate a form of LDL recognized by the acetyl LDL receptor. Thus even small degrees of lysine modification may suffice to generate immune complex, leading to accelerated uptake by macrophages' (Steinberg *et al.*, 1989). We concur with this view and wonder whether or not dietary lipid oxidation products might be able to alter lysine residues to the extent that immunological properties are altered.

Ylä-Herttuala *et al.* (1989) demonstrated that LDLs isolated from athero-sclerotic lesions exhibit physical and chemical properties resembling those of oxidatively modified LDL (electrophoretic mobility, density, etc.) and different from those of plasma LDL. Immunological data have been reported supporting the hypothesis that lesion LDL is similar to oxidatively modified LDL. Also, lesion LDL and oxidatively modified LDL both produce greater stimulation of cholesterol esterification and were degraded more rapidly by macrophages compared to plasma LDL. Lesion LDL and oxidatively modified LDL were shown to be chemotactic for monocytes; plasma LDL was not.

Another line of evidence supporting the idea that oxidative modification of LDL is an important step in atherosclerosis is the presence of 'ceroid', an autofluorescent material noted in atherosclerotic intima, specifically in macrophages of atherosclerotic plaque (Ball *et al.*, 1987). The presence of ceroid records previous oxidative events.

Other, nonoxidative modifications of LDL are possible, including glycated LDL, discussed briefly by Steinberg *et al.* (1989), which may lead to accelerated macrophage uptake. For a comprehensive treatise on the subject of protein glycation in ageing, diabetes, atherosclerosis and an interesting discussion of 'autoxidative glycosylation', the reader is referred to Wolff *et al.* (1989).

Dietary lipid oxidation products

The area of research investigating the possible role of dietary lipid oxides in CHD has been one of low public profile. Nevertheless, an impressive number of publications have reported a great amount of data on this subject. The number of review articles published is quite large, indicating a great deal of interest on the part of biologists, food scientists, nutritionists and chemists.

The chemical structures of lipid oxidation products which commonly have been or are now being studied in relation to CHD (and other health effects) are shown in Figure 3. Also shown are some of the cyclic dimers and trimers formed in heated fats.

The investigations have focused primarily on fatty acid hydroperoxides and cholesterol oxides. Because of the central role thought to be played by cholesterol in CHD, cholesterol oxidation products have received the most attention and, therefore, are reviewed first. Fatty acid hydroperoxides and other peroxides and secondary products may be as important as cholesterol oxidation products, but methods for determining peroxides have been slower to develop. Heavy reliance on the thiobarbituric acid (TBA) method for peroxide determination, a very non-specific technique (Csallany *et al.*, 1984), limits what can be said about many of these studies.

Cholesterol oxidation products

A historical view of the cholesterol–atherosclerosis connection provides a fascinating account of how a single flawed experiment and equally flawed sequels can mislead medical science and the public. The relationship of these

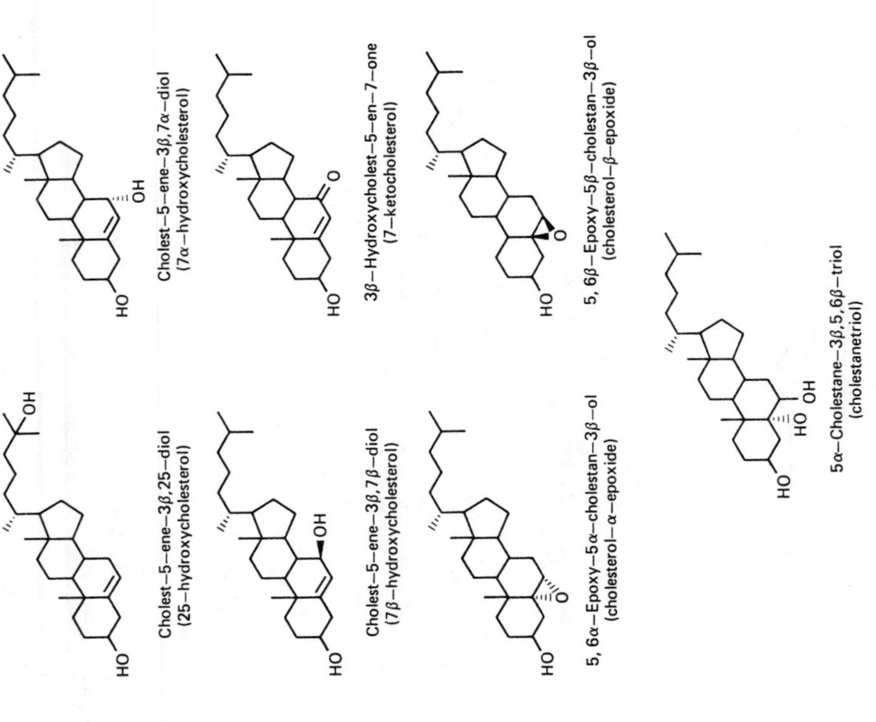

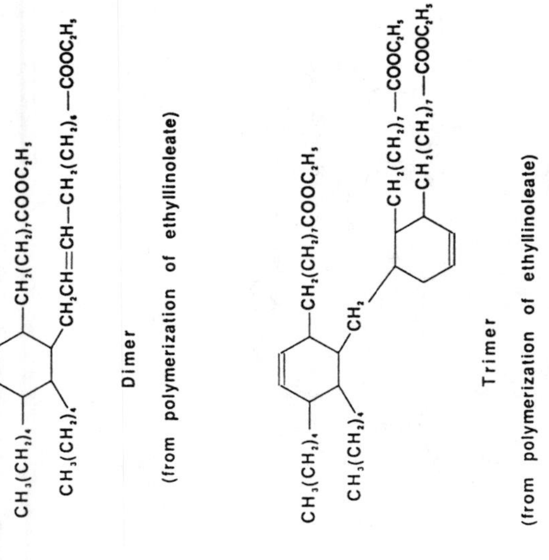

Figure 3 Names (IUPAC and common) and structures of cholesterol and lipid oxidation products

Dimer

(from polymerization of ethyllinoleate)

Trimer

(from polymerization of ethyllinoleate)

Cholest—5—ene—3β,7α—diol
(7α—hydroxycholesterol)

3β—Hydroxycholest—5—en—7—one
(7—ketocholesterol)

5, 6β—Epoxy—5β—cholestan—3β—ol
(cholesterol—β—epoxide)

Cholest—5—ene—3β,25—diol
(25—hydroxycholesterol)

Cholest—5—ene—3β,7β—diol
(7β—hydroxycholesterol)

5, 6α—Epoxy—5α—cholestan—3β—ol
(cholesterol—α—epoxide)

5α—Cholestane—3β,5,6β—triol
(cholestanetriol)

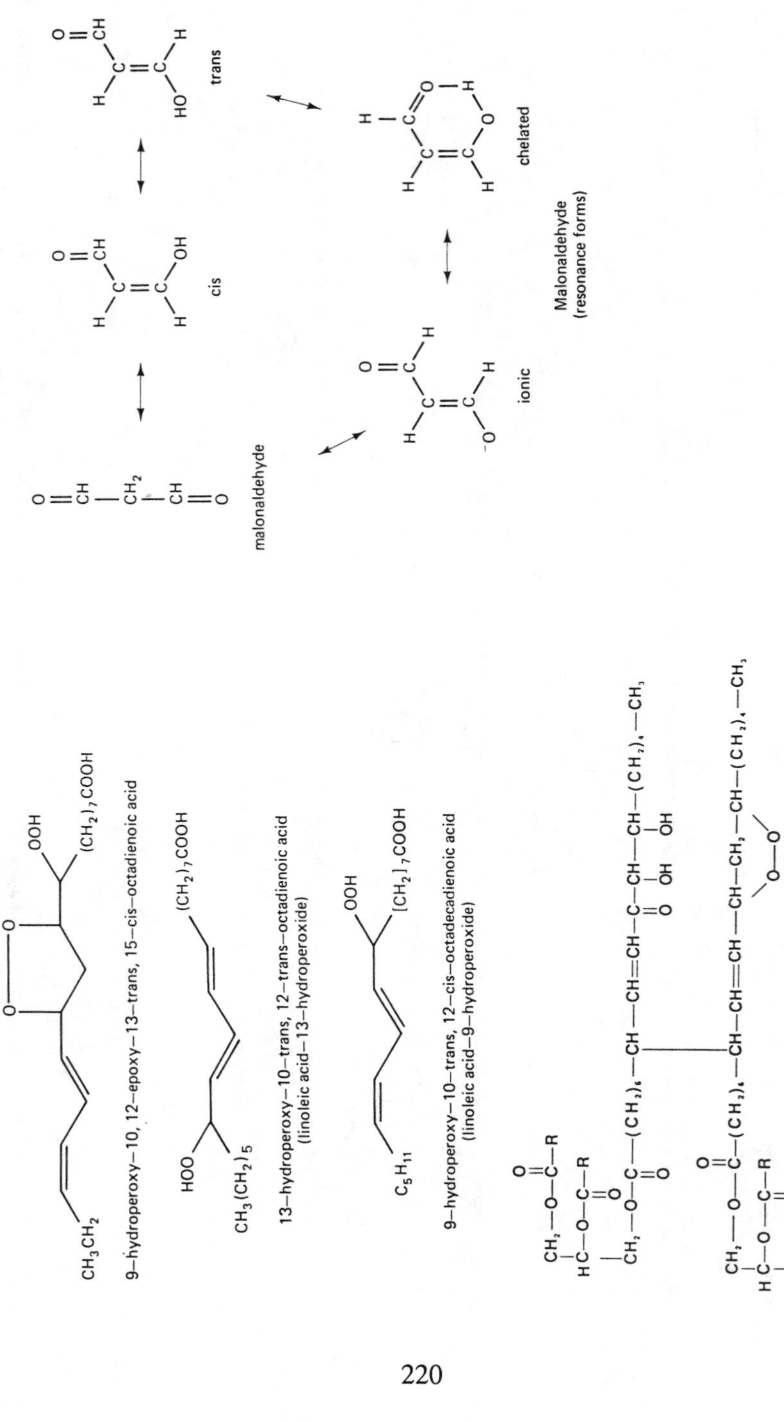

Figure 3 (continued)

events to the popularity of the lipid hypothesis of atherosclerosis over the past 50 years is also interesting.

In 1913, Anitschkow reported on one of the earliest studies of feeding cholesterol dissolved in vegetable oil to rabbits. He noted that cholesterol induced atherosclerosis. This type of experimental protocol has been employed frequently in animal models since Anitschkow's time. It is apparent that the countless publications in the scientific literature have had a great impact on how the medical community views cholesterol in the human diet. Whether one supported the injury hypothesis or the lipid hypothesis, cholesterol 'had become inextricably linked to atherosclerosis' (Addis and Park, 1989). Cholesterol was injurious to the artery and also was hypercholesterolaemic in the diet; therefore, both aspects of atherosclerosis were satisfied.

Unfortunately, researchers were slow to recognize the obvious, that cholesterol, an unsaturated lipid, is susceptible to autoxidation. The atherogenicity of cholesterol is thought to be due to contaminating cholesterol oxidation products. Pure cholesterol is not atherogenic, even in a sensitive animal such as the rabbit (Taylor *et al.*, 1979). Evidence obtained from human studies indicates a weak response to dietary cholesterol (Addis and Park, 1989). If humans are maintained on diets low in fat and saturated fat and high in fibre, long-term effects on plasma cholesterol levels (>8 weeks) of impressively large differences in dietary cholesterol are negligible, even in hypercholesterolaemic subjects (Edington *et al.*, 1987). Unfortunately, it is not likely that the AHA and NHLBI will soon recognize these foregoing facts about dietary cholesterol in humans, given the reluctance of these groups to recognize research which does not fit the AHA–NHLBI hypothesis on CHD (Smith, 1988). Of course, the foregoing comments on the benign nature of cholesterol in the diets of humans do not apply to cholesterol oxides. Our intent here is to focus attention on the difficulty in interpreting data on atherosclerosis obtained from studies which employed impure cholesterol sources such as powdered eggs, dried egg yolk or improperly stored USP cholesterol. Dried egg yolk in particular frequently contains high levels of both cholesterol oxidation products and cholesterol (Addis and Park, 1989).

Most of the research on cholesterol oxides has focused on early atherosclerosis, or arterial injury. Biological activities of cholesterol oxides possibly relevant to CHD include atherogenicity, angiotoxicity, cytotoxicity and enzyme effects. Cholesterol appears to be free of the effects of toxicity and is minimally able to influence activity of most enzymes studied, compared with cholesterol oxides and other oxysterols (Smith, 1987). However, a connection between the cytotoxic and, therefore, atherogenic effects of oxysterols and the initiation of atherosclerosis has been made which supports both the role of oxysterols in CHD and the injury hypothesis at the same time.

Structures of the most frequently studied cholesterol oxides are shown in Figure 3. Cholestanetriol and 25-hydroxycholesterol have been established by early studies to be the most atherogenic of the oxysterols studied (Taylor *et al.*, 1979). Peng *et al.* (1985a) attempted to describe the ultrastructural details of endothelial damage caused by cholesterol oxidation products. Three groups of New Zealand male rabbits were fed a cholesterol-free rabbit chow. The three groups were employed as follows: (a) 2.5 mg kg^{-1} of 25-hydroxycholesterol ($n=6$); (b) 2.5 mg kg^{-1} of cholestanetriol (triol) ($n=6$); and (c) a control group ($n=6$) receiving vehicle only. Sterols were dissolved in 0.3 ml ethanol, then added to 3 ml of the 'rabbit's own serum' which was obtained prior to the experiment, and infused into the rabbits via an ear vein by slow drip. Animals were killed after 24 h. Scanning electron microscopy (SEM) and transmission electron microscopy (TEM) were used to evaluate the degree of endothelial damage. SEM revealed endothelial lesions resembling balloon-like protrusions and crater-like defects in oxysterol treated rabbits. TEM demonstrated subendothelial oedema and intracytoplasmic vacuoles in the endothelium. Control rabbits displayed far less endothelial damage. The results demonstrated a remarkably acute (24 h) injury to the endothelium and, therefore, were consistent with many previous studies of endothelial injury resulting from oxysterols (Addis, 1986; Addis and Park, 1989).

Peng *et al.* (1985a) made several other observations which emphasized that the endothelial injury noted by them displayed numerous pathological characteristics which are consistent with the response-to-injury hypothesis of atherosclerosis. Injured aortic areas displayed adhering platelets, erythrocytes and leukocytes. Microthrombi, essentially aggregates of platelets and erythrocytes, were noted at sites of endothelial injury. Injury was assessed primarily by noting 'balloons and craters'. The number of craters was significantly ($p < 0.05$) greater in triol and 25-hydroxycholesterol treated rabbits (13.6 ± 1.5 and 6.6 ± 0.6, respectively) compared with controls (2.0 ± 0.4). Balloon-like lesions numbered 4.5 ± 1.3 ($p < 0.05$) and 2.2 ± 0.7 ($p < 0.01$) for triol and 25-hydrocholesterol treated rabbits, respectively, compared with 0.8 ± 0.3 in the controls. Only craters or balloons larger than 5 μm in diameter were counted.

TEM studies revealed that the oxysterol treated rabbits experienced subendothelial oedema or separation from subendothelial attachments, phenomena rarely seen in control rabbits (Peng *et al.*, 1985a). Balloons and craters are common responses to injury of the endothelia of arteries in several species (Peng *et al.*, 1985a).

Several possibilities exist with regard to the mechanism of oxysterol induced arterial endothelial damage. Firstly, cholesterol oxides are far more inhibitory to cholesterol biosynthesis by cells than cholesterol itself. Inhibition of the rate-limiting step in cholesterol biosynthesis, 3-hydroxy-3-methylglutaryl coenzyme A (HMGCoA) reductase, may render cells deficient in cholesterol, a key cellular component (Smith and Johnson, 1989), thereby exerting cellular injury.

Table 3 Effects of cholesterol oxidation products on cholesterol and fatty acid synthesis in cultured aortic smooth-muscle cells[1]

Sterol [2]	Change in synthesis[3]	
	Cholesterol	*Fatty acids*
Control (vehicle)		
25-Hydroxycholesterol	−82	+46
20α-Hydroxycholesterol	−78	+10
7-Ketocholesterol	−69	+19
7β-Hydroxycholesterol	−56	+102
7α-Hydroxycholesterol	−51	+94
Cholesterol-α-epoxide	−44	+68
Cholestanetriol	−34	+42
Purified cholesterol	−22	+35

[1] Source: modified from Peng *et al.* (1985b)
[2] Sterols at 3 μg ml^{-1} medium
[3] Compared with controls

Secondly, the inhibition of cholesterol uptake from exogenous sources could conceivably occur. This possibility was studied by Peng *et al.* (1985b). New Zealand white male rabbits were used as a source of aortic smooth-muscle cells which were grown in culture. Cholesterol-4-^{14}C was dissolved in ethanol and dispersed in culture medium containing 0–100 μg ml^{-1} oxysterols. The results showed that oxysterols strongly inhibited cholesterol uptake. The effects of oxysterols on biosynthesis of cholesterol and fatty acids from ^{14}C labelled sodium acetate are summarized in Table 3. Oxysterols clearly inhibited cholesterol biosynthesis with cholesterol exhibiting the lowest degree of inhibition of the eight sterols (seven oxysterols) tested. Both cholesterol and oxysterols appeared to increase fatty acid synthesis (Peng *et al.*, 1985a). Two possible explanations for the observed reduction in cholesterol uptake are suggested:

(1) the inhibition of cholesterol biosynthesis by cholesterol oxidation products may cause membrane cholesterol levels to decline, and the functionality, including receptor-dependent processes, could be adversely affected; or

(2) cholesterol oxides may compete with cholesterol for cell-surface binding sites (Peng *et al.*, 1985b).

Other potentially important effects of cholesterol oxides include the ability of 25-hydroxycholesterol and triol to inhibit 5′-nucleotidase activity (Peng *et al.*,

1985c). Triol, incubated for 48 h with cultured aortic smooth-muscle cells also significantly inhibited Na^+–K^+-adenosine triphosphatase (ATPase) activity.

Cultured aortic smooth-muscle cells were also employed by Peng and Morin (1987) in a study of the effects of oxysterols on membrane function. Na^+–K^+-ATPase and 5'-nucleotidase were measured cytochemically using TEM. Cells incubated with triol and 25-hydroxycholesterol ($10 \mu g \, ml^{-1}$) for 24 and 48 h displayed marked inhibition of both enzymes. Carrier-mediated hexose transport was also studied using 2-deoxy-D-[^{3}H] glucose. Triol caused a rapid inhibition of hexose transport; the effect was reversible. However, 25-hydroxycholesterol did not alter transport of 2-deoxy-D-glucose after up to 8 h incubation. Peng and Morin (1987) speculated that the rapid inhibition of transport observed with triol indicated that triol quickly inserts into the membrane, whereas the effects of 25-hydroxycholesterol, if any, are seen later than 8 h because the primary mechanism of 25-hydroxycholesterol may involve inhibition of cellular cholesterol biosynthesis.

An interesting study by Hennig and Boissonneault (1987) demonstrated impaired barrier functions in cultured endothelial cell monolayers exposed to triol ($20 \mu M$ for 24 h). No effect was observed with cholesterol at levels as high as $130 \mu M$. Altered morphology was detected in monolayers incubated with triol. Adding cholesterol or vitamin E to the incubation medium did not reverse the effects of triol. Insertion of triol into the endothelial cell membrane may occur and result in altered permeability. Leakage of lactate dehydrogenase from monolayers was noted after 24 h of incubation with triol. Hennig and Boissonneault (1987) concluded that dietary cholesterol oxides may be an important risk factor for CHD.

Triol was also the subject of an investigation by Jacobson *et al.* (1985) who fed by gavage to white Carneau pigeons' diets of either 0.05% pure cholesterol or 0.05% cholesterol plus triol at 0.3% of cholesterol (0.16 mg triol plus 51.9 mg cholesterol). Pigeons fed triol displayed 87% greater lumenal stenosis ($p < 0.01$) and 42% greater aortic calcium accumulation ($p < 0.02$) than the controls. Jacobson *et al.* (1985) stated that the level of triol used (0.3% of cholesterol) approximated the intake of humans, but adequate data on this question are lacking. Most studies on food composition appear to suggest very limited quantities of triol and 25-hydroxycholesterol (Addis, 1986; Addis and Park, 1989). However, the results of Jacobson *et al.* (1985) are impressive because the levels of both cholesterol and triol fed represented a reasonable attempt to be realistic and also represented United States Pharmacopea (USP) cholesterol, in terms of oxidation product levels. USP cholesterol is frequently employed in experiments of 'cholesterol-induced' atherogenesis without regard to contamination by cholesterol oxides (Taylor *et al.*, 1979). Jacobson *et al.* (1985) stated that their results 'call for reinterpretation of data from studies using animal models fed USP cholesterol and of human epidemiological data not accounting for cholesterol oxide intake'.

Matthias *et al.* (1987) reported triol induced aortic smooth-muscle-cell toxicity and damage to the endothelial cells of rats, a species relatively resistant to atherosclerosis. Cholesterol administered at the same levels displayed no significant cytotoxic effects and no potentiation or diminishment by cholesterol of triol cytotoxicity was seen.

Most research dealing with the atherogenicity of oxysterols has focused on arterial injury. However, a very interesting recent study indicates that dietary oxysterols cause a greater elevation of plasma cholesterol than purified cholesterol in the rabbit (Kosykh *et al.*, 1989). All animals received a laboratory rabbit chow plus 0.5 ml day^{-1} olive oil. Commercial cholesterol containing 5% oxysterols was fed in olive oil (0.2 g cholesterol/kg body weight) to one group; another group received 0.2 g cholesterol/kg body weight purified cholesterol; a third group received olive oil without cholesterol or oxysterols. After six weeks the animals were killed and blood and hepatocytes were collected. Rabbits fed commercial cholesterol exhibited a five-fold increase in the serum cholesterol concentration compared with rabbits fed purified cholesterol. The values were 60 ± 8, 180 ± 30 and 900 ± 140 mg dl^{-1} for control, purified cholesterol and commercial cholesterol diets, respectively. Cholesteryl ester levels in hepatocytes from the commercial cholesterol group were greatly increased over the control and purified cholesterol groups: the values were 39.2 ± 5.6, 91.4 ± 12 and 94.9 ± 120 μg lipid/mg cell proteins for control, purified cholesterol and commercial cholesterol, respectively. Increased secretion of very low-density lipoprotein (VLDL) by hepatocytes of oxysterol fed rabbits is the likely explanation for the increased plasma cholesterol seen in rabbits fed oxysterol.

Morin and Peng (1989) studied the effects of 25-hydroxycholesterol and cholestanetriol on enzymes that affect the rate of accumulation of cholesterol esters in cultured rabbit aortic smooth-muscle cells. Imbalances stimulated by 25-hydroxycholesterol were noted which favoured a net accumulation of cholesterol ester, an important step in the formation of plaque.

For a more complete review of the recent literature of oxysterols and *in vivo* and *in vitro* cytotoxicity and atherogenicity, the reader is referred to Smith and Johnson (1989). In general, the vast majority of the studies in this area of research suggest that oxysterols are far more atherogenic than the native sterol counterpart and that the increased atherogenicity seen in the case of oxysterols is independent of any increase in serum cholesterol. This conclusion is consistent with the idea that oxysterols appear to be most active in the early stages of atherosclerosis, based on the available evidence. As a corollary to this, cholesterol in the diet of humans can neither be atherogenic nor hypercholesterolaemic (intake of 200–750 mg day^{-1}) and food technology research in the future should focus on prevention of lipid oxidation instead of cholesterol removal (Addis and Park, 1989). Of course, there are two sides to every scientific argument. Several publications have reported that oxysterols are not atherogenic but may even have beneficial effects! These are discussed later in this chapter. First, however, it is important to broaden the view of this subject to include other lipids and oxidation products derived from them. As was discussed by Addis (1986), human diets rarely contain cholesterol oxides without other lipid oxidation products, including malonaldehyde, fatty acid hydroperoxides, and secondary degradation products. To these groups, thermally altered and thermally oxidized lipids may also be added. Figure 3 shows some examples of these types of compound.

Other lipid oxidation and thermal-degradation products

Although some indication of endothelial injury is evident in the case of intravenously administered fatty acid hydroperoxides, most of the published research has dealt with acceleration of foam cells formation, often increasing binding between LDL and smooth-muscle cells. Malonaldehyde has received little attention in relation to CHD but should be studied because improved methodology exists (Csallany *et al.*, 1984). Products such as those that are uniquely produced by deep-fat frying should be investigated in relation to CHD, including the foregoing groups of compounds as well as thermal-oxidation products and compounds produced by purely thermal (nonoxidative) mechanisms.

Methodological limitations have hampered definitive research into mechanisms whereby dietary lipid oxidation products can affect atherosclerosis or exert other health-related effects. Most of the early literature reported research results based on the thiobarbituric acid (TBA) test and has reported results in terms of parts per million of malonaldehyde. However, it is far more accurate to use the expression 'thiobarbituric reactive substances' (TBARS) because many more compounds than malonaldehyde react with TBA. Csallany *et al.* (1984) noted that the TBA assay greatly overestimates the malonaldehyde present (as determined by size-exclusion HPLC). Therefore, the TBA, or more correctly TBARS, test provides a generalized observation of total lipid oxidation products present but cannot differentiate between fatty acids and sterol hydroperoxides or detect many of the secondary breakdown products, including all the commonly studied cholesterol oxides (alcohols) and many of the secondary and tertiary fatty acid breakdown products. It is common knowledge that the TBARS test, a simple and useful test for rancidity of foods, can be misleading over a long shelf-life study or a shorter term study of thermal oxidation of frying oil. Therefore, low values, while correctly indicating low peroxide content, do not prove that peroxides at a previous time had not been present at high levels and that at the time of the low TBARS value secondary lipid oxidation products, some of which are extremely active biologically, are not present. For these reasons, the reader is cautioned about the results reviewed here and how many conclusions can be safely drawn.

On the other hand, the reader is invited to consider the many new techniques now available for the quantification of specific lipid oxidation products and secondary degradation products (Pryor, 1987, 1989). Of particular interest are methods now available for the quantification of lipid peroxides, including fatty acid hydroperoxides (Funk, 1987; Iwaoka *et al.*, 1987; Matsushita *et al.*, 1987; Pendleton and Lands, 1987; Terao and Matsushita, 1987; van Kuijk and Dratz, 1987; Wendel, 1987; Yamamoto and Ames, 1987). Also recommended are methods for conjugated dienes (Corongiu *et al.*, 1989), malonaldehyde by GLC (Dennis and Shibamoto, 1989), and several other recently developed methods including those described by Dillard and Tappel (1989), Esterbauer and Zollner (1989), Kosugi and Kikugawa (1989), Miyazawa (1989) and Piretti and Pagliuca (1989). Pryor (1989) states the need for single research groups to use *several* of the newer more sensitive and specific techniques available, and we concur with this view.

Yagi and co-workers have contributed much to the literature concerning the possible atherogenic effects of fatty acid hydroperoxides. The earliest of these studies employed TBA methodology and reported that serum peroxide levels increased with age, and that levels in diabetics with angiopathy exceeded levels in diabetics without angiopathy. Subsequently, studies were done which showed that linoleic hydroperoxide induced endothelial damage and accelerated uptake of LDL by cultured arterial smooth-muscle cells.

Yagi *et al.* (1987) studied the formation of 'foam' cells from cultured aortic smooth-muscle cells and macrophages as influenced by LDL and linoleic acid hydroperoxide. In the study, rabbit aortic smooth-muscle cells were grown in RPMI 1640 medium, 10% fetal calf serum at 37°C. Chylomicrons, VLDL and LDL were obtained from rabbits by sequential ultracentrifugation; linoleic acid hydroperoxide (Figure 3) was prepared from soya-bean lipoxygenase so that the resulting product (13S)-13-hydroperoxy-*cis*-9,*trans*-11-octadecadienoic acid was 96% pure (Gardner, 1989). Incubation of aortic smooth-muscle cells with lineolic acid hydroperoxide and then LDL, led to foam cell production. Both the peroxide and LDL needed to be present. Similar results were seen with monocyte-macrophages. Pretreatment of LDL with linoleic acid hydroperoxide (5 mmol ml^{-1} at 4°C for 2 days) also stimulated foam cell formation. However, control treatment with linoleic acid when conducted on LDL did not result in foam cell formation. VLDL and chylomicrons, when pretreated with peroxide, also showed stimulation of foam cell formation. These results strengthen the hypothesis that lipid peroxides are able to promote atherosclerotic plaque accumulation.

In a sequel to the foregoing study, Sasaguri *et al.* (1988) noted that the phagocytotic activity of macrophages was not inhibited by the presence of linoleic acid hydroperoxide up to $5 \, mmol \, ml^{-1}$, the concentration at which cultured endothelial cells are injured. At $14 \, mmol \, ml^{-1}$ linoleic acid hydroperoxide, macrophages experience observable indication of cellular damage yet 'retained phagocytic activity to a considerable effect'. Thus it seems that macrophages which have phagocytosed 'denatured LDL' (produced by peroxide treatment), become degenerated macrophages which adhere to the injured site and stimulate progression of atherosclerosis, probably by inflammation (Sasaguri *et al.*, 1988).

The results described above and the research described below raise interesting questions about dietary recommendations. Early dietary recommendations (namely, to increase intake of polyunsaturates and reduce intakes of saturates) resulted in greater exposure of consumers to lipid oxidation products. Furthermore, many erroneous conclusions were made about the cholesterolaemic effects of polyunsaturates, monounsaturates, saturates and cholesterol itself and revisions, based on new data, appear to be in order (Addis and Park, 1989). An important area of research needs to be addressed in this regard. In 1971, Carroll and Khor demonstrated a higher tumour incidence in rats fed vegetable fats than in rats fed animal fats. Likewise, it is possible to assemble an impressive arsenal against vegetable oils rather than in favour of them insofar as CHD is concerned. Vegetable oils generally are high in ω-6 fatty acids, oxidize readily, promote *in vivo* lipid peroxidation and antioxidant vitamin depletion, lower HDL along with LDL and are usually hydrogenated, forming *trans* fatty acids (Addis and Park, 1989).

Fish oils and high-monounsaturate oil (rapeseed) are becoming popular. Fish oils, high in ω-3 fatty acids, would appear to help slow monocyte and platelet activity. However, the extreme susceptibility of fish oils to autoxidation may also result in untoward effects. Thiery and Seidel (1987) noted the unexpected enhancement of atherosclerosis in rabbits given fish oils. Three groups of rabbits were used (I, basal diet; II, basal diet + 1.5% cholesterol; III, basal diet + 1.5% cholesterol + 2 ml Maxepa per day orally by intrabuccal gavage). The duration of the experiment was 5 months. Atherosclerosis was assessed by determining the sudanophilic surface of the aortae. Group I exhibited the least, group III the most and group II was intermediate in this particular measure of atherosclerosis. Serum cholesterol did not differ among the three groups. Platelet half-life was reduced by cholesterol and the serum peroxide level was increased markedly by fish oil feeding. Thiery and Seidel (1987) speculated that malonaldehyde modification of LDL may have been responsible for the increased atherosclerosis seen in these animals.

Further evidence of deleterious effects of lipid peroxides on atherosclerosis and potentially on CHD, especially myocardial infarction as induced by thrombosis, is provided by the finding that linoleic acid hydroperoxide inhibits prostacyclin production in cultured endothelial cells (Sasaguri *et al.*, 1985). If such an effect occurred in humans (*in vivo*), it could mean that peroxides not only accelerate atherosclerosis but also stimulate thrombosis (Addis and Park, 1989).

Deep-fat-fried foods represent another potentially important source of lipid oxidation products in the diet of modern man. In this case, thermal oxidation and thermal rearrangement of lipids result in a somewhat different mix of products, but the possible detrimental effects on atherosclerosis may be similar. A study by Naruszewicz *et al.* (1987) suggested that consumption of thermally oxidized soya-bean oil increases the uptake and degradation of chylomicrons (which possessed dietary oxidation products postprandially). In this study, human subjects were challenged with 100 g fresh oil (peroxide value 1.6 meq kg^{-1}) on the first day and with 100 g thermally oxidized (220°C for 7 h) oil (peroxide value 4.8 meq kg^{-1}) on the second day. Chylomicrons were obtained 4 h postprandially by preparative ultracentrifugation, labelled with ^{125}I and incubated with cultured murine peritoneal macrophages for 5 h at 37°C. Humans ingesting thermally oxidized soya-bean oil exhibited marked elevation of plasma TBARS (five- to seven-fold increase over fasting levels in some cases). Plasma cholesterol levels were largely unaffected and triglycerides increased as would be expected after oil feeding. Elevations in plasma TBARS after ingestions of fresh oil were minimal, reflecting the lower degree of oxidation noted in the fresh oil.

Increased degradation by mouse macrophages was noted for chylomicrons with increased peroxide levels, compared with control chylomicrons obtained after fresh oil ingestion. Naruszewwicz *et al.* (1987) also obtained evidence that the acetyl-LDL receptor and the β-VLDL receptor on macrophages are involved in the uptake and degradation of chylomicrons with elevated peroxide levels. As is noted later in this chapter, numerous other effects on the health of experimental animals have been reported when animals are fed heated oils.

Absorption and plasma lipid oxidation products

Although the results obtained by Naruszewicz *et al.* (1987) clearly demonstrated the absorption of lipid oxidation products, as revealed by the TBARS test, many critical questions remain. Research on the possible postprandial absorption of many specific lipid oxidation products is extremely limited. Indeed, the prevailing early scientific opinion was that linoleic acid hydroperoxide is not absorbed as the hydroperoxide (Meade, 1962). Bascoul *et al.* (1986) demonstrated the absorption of cholesterol-α-epoxide in the rat. Clearly the advent of the development of a specific and sensitive methodology for quantification of lipid oxidation products in food and biological fluids and tissues should stimulate much new research on absorption. Although the use of the TBA test to quantify TBARS has served researchers well in the past, clearly future research done in the area of lipid oxidation products and health requires the use of more sophisticated techniques (reviewed by Csallany *et al.*, 1984) because of the lack of specificity of TBARS.

The TBARS assay may be employed in combination with more modern methodology but should no longer be used by itself. Based on the scientific literature reviewed, it is apparent that at least some of the lipid oxidation products are absorbed and are similar to, if not the same as, the aldehydic compounds believed to participate in the modification of LDL. Therefore, the dietary occurrence of such products of lipid oxidation may be important in atherosclerosis and perhaps in other health problems as well. Although the presence of lipid oxidation products in human plasma has been reported for some time, their origins are, in many cases, still unknown. In addition, unabsorbed lipid oxidation products may have deleterious effects on the gastrointestinal mucosa. Therefore, lack of absorption does not indicate lack of health effects.

In addition to the study by Naruszewicz *et al.* (1987), several other studies have been conducted on the absorption of oxidized lipids. Glavind *et al.* (1971) could not detect lymphatic methyllinoleate hydroperoxide after it had been administered intragastrically to rats. The authors concluded that methyllinoleate hydroperoxide is converted to the hydroxyoctadecadieneoate, which is partially recovered in the lymph.

Piché *et al.* (1988) obtained indirect evidence of malonaldehyde absorption by measuring urinary malonaldehyde in subjects consuming (1) either control or unstabilized (no preservatives) cod-liver oil, or (2) either control or stabilized cod-liver oil. The results demonstrated a clear increase ($p < 0.01$) in urinary malonaldehyde excretion after the first comparison but not the second. The authors concluded that the unpreserved cod-liver oil contained malonaldehyde, and that consumption results in absorption and urinary excretion of malonaldehyde. They also expressed concern about adverse health effects of consumption of highly polyunsaturated and unstabilized oils which not only expose consumers to exogenous xenobiotics such as malonaldehyde, but also, over time, tend to reduce tissue levels of antioxidants, thereby promoting *in vivo* lipid oxidation and further exposure to oxidation products.

Kanazawa *et al.* (1985) demonstrated in rats the absorption of secondary autoxidation products, but not hydroperoxides, and the excretion of some secondary products in the faeces and the uptake of some secondary products by the liver. Evidence of hepatotoxicity was reported.

Several reports of oxysterols in human blood samples have appeared in the literature. Gray *et al.* (1971) reported the finding of impressively high levels of cholesterol-α-epoxide in sera from hyperlipidaemic humans. Brooks *et al.* (1983) reported a 'profile' of several oxysterols in human blood samples. Recently, our laboratory adapted the procedures developed by Park and Addis (1985) for the analysis of cholesterol oxidation products in food products to the analysis of plasma lipoproteins of fasted humans (Addis *et al.*, 1989). No attempt was made to control overall food-consumption patterns, antioxidant intake or other potentially important factors such as smoking. All three lipoproteins (HDL, LDL and VLDL) contained, in some subjects, appreciable levels of cholesterol-α and β-epoxide, 7β-hydroxycholesterol and 7-keto-cholesterol with lesser quantities of cholestanetriol and 25-hydroxycholesterol. The newer procedures for cholesterol oxide analysis in lipoproteins permit critical experiments to be conducted on the possible roles of dietary and *in vivo* produced cholesterol oxides in CHD and the possible effects of dietary antioxidant status (Addis *et al.*, 1989).

Recent research has clearly demonstrated the chylomicron-associated absorption of cholesterol oxidation products in humans (Emanuel, 1989). Humans fed a meal consisting primarily of powdered eggs with high levels of cholesterol oxides displayed a pronounced postprandial increase in chylomicron and plasma cholesterol oxides. Subjects consuming fresh eggs (containing only trace amounts of cholesterol oxides) displayed only minor increases in postprandial plasma cholesterol oxides.

There are significant variations among human subjects with respect to the pattern of the rise in cholesterol oxide concentration vs. postprandial time. The cholesterol oxides are rapidly cleared from the plasma by a mechanism which is not fully understood (Emanuel, 1989).

The foregoing studies on the absorption of lipid oxidation products indicate that most are readily absorbed. However, data are needed concerning the absorption in humans of fatty acid hydroperoxides, postulated to be important in atherosclerosis and CHD (Yagi, 1988). The issue is a complex one because of the large number of fatty acid hydroperoxide isomers which can be formed. In addition, quantitative data are needed concerning the efficiency of absorption and the ultimate fate of oxidation products. The possibility that fibre may reduce absorption of lipid oxidation products has been suggested as a potentially fruitful area of research (Addis and Park, 1989).

The observations made on the absorption of lipid oxidation products and the possibility that *in vivo* lipid oxidation may also be involved in atherosclerosis and CHD suggest that antioxidant status may be important. Szczeklik *et al.* (1985) used type II and type IV hyperlipoproteinaemic subjects to study the effects of dietary vitamin E on plasma lipid peroxides, prostacyclin generation and platelet aggregability. Dietary tocopherol increased serum tocopherol levels, but total lipids, cholesterol, triglycerides, ceruloplasmin and transferrin levels remained unchanged. Tocopherol depressed plasma lipid peroxides and mildly suppressed platelet activity. As part of the same study Szczeklik *et al.* (1985) fed an atherogenic diet to rabbits and noted an increase in serum lipid peroxides and a 90% decrease in arterial synthesis of prostacyclin. Supplementation of the atherogenic diet with tocopherol prevented the increase in serum lipid peroxides and prevented loss of arterial prostacyclin synthesis.

231

Children from families with a history of CHD exhibit elevated serum peroxide levels and lower HDL values than children from control families (Szamosi *et al.*, 1987).

Clearly there is an urgent need for definitive studies on the use of antioxidants in foods from the standpoints of protecting foods and protecting tissues of the subject consuming such foods, and possible benefits to be derived therefrom in terms of prevention of CHD. The large number of sensitive techniques developed recently should make such studies possible. Furthermore, the inappropriateness of feeding powdered eggs or oxidized cholesterol to rabbits or monkeys and making recommendations to the public about fresh meat, dairy products and eggs has never been clearer (Addis and Park, 1989).

Dietary oxidation products, atherogenesis and mLDL

It appears possible at this time to postulate and hypothesize mechanisms whereby dietary lipid oxidation products could accelerate atherosclerotic arterial changes and contribute to CHD (Figure 2). A key facet of the hypothesized mechanisms involves the modification of LDL to mLDL. The possibility exists that lipid oxides from the diet increase LDL uptake by the artery and that, once in the artery, these more polar oxidation products accelerate the interactions between macrophages and a 'slightly modified' LDL (LDL-LOPS in Figure 2). Such an interaction could occur if the lipid oxidation products caused LDL-LOPS to be chemotactic for macrophages, which would, along with endothelial cells and smooth-muscle cells, cause further oxidation to mLDL and rapid uptake by macrophages. Therefore, the significance of dietary lipid oxidation products may extend well beyond the arterial injury phenomenon reported earlier (Taylor *et al.*, 1979; Peng *et al.*, 1985a).

Opposing viewpoints

Unanimity is rarely achieved in active areas of scientific research and the potential role of cholesterol oxides in atherosclerosis is no exception. The viewpoint that takes cholesterol as the primary atherogenic agent and has oxysterols playing a role as inhibitors of atherosclerosis has been expressed in a few publications. Krut (1982a) demonstrated that phosphatidylcholine is limited in its capacity to maintain the solubility of cholesterol in a supersaturated solution of cholesterol in triglyceride oil, but that small quantities of oxysterols added in combination with phosphatidylcholine maintain cholesterol in solution. Similar effects have been reported in aqueous media. Dihydroxy derivatives (7α, 7β- and 25-hydroxycholesterol) are the most effective in terms of solubilizing cholesterol. Krut (1982a) claimed that his findings indicate a possible role for oxysterols in inhibiting atherosclerosis, by preventing the crystallization of cholesterol in tissues.

A subsequent study (Krut, 1982b) employed the technique of subcutaneously implanting cholesterol in rats and measuring rates of clearance as a function of oxysterol content. Again, solubilization of cholesterol by oxysterols was seen. Implants containing oxysterols dissolved more rapidly than those containing only cholesterol; the latter required some phospholipid for clearance to occur. Krut (1982b) stated that 'oxidation products of cholesterol form readily in foods of animal origin when suitably exposed to light and air. It is suggested that technology designed to prevent spoilage of foods has inadvertently resulted in the elimination from the Western diet of compounds which prevent accumulations of cholesterol in the arterial wall.

The results obtained by Krut (1982a,b) would appear to support a very simplistic view of atherosclerosis, not at all consistent with the complex pathology discussed earlier (Faggiotto *et al.*, 1984; Faggiotto and Ross, 1984) and recent data on mLDL (Steinberg *et al.*, 1989). In addition, the statement concerning advances in food technology adversely affecting atherosclerosis are not supported at all by epidemiological data because CHD rates have been declining since 1962 (Smith, 1988), coinciding with increased use of vacuum packaging, antioxidants and other techniques which retard rancidity. It would appear that the reports of Krut (1982a,b) may have little relevance to CHD pathology.

Higley *et al.* (1986) also showed what appeared to be evidence of oxysterols 'protecting' rabbits from cholesterol induced atherosclerosis. The methodology and results of Highley *et al.* (1986) have been reviewed in great detail by Addis and Park (1989) who concluded that the study, although carefully conducted in many respects, suffered from the facts that it excluded cholestanetriol and 25-hydroxycholesterol from the oxysterol mixture and also did not monitor early stages of arterial injury, phenomena which are well-known to be caused by oxysterols. Instead, atherosclerosis was determined after 11 weeks of dietary treatment. Dietary cholesterol fed to rabbits is strongly hypercholesterolaemic, but plasma lipid levels were not monitored. The choice of experimental animals used and other factors discussed earlier make the results of Higley *et al.* (1986) difficult to interpret.

Tipton *et al.* (1987) reported that cholesterol hydroperoxides inhibit atherogenesis in the rabbit but, like Higley *et al.* (1986), waited far beyond the arterial-injury phase (56–61 days) to determine the atherogenic effects in rabbit aortae. Peng *et al.* (1985a) note atherogenic changes within 24 h of oxysterol administration. Hydroperoxides of cholesterol have not been characterized by previous researchers with regard to affects on atherogenesis; studies have concentrated on oxysterols. In the observations reported in Krut (1982a,b), Higley *et al.* (1986) and Tipton *et al.* (1987), there are inconsistencies which emphasize the complex nature of the relationship between dietary cholesterol oxides and atherosclerosis.

Cytotoxicity, membrane and enzyme effects

The literature on cytotoxicity and membrane effects of oxysterols is extensive, that for enzyme effects less so, but all have been expertly reviewed by Smith and Johnson (1989) who stated that the cytotoxicities of oxysterols 'are on balance their predominant biological characteristic'. Again, we emphasize the need to seek and be aware of interrelationships among all the potentially health-related effects.

Both the *in vivo* and *in vitro* effects of oxysterols have been documented extensively, but the interpretation of the *in vitro* findings to living organisms is difficult. Cellular *in vivo* effects include reduction or cessation of growth, loss of weight, diminished appetite and pathological changes (Smith and Johnson, 1989). Other effects noted in the literature include necrosis and acute inflammation (subcutaneous implants), nuclear aberrations, toxicity to micro-organisms and lethality: $LD_{50} = 0.3$ mmol kg^{-1} in Swiss mice for the 3,7-dihemisuccinate derivative of 7α-hydroxycholesterol (Smith and Johnson, 1989). However, Naber *et al.* (1985) found little evidence of health effects of cholesterol oxidation products on laying hens. Three groups of hens were fed either a control diet, 0.5% pure cholesterol, or 0.5% cholesterol oxides. Eggs produced by the latter group displayed modest but significant ($p < 0.01$) reductions in yolk cholesterol content. Conversion of 1-^{14}C-acetate into cholesterol was also reduced by cholesterol oxides to a greater extent than by pure cholesterol.

In vitro toxicities of oxysterols are extremely diverse. A sampling of the effects noted in the literature include fibroblast toxicity, cell-growth inhibition, lipid accumulation, reduced protein levels, lethality to many cell types, impairment of synchronous beating in rat myocardial cells, inhibition of cellular proliferation, increase in thrombin-induced platelet aggregation, and toxicity to many cells at concentrations as low as $2 \mu g$ ml^{-1} (Smith and Johnson, 1989). Stereochemical effects have been noted as 7β-hydroxycholesterol was found to be eight-fold more toxic than 7α-hydroxycholesterol on Chinese hamster embryo cells as measured by relative plating efficiency (Chan and Chan, 1980).

The mechanisms of cytotoxicity are varied but prominent, among them are insertion into membranes and enzyme effects. In addition, these two mechanisms are often closely related.

Cellular membranes play a critical role in the survival of the cell. In addition to encapsulating the cellular contents, the membrane is necessary for reproduction, locomotion, exclusion of toxic substances, accumulation of nutrients, and disposal of harmful waste products. The lipid composition of membranes varies according to cell type. Major lipids comprising eukaryotic cell membranes include phosphatidylcholine, phosphatidylethanolamine and cholesterol.

Membrane fluidity regulates cellular processes such as proliferation, fusion and endocytosis. Fluidity of membranes is affected by long-chain fatty acids, unsaturated fatty acids, cholesterol and divalent cations such as Ca^{2+} and Mg^{2+}. A decrease in fluidity is associated with saturated long-chain fatty acids; divalent cations, which presumably form ionic bonds between neighbouring phospholipid head-groups resulting in stabilization; and cholesterol, which intercalates among the fatty acyl chains of the phospholipids, restricting their movement.

The activities of membrane-bound enzymes have been shown to be affected by changes in the fluidity of cholesterol enriched membranes (Graham and Green, 1970; Farias *et al.*, 1975; Houslay *et al.*, 1981).

Hydroxylated sterols have been found to act as potent inhibitors of *de novo* sterol synthesis (by inhibiting HMGCoA reductase), but the exact mechanism by which they act is unknown because HMGCoA reductase inhibition is demonstrable only in intact cells and not in the isolated enzyme. In addition, steps involving side-chain transformation are inhibited by oxysterols (Smith and Johnson, 1989). Richert *et al.* (1984) observed that 25-hydroxycholesterol and 7β-hydroxycholesterol greatly reduced membrane fluidity and strongly inhibited HMGCoA reductase activity in HTC hepatoma cells. However, the hydrophilic compound 7β-hydroxycholesterol-sodium-3,7-bis(hemisuccinate) did not affect membrane fluidity and, consequently, did not inhibit HMGCoA reductase. These findings are also consistent with the fact that 25-hydroxycholesterol requires intact cells for the inhibition of HMGCoA reductase (Kandutsch and Chen, 1973, 1974; Sinensky *et al.*, 1979). Smith and Johnson (1989) reviewed several other enzymes that are affected by oxysterols, including acylcholesterol:acylcoenzyme A O-transferase (ACAT), side-chain cytochrome P-450$_{sc}$, cholesterol 7α-hydroxylase, cholesterol 5,6-epoxide hydrolase and the 4- and 14-methylsterol oxidases.

Hydroxylated sterols have been found not only to inhibit sterol synthesis, but also to inhibit DNA synthesis, to alter membrane permeability, and to change the membrane stability of cells.

Unlike HMGCoA reductase activity, which is affected by membrane fluidity, DNA synthesis apparently is not. 7β-Hydroxycholesterol and its water-soluble derivative 7β-hydroxycholesterol-sodium-3,7-bis(hemisuccinate) both inhibit DNA synthesis, in HTC cells, to the same extent, although their effects are diminished by the presence of lipoproteins (Richert *et al.*, 1983).

Oxysterols inserted into membranes have profound effects on membrane permeability. Holmes and Yoss (1984) found that 25-hydroxycholesterol increased the permeability of Ca^{2+} in liposomes at concentrations as low as 1 mol%. Cholesterol had no effect on permeability. The greatest permeability to Ca^{2+} was seen when zwitterionic phosphatidylcholine and phosphatidylethanolamine were predominant in the liposome membrane. Permeability to Ca^{2+} was observed to a reduced extent when acidic phospholipids, phosphatidylinositol and phosphatidylserine predominated. Translocation across the membrane was not limited to Ca^{2+}. Other divalent cations, such as Mn^{2+}, Mg^{2+}, Sr^{2+} and Ba^{2+}, and Na^+ were also found to cross the membrane. However, the mechanism of this translocation is unknown. Oxysterols do not act as ionophores, but more likely cause a general perturbance of the membrane.

Glucose permeability to membranes is also affected by insertion of oxysterols (Theunissen *et al.*, 1986). The 7-oxygenated sterols along with 25-hydroxycholesterol were found to be perpendicularly oriented at the membrane interphase. A condensing effect on mixed monolayers of dioleoylphosphatidylcholine was seen in the order 7-ketocholesterol > 7β-hydroxycholesterol > 7α-hydroxycholesterol. Glucose permeability to these liposomes decreased in the same order. 25-Hydroxycholesterol, however, acted as a spacer molecule and showed no condensing effect. Similarly, glucose permeability was greatly increased reaching a maximum at 2.5 mol% 25-hydroxycholesterol.

The above-described effects in liposomes may result from the fact that oxygenated sterols influence the gel to liquid crystalline and bilayer to hexagonal phase transitions. The 7-oxygenated sterols lower the temperature of the phase transition in dipalmitoylphosphatidylcholine liposomes more than pure cholesterol (Egli *et al.*, 1984). Cholesterol lowers the bilayer to hexagonal phase transition temperature of phosphatidylethanolamines at mole fractions of about 0.1 (Epand and Bottega, 1987). However, oxysterols also influence this transition temperature. 7α-Hydroxycholesterol has a greater effect than pure cholesterol in lowering the bilayer to hexagonal phase transition, presumably because of its greater solubility in the lipid bilayer. Triol, on the other hand, because of its larger head-group, raises the bilayer to hexagonal phase transition temperature.

Oxysterol incorporation into some membranes may actually improve their stability. Incubation of L cells and Hela cells with 25-hydroxycholesterol made them resistant to streptolysin O, a cytolytic toxin (Duncan and Buckingham, 1980. The cells were also more resistant to saponin and digitonin, other agents which are known to interact with membrane cholesterol. This implies that replacing membrane cholesterol with oxysterols may cause an increased resistance to these cytotoxins. Reduced erythrocyte osmotic fragility is seen after incubation with 25 μM 7α-hydroxycholesterol, resulting from the expansion of cell surface area without changes in the mean cell volume (Streuli *et al.*, 1981).

Evidence of membrane damage induced by linoleic acid hydroperoxide has been obtained. Yagi (1987) reported that linoleic acid hydroperoxide injected into rabbits caused endothelial cell membrane damage, whereas linoleic acid injection caused minimal damage. Sevanian *et al.* (1988) demonstrated that linoleic acid hydroperoxide was considerably more toxic to bovine endothelial cells than were several cholesterol oxides.

Although the research completed on atherogenesis, cytotoxicity, enzyme and membrane effects is extremely extensive, it is difficult to draw solid conclusions on definite health effects mediated by these mechanisms. It is certain, however, that the potential for adverse effects in certain areas of health such as CHD are very great and are promising enough for so many health effects other than CHD that the entire area of oxysterol research demands increased attention (addressing, for example, the implications of the accumulation of oxysterols in cells and membranes and the potential long-term effect on various degenerative processes that oxysterols may pose). Much more data are needed on half-life, turnover and detoxification mechanisms for oxysterols. These issues are crucial to understanding the relevance of oxysterols to degenerative diseases such as CHD and cancer.

Mutagenesis and carcinogenesis

Early research results on oxysterol carcinogenicity were ambivalent (Addis *et al.*, 1983). Specific oxysterols are now known to be mutagenic and may be carcinogenic, but cholesterol is neither (Smith and Johnson, 1989). Cholesterol-α-epoxide mutagenicity has been demonstrated in V-79 Chinese hamster lung fibroblasts (Sevanian and Peterson, 1984) and in C3H-10T1/2 mouse embryo cells (Raaphorst *et al.*, 1987). The latter study also showed that cholesterol-β-epoxide is able to induce a greater degree of cell transformation than is the α-isomer. The *in vivo* evidence for the carcinogenicity of these compounds is ambivalent. Evidence favouring the view of α- and β-epoxide carcinogenicity includes the research of Gruenke *et al.* (1987) which indicated a relationship between α- and β-epoxide levels in nipple aspirates and factors which are known correlates with breast cancer. The origin of the epoxides was unknown. It is suggested that diet may be one possibility. Ames (1983), in a comprehensive review of dietary carcinogens and anticarcinogens, listed rancid fat as one category of carcinogen.

Diet is believed to be a significant factor in human colon cancer and some research suggests the involvement of cholesterol oxidation products (Suzuki *et al.*, 1986). 5α-Cholest-4-en-3-one and cholest-4-en-3-one were isolated from human faeces and assayed for carcinogenic potential by determining nuclear aberrations in mouse colons. Data for these cholesterol oxidation products were comparable with the known colon carcinogen, 2′,3-dimethyl-4-aminobiphenyl (Suzuki *et al.*, 1986).

Although data are limited with respect to possible carcinogenesis from dietary lipid oxidation products, the broader area of *in vivo* peroxidation and antioxidants in relation to carcinogenesis is well developed and may provide clues about dietary effects, assuming badly needed data on absorption of lipid oxidation products can be demonstrated. (Even in the absence of significant absorption, dietary oxidation products may pose a risk to intestinal mucosa.) Cerutti (1985) reviewed the literature on pro-oxidant states and tumour promotion. Active oxygen species as well as organic peroxides may function as weak initiators and as promoters of carcinogenesis; many antioxidants are anticarcinogens. This general relationship is also true as far as dietary carcinogens and anticarcinogens are concerned (Ames, 1983).

Malonaldehyde mutagenicity and carcinogenicity has been established (Basu and Marnett, 1983; Addis *et al.*, 1983). Basu *et al.* (1988) have demonstrated the formation of covalent adducts between guanine and guanine nucleosides on the one hand and malonaldehyde on the other, including an oxadiazabicyclo[3.3.1]nonene which was formed by the addition of a second malonaldehyde molecule to the initial adduct. According to Basu *et al.* (1988), the formation of multimeric adducts is 'unique to malonaldehyde among all known chemical mutagens and carcinogens'. A key factor in multimeric adduct formation is the ability of malonaldehyde to act as a nucleophile and as an electrophile. The ability of malonaldehyde to form multimeric adducts is related to its ability to induce frameshift mutagenesis in bacteria (Basu *et al.*, 1988).

Numerous other secondary lipid oxidation products have been shown to produce fluorescence when reacted with DNA in the presence of metals and reducing agents (Fujimoto *et al.*, 1984). Therefore, there is a clear need for the development of two areas of research:

(1) accurate quantification of the levels of lipid oxidation products in foods; and

(2) measurement of postprandial absorption in humans.

This information is needed to further our knowledge of the potential role of oxidation products in human cancer.

Potential problem foods

A 'problem food' is defined here as any food which is currently, or has been in the past, responsible for the exposure of a large segment of the population to significant levels of lipid oxidation or degradation products. Inherent in this definition are the concepts of high frequency of consumption and relatively high levels of lipid oxidation (i.e. ≥ 10 ppm vs. trace) in the food. Of course, at this time it is impossible to be sure that a 'problem food' actually exists, let alone try to identify it. Much further research on food analysis, absorption by humans and toxicology is needed. Our main purpose is to suggest as future research areas foods (and processes) which appear to be potential problems. There is yet another way to view problem foods as discussed here. The AHA and NHLBI have done much to promote a 'prudent diet', which limits consumption of eggs, meat and dairy products. Based on the research reviewed in this chapter, limitations on 'problem foods' makes at least as much sense as limiting consumption of fresh meats, for example, in a prudent diet. Finally, it must be realized that problem foods of yesterday are not necessarily problem foods of tomorrow. There is some evidence that changes have been made by the industry to lessen the exposure of consumers in some cases.

In our opinion, there are two major categories of 'problem foods' which should receive the highest priority for future research: heated fats and powdered eggs. In the case of heated fats it matters little whether a vegetable shortening, an animal fat or a combination of the two is used because the primary products formed would be fatty acid degradation products, cholesterol oxides and a mixture, respectively.

Heated fats

Health concerns have been raised about heated fats since the inception of deep-frying. Both saturated and unsaturated triaclyglycerols undergo both oxidative and nonoxidative (thermolytic) degradation (Nawar and Witchwoot, 1980). Saturated fats are more stable, but potentially significant thermolytic and oxidative products can occur, particularly in abused oil. Unsaturated fats degrade rapidly, although hydrogenated fats somewhat less so. Some of the compounds formed in heated oils are shown in Figure 3. Cholesterol present in heated tallow degrades initially to 7-ketocholesterol, 7α-hydroxycholeste-rol, 7β-hydroxycholesterol and α-epoxide (Park and Addis, 1986a), and subsequently to derivatives which have not yet been identified. Antioxidants (α-tocopherol plus ascorbyl palmitate) slow but do not stop the cholesterol degradation reactions (Park and Addis, 1986b). Bascoul *et al.* (1986) reported that heated tallow formed all the products found by Park and Addis (1986a) plus β-epoxide, cholestanetriol and 20- and 25-hydroxycholesterol. Unfortu-nately, Bascoul *et al.* (1986) used hot saponification and reported the artifact 3,5-cholestadiene-7-one. Variable but significant levels of cholesterol oxides were found in French fries from fast-food restaurants. In one restaurant, total cholesterol oxides reached 50 ppm, α- plus β-epoxides reaching 42 ppm. In another restaurant, variable levels were also seen, but it is perhaps significant

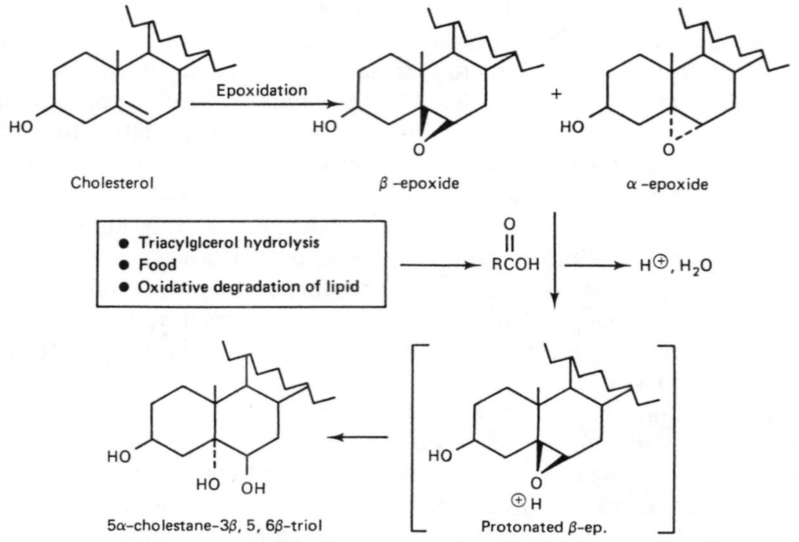

Figure 4 Formation of cholestane-$3\beta,5,6\beta$-triol. The suggested reaction probably occurs in deep-fat fryers in restaurants and could result in contamination of French fries with triol. The structure of cholestanetriol was confirmed by mass spectroscopy

that the highly atherogenic cholestanetriol was noted fairly consistently in daily samples.

Restaurants are reluctant to use the available quality-control devices to monitor oil quality. According to Gray and Morton (1981) the primary end-point selected as an indicator that the oil has reached the end of its 'fry-life' is foaming, a characteristic of heated fats that occurs with extensive polymer formation. Because polymer formation is preceded by extensive chemical degradation of the oil, a large build-up of potentially toxic compounds can occur. Recent studies emanating from the authors' laboratory indicated that measurements of polarity are highly significantly correlated to the cholesterol oxide levels of a 90/10 tallow/cottonseed shortening used to fry French fries under laboratory conditions.

Based on the extensive degradation of cholesterol in heated tallow, both in restaurants and in laboratory investigations, one can only imagine the complex mixture of potentially toxic compounds formed by hydrogenated vegetable shortenings and, even worse from the oxidation standpoint, lightly hydrogenated vegetable oils. Indeed, some highly complicated triglyceride polymers have been reported in heated fats (Ohfugi and Kaneda, 1973). Clearly there is an urgent need for investigations, using the improved analytical and toxicological methods available, of the heated-fats and -oils issue.

The literature on the toxicology of heated fats is extensive but much of the research conducted to date has at least two important shortcomings, especially the early research on the subject. Toxicological end-points were often crude and almost never included atherosclerosis. The possible link between consumption of heated fats and CHD must be vigorously explored. Secondly, heated fats used for early studies were often heated far more extensively than would occur in a restaurant. On the surface, one might assume that such a practice would tend to overestimate the problem of heated-fat toxicity, but in fact just the opposite might be true. As oils are heated, polymer formation occurs following the formation of oxidation products and these polymers are not well absorbed. Therefore, in the absence of untoward effects on the intestinal mucosa they are probably minimally toxic. This is clearly not the case for the aldehydes, hydroperoxides, lipid peroxides, dimers, cyclic compounds and, in particular, malonaldehyde, which are formed prior to polymers. For tallow, the analogous situation may exist. Cholesterol oxides, shown to be toxic in many studies, form fairly rapidly but eventually break down to other unknown and possibly less (or more) toxic compounds (Park and Addis, 1986a,b). Several early studies are recommended to the reader, including Morris *et al.* (1944), Lane *et al.* (1950), Crampton *et al.* (1956), Nishida *et al.* (1958), Perkins and Kummerow (1959) and Poling *et al.* (1969). Various forms of toxicity and some carcinogenicity were reported by the authors and loss of nutritional values was consistently reported, but at least one group (Poling *et al.*, 1969) concluded that levels of exposure of humans to toxic compounds in heated fats were insignificant.

Alexander (1983) summarized the biological effects of heated fats in experimental animals to include 'depression of growth, diminished feed efficiency, increased liver size, fatty necrosis of the liver and numerous other organ lesions'. Heated oils were found to induce damage to interstitial tissues and blood vessel walls, including vascular endothelium.

A more recent study by Alexander *et al.* (1987) confirmed the deleterious effects of heated oils in the rat. Male weanling rats were given diets of 15% fresh or laboratory-heated corn oil or fresh, laboratory-heated, or 'commercial-pressure deep-fry peanut oil'. The rats given heated corn oil or heated peanut oil exhibited diarrhoea, dermatitis, seborrhoea and hair loss. Commercial-pressure deep-fry peanut oil caused liver damage, toxicity to the thymus, and to testes and epididymis, the latter effects causing complete cessation of spermatogenesis.

Powdered eggs

The other major problem food is, and has been for some time, powdered eggs. Interestingly, as this is written, the importance of powdered eggs as a source of cholesterol oxides in the human diet may be decreasing for a number of reasons. Powdered eggs are being used with less frequency in traditional products because of the cholesterol controversy and perhaps because of the cholesterol oxidation product problem. In addition, powdered eggs are possibly produced with less cholesterol oxidation product formation as processors nowadays change methods of spray-drying of eggs and yolks.

Several studies have been completed on cholesterol oxides in powdered eggs. These include the studies reported by Tsai and Hudson (1985), Missler *et al.* (1985), Morgan and Armstrong (1987) and Sander *et al.* (1989a). In general, gas-fired dryers are more detrimental than steam-injected dryers. Cholesterol oxidation increases with time and H_2O_2 treatment increased cholesterol autoxidation. Sander *et al.* (1989a) reported > 150 ppm total epoxides in some powdered-egg samples but little or no triol and 25-hydroxy-cholesterol was seen.

Powdered eggs are a frequently used source of cholesterol for the inducement of atherosclerosis in animals. The atherosclerosis seen in animals from such experiments is invariably attributed to hypercholesterolaemia, which in turn is attributed to dietary cholesterol. The results are then applied to humans to make dietary recommendations.

However, the following questions could be asked. Is the atherosclerosis seen as the result of hypercholesterolaemia or arterial injury or both? Is it cholesterol or cholesterol oxides or both that are the atherogenic factors? Finally, how applicable are these findings to humans, who are not as responsive to dietary cholesterol in terms of developing hypercholesterolaemia as rabbits? Clearly more research is needed to answer these questions.

Other problem foods

In our opinion, deep-fat-fried foods and powdered eggs are in a class by themselves as far as lipid oxidation products are concerned. However, other areas of concern exist.

Freeze-dried meats, dehydrated cheddar, blue, parmesan and romano cheese powders, as well as sour cream and butter powders, all contain variable but possibly significant quantities of cholesterol oxides (Sanders *et al.*, 1989a). Fresh dairy products contain minimal cholesterol oxides however. Long-term heat treatment of butter oil can cause extensive oxidation of cholesterol (Sander *et al.*, 1989b). Precooked intact beef muscle contains little or no cholesterol oxides; but approximately 2% of the cholesterol in com-

Table 4 TBA values and 7-ketocholesterol of raw (a) and cooked (b) ground-beef patties stored at 4°C for 0, 2 and 4 days. TBA values[a] are expressed in mg MDA kg^{-1} tissue. For 7-ketocholesterol[b], each value represents duplicate HPLC determinations on two lipid extracts of each muscle. ND means not detected. Adapted from De Vore (1988)

a) TBA values and 7-ketocholesterol of raw ground-beef patties

Muscle sample	*TBA value[a]* (mg kg^{-1}) Storage days			*7-ketocholesterol[b]* (μg 100 g^{-1}) Storage days		
	0	2	4	0	2	4
1	0.1	1.3	1.9	25.6	37.5	60.4
2	0.2	0.6	1.1	trace	13.1	46.0
3	0.2	0.7	1.4	ND[d]	32.5	—
4	0.2	0.5	0.9	11.3	12.1	20.6
Overall means	0.2	0.8	1.3	9.65	23.8	42.3

b) TBA values and 7-ketocholesterol of cooked ground-beef patties

Muscle sample	*TBA value[a]* (mg kg^{-1}) Storage days			*7-ketocholesterol[b]* (μg 100 g^{-1}) Storage days		
	0	2	4	0	2	4
1	0.1	4.9	8.6	18.2	275.0	392.0
2	0.1	5.8	10.7	trace	264.7	622.2
3	0.2	7.4	17.4	ND[d]	390.6	—
4	0.1	5.1	9.2	ND	181.1	440.0
Overall means	0.1	5.8	9.5	6.33	277.9	484.7

minuted precooked beef has been noted to be oxidized (Park and Addis, 1987). In comminuted precooked turkey however, the amount of cholesterol that had undergone oxidation was approximately 3%. As rancidity development advanced in comminuted and cooked meat during storage, the oxidation of cholesterol became apparent (Park and Addis, 1987).

In addition to cholesterol, the structural membranes of muscle foods contain appreciable quantities of polyunsaturated fatty acids (PUFA). The TBA test has been adapted by food scientists to estimate oxidation of PUFA in meat. The 'TBA value' is used as an index of lipid oxidation in meat. Values of absorbance measurements at 532 nm, for example, are multiplied by a factor and then expressed as milligrams of malondialdehyde per kilogram of meat (Witte *et al.*, 1970; Govindarajan *et al.*, 1977). Studies which examined the levels of TBA values and the presence of 7-ketocholesterol (one of the products occurring in oxidatively modified low density lipoproteins, see Table 2) have concluded that after four days of storage, significant levels of TBA values and 7-ketocholesterol were observed in the raw ground-beef patties (De Vore, 1988) (Table 4a). Levels were much higher in cooked patties (Table 4b). The correlation coefficient of TBA values with 7-ketocholesterol for raw ground-beef stored over the 4 days at 4°C was 0.82 ($p < 0.0018$). For TBA values and 7-ketocholesterol using cooked ground-beef stored similarly, the correlation coefficient was 0.98 ($p < 0.0001$) (De Vore, 1988). Given the quantity of ground-beef consumed, the foregoing studies suggest the need for further research on antioxidants, packaging systems and other approaches in order to lessen the exposure of humans to lipid oxidation products in ground-beef.

Further research needs to be completed on precooked meat products of all types because of the increasing popularity of these products. In addition, methods need to be developed to quantify fatty acid degradation products in meats, especially precooked products.

Summary and conclusions

There are manifold ramifications of ongoing research on foods on the possible health aspects of lipid oxidation products in food. Some of these aspects are briefly outlined in this section and a brief appraisal is given of the regulatory aspects of rancidity in foods and heated oils. The reader is referred to Addis and Park (1989) for suggestions for future research in this area.

There is, at the present time, little in the way of regulation of foods with regard to rancidity in the USA (Firestone and Summers, 1989). Certainly the presence of toxic xenobiotics will be a sufficient basis for FDA regulatory action against fats and oils, but the issue of process-induced deleterious substances, which would include lipid oxidation products, is not as clear cut and no Federal regulation currently exists for control of rancidity. However, two municipalities, Chicago and San Francisco, do list rancidity as one factor which must be controlled in frying oils (Firestone, 1989).

In Europe, the laws are very explicit with regard to oxidation products in frying oils. Belgium, France, Germany, Spain and Switzerland restrict polar compounds to 25–27% as determined by IUPAC method 2.507 (Firestone, 1989).

Scandinavian countries do not have specific regulations but food inspectors employ a wide variety of tests to determine if oils should be discarded. These include 'food oil sensor', free fatty acids, smokepoint, taste, odour, foam and acid value. There is much current research concerning which method is the best for evaluating oils. Clearly, the area of heated-fats research is ripe for harvest in terms of research on toxicity, oil degradation, antioxidants, filtration and methods of evaluation. These comments apply equally well to the many other ramifications of food lipid oxidation products. It is difficult to overestimate the potential importance, both from the scientific and health standpoints, of lipid oxidation products and it seems appropriate to attempt to discuss some of the broad significance of this exciting area of research.

To begin with, it seems appropriate to consider some of the most fundamental ideas on CHD and challenge them based on the new findings on lipid oxidation products. It appears that dietary (pure) cholesterol is neither angiotoxic nor hypercholesterolaemic and, therefore, cannot initiate or promote CHD. It is tempting to speculate that lipid oxidation product consumption patterns may partially explain why some persons with low serum cholesterol are susceptible to CHD, while others with high serum cholesterol appear to escape the disease. The role of smoking, perhaps the single most important risk factor in CHD, may be linked to *in vivo* oxidation of blood and tissue lipids. Research is urgently needed on this point.

Lipid oxidation products in food represent 'process-induced' toxicants and, therefore, are contrasted to the usual xenobiotic contaminant. Because such oxidation products are endogenously produced, as opposed to being derived from exogenous sources, the regulatory status is uncertain in the USA. Nevertheless, the FDA has established a program in 'process-induced' phenomena, indicating possible future regulatory interest. Heated oils would probably be targeted for early consideration of regulatory activity based on activities in Europe. Interestingly, the recent popularity of a more polyunsaturated-type of frying oil will likely produce greater oxidation problems than use of tallow or shortening.

There may be a connection between dietary lipid oxidation products and mLDL and between both of these and the consumption of dietary antioxidants. The potential benefits of antioxidants would appear to be very great if the conversion of LDL to mLDL can be slowed by antioxidants.

Future research needs

The future research needs of the health effects of lipid oxidation products are very great. Because of the highly significant new findings in CHD research as well as the highly specific and sensitive procedures now available for the quantification of lipid oxidation products, some extremely important advances are anticipated in CHD research. It is clear that much more data are needed on the absorption and transport of lipid oxidation products in both animal models and humans. Are fatty acid hydroperoxides absorbed? What percentages of the various oxysterols are absorbed and what factors influence the efficiency of absorption of oxysterols? Once absorbed, what factors influence the rate of clearance of oxides from the circulation and is there any connection to atherosclerosis? Is the rate of formation of mLDL influenced by dietary lipid oxidation products? Research is urgently needed to understand the complete metabolism of oxysterols, including absorption, transfer among lipoproteins in the blood and the assimilation into various tissues.

Oxysterols appear to raise serum cholesterol to a greater extent than cholesterol itself. Are other oxidation products also more hypercholesterolaemic than their native counterparts? Fatty acid degradation products inhibit prostacyclin synthesis, a factor favouring thrombosis/spasm. Do cholesterol oxides have similar effects?

French-fried foods are a major source of dietary oxidation products. Clearly more research is needed on the detailed content of all the various lipid oxidation products in such foods. An assessment is needed of the toxicology of these oxidation products using appropriate animal models, relevant combinations and levels of oxides and appropriate experimental treatment durations. In addition, a similar assessment is needed of the dimers, trimers and polymers produced by the thermal degradation of fats. There would also appear to be an urgent need for research on improved methods of monitoring oil quality and improved handling and filtration (clear-up) of oils and shortenings used for deep-frying.

From the standpoint of public health (CHD) a major question is related to whether or not it is advisable to change to unhydrogenated or lightly hydrogenated vegetable oils (substituted for animal fats) which are very susceptible to degradation. This question is especially pertinent in the USA where essentially no laws regarding oil quality exist and where effective methods for oil-quality assessment are largely ignored.

The other health-related research in relation to lipid oxidation products includes studies on the possible carcinogenic effects, the long-term effects on membranes, the possible accumulation in tissues, the enzyme effects and the possible clinical manifestation of these phenomena. Progress will likely be slower than in CHD research because less is known about cancer, ageing and other diseases which might be adversely affected by lipid oxidation products.

Much research is needed on improvements in methods for retarding the rancidity in foods. Powdered eggs should receive top priority in this regard. Also, fats and oils used for frying and deep-frying, precooked (uncured) meats and powdered products of all types need scrutiny. Freeze-dried products need much research.

In terms of broad scientific interest, the potential health effects of dietary lipid oxidation products are not going to be elucidated by the efforts of a single scientific field such as food chemistry or medicine. Only through cooperative research investigations among nutritionists, toxicologists, medical researchers and food chemists can truly significant advances be made. It is our hope that this treatise has helped to stimulate such cooperation.

Acknowledgements

Published as Paper No. 17,961 of the contribution series of the Minnesota Agricultural Experiment Station based on research conducted under Project No. 18–23, supported by Hatch funds. The authors thank R.J. Epley and C.A. Hassel for their helpful suggestions.

References

Addis, P.B. (1986). *Food Chemical Toxicology*, **24**, 1021–30

Addis, P.B. and Park, S.W. (1989). in Taylor, S.L. and Scanlan, R.A. (Eds), *Food Toxicology. A Perspective on the Relative Risks*, pp.297–330, New York: Marcel Dekker

Addis, P.B., Csallany, A.S. and Kindom, S.E. (1983). in Finley, J.W. and Schwass, D.E. (Eds), *Xenobiotics in Foods and Feeds*, ACS Symposium Series 234, pp.85–98, Washington, D.C.: American Chemical Society

Addis, P.B., Emanuel, H.A., Bergmann, S.D. and Zavoral, J.H. (1989). *Free Radical Biology and Medicine*, **7**, 179–82

Alexander, J.C. (1983). in Finley, J.W. and Schwass, D.E. (Eds), *Xenobiotics in Foods and Feeds*, ACS Symposium Series 234, pp.129–48, Washington, D.C.: American Chemical Society

Alexander, J.C., Valli,VE. and Channin, B.E. (1987). *Journal of Toxicology and Environmental Health*, **21**, 295–309

Ames, B.N. (1983). *Science*, **221**, 1256–64

Ball, R.Y., Carpenter, K.L.H. and Mitchinson, M.J. (1987). *Archives of Pathology and Laboratory Medicine*, **111**, 1134–40

Bascoul, J., Domerue, N., Olle, M. and Crastes de Paulet, A. (1986). *Lipids*, **21**, 383–7

Basu, A.K. and Marnett, L.J. (1983). *Carcinogenesis*, **4**, 331–3

Basu, A.K., O'Hara, S.M., Valladier, P., Stone, K., Mols, O. and Marnett, L.V. (1988). *Chemical Research in Toxicology*, **1**, 53–9

Brooks, C.J.W., McKenna, R.M., Cole, W.J., MacLacklan, J. and Laurie, T.D.V. (1983). *Biochemical Society Transactions*, **11**, 700–1

Brown, M.S. and Goldstein, J.L. (1976). *Science*, **191**, 150–4

Carroll, K.K. and Khor, H.T. (1971). *Lipids*, **6**, 415–20

Cerutti, P.A. (1985). *Science*, **227**, 375–81

Chan, J.T. and Chan, J.C. (1980). *Photobiochemistry and Photobiophysics*, **1**, 113–17

Corongiu, F.P., Banni, S. and Dessi, M.A. (1989). *Free Radical Biology and Medicine*, **7**, 183–6

Crampton, E.W., Common, R.H., Pritchard, E.T. and Farmer, F.A. (1956). *Journal of Nutrition*, **60**, 13–24

Csallany, A.S., Guan, M.D., Manwaring, J.D. and Addis, P.B. (1984). *Analytical Biochemistry*, **142**, 277–83

Dennis, K.J. and Shibamoto, T. (1989). *Free Radical Biology and Medicine*, **7**, 187–92

De Vore, V.R. (1988). *Journal of Food Science*, **53**, 1058–61

Dhopeshwarkar, G.A. (1981). *Progress in Lipid Research*, **19**, 107–18

Dillard, C.J. and Tappel, A.L. (1989). *Free Radical Biology and Medicine*, **7**, 193–6

Duncan, J.L. and Buckingham, L. (1980). *Biochimica et Biophysica Acta*, **603**, 278–87

Edington, J., Geekie, M., Carter, R., Benfield, L., Fisher, K., Ball, M. and Mann, J. (1987). *British Medical Journal*, **294**, 333–6

Egli, U.H., Streuli, R.A. and Dubler, E. (1984). *Biochemistry*, **23**, 148–52

Emanuel, H.A. (1989). M.Sc. Thesis, University of Minnesota, Minneapolis, Minnesota

Epand, R.M. and Bottega, R. (1987). *Biochemistry*, **26**, 1820–5

Esterbauer, H. and Zollner, H. (1989). *Free Radical Biology and Medicine*, **7**, 197–204

Faggiotto, A. and Ross, R. (1984). *Arteriosclerosis*, **4**, 341–56

Faggiotto, A., Ross, R. and Harker, L. (1984). *Arteriosclerosis*, **4**, 323–40

Farias, R.N., Bloj, B., Morero, R.D., Siñeriz, F. and Trucco, R.E. (1975). *Biochimica et Biophysica Acta*, **415**, 231–51

Finocchiaro, E.T. and Richardson, T. (1983). *Journal of Food Protection*, **46**, 917–25

Firestone, D. (1989). *Proceedings of Deep Frying of Foods: Science and Practice*, University of California, Davis, CA

Firestone, D. and Summers, J.L. (1989). *Proceedings of Deep Frying of Foods: Science and Practice*, University of California, Davis, CA

Fujimoto, K., Neff, W.E. and Frankel, E.N. (1984). *Biochimica et Biophysica Acta*, **795**, 100–7

Funk, M.O. (1987). *Free Radical Biology and Medicine*, **3**, 319–22

Gardner, H.W. (1989). *Free Radical Biology and Medicine*, **7**, 65–86

Glavind, J., Christensen, F. and Sylven, C. (1971). *Acta Chemica Scandinavica*, **25**, 3220–6

Goldstein, J.L., Ho, Y.K., Basu, S.K. and Brown, M.S. (1979). *Proceedings of the National Academy of Sciences of the U.S.A.*, **76**, 333–7

Govindarajan, S., Hultin, H.O. and Kotula, A.W. (1977). *Journal of Food Science*, **42**, 571–7

Graham, J.M. and Green, C. (1970). *European Journal of Biochemistry*, **12**, 58–66

Gray, J.I. and Morton, I.D. (1981). *Journal of Human Nutrition*, **35**, 5–23

Gray, M.F., Lawrie, T.D.V. and Brooks, C.J.W. (1971). *Lipids*, **6**, 836–43

Gruenke, L.D., Wrensch, M.R., Petrakis, N.L., Miike, R., Ernster, V.L. and Craig, J.C. (1987). *Cancer Research*, **47**, 5483–7

Heinecke, J. (1987). *Free Radical Biology and Medicine*, **3**, 65–73

Hennig, G. and Boissonneault, G.A. (1987). *Atherosclerosis*, **68**, 255–61

Higley, N.A., Beery, J.T., Taylor, S.L., Porter, J.W., Dziuba, J.A. and Lalich, J.J. (1986). *Atherosclerosis*, **62**, 91–104

Hoff, H.F., O'Neil, J., Chisholm, III, G.M., Cole, T.B., Quehenberger, O., Esterbauer, H. and Jürgens, G. (1989). *Arteriosclerosis*, **9**, 538–49

Holmes, R.P. and Yoss, N.L. (1984). *Biochimica et Biophysica Acta*, **770**, 15–21

Houslay, M.D., Dipple, I. and Gordon, L.M. (1981). *Biochemical Journal*, **197**, 675–81

Iwaoka, T., Tabata, F. and Takahashi, T. (1987). *Free Radical Biology and Medicine*, **3**, 329–34

Jacobson, M.S., Price, M.G., Shamoo, A.E. and Heald, F.P. (1985). *Atherosclerosis*, **57**, 209–17

Jurgens, G., Hoff, H.F., Chisolm, III, G.M. and Esterbauer, H. (1987). *Chemistry and Physics of Lipids*, **45**, 315–36

Kandutsch, A.A. and Chen, H.W. (1973). *The Journal of Biological Chemistry*, **248**, 8408–17

Kandutsch, A.A. and Chen, H.W. (1974). *The Journal of Biological Chemistry*, **249**, 6057–61

Kosugi, H. and Kikugawa, K. (1989). *Free Radical Biology and Medicine*, **7**, 205–8

Kosykh, V.A., Lankin, V.Z., Podrez, E.A., Novikov, D.K., Volgushev, S.A., Victorov, A.V., Repin, V.S. and Smirnov, V.N. (1989). *Lipids*, **24**, 109–15

Krut, L.H. (1982a). *Atherosclerosis*, **43**, 95–104

Krut, L.H. (1982b). *Atherosclerosis*, **43**, 105–18

Lane, A., Blickenstaff, D. and Ivy, A.C. (1950). *Cancer*, **3**, 1044–51

Leaf, A. and Weber, P.C. (1987). *American Journal of Clinical Nutrition*, **45**, 1048–53

Leaf, A. and Weber, P.C. (1988). *The New England Journal of Medicine*, **318**, 549–

Matsushita, S., Terao, J. and Shibata, S.S. (1987). *Free Radical Biology and Medicine*, **3**, 335–6

Matthias, D., Becker, C.H., Gödicke, W., Schmidt, R. and Ponsold, K. (1987). *Atherosclerosis*, **63**, 115–24

Mead, J.F. (1962). in Schulz, H.W., Day, E.A. and Sinnhuber, R.O. (Eds), *Symposium on Foods: Lipids and Their Oxidation*, pp.360–3, Westport, CT: The, A.V.I., Publishing Company

Missler, S.R., Wasilchuk, B.A. and Merrit Jr., C. (1985). *Journal of Food Science*, **50**, 595–8, 646

Miyazawa, T. (1989). *Free Radical Biology and Medicine*, **7**, 209–18

Morgan, J.N. and Armstrong, D.J. (1987). *Journal of Food Science*, **52**, 1224–7

Morin, R.J. and Peng, S-K. (1989). *Lipids*, **24**, 217–20

Morin, R.J., Zemplényi, T. and Peng, S-K. (1987). *Pharmacologic Therapy*, **32**, 237–83

Morris, H.P., Larsen, C.D. and Lippincott, S.W. (1944). *Journal of the National Cancer Institute*, **4**, 285–303

Naber, E.C., Allred, J.B., Winget, C.J. and Stock, A.E. (1985). *Poultry Science*, **64**, 675–80

Naruszewicz, M., Wozny, E., Mirkiewicz, E., Nowicka, G. and Szostak, W.B. (1987). *Atherosclerosis*, **66**, 45–53

Nawar, W.W. and Witchwoot, A. (1980). in Simic, M.G. and Karel, M. (Eds), *Autoxidation in Food and Biological Systems*, pp.207–22, New York: Plenum Press

Nishida, T., Takenaka, F. and Kummerow, F.A. (1958). *Circulation Research*, **6**, 194–202

Ohfuji, T. and Kaneda, T. (1973). *Lipids*, **8**, 353–9

Palinski, W., Rosenfeld, M.E., Ylä-Herttuala, S., Gurtner, G.C., Socher, S.S., Butler, S.W., Parthasarathy, S., Carew, T.E., Steinberg, D. and Witztum, J.L. (1989). *Proceedings of the National Academy of Sciences of the USA*, **86**, 1372–6

Park, S.W. and Addis, P.B. (1985). *Journal of Food Science*, **50**, 1437–41, 1444

Park, S.W. and Addis, P.B. (1986a). *Journal of Agricultural and Food Chemistry*, **34**, 653–9

Park, S.W. and Addis, P.B. (1986b). *Journal of Food Science*, **51**, 1380–1

Park, S.W. and Addis, P.B. (1987). *Journal of Food Science*, **52**, 1500–4

Pendleton, R.B. and Lands, W.E.M. (1987). *Free Radical Biology and Medicine*, **3**, 337–40

Peng, S.K. and Morin, R.J. (1987). *Artery*, **14**, 85–99

Peng, S.K. and Taylor, C.B. (1983). in Perkins, E.G. and Visek, W.J. (Eds), *Dietary Fats and Health*, pp.919–33, Champaign, IL: American Oil Chemists Society

Peng, S.K., Taylor, C.B., Hill, J.C. and Morin, R.J. (1985a). *Atherosclerosis*, **54**, 121–33

249

Peng, S.K., Morin, R.J., Tham, P. and Taylor, C.B. (1985b). *Artery*, **13**, 144–64
Peng, S.K., Hill, J.C., Morin, R.J. and Taylor, C.B. (1985c). *Proceedings of the Society for Experimental Biology and Medicine*, **180**, 126–32
Perkins, E.G. and Kummerow, F.A. (1959). *Journal of Nutrition*, **68**, 101–8
Piche, L.A., Draper, H.H. and Cole, P.D. (1988). *Lipids*, **23**, 370–1
Piretti, M.V. and Pagliuca, G. (1989). *Free Radical Biology and Medicine*, **7**, 219–22
Poling, C.E., Eagle, E., Rice, E.E., Durand, A.M.A. and Fisher, M. (1969). *Lipids*, **5**, 128–36
Pryor, W.A. (1987). *Free Radical Biology and Medicine*, **3**, 317–18
Pryor, W.A. (1989). *Free Radical Biology and Medicine*, **7**, 177–8
Raaphorst, G.P., Azzam, E.I., Langlois, R. and Van Lier, J.E. (1987). *Biochemical Pharmacology*, **36**, 2369–72
Richert, L., Bergmann, C., Beck, J-P., Rong, S., Luu, B. and Ourisson, G. (1983). *Biochemical and Biophysical Research Communications*, **117**, 851–8
Richert, L., Castagna, M., Beck, J-P., Rong, S., Luu, B. and Ourisson, G. (1984). *Biochemical and Biophysical Research Communications*, **120**, 192–8
Ross, R. (1981). *Arteriosclerosis*, **1**, 293–311
Ross, R. (1986). *The New England Journal of Medicine*, **314**, 488–500
Sander, B.D., Addis, P.B., Park, S.W. and Smith, D.E. (1989a). *Journal of Food Protection*, **52**, 109–14
Sander, B.D., Smith, D.E., Addis, P.B. and Park, S.W. (1989b). *Journal of Food Science*, **54**, 874–9
Sasaguri, Y., Morimatsu, M., Nakashima, T., Tokunaga, O. and Yagi, K. (1985). *Biochemistry International*, **11**, 517–21
Sasaguri, Y., Morimatsu, M., Nakano, R., Tokunaga, O. and Yagi, K. (1988). *Journal of Clinical and Biochemical Nutrition*, **5**, 117–26
Sevanian, A. and Peterson, A.R. (1984). *Proceedings of the National Academy of Sciences of the U.S.A.*, **81**, 4198–202
Sevanian, A., Peterson, H. and Coates, T. (1988). *Proceedings of the 8th International Symposium of Atherosclerosis*, Rome: Pekno Press, pp.103–18
Simic, M.G. and Karel, M. (1980). *Autoxidation in Food and Biological Systems*, New York: Plenum Press
Sinensky, M., Duwe, G. and Pinkerton, F. (1979). *The Journal of Biological Chemistry*, **254**, 4482–6
Smith, L.L. (1981). *Cholesterol Autoxidation*, New York: Plenum Press
Smith, L.L. (1987). *Chemistry and Physics of Lipids*, **44**, 87–125
Smith, R.L. (1988). *Diet Blood Cholesterol and Coronary Heart Disease: a Critical Review of the Literature*, Santa Monica: Vector Enterprises
Smith, L.L. and Johnson, B.H. (1989). *Free Radical Biology and Medicine*, **7**, 285–332
Steinberg, D., Parthasarathy, S., Carew, T.E., Khoo, J.C. and Witztum, J.L. (1989). *The New England Journal of Medicine*, **320**, 915–24
Steinbrecher, U.P., Fisher, M., Witztum, J.L. and Curtiss, L.K. (1984). *Journal of Lipid Research*, **25**, 1109–16
Streuli, R.A., Kanofsky, J.R., Gunn, R.B. and Yachnin, S. (1981). *Blood*, **58**, 317–25
Suzuki, K., Bruce, W.R., Baptista, J., Furrer, R., Vaughan, D.J. and Krepinsky, J.J. (1986). *Cancer Letters*, **33**, 307–16
Szamosi, T., Gara, I., Venekei, I., Javor, A., Ceskel, R. and Knoll, J. (1987). *Atherosclerosis*, **68**, 111–15

Szczeklik, A., Gryglewski, R.J., Domagala, B., Dworski, R. and Basista, M. (1985). *Thrombosis and Haemostasis*, **54**, 425–30

Taylor, C.B., Peng, S.K., Werthessen, N.T., Tham, P. and Lee, K.T. (1979). *American Journal of Clinical Nutrition*, **32**, 40–57

Terao, J. and Matsushita, S. (1987). *Free Radical Biology and Medicine*, **3**, 345–8

Theunissen, J.J.H., Jackson, R.L., Kempen, H.J.M. and Demel, R.A. (1986). *Biochimica et Biophysica Acta*, **860**, 66–74

Thiery, J. and Seidel, D. (1987). *Atherosclerosis*, **63**, 53–6

Thomas, W.A. and Kim, D.N. (1983). *Laboratory Investigation*, **48**, 245–55

Tipton, C.L., Leung, P.C., Johnson, J.S., Brooks, R.J. and Beitz, D.C. (1987). *Biochemical and Biophysical Research Communications*, **146**, 1166–72

Tsai, L.S. and Hudson, C.A. (1985). *Journal of Food Science*, **50**, 229–31, 237

Van Kuijk, F.J.G.M. and Dratz, E.A. (1987). *Free Radical Biology and Medicine*, **3**, 349–54

Wendel, A. (1987). *Free Radical Biology and Medicine*, **3**, 355–8

Witte, V.C., Krause, G.F. and Bailey, M.E. (1970). *Journal of Food Science*, **35**, 582–5

Wolff, S.P., Bascal, Z.A. and Hunt, J.V. (1989). in Baynes, J.W. and Monnier, V.M. (eds), *The Maillard Reaction in Aging, Diabetes and Nutrition*, pp. 259–75, New York: Alan R. Liss

Yagi, K. (1987). *Chemistry and Physics of Lipids*, **43**, 337–51

Yagi, K. (1988). in Ando, W. and Moro-oka, Y. (Eds), *The Role of Oxygen in Chemistry and Biochemistry*, Vol.33, pp. 383–90, Amsterdam: Elsevier

Yagi, K., Inagaki, T., Sasaguri, Y., Nakano, R. and Nakashima, T. (1987). *Journal of Clinical and Biochemical Nutrition*, **3**, 87–94

Yamamoto, Y. and Ames, B.N. (1987). *Free Radical Biology and Medicine*, **3**, 359–62

Ylä-Herttuala, S., Palinski, W., Rosenfeld, M.E., Parthasarathy, S., Carew, T.E., Butler, S., Witztum, J.L. and Steinberg, D. (1989). *Journal of Clinical Investigation*, **84**, 1086–95

Discussion

Dr Katan: As you know, I share your interest in oxysterols, although we have done much less on them than you have. I wonder if we already have the evidence that oxysterols promote atherosclerosis. Has any one fed oxysterols to animals and shown that they produced more atherosclerosis mg per mg than cholesterol does?

Dr Addis: Yes, there have been a number of early studies by the workers at Albany. It was Bruce Taylor and S.K. Peng (now at UCLA). They compared equal levels of oxysterols and purified cholesterol. Also, cholestanetriol was fed to the White Carneau pigeon by Jacobson's group. Triol accelerated atherosclerosis.

Dr Katan: But, were the oxysterols fed or were they ingested? I remember their studies on isolated cells.

Dr Addis: Some were injection studies and some were feeding studies.

Dr Stehbens: Although I approve of your usage of the word atherogenic, I do not believe that cholesterol feeding produces atherosclerosis. I think it is a fat storage disease. But, when you have substances such as these oxidation products, they are also cytotoxic. You are adding another aspect, in that you are damaging the tissue in the first instance, and then you have the sterol effect with a fat storage phenomenon superimposed. This would be aggravated by the oxidation product primarily because trauma also localizes the accumulation of lipid in fat storage disorders. But, I think the problem with cytotoxic substances is that they should not be called atherogenic at this stage. It is also important to know whether or not they produce a cytotoxic effect on other cells throughout the body, including the central nervous system. It is a non-specific cellular toxicity.

Dr Addis: Yes, however, the hypothesis includes the fact that the cytotoxicity is the basis for beginnings of the atherogenic effects seen. In other words, the cytotoxicity of the endothelial cells is the initiating factor in atherosclerosis in this case.

Dr Stehbens: But, I do not believe they should be called atherogenic because they are not atherogenic unless they actually produce the full-fledged story of atherosclerosis, including its complications. I would feel more comfortable if you called them angiotoxic or cytotoxic.

Dr Addis: I agree, angiotoxic is a better term.

Dr Navab: I would like to respond to Dr Katan's questions concerning cytotoxicity. We have studied a number of experiments that fed various strains of mice 0.2% cholesterol. After 6 weeks of feeding, fatty livers are seen. There is variability, but in some of the mice we see 50–100-fold induction of message for monocyte chemotactic protein, the homologue in mice which is the JE gene. There may also be mild symptoms of cytotoxicity and/or cytokine induction. This may be one of the specific effects of feeding 0.2% cholesterol after 6 weeks after seeing such dramatic induction of monocyte chemotactic gene in the liver.

Dr Connor: In conjunction with oxysterols, I wanted to mention some experiments done a long time ago in the White Carneau pigeon, which has genetic hypercholesterolaemia. These studies were done with a drug, cholestanetriol, which lowered the plasma cholesterol levels in these pigeons from approximately 348 mg/dl to 230 mg/dl. I think we have to appreciate the fact that some of these oxysterols may prevent cholesterol absorption and therefore might have a beneficial effect. I am not suggesting that the ones you talked about would have had that effect, but certainly cholestanetriol did.

Dr Addis: In response, I would have to point out Dr Jacobson's work (Jacobson *et al.* (1985). *Atherosclerosis*, **57**, 209) which showed the effects of feeding that same animal model cholesterol and cholestanetriol in appropriate quantities. He found levels of cholesterol which were appropriate in reflecting human consumption and, although at the time he had no idea of the triol consumption in our diet because he did not have the food analysis conducted, it was a very modest level of triol. Jacobson's group showed very clear effects as far as angiotoxicity of triol and also indications of atherosclerosis. He showed plaque build-up was accelerated by triol. I just might say that oxysterols are very capable angiotoxic substances regardless of cholesterol levels. Because they are cytotoxic, they do not depend on raising the cholesterol levels to induce angiotoxicity.

Dr Dietschy: Would you comment briefly on the methodology? To pick these up and quantitate them in the diets, is it gas–liquid chromatography or mass spectrometry and how does one do this easily?

Dr Addis: It is not an extremely difficult technique. However, it is a fairly time consuming one because there are two things which we insist upon: one is cold saponification of the lipids because hot saponification has been shown in our lab, and in others, to produce artifacts. The other thing is, when analyzing any experiment, or the first time through an experiment, or in food analysis, you must use mass spectral confirmation. The reason for this is because the peaks that you see on a chromatogram, even if perfectly amplified with appropriate standards, still may be different compounds. We have had examples of this in our own research. So, it is very important to do a mass spectral identification. Basically what we do is a Folch extraction, cold saponification for about 20 hours and then we go through a number of clean-up steps. I will be glad, if anyone is interested, to send you the detailed methodology.

15

Regulation of the concentration of cholesterol carried in low density lipoproteins in the plasma*

J.M. DIETSCHY

There are a number of risk factors that are now known to be associated with the development of atherosclerosis and, hence, with the clinical syndromes of myocardial infarction, cerebral infarction and peripheral vascular disease. These factors are diverse and include such things as smoking, hypertension, elevated levels of low density lipoproteins (LDL), reduced levels of high density lipoproteins (HDL) and even the presence of unusual lipoprotein fractions in the plasma such as oxidized LDL or Lp(a). However, of these various risk factors, the association of atheroma formation with plasma LDL-cholesterol concentrations has received the most attention[1]. In young people, for example, there is a direct relationship between the presence of early atherosclerotic lesions and levels of plasma LDL-cholesterol, and in adults there is a similar relationship between the incidence of atherosclerotic complications and this lipoprotein fraction[2,3]. More recently, it has also been shown that lowering the levels of LDL-cholesterol is associated with a lower incidence of disease associated with atherosclerosis and even with regression of the atherosclerotic lesion itself[4]. Thus, there is now considerable interest in identifying those individuals in the general population who have elevated plasma LDL-cholesterol levels so that they can be appropriately treated with dietary or pharmacological manipulations.

At the same time that these epidemiological data have been evolving, a great deal of new information has also become available on the mechanisms of regulation of LDL-cholesterol concentrations in plasma and how these mechanisms may be altered to cause hypercholesterolaemia. Thus, this review has

* Portions of this article were previously published in *Hospital Practice*, 25, 67–78, 1990 and the *Proceedings from the Scientific Conference on the Effects of Dietary Fatty Acids on Serum Lipoproteins and Hemostasis*, pp. 67–75, 1989. (Dallas: American Heart Association).

three sections. The first outlines the essential features of the normal physiology of the LDL particle, the second deals with quantitative aspects of the regulation of LDL levels and the third reviews, insofar as data are available, the dietary mechanisms that result in elevation of the plasma LDL-cholesterol level.

Normal physiology of the LDL particle

In general, lipoproteins function to carry insoluble substances such as triacylglycerol, cholesterol and fat-soluble vitamins between different compartments in the body. Each major lipoprotein fraction consists of a hydrophobic core made up primarily of triacylglycerol and/or cholesteryl esters and a surface coat of unesterified cholesterol and phospholipid. Specific apolipoprotein molecules (apo A, B, C and E) are embedded in this surface coat, and these act to target the particular particle to a specific metabolic and transport pathway[5].

As shown in Figure 1, triacylglycerol of dietary origin and cholesterol of both dietary and biliary origins are absorbed into the enterocyte and incorporated into the nascent chylomicron (CM) particle. When secreted into the intestinal lymph this particle contains only members of the apo A and apo B families of apolipoproteins. After mixing with HDL in the lymph and plasma, however, it also acquires apolipoproteins of the C and E classes. This mature CM is then circulated to the capillary beds of muscle and adipose tissue where one of the apo C proteins interacts with a specific enzyme, lipoprotein lipase, to bring about the hydrolysis and removal of much of the triacylglycerol core.

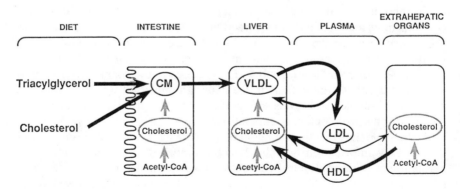

Figure 1 The role of the major lipoprotein classes in cholesterol transport. This diagram shows the general pathways by which cholesterol is transported in the major lipoprotein classes between the tissue compartments of the body. Although not shown in this diagram, CM and VLDL are also important in delivering triacylglycerol from the intestine and liver, respectively, to peripheral muscle and adipose tissue

The fatty acids derived from this reaction are then oxidized for energy production (in muscle) or are stored as triacylglycerol (in adipose tissue). At some point in this process the particle is released back into the circulation and is now designated a chylomicron remnant. This remnant is immediately recognized, apparently through the apo B and apo E on its surface, by a remnant receptor on the sinusoidal membrane of the hepatocyte and taken up into the liver[6]. In this manner most of the cholesterol and a portion of the triacylglycerol that was absorbed from the intestinal lumen is delivered to the liver.

As also shown in Figure 1, both the intestine and liver are capable of synthesizing significant amounts of cholesterol, and this process is under tight feedback regulation. Thus, the absorption of increasing amounts of dietary cholesterol is associated with progressive suppression of synthesis in these organs so that net cholesterol availability in the liver cell tends to remain relatively constant, even in the face of variable dietary sterol intake[7].

The liver makes a second lipoprotein particle, very low density lipoprotein (VLDL), that primarily functions to transport triacylglycerol out of the liver to the peripheral organs of utilization and storage. The hepatocyte continuously accumulates triacylglycerol from the uptake of plasma free fatty acids, from uptake of the chylomicron remnant and from *de novo* synthesis of free fatty acids from acetyl-CoA. Once secreted, the triacylglycerol core of the VLDL particle is largely removed by lipoprotein lipase in the capillary beds of muscle and adipose tissue in a manner that is essentially identical to that described for the metabolism of the chylomicron. A partially metabolized or remnant VLDL particle is also formed that is cleared from the plasma by receptors in the liver. However, unlike the CM, a portion of the VLDL pool is further metabolized to a smaller, more dense lipoprotein that contains predominantly cholesteryl esters and little triacylglycerol, and that has only one apolipoprotein, i.e. apo B-100. This is the LDL particle. Little, if any, LDL is normally directly secreted by the liver into the plasma; rather, most is derived from the metabolism of VLDL[8]. This LDL particle is then removed from the plasma space by receptor-dependent and receptor-independent mechanisms that are located both in the liver and in extrahepatic organs.

As also indicated in Figure 1, most extrahepatic organs also have significant rates of cholesterol synthesis and, in addition, take up small amounts of LDL-cholesterol. Since these organs do not accumulate sterol, an amount of cholesterol equal to the sum of these two processes must be removed each day and carried back to the liver for excretion in the bile. Presumably, it is the HDL particle that subserves this role of reverse cholesterol transport.

From these considerations, it is apparent that the steady-state concentration of LDL-cholesterol in the plasma is determined by the rate at which VLDL is converted to LDL, i.e. the LDL-cholesterol production rate, and by the rate at which this lipoprotein fraction is removed from the plasma by the various tissues. Since the discovery of the LDL receptor by Brown and Goldstein[9], two different mechanisms have been identified in the whole animal and in man that are responsible for this removal process. The first transport mechanism is recognized as being receptor-dependent and is a saturable uptake process mediated by LDL receptors situated on the surface of a variety of cell types. The second transport mechanism is receptor-independent and non-saturable, and is also located in many different organs[10-12].

Quantitative considerations in the regulation of LDL-cholesterol levels

There are now a variety of data that deal with the quantitative importance of each of these two transport processes in normal animals and in man. As illustrated in the first column of Figure 2, for example, the majority of the LDL-cholesterol that is removed from the plasma is transported out by means of the receptor-dependent process. Thus, in every species in which data are available, and these include hamster, rat, mouse, rabbit, dog, cynomolgus monkey and man, approximately 60–80% of the plasma pool of LDL-cholesterol is taken up and degraded by the receptor-dependent process.

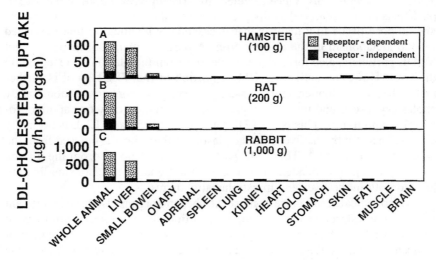

Figure 2 The distribution of receptor-dependent and receptor-independent LDL transport activity in several animal species. The first column shows the relative importance of the receptor-dependent and receptor-independent mechanisms for the uptake and degradation of LDL-cholesterol in the whole animal. The other columns quantify the distribution of these two transport activities in the major whole organs of these same animals

The tissues in which this transport activity is located are also illustrated in Figure 2. The liver and small bowel clearly account for the clearance of most of the LDL-cholesterol that is removed from the plasma space and degraded each day. Of the receptor-dependent transport activity that can be identified in the whole animal, nearly 90% is located in these same two organs. In contrast, the receptor-independent process, which in the whole animal accounts for the clearance of 20–40% of the plasma LDL-cholesterol pool, is distributed in many tissues, although about 30% of this activity is still found in the liver. It should be noted that the receptor-dependent transport process is regulable by diet and pharmaceutical agents while the receptor-independent process apparently is not. Under circumstances where receptor-dependent LDL transport is very low, the receptor-independent process becomes the predominantly mechanism for removing LDL-cholesterol from the plasma, and the site of this degradation is shifted away from the liver to the extrahepatic organs.

Thus, in general terms, the plasma LDL-cholesterol concentration is determined by the rate of entry of LDL into the plasma space relative to the rate at which it is removed by both the receptor-dependent and receptor-independent transport processes localized predominantly in the liver, but also in extrahepatic organs. Each of these processes can be expressed in more quantitative terms as shown in Figure 3.

The rate of input of LDL into the vascular space is given by the LDL-cholesterol production rate (J_t) and in the young, healthy human subject this rate constant equals approximately 0.58 mg/h per kg of body weight. The rate of output of LDL-cholesterol from the vascular space is determined by both the receptor-dependent and receptor-independent transport processes. Removal of LDL by the receptor-dependent process involves interaction of the LDL molecules with a finite number of receptors, so this process is saturable. The rate of such transport, therefore, must be described in terms of two parameters, the maximal transport velocity that can be achieved when all receptors are saturated (J^m) and the concentration of plasma LDL-cholesterol that is necessary to achieve half of this maximal transport velocity (K_m). J^m is a function of total LDL receptor activity in the whole animal while K_m reflects the functional affinity of the LDL particles for these receptors. Thus, in man the maximal rate of receptor-dependent LDL-cholesterol transport that is achievable equals about 0.78 mg/h per kg. However, since the plasma LDL-cholesterol concentration is only about 75 mg/dl in such young subjects while the K_m value is approximately 90 mg/dl, the absolute rate of receptor-dependent LDL-uptake found in these young subjects is only about 0.35 mg/h per kg.

In contrast to the receptor-dependent system, the receptor-independent clearance of LDL-cholesterol is a linear function of the plasma LDL-cholesterol concentration and, therefore, is described by a simple proportionality

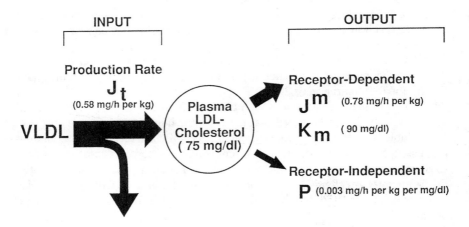

Figure 3 The four rate constants that determine the steady-state plasma LDL-cholesterol concentration. The plasma concentration of LDL-cholesterol is determined by the rate at which LDL-cholesterol is formed from VLDL and enters the plasma space (J_t) and by the rate at which this particle is removed from the plasma and degraded through the receptor-dependent and receptor-independent transport mechanisms. The receptor-dependent process is saturable and so is described in terms of the maximal achievable rate of transport (J^m) and the concentration of plasma LDL-cholesterol necessary to achieve half of this maximal transport velocity (K_m). The receptor-independent transport process is a linear function of the LDL-cholesterol concentration and so is described by a simple proportionality constant (P). The values shown for these four rate constants are those that are appropriate for young, healthy human subjects

constant. In man this constant equals approximately 0.003 mg/h per kg per mg/dl of LDL-cholesterol. The absolute rate of LDL-cholesterol uptake by this process equals the product of this proportionality constant times the concentration of LDL-cholesterol in the plasma or about 0.23 mg/h per kg. Thus, in these young, healthy subjects where the steady-state LDL-cholesterol concentration equals about 75 mg/dl, the rate of LDL-cholesterol entry into the plasma space equals 0.58 mg/h per kg while the rate of removal by the receptor-dependent process equals 0.35 mg/h per kg (61% of the total removal) and by the receptor-independent process equals 0.23 mg/h per kg. In this steady-state, the rate of entry equals the rate of removal of LDL-cholesterol.

Experimental means are now available for measuring these rate constants directly in the experimental animal or indirectly in man. These rate constants for four species are shown in Table 1. As is apparent, in the absence of dietary lipids (except in the case of man) the rate of LDL-cholesterol production varies from 3.11 mg/h per kg in the hamster to only 0.58 mg/h per kg in man. The

Table 1 Values for the four major rate constants regulating LDL-cholesterol levels in four different species

| Species | Production rate J_t (mg/h per kg) | Receptor-dependent transport | | Receptor-independent transport |
		J^m (mg/h per kg)	K_m (mg/dl)	P (mg/h per kg per mg/dl)
Hamster	3.11	4.85	91	0.012
Rat	2.18	4.06	97	0.006
Rabbit	1.67	2.13	90	0.009
Man	0.58	0.78	90	0.003

The values for the four rate constants in the hamster, rat and rabbit were determined by direct measurements in animals that had been maintained on a diet essentially free of cholesterol and triacylglycerol[13]. The values in man have been estimated indirectly as described elsewhere[14].

maximal rate of receptor dependent LDL-cholesterol uptake (J^m) is higher than these production rates and the K_m values in all species are approximately 90–100 mg/dl. Thus, since the plasma LDL-cholesterol concentration in essentially all species (on a low cholesterol, low triacylglycerol diet) is below these K_m values, the receptor-dependent LDL transport system is always operating well below maximal achievable velocities. The proportionality constant for the receptor-independent transport process also varies inversely with animal size. Thus, in every species the total rate of LDL-cholesterol removal from the plasma equals the rate of LDL-cholesterol production in the steady-state and, furthermore, the relative importance of these two transport processes is essentially the same in every species, at least under conditions where there is essentially no cholesterol or triacylglycerol in the diet.

While the value of these four kinetic parameters varies among different animal species, it is clear that any alteration in the plasma LDL-cholesterol concentration in any animal model or in man must be explained in terms of a change in J_t, J^m, K_m or P. Intuitively, one can easily appreciate from Figure 3 that an increase in LDL-cholesterol production rate (J_t) or a reduction in whole-body LDL receptor activity (J^m) would very likely lead to an elevation of the plasma cholesterol concentration.

The manner in which a change in these parameters affects the circulating levels of LDL-cholesterol is illustrated in more quantitative terms in Figure 4. The solid curve shows the total rate at which LDL-cholesterol is removed from the plasma at levels of plasma LDL-cholesterol varying from 0 to 350 mg/dl. The shape of this curve is dictated by the saturable receptor-dependent component of this removal process and by the linear receptor-independent process. The data point labelled **a** represents a normal animal with a LDL-cholesterol production rate of 1 mg/h per kg and an identical removal

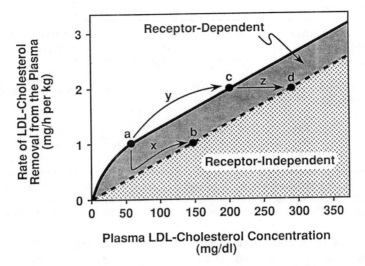

Figure 4 Theoretical curves illustrating the effects of altering either the LDL-cholesterol production rate or receptor-dependent LDL transport. In these examples, the values for P and K_m have been kept constant while J_t and J^m have been varied. Point **a** represents a normal animal with a LDL-cholesterol production rate of 1.0 mg/h per kg and where approximately 65% of LDL-cholesterol removal from the plasma is accomplished by the receptor-dependent process. Point **b** shows the effects of eliminating all receptor-dependent LDL transport from the animal while point **c** shows the effects of doubling the LDL-cholesterol production rate. Point **d** illustrates the shift in the plasma LDL-cholesterol concentration when J_t is doubled at the same time that J^m is set equal to zero

rate. As is apparent, about 65% of this removal is accomplished through receptor-dependent transport while 35% takes place through the receptor-independent process. Under these conditions the plasma LDL-cholesterol concentration equals 50 mg/dl.

If, in this example, all receptor-dependent LDL transport were suddenly lost, i.e. J^m drops to zero, the rate of LDL-cholesterol removal would immediately decrease to only 35% of its initial value (illustrated by arrow **x**). Since the rate of LDL-cholesterol entrance into the plasma is now nearly three times the rate of removal, the plasma LDL-cholesterol concentration would necessarily increase until the velocity of removal by the receptor-independent process reached 1.0 mg/h per kg (point **b**). At this point the animal is back in a new steady-state where the rate of LDL removal equals the rate of LDL production. However, to achieve this state the plasma LDL-cholesterol concentration had to rise to approximately 150 mg/dl, and the receptor-independent transport process accounts for 100% of LDL removal and degradation.

Point **c** illustrates a second example where the LDL-cholesterol production rate has been doubled under circumstances where the other three kinetic constants have been kept constant. Again, since the rate of LDL entry now exceeds the rate of LDL removal, the plasma LDL-cholesterol concentration will necessarily increase (along arrow **y**) until point **c** is achieved. At this point, the rate of LDL entry and removal equals 2.0 mg/h per kg and the new steady-state LDL-cholesterol concentration equals approximately 200 mg/dl. Even though total body receptor activity has been kept constant in this example, in this new steady-state only about 30% of LDL-cholesterol removal from the plasma is receptor-dependent. Finally, point **d** represents the more complex situation where the LDL-cholesterol production rate has been doubled at the same time that all receptor-dependent LDL transport has been deleted. Once again, the animal will come into a new steady-state where the two-fold increase in J_t is balanced by a marked increase in the removal of LDL by the receptor-independent transport process. In order to achieve this high rate of removal, however, the plasma LDL-cholesterol concentration must reach nearly 300 mg/dl.

It is now clear that in virtually all mammalian species, in newborn man and in human populations that live on diets containing little cholesterol and triacylglycerol, the steady-state LDL-cholesterol concentration in plasma is well below 100 mg/dl. The significantly higher levels that are routinely found in Western human populations must be explained in terms of either environmental or genetic effects on one of these four rate constants that dictate plasma LDL-cholesterol levels.

Dietary effects on these parameters of LDL-cholesterol metabolism

While it is theoretically possible that alterations in any of the four rate constants could account for changes in plasma cholesterol levels, recent data have shown that most dietary effects are mediated through changes in only two of these constants, i.e. the LDL-cholesterol production rate and the level of receptor-dependent LDL transport. Once the absolute values of these rate constants have been measured in a particular animal species or in man, it is possible to calculate how a change in either J_t or J^m will alter the steady-state plasma LDL-cholesterol concentration. Such data can then be plotted and provide a graphic display of how changes in these two parameters of LDL metabolism alter steady-state plasma levels.

Such a graphic presentation is shown in Figure 5 where the values of P and K_m have been kept constant while the values for LDL production and receptor-dependent transport have been systematically varied. For simplicity,

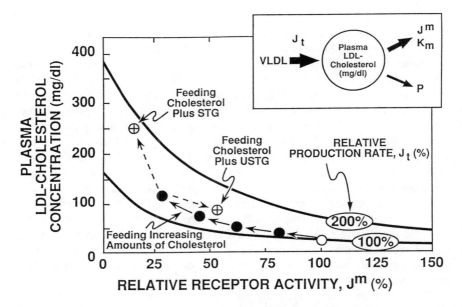

Figure 5 The effect of varying the amount of receptor-dependent LDL transport or the LDL-cholesterol production rate on the steady-state plasma LDL-cholesterol concentration. In this diagram, the plasma LDL-cholesterol concentration is shown under circumstances where there has been a systematic alteration in the LDL-cholesterol production rate (J_t) and the maximal rate of receptor-dependent LDL transport (J^m) but where the values of K_m and P have been kept constant. For simplicity, the values of J_t and J^m are expressed as relative activities where 100% is taken as the level of receptor-dependent transport and LDL-cholesterol production in an animal on a diet free of cholesterol and triacylglycerol. Such an animal or man is represented by the open circle. It should be emphasized that the exact shape of these curves is determined by the specific values for the four kinetic constants that are appropriate for any given animal species. Superimposed upon these theoretical curves are the usual results obtained when increasing amounts of cholesterol are fed (solid circles) and when triacylglycerols containing either predominantly saturated (STG) or unsaturated (USTG) fatty acids are added to one of these diets containing a fixed amount of cholesterol

J^m is plotted along the horizontal axis as the relative amount of receptor-dependent LDL transport, while the two solid lines show the relationship between receptor activity and the plasma LDL-cholesterol concentration at two different rates of LDL-cholesterol production. The open circle represents the situation in a normal animal fed no dietary lipids that has a plasma LDL-cholesterol concentration of approximately 25 mg/dl. The amount of receptor activity in this control animal has been assigned a value of 100%, as has the rate of LDL-cholesterol production.

There are several features concerning the relationships shown in this figure that deserve emphasis. First, when the production rate is kept constant at 100%, loss of receptor activity has relatively little effect on the LDL-cholesterol concentration until only about 50% of the receptor activity remains. As further loss of receptors occurs there is a relatively abrupt increase in the LDL-cholesterol concentration to about 170 mg/dl. Second, in the presence of high receptor activity, doubling the production rate also has a relatively small effect on the plasma cholesterol concentration. At 100% receptor activity, for example, a two-fold increase in the production rate increases the LDL-cholesterol level in this example to only about 75 mg/dl. Third, the effect of increased LDL production is very sensitive to the amount of receptor activity present in the animal. In the presence of 100% receptor activity, doubling the production rate raises the LDL-cholesterol concentration by only 50 mg/dl. When only 25% of the receptor activity is present, however, this same increase in the LDL production rate causes the LDL-cholesterol concentration to increase by 150 mg/dl. Thus, any genetic or environmental factor that results in loss of receptor activity coupled with an increase in production rate is likely to markedly increase the LDL-cholesterol concentration in the new steady-state.

One of the most important environmental factors to do this is dietary cholesterol. In the absence of sterol in the diet there are significant rates of cholesterol synthesis in the liver and extrahepatic tissues, although in species such as man and several other primates, hepatic sterol synthesis rates are much lower than in many of the extrahepatic organs. When cholesterol is fed and reaches the liver in the CM remnant (Figure 1) there is suppression of hepatic sterol synthesis, accumulation of cholesteryl esters and suppression of receptor-dependent LDL transport[15]. Thus, as also shown in Figure 5, in the whole animal, feeding increasing amounts of cholesterol is associated with a modest increase in the plasma LDL-cholesterol concentration. This increase results primarily from loss of receptor activity, although there is also a small increase in the LDL-cholesterol production rate (the solid points in Figure 5). These effects are clearly dose-dependent in that the more cholesterol that is fed, the greater is the loss of receptor activity and the increase in the plasma LDL-cholesterol concentration. Nevertheless, cholesterol feeding alone in many animal species and in man has only modest effects on plasma cholesterol levels.

The second environmental factor that markedly alters plasma cholesterol levels is dietary triacylglycerol. While the daily intake of cholesterol in many Western diets is only a few hundred milligrams, the daily intake of triacylglycerol often is in the range of 100–150 g. When triacylglycerol is fed along with small amounts of cholesterol there is an increase in the rate of hepatic cholesterol synthesis and very significant effects on hepatic receptor activity. If the triacylglycerol contains saturated fatty acids, there is significant further suppression of receptor activity, but if the predominant fatty acids are unsaturated, then there is actually restoration of receptor-dependent LDL transport. The saturated fatty acids also increase the production rate[16,17].

The overall effect of these complex changes in the whole animal or man is also illustrated diagrammatically in Figure 5. The superimposition of saturated triacylglycerols (STG) on the cholesterol-containing diet markedly elevates the plasma LDL-cholesterol concentration because of further loss of receptor activity and a significant increase in the LDL-cholesterol production rate. In contrast, triacylglycerols containing unsaturated fatty acids (USTG) slightly reduce the plasma LDL-cholesterol concentration. It should be apparent from this diagram that changing from a diet containing predominantly saturated fatty acids to one containing predominantly unsaturated fatty acids will markedly lower the plasma LDL-cholesterol concentration even when the total triacylglycerol and cholesterol content are kept constant. Alternatively, simply reducing the amount of saturated triacylglycerol in the diet will also lower the plasma LDL-cholesterol concentration even when the composition of this triacylglycerol remains unaltered.

Further work in this important area must deal with a number of questions concerning how these dietary effects are influenced by the composition of the triacylglycerol in the diet. For example, in the saturated fatty acid series, which specific fatty acids exert these effects on LDL-cholesterol production rates and receptor activities? Which of the unsaturated fatty acids are active in restoring LDL-cholesterol receptor-dependent transport? Does the position of the individual fatty acid on the triacylglycerol molecule affect how these fatty acids alter hepatic LDL metabolism? Finally, it will also be of considerable importance to understand at the cellular level how the uptake of both cholesterol and fatty acids alters regulation of these parameters of LDL-cholesterol metabolism.

Acknowledgements

The general principles and data presented in this paper were derived from studies supported in this laboratory by US Public Health Service research grant HL-09610 and by grants from the Moss Heart Fund and American Heart Association.

References

1. The Expert Panel. (1988). Report of the National Cholesterol Education Program Expert Panel on Detection, Evaluation, and Treatment of High Blood Cholesterol in Adults. *Arch. Intern. Med.*, **148**, 36–69

2. Newman III, W.P., Freedman, D.S., Voors, A.W., Gard, P.D., Srinivasan, S.R., Cresanta, J.L., Williamson, G.D., Webber, L.S. and Berenson, G.S. (1986). Relation of serum lipoprotein levels and systolic blood pressure to early atherosclerosis. The Bogalusa Heart Study. *N. Engl. J. Med.*, **314**, 138–44

3. Castelli, W.P., Garrison, R.J., Wilson, P.W.F., Abbott, R.D., Kalousdian, S. and Kannel, W.B. (1986). Incidence of coronary heart disease and lipoprotein cholesterol levels. The Framingham Study. *J. Am. Med. Assoc.*, **256**, 2835–8

4. Blankenhorn, D.H., Nessim, S.A., Johnson, R.L., Sanmarco, M.E., Azen, S.P. and Cashin-Hemphill, L. (1987). Beneficial effects of combined colestipol-niacin therapy on coronary atherosclerosis and coronary venous bypass grafts. *J. Am. Med. Assoc.*, **257**, 3233–40

5. Havel, R.J. (1986). Functional activities of hepatic lipoprotein receptors. In Berne, R.M. (ed.). *Annual Review of Physiology*, Vol. 48, pp. 119–34. (Palo Alto: Annual Reviews)

6. Kita, T., Goldstein, J.L., Brown, M.S., Watanabe, Y., Hornick, C.A. and Havel, R.J. (1982). Hepatic uptake of chylomicron remnants in WHHL rabbits: a mechanism genetically distinct from the low density lipoprotein receptor. *Proc. Natl. Acad. Sci. USA*, **79**, 3623–7

7. Turley, S.D. and Dietschy, J.M. (1988). The metabolism and excretion of cholesterol by the liver. In Arias, I.M., Jakoby, W.B., Popper, H., Schachter, D. and Shafritz, D.A. (eds). *The Liver: Biology and Pathobiology*, 2nd edn., pp. 617–41. (New York: Raven Press)

8. Yamada, N., Shames, D.M., Stoudemire, J.B. and Havel, R.J. (1986). Metabolism of lipoproteins containing apolipoprotein B-100 in blood plasma of rabbits: Heterogeneity related to the presence of apolipoprotein E. *Proc. Natl. Acad. Sci. USA*, **83**, 3479–83

9. Brown, M.S. and Goldstein, J.L. (1986). A receptor-mediated pathway for cholesterol homeostasis. *Science*, **232**, 34–47

10. Spady, D.K., Bilheimer, D.W. and Dietschy, J.M. (1983). Rates of receptor-dependent and -independent low density lipoprotein uptake in the hamster. *Proc. Natl. Acad. Sci. USA*, **80**, 3499–503

11. Spady, D.K., Turley, S.D. and Dietschy, J.M. (1985). Receptor-independent low density lipoprotein transport in the rat in vivo. Quantitation, characterization, and metabolic consequences. *J. Clin. Invest.*, **76**, 1113–22

12. Spady, D.K., Huettinger, M., Bilheimer, D.W. and Dietschy, J.M. (1987). Role of receptor-independent low density lipoprotein transport in the maintenance of tissue cholesterol balance in the normal and WHHL rabbit. *J. Lipid Res.*, **28**, 32–41

13. Dietschy, J.M., Spady, D.K. and Meddings, J.B. (1988). A quantitative approach to low density lipoprotein metabolism in man and in various experimental animals. In Suckling, K.E. and Groot, P.H.E. (eds). *Hyperlipidaemia and Atherosclerosis*, pp. 17–32. (London: Academic Press)

14. Meddings, J.B. and Dietschy, J.M. (1986). Regulation of plasma levels of low-density lipoprotein cholesterol: interpretation of data on low-density lipoprotein turnover in man. *Circulation*, **74**, 805–14

15. Spady, D.K. and Dietschy, J.M. (1988). Interaction of dietary cholesterol and triglycerides in the regulation of hepatic low density lipoprotein transport in the hamster. *J. Clin. Invest.*, **81**, 300–9

16. Spady, D.K. and Dietschy, J.M. (1985). Dietary saturated triacylglycerols suppress hepatic low density lipoprotein receptor activity in the hamster. *Proc. Natl. Acad. Sci. USA*, **82**, 4526–30
17. Woollett, L.A., Spady, D.K. and Dietschy, J.M. (1989). Mechanisms by which saturated triacylglycerols elevate the plasma low density lipoprotein-cholesterol concentration in hamsters. Differential effects of fatty acid chain length. *J. Clin. Invest.*, **84**, 119–28

Discussion

Dr Wood: I wonder if you could expand on your statement that cholesterol turns off the receptors; could you give us some idea of how you think that might occur?

Dr Dietschy: Everyone talks about a 'regulatory' pool, yet we know very little about the details of this process. Cholesterol is insoluble and is a structural component of membranes so that it is difficult to understand how the cell 'senses' the level of sterol. It is reasonable to assume that some 'regulatory' pool of cholesterol exists in the cell and is in equilibrium with the sterol regulatory elements on the genes that regulate receptor activity and HMG CoA reductase activity. It is possible that the entrance of various fatty acids into the cell disrupt this equilibrium in such a way that receptors are either inappropriately turned on or turned off. However, at this time, this is pure speculation.

Dr Clandinin: I would be interested in hearing your comments on how you are able to control for the fact that when you feed a highly saturated triglyceride from 18:0 or 16:0 that these are very poorly absorbed and therefore the flux of lipid would be much different from that with some of the other comparisons.

Dr Dietschy: We were aware of these problems at the start of these experiments. Indeed, the triacylglycerols with the longer chain-length saturated fatty acids did cause steatorrhea. Therefore, the experiments that I have just shown were undertaken using diets containing a constant 10% of olive oil. Under these circumstances net sterol balance appeared to be similar for all saturated fatty acids. In addition, analysis of the lipids in the liver cell showed that there was an equal enrichment of the 18:0 fatty acid when this lipid was fed as was seen with the shorter chain-length saturated fatty acids. Thus, these data suggested that, under the conditions of these particular experiments, all of the saturated fatty acids were being absorbed essentially to the same degree and were reaching the liver.

Dr Clandinin: We have considered this approach too and I have no doubt that you find those fatty acids reflected in most of the things that you measure. But, I would add one word of caution that many of these triglycerides are unusual. They may in fact be digested quite differently than a normal dietary triglyceride. Even the fact that they are all saturated presents certain problems for the enterocyte and processing which may cause them to be handled in a somewhat different form.

269

Dr Dietschy: Yes, I agree with what you have said, but the fact remains, when you feed them, they do reach the liver. They become incorporated into the cholesteryl esters and into the triacylglycerol fraction. Thus, whatever the nature of the differences in absorption, these particular fatty acids do reach the liver and result, either directly or indirectly, in changes in LDL metabolism.

Dr Katan: Apparently, the saturated fatty acids simultaneously depress the number of receptors and increase the production of LDL. Would you care to speculate on where these two processes are coupled, or is it just an accident that they do both? They seem to be fairly far removed from each other.

Dr Dietschy: In many situations these two processes do seem to be coupled. In general, when receptor activity in the liver goes up there is a reduction in the LDL-cholesterol production rate. While the nature of this coupling is poorly understood at this time, it is possible that it is related to the percentage of the VLDL pool that is converted to LDL in these various situations. Evidence suggests that intermediate density lipoproteins are also cleared from the plasma by the LDL receptor. Thus, if receptor activity is suppressed, more of this intermediate density pool may be converted to LDL. The exact mechanisms for this apparent coupling remain to be elucidated, however.

Dr Ueshima: We Japanese eat a lot of fish; have you ever examined LDL receptor activity when you feed fish?

Dr Dietschy: We have not, but Dr David Spady has done such experiments. When the diet contains a relatively large quantity of fish oil, hepatic LDL receptors are turned on, at least in the rat. This does not necessarily mean, however, that the relatively small amounts of fish oil taken as supplements to the human diet have any important physiological effect.

Dr Gold: I wonder, Dr Dietschy, if you would make mention of physiological effects of fatty acids with either *cis* or *trans* double bonds. Have those been done yet?

Dr Dietschy: While we intend to look at the effects of *cis* and *trans* fatty acids in the near future, these have not yet been done. However, there are data published from other laboratories which suggest that *trans* fatty acids may raise the circulating LDL cholesterol level. The mechanisms involved in this elevation, however, are not yet understood.

Dr Vega: In the studies of the hyperresponders to dietary cholesterol, have you looked at these animals for their absorption or responsiveness to plant sterols, β-sitosterol? Are they also hyperresponders?

Dr Dietschy: No, we have specifically not evaluated these responding and non-responding monkeys to different plant sterols.

Dr Kubow: Could you comment on your results with the position of distribution of fatty acids on the triacylglycerol molecule?

Dr Dietschy: These studies are now just being done and we do not yet have any definitive results. Both pancreatic lipase and lipoprotein lipase appear to have their primary enzymatic activities in attacking 1 and 3 positions of the triacylglycerol molecule. At least in theory, therefore, the fatty acid in the 2 position might be preferentially delivered to the liver. Whether or not this is true, however, remains to be seen.

Dr Clandinin: We have tested whether it matters if you have 16:0 in the beta position for absorption of the fats. Both in the animal and in the human we can find no apparent difference attributable to having 16:0 in the 1 or 3 or in the 2 position.

Dr Dietschy: But if the fatty acid is left in the 2 position and if lipoprotein lipase also preferentially attacks the 1 and 3 position fatty acids, then one might imagine that there would be preferential delivery to the liver of the fatty acid in this position. This remains speculative at this time.

Dr Hayes: Would you comment on the striking ability of oleic acid to increase LDL receptor activity? Do you have any mechanism in mind?

Dr Dietschy: There is no question, based upon studies by Dr Laura Woollett, that the 18:1 fatty acid is much more active than the 18:2 fatty acid in restoring LDL receptor activity. For a given level of dietary cholesterol intake the steady-state cholesteryl ester content of the liver cell is always significantly higher after feeding the 18:1 fatty acid, compared to the 18:2 lipid. It is conceivable that this partitioning of the cholesterol into the ester pool leads to a significant lowering of the regulatory pool of cholesterol in the liver cell and a disproportionate restoration of receptor activity. However, at this time this mechanism is clearly speculative.

Dr Katan: I have been asked by the organizers to comment on our *trans* fatty acid studies, so this is not really a question relating to your beautiful studies.

271

We published a study last year showing that transmonounsaturates raised LDL cholesterol and lowered HDL cholesterol. Recently, Peter Zoch in my group has done another study with a lower level of *trans* fatty acids, which more or less confirmed this. So, it looks as if the *trans* fatty acids really fall into the saturate class as far as LDL is concerned. However, there is one thing that I would like to set straight. There has been some media to-do about our study where our results were translated into foods by equating saturates with butter and *trans* with margarine. That is a fairly serious mistake. Butter does not equal saturates – butter contains about 60% saturates – and margarine does not equate *trans*. The *trans* fatty acid content of margarines ranges from 0 to 30% in the United States and 0–50% in my country. Depending on the type of margarine you choose, you can either choose something with less *trans* fatty acids than butter, because butter has about 5% *trans* produced by biohydrogenation in the rumen of the cow, or you can have a margarine that has a lot more *trans*. So, I think this really speaks to the issue of margarine composition and that has been something that has been studied carefully in the Canada. So, if you are worried about *trans* fatty acids, you should carefully choose your margarine. Depending on which one you choose in Canada, you can minimize or maximize your *trans* fatty acid intake. Finally, a recent study in Britain suggested that the major source of *trans* fatty acid in that country was milk fat and the body fat of ruminants, of cows and sheep, so we should not neglect that source of *trans* fatty acids. People consume a lot of beef and pork and a lot of cheese and milk and this can be an appreciable source of *trans* fatty acids.

Dr Dietschy: This is a very important issue. We are only now about to study, using our hamster model, the effect of the *cis* and *trans* 18:1 fatty acids. It will be of great interest to know if we can enrich the hepatic lipids with these two fatty acids and if this enrichment is associated with similar or different metabolic effects on LDL metabolism.

Dr Kubow: But, then how do we explain an absence of an effect of stearic acid? Do you believe that the stearic acid is immediately whished away and turned into oleic acid, is the evidence for that hardy enough?

Dr Dietschy: In all of our studies with the saturated fatty acids, the level of 18:0 fatty acid remains essentially unchanged. In particular, after feeding the 18:0 fatty acid there is no change in the relative abundance of the 18:1 fatty acid. Thus, at the moment, we have no explanation for the absence of a suppressive effect of the 18:0 saturated fatty acid on receptor activity.

Dr Connor: I wanted to ask you about saturated fatty acids of slightly higher chain length, arachidic and behenic and C:20 and C:22.

Dr Dietschy: We have not yet done anything with these types of fatty acids.

Dr Connor: Do you think they would fade off like stearic acid?

Dr Dietschy: I presume they would, but there also would be a significant problem with absorption. At the moment, I know of no data that bear on this point.

Dr Katan: I do not know if you can get quantities of margaric acid, C:17; it would certainly be interesting to use margaric acid to differentiate between different structural mass actions and physiological actions. I am assuming that C17:0 is not metabolized well in man and it should have properties in between the two.

Dr Connor: I think that would be a very interesting experiment. What about α-linolenic acid?

Dr Dietschy: We have not done that. There is an infinite number of possibilities as you realize.

16
Plasma cholesterol responsiveness to saturated fatty acids[1-3]

S.M. GRUNDY and G.L. VEGA

Introduction

The feeding of dietary cholesterol to laboratory animals, particularly non-human primates, has revealed a variability in response for plasma cholesterol levels[1-4]. Within a given species of primates, some animals are hyperresponders because they develop severe hypercholesterolemia when dietary cholesterol is increased, whereas others are poor responders and show much less of an increment in cholesterol levels. The extremes of response within a continuum were shown to be genetically determined although the mechanisms responsible for these extreme differences remain in dispute. In laboratory animals the greatest range in responsiveness in plasma concentrations of cholesterol appears to be caused by increasing dietary cholesterol; the changes in cholesterol concentrations resulting from changes in other nutrients (e.g. saturated fatty acids) are less[5].

In humans high-cholesterol diets do not produce the great range in response in concentrations of plasma cholesterol noted for non-human primates[6-8]. The data from previous studies[6-11] suggest that some individuals respond more to dietary cholesterol than others but even if this is true, the extremes of plasma cholesterol increase are much less in humans than in other primates. In humans

[1]From the University of Texas Health Science Center at Dallas (SMG), Center for Human Nutrition and the Veterans Administration Medical Center, Dallas, TX.
[2]Supported in part by the Veterans Administration, grant HL-29252 from the National Institutes of Health, the Southwestern Medical Foundation, and the Moss Heart Foundation, Dallas, TX.
[3]Address reprints to Scott M. Grundy, MD, PhD, University of Texas Health Science Center at Dallas, Center for Human Nutrition, 5323 Harry Hines Boulevard, Dallas, TX 75235.
First Published in *Am. J. Clin. Nutr.*, 1988;47:822–4, ©1988 American Society for Clinical Nutrition. Reproduced with permission.

the dietary factor having the greatest effect on the plasma cholesterol appears to be saturated fatty acids[7,11,12]. In previous studies Keys *et al.*[13,14] examined inherent differences in responsiveness to different kinds of fatty acids in the diet. These workers pointed out that considerable variation in response exists; they examined possible mechanisms for these differences and noted that individuals having the highest cholesterol levels from saturated fatty acids tended to have the greatest reductions in cholesterol concentrations. Thus, they recognized that equations developed to predict plasma cholesterol responses to changes in diet composition apply more to groups than to individuals. A recent report by Zanni *et al.*[15] noted a similar variability in dietary responsiveness in women. In the present report, we further examine the question of individual variation in response to saturated fatty acids as compared with unsaturated fatty acids.

Methods

Studies of the relative effects of saturated fatty acids and unsaturated fatty acids on plasma concentrations and composition of lipoproteins were carried out in our laboratory[16-18]. These studies employed liquid-formula diets in which the types of fat in the formula mix was the only variable. Four studies can be identified from these investigations. Study 1[16] compared high-linoleic acid safflower oil and lard in 10 patients. Study 2[17] compared high-linoleic acid safflower oil and palm oil in 12 patients. Study 3[17,18] was carried out in 17 patients and compared high-oleic safflower oil and palm oil. Finally, study 4[18] included seven patients and used high-oleic safflower oil vs coconut oil. The subjects of these investigations generally had high-normal concentrations of plasma triglycerides but their plasma total cholesterol covered a broad range of concentrations. In study 1[16] the diet high in saturated fatty acids was always fed first whereas in the other three[17,18] the order of the different fats was randomized. In all studies each response represents the mean of six measurements taken after patients had achieved a steady state on a particular diet regimen.

Results

The results for the four studies are summarized in Table 1 and are shown for individual patients in Figures 1 and 2. Figure 1 compares responses in plasma total cholesterol and LDL cholesterol with the feeding of polyunsaturated fatty acids (High Poly) and saturated fatty acids (High Sat); Figure 2 compares monounsaturated fatty acids (High Mono) and saturated fatty acids (High Sat). In study 1, patients generally had higher cholesterol levels than in study 2

(Table 1) and the average changes in total cholesterol and LDL cholesterol were greater in study 1. However, in both studies the variability in response for individual patients was considerable as shown by the large standard deviations and ranges of the change. A similar variability in response was noted for the comparison of monounsaturated fatty acids and saturated fatty acids. As shown in both figures, some patients had a striking increase in cholesterol levels for dietary saturated fatty acids but others definitely had lesser responses. The individual results indicate that the greatest responses generally occurred in those having higher levels of cholesterol for dietary saturated fatty acids but this was not invariably true. The patterns of response were similar for patients receiving polyunsaturated fatty acids and for those receiving monounsaturated fatty acids.

Table 1 Summary of studies of dietary responsiveness*

	Total cholesterol mg/dl (mmol/l)	LDL cholesterol mg/dl (mmol/l)
Study 1[16] (*n*=10)		
High Poly	223 ± 60 (5.77 ± 1.55)	156 ± 63 (4.03 ± 1.63)
High Sat (lard)	296 ± 77 (7.65 ± 1.99)	212 ± 79 (5.48 ± 2.04)
Change	73 ± 25 (1.89 ± 0.65)	56 ± 26 (1.45 ± 0.67)
Range	1–123 (0.03–3.18)	−7 to 105 (−0.18 to 2.71)
Study 2[17] (*n*=12)	191 ± 42 (4.94 ± 1.09)	136 ± 42 (3.52 ± 1.09)
High Sat (palm oil)	227 ± 51 (5.87 ± 1.32)	165 ± 49 (4.27 ± 1.27)
Change	37 ± 20 (0.96 ± 0.52)	30 ± 20 (0.78 ± 0.52)
Range	3–84 (0.08–2.17)	−2 to 67 (−0.05 to 1.73)
Study 3[17,18] (*n*=17)	195 ± 27 (5.04 ± 0.70)	129 ± 30 (3.34 ± 0.78)
High Mono		
High Sat (palm oil)	227 ± 46 (5.87 ± 1.19)	163 ± 43 (4.22 ± 1.11)
Change	37 ± 23 (0.96 ± 0.59)	30 ± 20 (0.78 ± 0.52)
Range	1–79 (0.03–2.04)	5–68 (0.13–1.76)
Study 4[18] (*n*=7)		
High Mono	219 ± 19 (5.66 ± 0.49)	146 ± 21 (3.78 ± 0.54)
High Sat (coconut oil)	254 ± 25 (6.57 ± 0.65)	178 ± 25 (4.60 ± 0.65)
Change	34 ± 17 (0.88 ± 0.44)	32 ± 15 (0.83 ± 0.39)
Range	8–53 (0.21–1.38)	6–51 (0.16–1.32)

*Mean ± SD. High Poly = high-linoleic safflower oil; High Sat = saturated fatty acids; High Mono = high-oleic safflower oil

Discussion

The findings reported herein have the limitation of containing retrospective data. The investigations were not carried out to determine the degree of responsiveness to saturated fatty acids, and a prospective study designed for this purpose will be required for proof. In particular, the saturated fatty acids were not provided from a single type of fat and different kinds of saturated acids may affect cholesterol levels differently[7,12]. No consistent response to fats having different patterns of saturated acids were observed but more

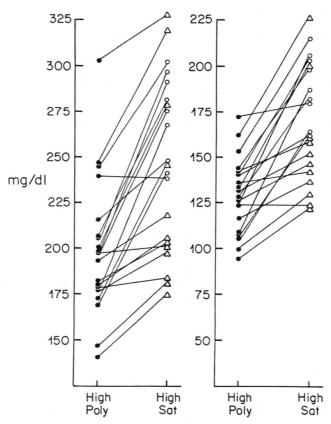

TOTAL CHOLESTEROL   LDL CHOLESTEROL

Figure 1 Effects of exchange of diets high in polyunsaturated fatty acids (High Poly) for saturated fatty acids (High Sat) on plasma total cholesterol and LDL cholesterol. The fat in the High Poly diet consisted entirely of high-linoleic safflower oil (solid circles). The fat of the High Sat diet was either lard (open circles) or palm oil (open triangles). (To convert mg/dl to mmol/l multiply by 0.02586.)

TOTAL CHOLESTEROL   LDL CHOLESTEROL

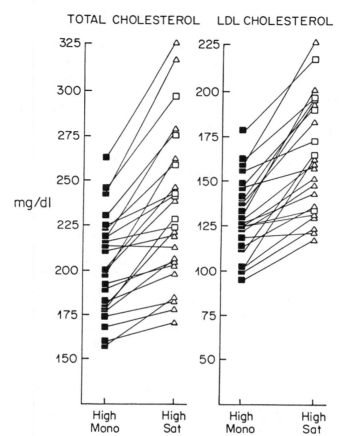

Figure 2 Effects of exchange of diets high in monounsaturated fatty acids (High Mono) for saturated fatty acids (High Sat) on plasma total cholesterol and LDL cholesterol. The fat in the High Mono diet consisted entirely of high-oleic safflower oil (solid squares). The fat of the High Sat diet was either coconut oil (open squares) or palm oil (open triangles). (To convert mg/dl to mmol/l, multiply by 0.02586.)

investigation on this point will be required. The sequence of the studies was not properly randomized in one of the investigations[16]. In spite of these limitations the variability in responsiveness is impressive and suggests strongly that the plasma-cholesterol response to saturated fatty acids is highly variable. Whether the pattern of response is genetically determined remains to be elucidated.

If future studies can confirm that response to saturated fatty acids is highly variable, the results could have significant clinical implications. A current debate centers on the question of whether the public health approach or the

279

high-risk strategy for cholesterol lowering is preferable for reducing coronary risk[19]. If it could be shown for example that individuals with higher cholesterol levels are more responsive to saturated fatty acids than are those with lower levels, as suggested by the current and previous studies[14], this would add support to the high-risk strategy particularly for the detection of elevated cholesterol levels. On the other hand, the data also imply that the composition of the diet may be more important in causation of primary hypercholesterolemia than has been generally realized. For this reason the data presented here point to the need for further investigations that are specifically designed to determine the range of responsiveness to dietary saturated fatty acids and the factors responsible for this variability.

References

1. Eggen, D.A. and Strong, J.P. (1972). Cholesterol metabolism in rhesus: extremes of response of serum cholesterol to atherogenic diet. *Circulation* (Suppl 2), **250**, 45–6

2. Eggen, D.A. (1974). Cholesterol metabolism in rhesus monkey, squirrel monkey and baboon. *J. Lipid Res.*, **15**, 139–45

3. Eggen, D.A. (1976). Cholesterol metabolism in nonhuman primates. In Goldsmith, E.I. and Moor-Jankowski, J. (eds), *Primates in Medicine*, pp. 267–99. (Basel: Karger)

4. Lofland, H.B. Jr., Clarkson, T.B., St Clair, R.W. *et al.* (1972). Studies on the regulation of plasma cholesterol levels in squirrel monkeys of two genotypes. *J. Lipid Res.*, **13**, 39–47

5. Strong, J.P. and McGill, H.C. Jr. (1967). Diet and experimental atherosclerosis in baboons. *Am. J. Pathol.*, **50**, 669–90

6. Keys, A., Anderson, J.T. and Grande, F. (1965). Serum cholesterol response to changes in the diet. II. The effect of cholesterol in the diet. *Metabolism*, **14**, 759–65

7. Hegsted, D.M., McGandy, R.B., Myer, M.L. and Stare, F.J. (1965). Quantitative effects of dietary fat on serum cholesterol in man. *Am. J. Clin. Nutr.*, **17**, 281–95

8. Mattson, F.H. (1972). Effect of dietary cholesterol on serum cholesterol in man. *Am. J. Clin. Nutr.*, **25**, 589–94

9. Beynen, A.C. and Katan, M.B. (1985). Reproducibility of the variations between humans in the response of serum cholesterol to cessation of egg consumption. *Atherosclerosis*, **57**, 19–31

10. Katan, M.B., Beynen, A.C., DeVries, J.H.M. and Nobels, A. (1986). Existence of consistent hypo- and hyperresponders to dietary cholesterol in man. *Am. J. Epidemiol.*, **123**, 221–34

11. McNamara, D.J., Kolb, R., Parker, T.S. *et al.* (1987). Heterogeneity of cholesterol homeostasis in man: response to changes in dietary fat quality and cholesterol quantity. *J. Clin. Invest.*, **79**, 1729–39

12. Keys, A., Anderson, J.T. and Grande, F. (1957). Prediction of serum cholesterol responses of man to change in fats in the diet. *Lancet*, **2**, 959–66

13. Keys, A., Anderson, J.T. and Grande, F. (1959). Serum cholesterol in man: diet fat and intrinsic responsiveness. *Circulation,* **19**, 201–14

14. Keys, A., Anderson, J.T. and Grande, F. (1965). Serum cholesterol response to changes in the diet. III. Differences among individuals. *Metabolism,* **14**, 766–75

15. Zanni, E.E., Zannis, V.I., Blum, C.B., Herbert, P.N. and Breslow, J.L. (1987). Effect of egg cholesterol and dietary fats on the lipids, lipoproteins, and apoproteins for normal women consuming natural diets. *J. Lipid Res.,* **28**, 518–27

16. Vega, G.L., Groszek, E., Wolf, R. and Grundy, S.M. (1982). Influence of polyunsaturated fats on composition of plasma lipoproteins and apolipoproteins. *J. Lipid Res.,* **23**, 811–22

17. Mattson, F.H. and Grundy, S.M. (1985). Comparison of dietary saturated, monounsaturated, and polyunsaturated fatty acids on plasma lipids and lipoproteins in man. *J. Lipid Res.,* **26**, 194–202

18. Grundy, S.M. (1986). Comparison of monounsaturated fatty acids and carbohydrates for plasma cholesterol lowering. *N. Engl. J. Med.,* **314**, 745–8

19. Grundy, S.M. (1986). Cholesterol and coronary heart disease. A new era. *J. Am. Med. Assoc.,* **256**, 2849–58

Discussion

Dr Hayes: I am interested in one of the earlier points you made in your discussion of palmitic acid vs. lauric vs. oleic in regard to cholesterolaemia. What was the dietary source of lauric acid and how did you control for other fatty acids?

Dr Vega: The study used liquid diets and so the fatty acids were analyzed by gas chromatography. I cannot remember the exact company they were obtained from but they were analyzed by fatty acids and they were liquid diets.

Dr Hayes: Was that trilaurin?

Dr Vega: Yes.

17

The role of n-3 fatty acids as modulators of n-6 fatty acid metabolism: health implications

P. BUDOWSKI

Introduction

It is useful to make a distinction between the different ways in which polyunsaturated fatty acids (PUFAs) exert their effects. PUFAs are first and foremost essential fatty acids (EFAs), as shown for linoleic acid as early as 1930[1]. The essentiality of PUFAs is a threshold effect in the sense that deficiency symptoms appear only when the dietary PUFA supply level remains below the minimum requirement which, for linoleic acid, is estimated at about 1 en%[2]. The cholesterol-lowering effect of PUFAs, on the other hand, is dose-dependent and is not generally viewed as being related to the EFA properties of PUFAs, although the late Hugh Sinclair maintained that atherosclerosis, coronary thrombosis and other modern diseases are the result of a *relative* EFA deficiency, i.e. a low ratio of EFAs in the body to saturated fatty acids and *trans* isomers[3-5]. Another example of a dose-dependent PUFA effect is provided by the production of eicosanoids formed from arachidonic acid (AA) and discussed in the section on unrestrained AA metabolism. This effect is well illustrated by a trial in which volunteers received a formula diet with different linoleic acid contents[6]: as the daily ingestion of linoleic acid was increased from 0 to 60 g, the excretion of prostaglandin metabolites in 24-h urine at the end of the two-week period rose markedly.

The latter example raises the intriguing question of an excessive production of AA-derived eicosanoids induced by the diet. This paper will discuss the concept of *unrestrained* AA metabolism and its possible detrimental consequences[7-10], the ways in which n-3 PUFAs attenuate such a process, and the origins and implications of the current imbalance between n-6 and n-3 PUFAs.

PUFA families

The most abundant PUFAs in Western diets are linoleic and α-linolenic acids, or 18:2n-6 and 18:3n-3, respectively. The shorthand notation shows the chain length, number of double-bonds and position of the double-bond proximal to the methyl terminus, as indicated in Scheme 1. These two fatty acids undergo alternating desaturation and chain elongation reactions (also shown in Scheme 1) in liver and other organs. Since the terminal segments of the fatty

---

Linoleic acid, 18:2n-6

$CH_3(CH_2)_4CH:CHCH_2CH:CH(CH_2)_7COOH$

└─ n-6 ─┘

α-Linolenic acid, 18:3n-3

$CH_3CH_2CH:CHCH_2CH:CHCH_2CH:CH(CH_2)_7COOH$

└─ n-3 ─┘

n-6 PUFA family

18:2n-6 → 18:3n-6 → 20:3n-6 → 20:4n-6 → 22:4n-6 → 22:5n-6

AA

n-3 PUFA family

18:3n-3 → 18:4n-3 → 20:4n-3 → 20:5n-3 → 22:5n-3 → 22:6n-3

EPA   DHA

Scheme 1 Chemical structures, shorthand notations and main desaturation–elongation pathways of linoleic and α-linolenic acids. Abbreviations: AA, arachidonic acid; EPA, eicosapentaenoic acid; DHA, docosahexaenoic acid

acid chains denoted by n-6 and n-3 remain unchanged during these conversion reactions, the two parent fatty acids give rise to two distinct PUFA families referred to as n-6 and n-3 PUFAs. AA (20:4n-6) constitutes the major conversion product within the n-6 series, whereas docosahexaenoic acid (DHA, 22:6n-3) is the usual end product in the n-3 family, accompanied, in fish and other marine organisms, by eicosapentaenoic acid (EPA, 20:5n-3).

The concept of unrestrained AA metabolism

AA plays a key role in the metabolism of n-6 PUFAs, as indicated in Scheme 2. It is a major constituent of membrane phospholipids and, as the free acid, serves as the main eicosanoid precursor. Eicosanoids comprise prostaglandins (PGs), thromboxanes (TXs), hydroperoxy- and hydroxyeicosatetraenoic acids (HPETEs and HETEs) and leukotrienes (LTs). They are locally acting potent physiological modulators which are being generated from AA present in a cellular free-fatty acid pool. AA is fed into the pool upon lipolytic release from membrane phospholipids, but there is also a direct link between the

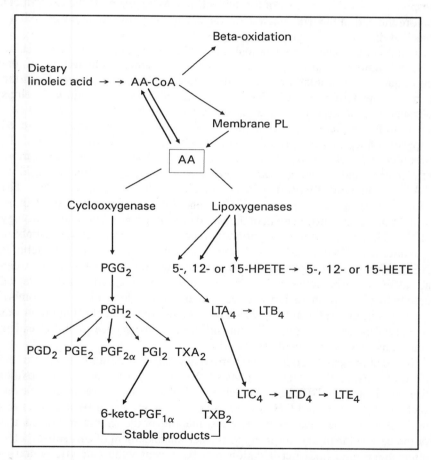

Scheme 2 Main metabolic pathways of arachidonic acid. Abbreviations: AA, arachidonic acid; PL, phospholipids; PGs, prostaglandins; TX, thromboxane; HPETEs, hydroperoxy-eicosatetraenoic acids; HETEs, hydroxyeicosatetraenoic acids; LTs, leukotrienes

dietary PUFA input and the free-fatty acid pool which bypasses membrane lipids. This is inferred from the rapid changes in eicosanoid formation or excretion in response to changes in dietary PUFA input in experimental animals[11,12] and healthy volunteers[13].

Detrimental effects of excessive AA metabolism have been described. For instance, intravenous AA led to rapid death of rabbits because of platelet aggregation in lung blood vessels[14], and intracarotid AA injection induced stroke in rats[15]. Sudden death in man associated with pulmonary aggregates has been attributed to excessive AA metabolism[16]. The ingestion of 6 g AA ethyl ester by four healthy males caused a pronounced increase in platelet response *ex vivo*[13], and two of the subjects had to be taken off the experiment before the end of the trial when their platelet aggregability was judged to have reached dangerously high levels.

Chick nutritional encephalomalacia (NE), also known as 'crazy-chick disease' among poultry growers, provides a dramatic illustration of the consequences of unrestrained AA metabolism. The name derives from the fact that the target organ in NE is the cerebellum which rapidly develops degenerative damage leading to ataxia and death. NE has been known as a vitamin E deficiency syndrome for over 60 years[17] and can be induced experimentally in young rapidly growing chicks by diets low in vitamin E, provided the diets also contain a source of linoleic acid[18]. AA is even more effective[19], and since chicks are efficient converters of linoleic acid to AA[20-22], the latter PUFA may be assumed to be the active agent in NE. The shorter bleeding times of ataxic chicks[21] and the protective action of dicoumarol[23] point to the involvement of the blood coagulation system in the aetiology of NE. This conclusion is supported by reports on the presence of thrombi in the microvasculature and of ischaemic–anoxic damage in the cerebella in NE[24]. Enhanced AA conversion to eicosanoids was shown by the elevated aortal PGE_2 formation[25] and increased lipoxygenase activity in the affected cerebella (S. Greenberg-Levy, unpublished). TXB_2 formation by thrombocytes in stimulated thrombocyte-rich plasma and in whole clotting blood was not significantly increased[25,26], nor did the cyclooxygenase inhibitor aspirin cause any drop in the incidence of NE[26].

In the above chick model, lipid peroxidation forms an important part of the picture[27]. Since the initial products of the AA cascade are hydroperoxides (i.e. PGG_2 and the HPETEs, see Scheme 2), damaging active oxygen species such as H_2O_2, O_2^- and OH^- would be formed as the result of side reactions in the AA cascade. Haemorrhages constitute one of the characteristic features of the cerebellar injury, resulting in further enhancement of this self-accelerating membrane lipid peroxidation process through the catalytic action of haemoglobin, hematin and free iron released from haemoglobin in the presence of peroxides[28].

That enhanced AA metabolism may result in peroxidative injury is also shown by the arteriolar damage, including endothelial lesions, caused by topical application of AA, PGG_2 or 15-HPETE to the brain surface of anaesthetized cats[29,30]. The vascular damage caused by AA was prevented by prior treatment of the animals with the cyclooxygenase inhibitor indomethacin, or the simultaneous application of the free-radical scavenger mannitol. Metabolites formed from PGG_2, such as PGH_2 and PGE_2, were inactive in this model, as was 20:3n-3 which is not a prostanoid precursor. No arteriolar abnormalities were observed when superoxide dismutase was applied together with PGG_2. These results leave little doubt that hydroperoxides formed initially in the AA cascade may cause severe damage to the cerebral microvasculature through the formation of active oxygen species.

Excessive eicosanoid production may lead to a variety of undesirable symptoms. An example relevant to human disease is provided by platelet TXA_2 formation. This prostanoid causes platelet aggregation and adhesion and has vasoconstrictive properties which are normally held in check by PGI_2 formed by the arterial endothelium[31]. When this delicate balance is disturbed, e.g. as the result of formation of minute amounts of peroxides which inhibit the biosynthesis of PGI_2, but not that of TXA_2[32,33], the tendency toward thrombosis is increased. Circulating peroxide-carrying lipoproteins have been reported to play a role in atherogenesis[34]. One of the effects of an overload of lipid peroxides could be a reduction of the PGI_2 producing capacity of the endothelium, resulting in enhanced platelet aggregation.

The involvement of PGs in immune-inflammatory reactions has long been known[35,36], but more recently, LTs are receiving increasing attention[37,38]. LTs are produced by leukocytes, lung and other cells and tissues. LTB_4 induces chemotaxis, chemokinesis, aggregation and adhesion of leukocytes, and causes generation of superoxide. This LT is therefore an important mediator of inflammation. The sulfur-containing leukotrienes, LTC_4, LTD_4 and LTE_4, exert spasmogenic effects on smooth muscle; they are potent bronchoconstricting agents and are believed to contribute to the symptoms of asthma and other hypersensitivity reactions. Like prostanoid production, LT formation must be regulated, and n-3 PUFAs play an important role in this respect.

The restraining action of n-3 PUFAs on AA metabolism

The inhibitory effect of α-linolenic acid on hepatic AA synthesis was inferred early from tissue fatty acid analyses in feeding trials with chicks and rats[39,40]. Experiments *in vitro* with liver microsomes[41] showed that the inhibition takes place mainly at the initial 6-desaturation reaction of linoleic acid (Scheme 1) which constitutes the rate-determining step in AA synthesis. There is also competition between long-chain n-3 PUFAs and AA for incorporation into the *sn*-2 position of phosphoglycerides[42,43], though this competition is subject to tissue specificity of acyl transferases and depends on the molecular phosphoglyceride species.

EPA and DHA are effective inhibitors of cyclooxygenase[44,45] at the initial step in the PG pathway (Scheme 2). EPA strongly binds to the cyclooxygenase but is a poor substrate for the enzyme[46], unless the 'peroxide tone' is elevated[47]. EPA-derived TXA$_3$, unlike TXA$_2$, is devoid of pro-aggregating and vasoconstrictor activities, while PGI$_3$ produces effects similar to those of PGI$_2$[48]. Therefore, EPA causes a shift in the TX–PGI balance which favours antithrombotic and vasorelaxing effects.

n-3 PUFAs also interfere with the 5-lipoxygenase pathway of AA oxygenation. For instance, EPA and DHA suppressed the formation of LTB$_4$, LTC$_4$ and 12-HETE by stimulated mouse peritoneal macrophages[49], and reduced LTB$_4$ synthesis by human neutrophils[50–52]. But EPA itself is readily converted to LTs of the 5-series *in vitro*[53,54], and a similar conversion has been reported for stimulated murine mastocyma cells[55] and activated human neutrophils after dietary supplementation with fish oil[50–52,56,57]. The neutrophil-aggregating and chemotactic activities of LTB$_5$ were lower by about one order of magnitude than those of LTB$_4$[51,57–60], while LTC$_5$ equalled LTC$_4$ in smooth-muscle contracting activity[59–61]. Unlike EPA, DHA was not readily oxygenated by 5-lipoxygenase from rat basophilic leukaemia-1 cells and only weakly interfered with LTB$_4$ biosynthesis, while the C$_{22}$ analog of LTC$_4$ was virtually devoid of spasmogenic activity[45].

The interference of n-3 PUFAs with the AA cascade is strikingly demonstrated in the chick NE model discussed in the previous section. Dietary α-linolenic acid, in contrast to linoleic acid, not only fails to cause any cerebellar damage, but also protects the chicks against the lethal effects of linoleic acid[21]. The opposing effects of the two PUFAs in this chick model create a paradox: the cerebellar injury involves peroxidation processes, but α-linolenic acid and its n-3 desaturation-elongation derivatives are known to be more susceptible to peroxidation than their n-6 counterparts. The paradox is resolved if α-linolenic acid is viewed as an inhibitor of the AA oxygenation cascade in which damaging active oxygen species are formed as by-products. In support of this view, it was shown that dietary supplementation with α-linolenic acid caused a reduction in TXB$_2$ production by thrombocyte-rich chick plasma, a decrease in aortal PGE$_2$ formation and a lowered response of thrombocytes to collagen[25]. The restraining action of α-linolenic acid on AA metabolism in this model had an overriding influence, counteracting the potentially damaging effect of the increased polyunsaturation and peroxidizability of the cerebellar lipids resulting from the partial replacement of AA by DHA[21,22].

In the context of heart disease, the attenuation of platelet AA metabolism and the resulting antiplatelet activity of n-3 PUFAs provided by fish oils are receiving much attention these days, but antiplatelet activity of dietary α-linolenic acid had been reported in rat models even before the days of the AA cascade[62–64]. Rats efficiently convert α-linolenic acid to long-chain n-3 fatty acids[20], so that the observed effects can be ascribed to the interference of α-linolenic acid and its long-chain n-3 derivatives with the metabolism of AA, as discussed above. Numerous reports attesting to the beneficial influence of dietary n-3 fatty acids from fish oils on cardiovascular diseases implicate a modification of the absolute and relative amounts of AA-derived prostanoids, although other atherogenic factors are favourably altered, including hepatic VLDL synthesis and secretion, platelet-activating factor, interleukin-1, tumour necrosis factor, platelet-derived growth factor, endothelial relaxing factor, erythrocyte deformability, blood viscosity and fibrinolytic factors (for reviews, see refs. 65–70). A recent report[71] described a reduction in superoxide production and chemiluminescence in stimulated human monocytes (believed to play a key role in atherogenesis) as the result of ingestion of n-3 fatty acids from codliver oil. Other chronic diseases in which eicosanoid production is believed to be favourably affected by n-3 fatty acids have been reviewed[67,72,73] and include immune-inflammatory conditions and some forms of cancer in animals. The effects of n-3 PUFAs on AA metabolism do not preclude other influences such as a modification of, and interaction with, hormonal factors, changes in membrane properties and enzyme and receptor functions.

The above examples illustrate the restraining action of n-3 fatty acids on AA metabolism. Do our habitual diets provide an appropriate balance of the two PUFA families to permit full expression of this important function of n-3 fatty acids?

The n-6:n-3 PUFA ratio in palaeolithic times

Humanity as a genus has existed for some two million years. During that period, the food available to early man underwent wide regional and temporal variations, nevertheless some central nutritional characteristics have been identified[74,75] which are in striking contrast to the nutrition pattern of today's affluent Western nations. Wild game and uncultivated plants contain far less fat than current Western diets[74]. That fat was at a premium in prehistoric times is shown, for instance, by an analysis of bone counts at the Garnsey bison kill sites in New Mexico[76], where hunters in the 15th century slaughtered their prey and discarded those parts of the animals that were lowest in fat.

Early man ate mainly structural lipids of low-fat foods such as fruits and berries, leafy plants and shoots, roots and tubers, seeds of non-cultivated plants, and the generally lean flesh and offal of wild animals. Structural lipids of plants and animals are rich in PUFAs, and the n-6 and n-3 fatty acids are on the whole well balanced, with seeds containing mainly linoleic acid, while chloroplasts are rich in α-linolenic acid. An analytical survey of 32 wild animal species in Africa[77] yielded mean ratios of 1 for the two PUFA families in brain phosphatidylethanolamine, the principal cerebral phospholipid, while the n-6:n-3 PUFA ratio in liver phospholipids ranged from 0.3 to 3.5 in all but one of the species examined. Muscle phospholipids of wild animals were reported to have n-6:n-3 ratios of 2–4. Therefore, during millions of years of evolution, *Homo* ate a variety of foods of vegetable and animal origin, with a low fat content and a good overall balance of n-6 and n-3 PUFAs.

Recent changes in the n-6:n-3 PUFA ratio

With the beginnings of agriculture and animal husbandry roughly 10 000 years ago, a gradual change in the food consumption pattern set in. Fat intake remained low, as most populations subsisted on simple fare made up mostly of grain and starchy foods which, even today, make up over 60% of the calorie intake in economically underprivileged countries[78]. Only the high and mighty 'lived off the fat of the land'. However, the change in nutritional pattern gathered momentum with the industrial revolution and the resulting improvements in the production, processing, transport, storage and distribution of foods. Stamler[78] has pointed out that grain, instead of being consumed directly, was being used more and more as fodder for 'corn–hog' and 'corn–steer' economies, so that fatty meat and animal fats became articles of mass consumption during the second half of last century. In addition to other well-known changes in dietary habits and lifestyle, fat consumption rose rapidly and approached, toward the close of the 19th century, the high levels characteristic of modern industrialized societies.

More recently, a change occurred in the nature of the fat consumed, a change which can be traced to several important innovations that took place at the turn of the century and which marked the beginnings of the modern vegetable oil industry. An account of these innovations is in order, as it will show how the current PUFA imbalance developed.

Oilseed extraction methods were revolutionized by V.D. Anderson's continuous screw press trade-named 'Expeller' and perfected in 1903[79]. Around the same time, David Wesson patented his steam–vacuum deodorization process which constitutes the crucial final stage in edible-oil refining even today. Both inventions together made possible the industrial production of cottonseed oil and later other seed oils for edible purposes (before that time, cottonseed was a valueless by-product of the fibre industry). After World War I, solvent extraction of oilseeds came into increasing use and rendered the large-scale production of vegetable oils more efficient. Catalytic hydrogenation, which had been discovered a few years earlier by P. Sabatier in France, began to be applied to the hardening of vegetable oils when the use of nickel as a catalyst was patented by Norman in Germany and Britain during the first years of this century. Liquid oils could now be converted to solid or semi-solid fats for shortenings and margarine stock which came to replace the more expensive animal fats. A special application of this process consists in the partial but selective hydrogenation of soybean oil in order to reduce its α-linolenic acid content while preserving most of its linoleic acid, thus yielding a liquid oil with much improved shelf life and organoleptic properties. For the same reason, the search is now on for new low-α-linolenic acid cultivars of soybeans[80], and similar efforts are being made with regard to rapeseed (canola) and linseed[81].

It cannot be overemphasized that these developments, together with the growth of large-scale cultivation of oilseed-yielding crops, have affected most of all the production of high-linoleic acid oils such as soybean, cottonseed and corn oils, as well as sunflower and safflower oils, among others. The increasing awareness of the public and the industry of the hypocholesterol-aemic action of polyunsaturated oils, and official recommendations concerning the P/S ratio during the last decades, undoubtedly gave additional impetus to these developments.

The national US supply of salad and cooking oils, for instance, increased from 1.9 g/person/day in 1909–13 to 29.1 g/person/day in 1980[82], causing a nearly threefold increase in the total dietary linoleic acid intake from 9.0 to 25.1 g/person/day during that period, while the supply of low-linoleic acid butter and lard decreased. Availability of α-linolenic acid increased lately[83] but remained very low, compared to the linoleic acid supply. A disproportion-ate rise in linoleic acid availability has also been reported in Britain[84] where vegetable oils partly replaced butter[85,86]. The ratio of linoleic to α-linolenic acid, which in practice represents the n-6:n-3 PUFA ratio, is generally estimated at 10 to 1[87]. The availability of long-chain derivatives of these parent fatty acids is lower by two orders of magnitude than that of linoleic acid[87].

An example of very high dietary linoleate level is provided by Israel, where linoleic acid consumption has been estimated at 8–9 en% from household expenditure and dietary recall studies[88,89]. Food balance sheets[90] show that linoleic acid-rich vegetable oils and margarines are the only separated fats available, apart from small amounts of butter, so that the total availability of fat of vegetable origin greatly exceeds that from animal sources. Five separate studies in which the fatty acid composition of subcutaneous fat obtained by needle biopsy was determined[91-95] yielded mean linoleic acid values exceeding 22% (of total fatty acids). The highest value was found in a study[93] in which *cis* and *trans* isomers were separated and in which a mean of 27.2% *cis,cis*-linoleic acid was found, with minor amounts of *trans* isomers. The mean value reported for α-linolenic acid in that study was 1.45%, indicating a wide discrepancy between the intakes of these two PUFAs. The adipose tissue linoleic acid content of Israelis is higher than the values reported for

US, Britain and many other countries and indicates a habitual linoleate consumption of up to 12 en%, using the mathematical relation between adipose and dietary linoleate[96].

Implications of the current PUFA imbalance

Under these conditions, the restraining action of n-3 PUFAs on AA metabolism does not receive its full expression. It is in this light that one should view the numerous reports on beneficial effects on cardiovascular diseases accruing from therapeutic doses of fish oils and the epidemiological surveys pointing to a lower mortality from heart disease of fish-eating populations[67–73].

Conversely, a large dietary excess of linoleic acid over α-linolenic acid is liable to interfere with the conversion of the n-3 parent fatty acid to DHA, whose role in the developing retina and brain has now been established in several animal species, including non-human primates[97]. An adequately balanced supply of n-6 and n-3 PUFAs would be of special importance to the newborn who requires both preformed AA and DHA[98].

Although interest at present is focused on health effects of n-3 fatty acids from fish and fish oil preparations, the possibility of increasing the consumption of α-linolenic acid in relation to the linoleate intake is of considerable nutritional significance. Arguments put forth against the nutritional effectiveness of α-linolenic acid from linseed oil, compared to long-chain n-3 PUFAs from fish oils, were based on early short-term trials in which little change in plasma and erythrocyte long-chain n-3 fatty acids were found upon linseed oil supplementation[99,100]. However, α-linolenic acid is readily converted to long-chain n-3 fatty acids, as shown by recent experiments in which volunteers received a bolus of deuterated α-linolenic acid[101]. Conversion of α-linolenic acid to long-chain n-3 fatty acids is also inferred from a study in which the ratio of derived PUFAs to parent PUFAs in human plasma was shown to be very much greater for the n-3 family than for the n-6 PUFAs[102]. Supplementation of a formula diet with α-linolenic acid in amounts ranging from 0 to 8 en% at a constant linoleic acid supply of 4 en% resulted in a nearly linear decrease in PG metabolite excretion in 24-h urine of healthy volunteers[6]. Platelet aggregation *ex vivo* in two healthy subjects decreased considerably after supplementation of the habitual diet with 60 ml linseed oil/day during 49–53 days[103]. Vegans seem to be doing very well without receiving any n-3 fatty acids other than α-linolenic acid from their diet[104]. Clearly, α-linolenic acid does affect the metabolism of AA.

The awakening interest in α-linolenic acid is reflected by a recent conference in which the nutritional significance of α-linolenic acid and of linseed and linseed oil as foods was discussed[105]. Improving the proportion of α-linolenic acid in the diet is obviously a question of long-term dietary habits, so as to reduce the large excess of linoleic acid over n-3 fatty acids in the body. Although the optimum dietary ratio of the two PUFAs for humans is not known, it would appear prudent to attempt to reduce the ratio from the present 10:1 proportion to less than 5:1[9].

Conclusions

Several conclusions can be drawn from this discussion.

(i) α-Linolenic acid, the parent fatty acid of the n-3 family, functions not only as an EFA but also acts as an important modulator of AA metabolism.

(ii) The diets of modern societies are unbalanced with respect to the two main PUFAs, with linoleic acid exceeding α-linolenic acid by about one order of magnitude.

(iii) Under these conditions, the modulating effect of α-linolenic acid on AA metabolism does not receive its full expression and the AA cascade becomes overactive.

(iv) The current PUFA imbalance is due to a rise in the production of high-linoleic acid oils and margarines and represents a late consequence of the industrial revolution which also caused, at a somewhat earlier stage, the sharp rise in the availability of animal fats, as well as numerous other changes in diet and lifestyle.

(v) Our genetic makeup is still virtually the same as in prehistoric *Homo sapiens*: we have not had time to adapt to these 'sudden' changes. The PUFA imbalance of modern diets should be taken into account when discussing the many changes that have brought about the diseases of civilization.

References

1. Burr, G.O. and Burr, M.M. (1930). On the nature and role of fatty acids in nutrition. *J. Biol. Chem.*, **86**, 587–621
2. Holman, R.T. (1968). Essential fatty acid deficiency. In Holman, R.T. (ed.). *Progress in the Chemistry of Fats and Other Lipids,* Vol. 9, pp. 274–348. (Oxford: Pergamon Press)
3. Sinclair, H.M. (1956). Deficiency of essential fatty acids and atherosclerosis etcetera. *Lancet,* **1**, 381–3
4. Sinclair, H.M. (1980). Prevention of coronary heart disease: the role of essential fatty acids. *Postgrad. Med. J.*, **56**, 579–84

5. Sinclair, H.M. (1984). Essential fatty acids in perspective. *Human Nutr. Clin. Nutr.*, **38C**, 245–60

6. Adam, O., Wolfram, G. and Zöllner, N. (1984). Wirkung der Linol- und Linolensäure auf die Prostaglandinbildung und Nierenfunktion beim Menschen. *Fette Seifen Anstrichmittel*, **86**, 180–3

7. Budowski, P. (1981). Nutritional effects of ω3-polyunsaturated fatty acids: review. *Isr. J. Med. Sci.*, **17**, 223–31

8. Budowski, P. (1985). Dietary linoleic acid should be balanced by alpha-linolenic acid; a discussion of the nutritional implications of the dietary ratio of polyunsaturated fatty acids. In Horwitz, C. (ed.) *Advances in Diet and Nutrition*, pp. 199–206. (London: John Libbey)

9. Budowski, P. and Crawford, M.A. (1985). Alpha-linolenic acid as a regulator of the metabolism of arachidonic acid: dietary implications of the ratio, n-6:n-3 fatty acids. *Proc. Nutr. Soc.*, **44**, 221–9

10. Budowski, P. (1989). Alpha-linolenic acid and the metabolism of arachidonic acid. In Galli, C. and Simopoulos, A. (eds). *Dietary w-3 and w-6 Fatty Acids: Biological Effects and Nutritional Essentiality, NATO-ASI Series: Series A: Life Sciences*, Vol. 171, pp. 97–110. (New York and London: Plenum Press)

11. Hassam, A.G., Willis, A.L., Denton, J.P., Stevens, P. and Crawford, M.A. (1979). The effect of essential fatty acid deficiency on the levels of prostaglandins and their fatty acid precursors in the rabbit. *Lipids*, **14**, 71–80

12. Ramesha, C.S., Gronke, R.S., Sivarajan, M. and Lands, W.E.M. (1985). Metabolic products of arachidonic acid in rats. *Prostaglandins*, **29**, 991–1008

13. Seyberth, H.W., Oelz, O., Kennedy, T., Sweetman, B.J., Danon, A., Frolich, J.C., Heimberg, M. and Oates, J.A. (1975). Increased arachidonate in lipids after administration to man: effects on prostaglandin biosynthesis. *Clin. Pharmacol. Ther.*, **18**, 521–9

14. Silver, M.J., Hoch, W., Kocsis, J.J., Ingerman, C.M. and Smith, J.B. (1974). Arachidonic acid causes sudden death in rabbits. *Science*, **183**, 1085–7

15. Furlow, T. and Bass, N. (1975). Stroke in rats produced by intracarotid injection of sodium arachidonate. *Science*, **187**, 658–60

16. Pirkle, H. and Carstens, P. (1974). Pulmonary platelet aggregates associated with sudden death in man. *Science*, **185**, 1062–4

17. Pappenheimer, A.M. and Goettsch, M. (1931). A cerebellar disorder in chicks apparently of nutritional origin. *J. Exp. Med.*, **53**, 11–16

18. Dam, H., Nielsen, G.K., Prange, I. and Søndergaard, E. (1958). Influence of linoleic and linolenic acids on symptoms of vitamin E deficiency in chicks. *Nature*, **182**, 802–3

19. Dam, H. and Søndergaard, E. (1962). The encephalomalacia-producing effect of arachidonic and linoleic acids. *Z. Ernaehrungswiss.*, **2**, 217–22

20. Budowski, P., Nachtomi, E. and Bartov, I. (1985). Fatty acid composition of four lipid classes in plasma of rats and chicks receiving linoleic and alpha-linolenic acids in their diets. In Halpern, J.A. (ed.) *Lipid Metabolism and Its Pathology*, pp. 169–77. (New York: Plenum Press)

21. Budowski, P., Hawkey, C.M. and Crawford, M.A. (1980). L'effet protecteur de l'acide α-linolénique sur l'encephalomalacie chez le poulet. *Ann. Nutr. Alim.*, **34**, 389–99

22. Budowski, P., Leighfield, M.J. and Crawford, M.A. (1987). Nutritional encephalomalacia in the chick: an exposure of the vulnerable period for cerebellar development and the possible need for both w6 and w3-fatty acids. *Br. J. Nutr.*, **58**, 511–20

23. Budowski, P., Bartov, I., Dror, Y. and Frankel, E.N. (1979). Lipid oxidation products and chick nutritional encephalopathy. *Lipids*, **14**, 768–72

24. Dror, Y., Budowski, P., Bubis, J.J., Sandbank, U. and Wolman, M. (1976). Chick nutritional encephalopathy induced by diet rich in oxidized oil and deficient in tocopherol. In Zimmerman, H.M. (ed.). *Progress in Neuropathology*, Vol. 3, pp. 343–57 (New York: Grune & Stratton)

25. Vericel, E., Budowski, P. and Crawford, M.A. (1991). Chick nutritional encephalomalacia and prostanoid production. *J. Nutr.*, **121**, 966–9

26. Bruckner, G., Infante, J., Combs, G.F. and Kinsella, J.E. (1983). Effects of vitamin E and aspirin on the incidence of encephalomalacia, fatty acid status and serum thromboxane levels in chicks. *J. Nutr.*, **113**, 1885–90

27. Budowski, P. and Mokadi, S. (1961). Detection of free-radical damage in the vitamin E-deficient chick. *Biochim. Biophys. Acta*, **52**, 609–11

28. Gutteridge, J.M.C. (1986). Iron promoters of the Fenton reaction and lipid peroxidation can be released from haemoglobin by peroxides. *FEBS*, **201**, 291–5

29. Kontos, H.A., Povlischock, J.T., Dalton, D.W., Magiera, C.J. and Ellis, E.F. (1980). Cerebral arteriolar damage by arachidonic acid and prostaglandin G_2. *Science*, **209**, 1242–5

30. Kontos, H.A. (1985). Oxygen radicals in cerebral vascular injury. *Circ. Res.*, **57**, 508–16

31. Higgs, E.A., Moncada, S. and Vane, J.R. (1981). The biological importance and therapeutic potential of prostacyclin. In Conn, H.L., DeFelice, E. and Cuo, P.T. (eds). *Prostaglandins, Platelets, Lipids*, pp. 1–102. (New York: Elsevier/North-Holland)

32. Moncada, S., Gryglewski, R.J., Bunting, S. and Vane, J.R. (1976). A lipid peroxide inhibits the enzyme in blood vessel microsomes that generates from prostaglandin endoperoxides the substance (prostaglandin X) which prevents platelet aggregation. *Prostaglandins*, **12**, 715–33

33. Salmon, J.A., Smith, D.R., Flower, R.J., Moncada, S. and Vane, J.R. (1978). Further studies on the enzymatic conversion of prostaglandin peroxide into prostacyclin by porcine aorta microsomes. *Biochim. Biophys. Acta*, **523**, 250–62

34. Bruckdorfer, K.R. (1989). The effects of plasma lipoproteins on platelet and vascular prostanoid synthesis. *Prostaglandins, Leukotrienes, Essential Fatty Acids*, **38**, 247–54

35. Ferreira, S.H. (1978). Participation of prostaglandins in inflammatory pain. In Vargaftig, B.B. (ed.) *Advances in Pharmacology and Therapeutics*, Vol. 4, pp. 63–9. (Oxford: Pergamon Press)

36. Kuehl, F.A. and Egan, R.W. (1980). Prostaglandins, arachidonic acid, and inflammation. *Science*, **210**, 978–84

37. Piper, P.J. (1984). The evolution and future horizons of research on the metabolism of arachidonic acid by 5-lipoxygenase. *J. Allergy Clin. Immunol.*, **74**, 441–4

38. Feuerstein, G. and Hallenbeck, J.M. (1987). Leukotrienes in health and disease. *FASEB J.*, **1**, 186–92

39. Machlin, L.J. (1962). Effect of dietary linolenate on the proportion of linoleate and arachidonate in liver fat. *Nature*, **194**, 868–9

40. Mohrhauer, H. and Holman, R.T. (1963). Effect of linolenic acid upon the metabolism of linoleic acid. *J. Nutr.*, **81**, 67–74

41. Brenner, R. and Peluffo, R.O. (1966). Effect of saturated and unsaturated fatty acids on the desaturation in vitro of palmitic, stearic, oleic, linoleic and linolenic acids. *J. Biol. Chem.*, **241**, 5213–19

42. Iritani, N. and Fujikawa, S. (1982). Competitive incorporation of dietary ω-3 and ω-6 polyunsaturated fatty acids into the tissue phospholipids in rats. *J. Nutr. Sci. Vitaminol.* (Tokyo), **28**, 621–9

43. Weaver, B.J. and Holub, R.J. (1985). The inhibition of arachidonic acid incorporation into human platelet phospholipids by eicosapentaenoic acid. *Nutr. Res.*, **5**, 31–7

44. Lands, W.E.M., Le Tellier, P.R., Rome, L.H. and Vanderhoek, J.Y. (1973). Inhibition of prostaglandin biosynthesis. *Adv. Biosci.*, **9**, 15–28

45. Corey, E.J., Shih, C. and Cashman, J.R. (1984). Docosahexaenoic acid is a strong inhibitor of PG but not LT biosynthesis. *Proc. Natl. Acad. Sci. USA*, **80**, 3581–4

46. Needleman, P., Raz, A., Minkes, M.S., Ferrendelli, J.A. and Sprecher, H. (1979). Triene prostaglandins: prostacyclin and thromboxane biosynthesis and unique biological properties. *Proc. Natl. Acad. Sci. USA*, **76**, 944–8

47. Culp, B.R., Titus, B.G. and Lands, W.E.M. (1979). Inhibition of prostaglandin biosynthesis by eicosapentaenoic acid. *Prostaglandins Med.*, **3**, 269–78

48. Weber, P.C., Fischer, S., von Schacky, C., Lorenz, R. and Strasser, T. (1986). Conversion of dietary eicosapentaenoic acid to prostanoids and leukotrienes. *Progr. Lipid Res.*, **23**, 273–6

49. Lokesh, B.R., Black, J.M., German, J.B. and Kinsella, J.E. (1988). Docosahexaenoic acid and other polyunsaturated fatty acids suppress leukotriene synthesis by mouse peritoneal macrophages. *Lipids*, **23**, 968–72

50. Lee, T.H., Hoover, R.L., Williams, J.D., Sperling, R.I., Ravalese, J.,III, Sour, B.W., Robinson, D.R., Corey, E.J., Lewis, R.A. and Austen, K.F. (1985). Effect of dietary enrichment with eicosapentaenoic and docosahexaenoic acids on *in vitro* neutrophil and monocyte leukotriene generation and neutrophil function. *N. Engl. J. Med.*, **312**, 1217–24

51. Prescott, S.M. (1984). The effect of eicosapentaenoic acid on leukotriene B production by human neutrophils. *J. Biol. Chem.*, **259**, 7615–21

52. Terano, T., Hirai, A., Tamura, Y., Yoshida, S., Salmon, J.A. and Moncada, S. (1986). Effect of eicosapentaenoic acid on eicosanoid formation by stimulated human polymorphonuclear leukocytes. *Progr. Lipid Res.*, **25**, 129–37

53. Hammerstrom, S. (1980). Leukotriene C_5: a slow-reacting substance derived from eicosapentaenoic acid. *J. Biol. Chem.*, **255**, 7093–4

54. Jakschik, B.A., Sams, A.R., Sprecher, H. and Needleman, P. (1980). Fatty acid structural requirement for leukotriene biosynthesis. *Prostaglandins*, **20**, 401–10

55. Murphy, R.C., Picket, W.C., Culp, B.R. and Lands, W.E.M. (1981). Tetraene and pentaene leukotrienes: selective production from murine mastocyma cells after dietary manipulation. *Prostaglandins*, **22**, 613–22

56. Strasser, S., Fischer, S. and Weber, P.C. (1985). Leukotriene B_5 is formed in human neutrophils after dietary supplementation with eicosapentaenoic acid. *Proc. Natl. Acad. Sci. USA*, **82**, 1540–3

57. Goldmann, D.W., Picket, W.C. and Goetzl, E.J. (1983). Human neutrophil chemotactic and degranulating activities of leukotriene B_5 derived from eicosapentaenoic acid. *Biochem. Biophys. Res. Commun.*, **117**, 282–8

58. Lee, T.H., Mencia-Huerta, J.M., Shih, C., Corey, E.J., Lewis, R.A. and Austen, K.F. (1984). Characterization and biological properties of 5,12-dihydroxy derivatives of eicosapentaenoic acid, including leukotriene B_5 and the lipoxygenase product. *J. Biol. Chem.*, **259**, 2383–9

59. Leitch, A.G., Lee, T.H., Ringel, E.W., Pricket, J.D., Robinson, D.R., Pym, S.G., Corey, E.J., Drazen, J.M., Austen, K.F. and Lewis, R.S. (1984). Immunologically induced generation of tetraene and pentaene leukotrienes in the peritoneal cavities of menhaden-fed rats. *J. Immunol.*, **132**, 2559–65

60. Terano, T., Salmon, J.A. and Moncada, S. (1984). Biosynthesis and biological activity of leukotriene B_5. *Prostaglandins*, **27**, 217–32

61. Lee, T.H., Lewis, R.A., Robinson, D., Drazen, J.M. and Austen, K.F. (1984). The effects of a diet enriched in menhaden fish oil on the pulmonary response to antigen challenge. *J. Allergy Clin. Immunol.*, **73**, 150

62. Nørdoy, A. (1965). The influence of saturated fat, cholesterol, corn oil and linseed oil on experimental venous thrombosis in rats. *Thromb. Diath. Haemorrh.*, **13**, 244–56

63. Nørdoy, A. (1965). The influence of saturated fat, cholesterol, corn oil and linseed oil on the ADP-induced platelet adhesiveness in the rat. *Thromb. Diath. Haemorrh.*, **13**, 543–9

64. Nørdoy, A., Hamlin, J.T., Chandler, A.B. and Newland, H. (1968). The influence of dietary fats on plasma and platelet lipids and ADP-induced platelet thrombosis in the rat. *Scand. J. Haematol.*, **5**, 458–73

65. Leaf, A. and Weber, P.C. (1988). Cardiovascular effects of n-3 fatty acids. *N. Engl. J. Med.*, **318**, 549–57

66. Fischer, S. (1989). Dietary polyunsaturated fatty acids and eicosanoid formation in humans. *Adv. Lipid Res.*, **23**, 169–98

67. Budowski, P. (1989). ω3-fatty acids in health and disease. *Wld. Rev. Nutr. Diet.*, **57**, 214–74

68. Kristensen, S.D., Schmidt, E.B. and Dyerberg, J. (1989). Dietary supplementation with n-3 polyunsaturated fatty acids and human platelet function: a review with particular emphasis on implications for cardiovascular disease. *J. Int. Med.*, **225** (Suppl. 1), 141–50

69. Kinsella, J.E., Lokesh, B. and Stone, R.A. (1990). Dietary n-3 polyunsaturated fatty acids and the amelioration of cardiovascular disease: possible mechanisms. *Am. J. Clin. Nutr.*, **52**, 1–28

70. Nicolisi, R.J. and Stucchi, A.F. (1990). n-3 Fatty acids and atherosclerosis. *Curr. Opin. Lipidol.*, **1**, 442–8

71. Fisher, M., Levine, P.H., Weiner, B.H., Johnson, M.H., Doyle, E.M., Ellis, P.A. and Hoogasian, J.J. (1990). Dietary n-3 fatty acid supplementation reduces superoxide production and chemiluminescence in a monocyte-enriched preparation of leukocytes. *Am. J. Clin. Nutr.*, **51**, 804–8

72. Lands, W.E.M. (1986). *Fish and Human Health*. (Orlando: Academic Press)
73. Kinsella, J.E. (1987). *Sea Foods and Fish Oils in Human Health and Disease*. (New York: Marcel Dekker)
74. Eaton, S.B. and Konner, M.J. (1985). Paleolithic nutrition: a consideration of its nature and current implications. *N. Engl. J. Med.*, **312**, 283–9
75. Eaton, S.B., Konner, M.J. and Shostak, M. (1988). Stone agers in the fast lane: chronic degenerative diseases in evolutionary perspective. *Am. J. Med.*, **84**, 739–49
76. Speth, J.D. (1983). *Bison Kills and Bone Counts: Decision Making by Ancient Hunters*, pp. 92–3. (Chicago: The University of Chicago Press)
77. Crawford, M.A., Casperd, N.M. and Sinclair, A.J. (1976). The long-chain metabolites of linoleic and linolenic acids in liver and brain in herbivores and carnivores. *Comp. Biochem. Physiol.*, **54B**, 395–401
78. Stamler, J. (1979). Population studies. In Levy, R., Rifkind, B., Dennis, B. and Ernst, N. (eds). *Nutrition, Lipids and Coronary Heart Disease*, pp. 25–88. (New York: Raven Press)
79. Kirschenbaum, H.G. (1960). *Fats and Oils*, 2nd edn. (New York: Reinhold)
80. Anon. (1982). Researchers report gains in hunt for low-linolenic soybeans. *J. Am. Oil Chem. Soc.*, **59**, 882A-4A
81. Fitch-Baumann, B. (1990). Low-linolenic acid flax: variation on familiar oilseed. *Inform*, 1, 934–51
82. Rizek, R.L., Welsh, S.O., Marston, R.M. and Jackson, E.M. (1983). Levels and sources of fat in the U.S. food supply and diets of individuals. In Perkins, E.G. and Visek, W.J. (eds). *Dietary Fats and Health*, pp. 13–43. (Champaign: American Oil Chemists' Society)
83. Hunter, J.E. (1990). n-3 Fatty acids from vegetable oils. *Am. J. Clin. Nutr.*, **51**, 809–14
84. Taylor, T.G., Gibney, M.J. and Morgan, J.B. (1979). Haemostatic function and polyunsaturated fatty acids. *Lancet*, **2**, 1378
85. Buss, D.H. (1988). Is the British diet improving? *Proc. Nutr. Soc.*, **47**, 295–306
86. James, W.P.T. (1985). Dietary trends in Britain. In Padley, P.B. and Podmore, J. (eds). *The Role of Fats in Human Nutrition*, pp. 9–22. (Chichester: Ellis Horwood)
87. Adam, O. (1989). Linoleic and linolenic acids intake. In Galli, C. and Simopoulos, A. (eds). *Dietary ω-3 and ω-6 Fatty Acids: Biological Effects and Nutritional Essentiality, NATO-ASI Series: Series A: Life Sciences*, Vol. 171, pp. 33–41. (New York and London: Plenum Press)
88. Bavly, S., Poznanski, R. and Kaufmann, N. (1980). *Levels of Nutrition in Israel 1975/76*. Published by the Ministry of Education and Culture, and The Hebrew University-Hadassah Medical School, Jerusalem
89. Kaufmann, N.A., Friedlander, Y., Halfon, S-T., Slater, P.E., Dennis, B.H., McClish, D., Eisenberg, S. and Stein, Y. (1982). Nutrient intake in Jerusalem – consumption in adults. *Isr. J. Med. Sci.*, **18**, 1183–97
90. Central Bureau of Statistics. *Food Balance Sheets*, Jerusalem, 1985/86
91. Blondheim, S.H., Horne, T., Davidovich, R., Kapitulnik, J., Segal, S. and Kaufmann, N. (1976). Unsaturated fatty acids in adipose tissue of Israeli Jews. *Isr. J. Med. Sci.*, **12**, 658–61
92. Schwartz, R.G., Horne, T. and Blondheim, S.H. (1979). Fatty acid saturation in subcutaneous fat of young Americans and Israelis. *Isr. J. Med. Sci.*, **15**, 778–81

93. Enig, M.G., Budowski, P. and Blondheim, S.H. (1984). Trans-unsaturated fatty acids in margarines and human subcutaneous fat in Israel. *Human Nutr. Clin. Nutr.*, **38C**, 223–30

94. Blondheim, S.H., Horne, T., Abu-Rabia, Y., Lehmann, E.E. and Heldenberg, D. (1982). Polyunsaturation of subcutaneous fat and concentration of serum lipids of Israeli Beduin Arabs. *Human Nutr. Clin. Nutr.*, **36C**, 449–57

95. Berry, E.M., Zimmerman, J., Peser, M. and Ligumsky, M. (1986). Dietary fat, adipose tissue composition and development of carcinoma of the colon. *J. Natl. Cancer Inst.*, **77**, 93–7

96. Beynen, A.C., Hermus, A.J.J. and Hautvast, J.G.A.J. (1980). A mathematical relationship between the fatty acid composition of the diet and that of adipose tissue in man. *Am. J. Clin. Nutr.*, **33**, 81–5

97. Neuringer, M., Connor, W.E., Lin, D.S., Barstad, L. and Luck, S.J. (1986). Biochemical and functional effects of prenatal and postnatal ω3 fatty acid deficiency in retina and brain in Rhesus monkey. *Proc. Natl. Acad. Sci. USA*, **83**, 4021–5

98. Clandinin, M.T. and Chappel, J.E. (1985). Long chain polyenoic essential fatty acids in human milk: are they of benefit to the newborn? In Schaub, J. (ed.) *Composition and Physiological Properties of Human Milk*, pp. 213–22. (New York: Elsevier Science Publishers)

99. Dyerberg, J., Bang, H.O. and Aagard, O. (1980). α-Linolenic and eicosapentaenoic acid. *Lancet*, **2**, 117–19

100. Sanders, T.A.B. and Roshanai, F. (1983). The influence of different types of ω3 polyunsaturated fatty acids on blood lipids and platelet function in healthy volunteers. *Clin. Sci.*, **64**, 91–9

101. Emken, E.A., Adlof, R.O., Rakoff, H. and Rohwedder, W.K. (1989). Metabolism of deuterium-labeled linolenic, linoleic, oleic, stearic and palmitic acid in human subjects. In Baillie, T.A. and Jones, J.R. (eds). *Synthesis and Application of Isotopically Labelled Compounds 1988*, pp. 713–16

102. Sieguel, E.L. and Maclure, M. (1987). Relative activity of unsaturated fatty acid pathways in humans. *Metabolism*, **36**, 664–9

103. Budowski, P., Trostler, N., Lupo, M., Vaisman, N. and Eldor, A. (1984). Effect of linseed oil ingestion on plasma lipid fatty acid composition and platelet aggregation in healthy volunteers. *Nutr. Res.*, **4**, 343–6

104. Sanders, T.A.B., Ellis, F.R. and Dickerson, J.W.J. (1978). Studies on vegans: the fatty acid composition of plasma choline phosphoglycerides, erythrocytes, adipose tissue and breast milk, and some indicators of susceptibility to ischaemic heart disease in vegans and controls. *Am. J. Clin. Nutr.*, **31**, 805–13

105. Third Toronto Workshop on Essential Fatty Acids: α-Linolenic Acid in Human Nutrition and Disease. May 17–18, 1991. University of Toronto

Discussion

Dr Kubow: How do you rationalize the decreased oxidation of LDL with the n-3 fatty acids when per carbon chain length, as compared to n-6, they have an increase in unsaturation? As well, animal studies have shown that feeding n-3 fats, as compared to n-6 fats, increase serum lipid peroxides.

Dr Budowski: Yes, I referred to this paradox. There is interference with the metabolism of arachidonic acid, even before the arachidonic cascade. In fact, the chicken model showed that there is less oxidation when linoleic acid is replaced by α-linolenic acid. If you prepare homogenates of tissues you will find that there is greater oxidizability but that is due to the fact that peroxidation occurs after homogenization. What you measure is not the actual peroxide content but the peroxidizability of the lipids. So I would say that the reason for the paradox is that α-linolenic acid or n-3 fatty acids interfere with the metabolism of arachidonic acid at various levels before and during the arachidonic acid cascade.

18

The ratio of polyunsaturates to saturates and its role in the efficacy of n-3 fatty acids

K.S. LAYNE, E.A. RYAN, M.L. GARG, Y.K. GOH, J.A. JUMPSEN and M.T. CLANDININ

Dietary n-3 fatty acids (eicosapentanoic and docosahexanoic acids) have recently been linked with reduction of various risk factors associated with coronary heart disease, diabetes, rheumatism, inflammatory bowel disease and psoriasis[1-3]. The high incidence of coronary heart disease in Western countries has prompted investigation of the effects of n-3 fatty acids on atherogenic risk factors. Although earlier reports focused on epidemiological evidence, it is clear that the mechanisms by which n-3 fatty acids exert their action require critical assessment.

In humans, the protective effects of marine lipids may be attributed to a variety of well established factors including shifts in eicosanoid metabolism leading to reduced platelet aggregation and thrombosis[4]. However, reports of n-3 fatty acid effects on circulating serum lipid and lipoprotein levels vary considerably. Generally, it has been found that plasma levels of triacylglycerol and very low density lipoprotein are reduced[5,6], while low density lipoprotein and high density lipoprotein levels may increase[7], decrease[8] or not change[9]. In the rat, we have found that dietary fat intake influences the efficacy of n-3 fatty acid action, therefore it seems that diets differing in polyunsaturated to saturated fatty acid (P/S) ratio may account for some of the inconsistency in serum lipid results previously observed for human subjects.

Effect of dietary n-3 fatty acids on cholesterol levels

Linseed oil contains α-linolenic acid (18:3n-3) which is the primary fatty acid in the n-3 fatty acid family. It is considered an essential fatty acid as it cannot be synthesized by animals or humans[10]. Long-chain fatty acids of the n-3 family (20:5n-3 and 22:6n-3) originate in the human diet predominantly from fish and fish oils. Recent studies have shown a striking inverse correlation between the consumption of fish rich in n-3 fatty acids and mortality from

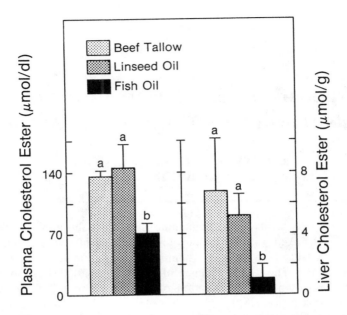

Figure 1 Effect of n-3 fatty acids on cholesterol ester content of rat plasma and liver. Animals were fed diets high in either saturated fat (beef tallow), linseed oil or fish oil for 28 days. Values are means±SD for six animals ($n=6$). Values without a common superscript are significantly different ($p < 0.05$) (Data adapted from ref. 12)

coronary heart disease[11]. To identify the specificity of n-3 fatty acid action, rats were fed diets high in either saturated fat (beef tallow), linseed oil (18:3n-3) or fish oil (20:5n-3 and 22:6n-3)[12]. It should be noted that in all animal work dietary 18:2n-6 levels were above those required for normal physiological function and growth. Feeding fish oil lowered the cholesterol ester content of rat plasma and liver, whereas feeding linseed oil had no significant effect when compared with the control group fed beef tallow (Figure 1). Similar reductions in hepatic and plasma triacylglycerol levels were found in the fish oil group (Figure 2). Animals fed diets high in either saturated fat, linseed oil or fish oil were challenged by a 2% dietary cholesterol load[13]. Cholesterol addition to the beef tallow and linseed oil diet increased plasma total cholesterol level, whereas cholesterol supplementation with fish oil had no significant effect (Figure 3). Cholesterol supplementation in all diets increased cholesterol content of the liver tissue; however, feeding cholesterol with fish oil appears to partially attenuate this effect (Figure 4).

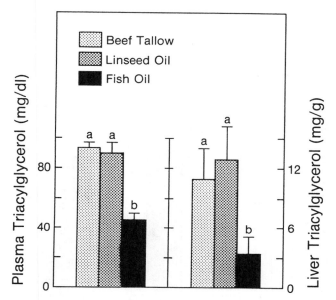

Figure 2 Effect of dietary n-3 fatty acids on triacylglycerol content of rat plasma and liver. Animals were fed diets high in either saturated fat (beef tallow), linseed oil or fish oil for 28 days. Values are means ± SD for six animals ($n = 6$). Values without a common superscript are significantly different ($p < 0.05$) (Data adapted from ref. 12)

Effect of dietary n-3 fatty acids on triacylglycerol levels

The effect of dietary linseed oil (18:3n-3) or fish oil (20:5n-3 and 22:6n-3) on serum and liver triacylglycerol levels in rats fed diets high in saturated fatty acids (beef tallow) versus low in saturated fatty acids (safflower oil) was studied[14]. Serum triacylglycerol levels were significantly reduced by fish oil when fed in combination with saturated fatty acids, while the combination of fish oil and safflower oil failed to do so (Figure 5). Hepatic triacylglycerol levels were also lowered by feeding fish oil with a diet high in saturated fat (Figure 6). All diets high in linoleic acid resulted in higher hepatic triacylglycerol levels when compared with diets high in saturated fat. These results suggest that long-chain n-3 fatty acids reduce serum and hepatic triacylglycerol levels more effectively when fed in combination with diets low in 18:2n-6 and high in saturated fatty acids.

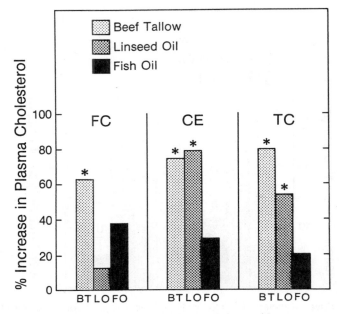

Figure 3 Effect of 2% dietary cholesterol and/or n-3 fatty acid on percentage increase in plasma cholesterol. Animals were fed diets high in either saturated fat (beef tallow), linseed oil or fish oil. Results indicate the percentage increase in plasma cholesterol levels in animals fed the above diets versus animals fed the diets supplemented with 2% cholesterol. Values are the mean±SD of six animals (n=6). Values with an asterisk displayed a significant percentage increase in plasma cholesterol when 2% cholesterol was added to the diet ($p < 0.05$) (Data adapted from ref. 13)

Conversion of 18:3n-3 to 20:5n-3

Since the hypocholesterolaemic and anti-thrombic attributes of n-3 fatty acids are demonstrated mainly by the long-chain fatty acids, it is important to determine the extent to which 18:3n-3 can be converted to 20:5n-3 and 22:6n-3 in animals and humans. Existing evidence suggests that both humans and animals possess limited ability to convert 18:3n-3 to 20:5n-3 and 22:6n-3, whereas 18:2n-6 is rapidly desaturated and elongated to 20:4n-6[15]. In growing rats we have found that conversion of 18:3n-3 to 20:5n-3 and inhibition of the conversion of 18:2n-6 to 20:4n-6 can be maximized by partial replacement of dietary 18:2n-6 by saturated fatty acids[16]. If this observation in animals is also valid in humans, then it may be desirable to not elevate the consumption of dietary 18:2n-6 and to include additional sources of 18:3n-3 in the diet.

Feeding 20:5n-3 and 22:6n-3 increases incorporation of these fatty acids into hepatic phospholipid at the expense of n-6 fatty acids[2]. Dietary 18:3n-3

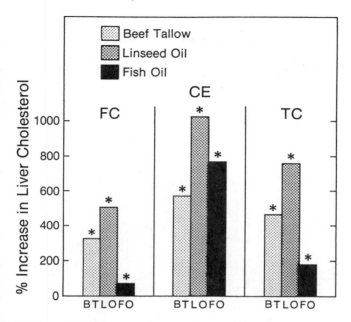

Figure 4 Effect of 2% dietary cholesterol and/or n-3 fatty acid on percentage increase in liver cholesterol. Animals were fed diets high in either saturated fat (beef tallow), linseed oil or fish oil. Results indicate the percentage increase in liver cholesterol levels in animals fed the above diets versus animals fed the above diets supplemented with 2% cholesterol. Values are the mean±SD of six animals ($n=6$). Values with an asterisk displayed a significant percentage increase in liver cholesterol levels when 2% cholesterol was added to the diet ($p<0.05$) (Data adapted from ref. 13)

is also incorporated into plasma and tissue lipids[13] and must compete with n-6 fatty acids for elongation and desaturation. Replacement of n-6 fatty acids (20:4n-6, 22:4n-6, 22:5n-6) by n-3 fatty acids (18:3n-3, 20:5n-3, 22:5n-3, 22:6n-3) in serum and liver lipid fractions is enhanced when linseed oil is fed with saturated fat (beef tallow) rather than when fed with linoleic acid (safflower oil)[16]. These results suggest that the cholesterol and arachidonate lowering effects of dietary α-linolenic acid may depend on the linoleic acid to saturated fatty acid ratio or 18:3n-3 to 18:2n-6 ratio.

Arachidonic acid and eicosanoid metabolism

Animals and humans are able to convert 20:4n-6 into a variety of biologically active metabolites which include prostaglandins, thromboxanes and leukotrienes, collectively known as eicosanoids[17]. The balance of these eicosanoid

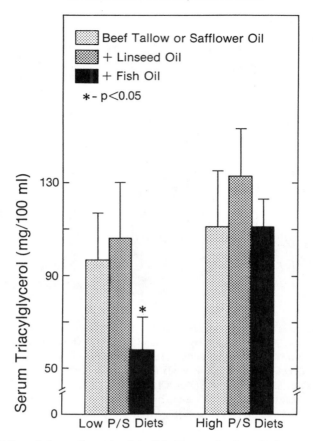

Figure 5 Effect of dietary linseed or fish oil fed in combination with low P/S (low 18:2n-6) versus high P/S diets on serum triacylglycerol levels in rats. Animals were fed diets either high in saturated fat (low P/S) or high in 18:2n-6 (high P/S) with and without addition of linseed or fish oil for 28 days. Values with an asterisk are significantly different from those without ($p < 0.05$) (Data adapted from ref. 14)

metabolites is important for regulation of physiological processes such as platelet function, inflammation, thrombosis[17,18] and many others. The profile of eicosanoids varies from cell to cell; blood platelets convert arachidonic acid to TXA_2, whereas vascular endothelium produces mainly PGI_2. TXA_2 is a potent vasoconstrictor which induces platelet aggregation and PGI_2 is the most potent vasodilator which inhibits platelet aggregation[17]. Balance between these two eicosanoids maintains normal haemostasis and any alteration in the TXA_2/PGI_2 ratio will affect thrombosis, haemostatic plug formation and atherogenesis[17].

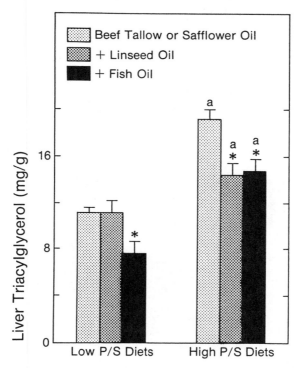

Figure 6 Effect of dietary linseed or fish oil fed in combination with low P/S (low 18:2n-6) versus high P/S diets on liver triacylglycerol levels in rats. Animals were fed diets either high in saturated fat (low P/S) or high in 18:2n-6 (high P/S) with and without addition of linseed or fish oil for 28 days. Values with an asterisk are significantly different from the beef tallow or safflower oil diets ($p < 0.01$). Values with superscript 'a' are significantly different from the corresponding values in the beef tallow diet ($p < 0.05$) (Data adapted from ref. 14)

Alteration in dietary fat may modify TXA_2/PGI_2 balance. Eicosapentanoic acid present in fish oil competes with arachidonic acid at the level of cyclo-oxygenase and inhibits TXA_2 and PGI_2 formation[19,20]. It appears that eicosapentanoic acid is converted to TXA_3, a weak pro-aggregating agent and PGI_3, a potent anti-aggregating agent[21]. Therefore, the overall effect of fish oil consumption is a decrease in platelet aggregation or increased bleeding time[22]. Since arachidonic acid availability is a key factor in eicosanoid formation, increased attention has been given to synthesis and incorporation of 20:4n-6 into phospholipid pools. N-3 fatty acids, particularly eicosapentanoic acid, are incorporated into plasma and tissue phospholipids at the expense of n-6 fatty acids[13]. We have recently shown that in rats 20:5n-3 is incorporated into plasma and tissue lipid pools to a greater extent when n-3 fatty acids are

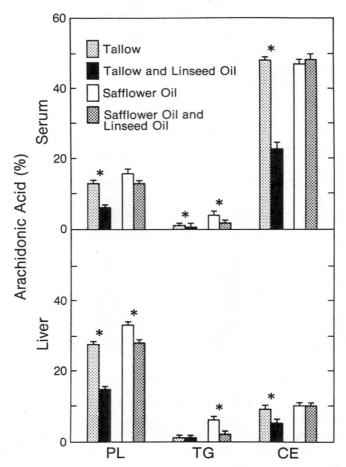

Figure 7 Effect of dietary 18:3n-3 in combination with a diet high in saturated fat versus low in saturated fat on 20:4n-6 content of rat serum and liver lipid fractions. PL, phospholipid; TG, triacylglycerol; CE, cholesterol ester. Animals were fed diets high in saturated fat versus 18:2n-6, with and without addition of 18:3n-3. Values are the mean±SD of five rats ($n=5$). Paired values with an asterisk are significantly different ($p < 0.05$) (Data adapted from ref. 16)

fed in combination with saturated fatty acid than with linoleic acid[23]. Consumption of linseed oil reduced the arachidonic acid content in serum and liver lipid fractions only when fed in combination with a diet high in saturated fat and low in 18:2n-6[16] (Figure 7). The decrease in phospholipid 20:4n-6 content may be partly due to a shift of 20:4n-6 from phospholipid to triacylglycerol and/or cholesterol ester pools in the same tissue[12]. This suggests that triacylglycerol and cholesterol esters may play a buffering role in the homeostatic maintenance of tissue phospholipid levels of 20:4n-6.

Effect of n-3 fatty acids on desaturase activity

Recently it has been shown that n-3 fatty acids decrease conversion of 18:2n-6 to 18:3n-6 by inhibiting Δ6-desaturase activity[24]. N-3 fatty acids may also reduce arachidonic acid formation by lowering Δ5-desaturase activity[25]. Although both linseed oil and fish oil reduce Δ6-desaturation, the decrease is significantly greater with fish oil suggesting that the mechanism for inhibition of desaturase activity by fish oil is different than that of linseed oil. It seems that 18:3n-3 may compete with 18:2n-6 for Δ6-desaturase activity while the fish oils may inhibit desaturation by other mechanisms[26].

The type of fat fed to the growing rat alters the efficacy of the n-3 fatty acid treatment. To examine the ability of n-3 fatty acids and P/S ratio to alter Δ6-desaturase activity, rats were fed diets enriched with linseed or fish oil in combination with a diet high in saturated fat (beef tallow) versus a diet low in saturated fat (safflower oil)[27]. The inhibition of Δ6-desaturase activity was greater when the diet contained 20:5n-3 and 22:6n-3 with beef tallow than 18:3n-3 with beef tallow or 20:5n-3 and 22:6n-3 with safflower oil (Table 1). Both linseed and fish oil inhibit conversion of 18:2n-6 to 18:3n-6 thus reducing the 20:4n-6 content in serum and hepatic phospholipids. This inhibition was evident only when n-3 fatty acids were fed with diets high in saturated fat indicating that low levels of 18:2n-6 in the high saturated fat diet offer less competition with 18:3n-3 for Δ6-desaturase activity and enhance the efficacy of the n-3 fatty acids. The optimum ratio of 18:2n-6 to saturated fatty acids

Table 1 Effect of dietary linseed oil and fish oil fed in combination with diets high in saturated fat versus 18:2n-6 on Δ6-desaturase activity in rat liver microsomes

Diet fat	Δ6-Desaturase activity
High in saturated fat	617 ± 84^a
plus 18:3n-3	218 ± 37^b
plus fish oil	141 ± 24^c
High in 18:2n-6	329 ± 38^d
plus 18:3n-3	240 ± 60
plus fish oil	263 ± 45^d

Values are the mean $\pm$ SD for five separate microsomal preparations ($n=5$) from each diet group.
[a,b,c]Values are significantly different within the high saturated fat diets ($p < 0.05$).
[d]Values are significantly different from the corresponding values in the high saturated fat fed animals ($p < 0.05$).

required for effective competition of 18:3n-3 with 18:2n-6 for Δ6-desaturation remains to be determined.

Effect of dietary n-3 fatty acids on lipoprotein metabolism in subjects consuming diets high or low in saturated fat

Results from the animal studies indicate that ability of n-3 fatty acids to alter eicosanoid metabolism and lower plasma triacylglycerol and cholesterol levels may depend on the dietary polyunsaturated to saturated fatty acid (P/S) ratio. Based on this, we have hypothesized that humans consuming a diet high in saturated fats (i.e. a low P/S diet) may display greater reductions in serum cholesterol and arachidonic acid levels from modest intakes of n-3 fatty acids when compared with individuals consuming higher dietary levels of linoleic acid.

To test this hypothesis a double-blind crossover study involving 32 normo-lipidaemic subjects was designed (Figure 8). Subjects were recruited on the basis of their normal dietary habits as determined by a 7-day food record and divided into two groups according to the P/S ratio of their diet (high, P/S = 0.75 versus low, P/S <0.56). All subjects provided an initial blood sample for baseline lipid and lipoprotein analysis and confirmation of a normal metabolic state. The experiment involved supplementation of three different purified triglyceride capsules (olive, linseed, and fish oil, the latter containing 32% C20 and C22 n-3 fatty acids) for a period of 3 months each. All subjects were supplemented with olive oil for the first 3-month period. Then, half of the subjects of each P/S group were randomly assigned to the n-3 fatty acid treatment and supplemented with 35 mg of n-3 fatty acid/kg body weight/day from either linseed or fish oil. All subjects completed the three oil treatment periods. After 3 months of capsule supplementation, blood samples were

Experimental Design of Clinical Trial

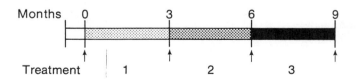

Figure 8 All subjects were supplemented with olive oil in treatment 1. Half of the subjects of each P/S group were randomly assigned to either fish oil or linseed oil for the second treatment and crossed over to the alternative oil for treatment 3. N-3 fatty acid doses were 35 mg of n-3 fatty acid/kg body weight/day. Arrows indicate times for completion of a 7-day diet record collection and blood sampling

Table 2 Effect of n-3 fatty acid intake on plasma total cholesterol, LDL cholesterol, HDL cholesterol and triacylglycerol levels in subjects consuming diets either high or low in saturated fatty acids

		Plasma fraction	
		LDL cholesterol (mmol/l)	Triacylglycerol (mmol/l)
Dietary group			
High P/S			
supplement:	None	2.32±0.25	0.95±0.09
	Olive oil	2.71±0.11	1.02±0.08
	Linseed oil	2.79±0.11	1.10±0.08
	Fish oil	2.92±0.13	0.75±0.09
Low P/S			
supplement:	None	2.27±0.18	0.97±0.12
	Olive oil	2.55±0.11	0.97±0.08
	Linseed oil	2.53±0.12	0.99±0.08
	Fish oil	2.74±0.11	0.65±0.08
Significant effects			
	Dietary group	$p < 0.003$	$p < 0.05$
	Oil supplement	$p < 0.0001$	$p < 0.0003$

Table 3 Effect of fish oil supplementation on lipoprotein 20:4n-6 and 20:5n-3 levels in normal subjects

		Phospholipid		Cholesterol ester	
Diet P/S ratio		20:4n-6	20:5n-3	20:4n-6	20:5n-3
		(% change from initial value)			
VLDL:	High	NS	180[**]	38[*]	260[***]
	Low	NS	190[**]	NS	200[***]
HDL:	High	NS	750[***]	−41[***]	550[***]
	Low	NS	540[***]	−33[***]	180[***]
LDL:	High	NS	600[***]	−27[*]	580[***]
	Low	NS	600[***]	−15[*]	540[***]

NS = non-significant percentage change from value observed before supplementation with fish oil.

[*] = $p < 0.05$, [**] = $p < 0.01$, [***] = $p < 0.001$ for percentage change from value observed before supplementation with fish oil.

drawn, 7-day diet records were collected and the subjects crossed over to the alternative treatment. Lab analyses were performed to determine total serum cholesterol and triacylglycerol levels (individual lipoprotein cholesterol levels) as well as fatty acid content of lipid classes (phospholipid, triacylglycerol, cholesterol ester, phosphatidylcholine, phosphatidylethanolamine) with each lipoprotein.

Analysis of serum total cholesterol, LDL cholesterol, HDL cholesterol and total triacylglycerol levels indicated that LDL cholesterol and total cholesterol are elevated by n-3 fatty acid supplementation (Table 2). For both the high and low P/S groups, total cholesterol and LDL cholesterol increased after all oil treatment periods when compared to initial values in the order: olive oil < linseed < fish oil. Total triacylglycerol levels were reduced by fish oil to a greater extent in the low P/S group than the high P/S group. This effect is apparently specific to fish oil as the olive oil and linseed oil treatments did not alter total serum triacylglycerol levels in either group of subjects.

Analyses of the fatty acid constituents of lipoprotein phospholipids and cholesterol esters (Table 3) indicates that feeding a low intake of n-3 fatty acids increases the 20:5n-3 level in all lipid classes examined, but only reduces the 20:4n-6 content in the HDL and LDL cholesterol ester fraction.

General conclusion

From both animal and human studies it is clear that there is considerable metabolic interaction between the effect of dietary C20 and C22 n-3 fatty acids and the metabolism of 18:2n-6. The efficacy of dietary ω-3 fatty acid intake is determined in part by this interaction and by the overall balance of dietary fatty acids fed. Thus one can envisage that potential beneficial metabolic effects of dietary n-3 fatty acids will be optimized by a dietary background that is low in competing substrates (i.e. low P/S) even though the overall level of n-3 fatty acid intake is relatively low.

Acknowledgements

This work was supported by funding from NSERC and the Canadian Dairy Bureau. The purified triglycerides utilized in the clinical feeding study were generously provided by CPL (Chromatography Purified Lipids) Company, Division LipidTeknik, Stockholm, Sweden. The authors are grateful for the competent laboratory assistance of A. Wierzbicki and I. Cheung.

References

1. Carroll, K.K. (1986). Review: Biological effects of fish oils in relation to chronic diseases. *Lipids*, **21**, 731–3
2. Garg, M.L., Thomson, A.B.R. and Clandinin, M.T. (1989). Effect of dietary fish oil on tissue lipid metabolism. In Chandra, R.K. (ed.) *Health Effects of Fish and Fish Oils*, pp. 53–79. (St. John's: ARTS Biomedical Publishers and Distributors)
3. Dyerberg, J. (1986). Unsaturated fatty acids and health. *N-3 News*, **1**, 1–4
4. Gibson, R.A. (1988). The effect of diets containing fish and fish oils on disease risk factors in humans. *Aust. N.Z. J. Med.*, **18**, 713–22
5. Bronsgeest-Schoute, H.C., Van Gent, C.M., Lutten, J.B. and Ruiter, A. (1981). The effects of various intakes of ω-3 fatty acids on blood lipid composition in healthy human subjects. *Am. J. Clin. Nutr.*, **34**, 1752–7
6. Nestel, P.J., Connor, W.E., Reardon, M.F., Connor, S., Wong, S. and Boston, R. (1984). Suppression by diets rich in fish oil of very low density lipoprotein in man. *J. Clin. Invest.*, **74**, 82–9
7. Sullivan, D.R., Sanders, T.A.B., Trayner, I.M. and Thompson, G.R. (1986). Paradoxical elevation of LDL apoprotein B levels in hypertriglyceridaemic patients and normal subjects ingesting fish oil. *Atherosclerosis*, **61**, 129–34
8. Illingworth, D.R., Harris, W.S. and Connor, W.E. (1984). Inhibition of low-density lipoprotein synthesis by n-3 fatty acids in humans. *Arteriosclerosis*, **4**, 270–5
9. Sanders, T.A.B., Vickers, M. and Haines, A.P. (1981). Effect on blood lipids and haemostasis of a supplement of cod liver oil, rich in eicosapentaenoic and docosahexanoic acids in healthy young men. *Clin. Sci.*, **46**, 601–11
10. Tinoco, J. (1982). Dietary requirements and functions of alpha-linolenic acid in animals. *Prog. Lipid Res.*, **21**, 1–45
11. Kromhout, D., Bosschieter, E.B. and De Lezenne Coulander, C. (1985). The inverse relation between fish consumption and 20-year mortality from coronary heart disease. *N. Engl. J. Med.*, **312**, 1205–9
12. Garg, M.L., Wierzbicki, A.A., Thomson, A.B.R. and Clandinin, M.T. (1989). Omega-3 fatty acids increase the arachidonic acid content of liver cholesterol ester and plasma triacylglycerol fractions in the rat. *Biochem. J.*, **261**, 11–15
13. Garg, M.L., Wierzbicki, A.A., Keelan, M., Thomson, A.B.R. and Clandinin, M.T. (1989). Fish oil prevents change in arachidonic acid and cholesterol content in rat caused by dietary cholesterol. *Lipids*, **24**, 266–70
14. Garg, M.L., Thomson, A.B.R. and Clandinin, M.T. (1989). Hypotriglyceridemic effect of dietary n-3 fatty acids in rats fed low versus high levels of linoleic acid. *Biochim. Biophys. Acta*, **1006**, 127–30
15. Zollner, N. (1986). Dietary linolenic acid in man – an overview. *Prog. Lipid Res.*, **25**, 177–80
16. Garg, M.L., Wierzbicki, A.A., Thomson, A.B.R. and Clandinin, M.T. (1989). Dietary saturated fat level alters the competition between α-linolenic acid and linoleic acid. *Lipids*, **24**, 334–9
17. Salmon, J.A. (1987). Role of arachidonic acid metabolites in inflammatory and thrombic responses. *Biochem. Soc. Trans.*, **15**, 324–6

18. Sammuelsson, B., Goldyne, M., Granstrom, B., Hamberg, M., Hammerstrom, S. and Malmster, C. (1978). Prostaglandins and thromboxanes. *Annu. Rev. Biochem.*, **47**, 997–1029

19. Siess, W., Scherer, B., Bohlig, B., Roth, P., Kurzmann, I. and Wever, P.C. (1980). Platelet-membrane fatty acids, platelet aggregation, and thromboxane formation during a mackerel diet. *Lancet*, **1**, 441–4

20. Culp, B.R., Ritus, B.G. and Lands, W.E.M. (1978). Inhibition of prostaglandin biosynthesis by eicosapentaenoic acid. *Prostagl. Med.*, **3**, 269–78

21. Needleman, P., Raz, A., Minkes, M.S., Ferrendell, J.A. and Sprecher, H. (1979). Triene prostaglandins: prostacyclin and thromboxane biosynthesis and unique biological properties. *Proc. Natl. Acad. Sci. USA*, **76**, 944–8

22. Dyerberg, J. and Jorgensen, K.J. (1982). Marine oils and thrombogenesis. *Prog. Lipid Res.*, **21**, 255–69

23. Garg, M.L., Wierzbicki, A.A., Thomson, A.B.R. and Clandinin, M.T. (1988). Fish oil reduces cholesterol and arachidonic acid content more efficiently in rats fed diets containing low linolenic to saturated fatty acid ratios. *Biochim. Biophys. Acta*, **962**, 337–44

24. Garg, M.L., Sebokova, E., Thomson, A.B.R. and Clandinin, M.T. (1988). Δ6-desaturase activity in liver microsomes of rats fed diets enriched with cholesterol and/or ω3 fatty acids. *Biochem. J.*, **249**, 351–6

25. Garg, M.L., Thomson, A.B.R. and Clandinin, M.T. (1988). Effect of dietary cholesterol and/or ω3 fatty acids on lipid composition and Δ5-desaturase activity of rat liver microsomes. *J. Nutr.*, **118**, 661–8

26. Brenner, R.R. and Pelufflo, R.D. (1967). Inhibiting effect of docosa-4,7,10,13,16,19-hexanoic acid upon the oxidative destruction of linoleic into α-linolenic acid and of α-linolenic into octadeca-6,9,12,15-tetraenoic acid. *Biochim. Biophys. Acta*, **137**, 184–6

27. Garg, M.L., Thomson, A.B.R. and Clandinin, M.T. (1990). Interaction of saturated, n-6 and n-3 polyunsaturated fatty acids to modulate arachidonic acid metabolism. *J. Lipid Res.*, **31**, 271–7

Discussion

Dr Budowski: In your animal experiments you mentioned saturated fatty acids and linoleic acid and showed that the activity of α-linolenic acid was different for these two types of fatty acids. I wonder how oleic acid would act in this respect. Would it act like saturated fatty acids or would it act like linoleic acid?

Dr Clandinin: I think that is a very good question. We have not looked at it in terms of plasma lipids but we have looked at it in terms of incorporation of fatty acids into membranes. I think, and this may relate a bit to what John Dietschy was saying this morning, one of the things that we find with membrane lipids is that the saturates remain relatively constant. You might trade the balance off between 16:0 and 18:0 a bit, but the monoenes can be manipulated quite a bit. How much they change really depends on the level of ω-6 and the level of ω-3 in the diet. Whether this has any bearing on or is reflected in plasma levels is not known.

Dr Vega: You mentioned during your talk that with the high P/S ratio an increase in the LDL cholesterol was noted in some groups and that there was a variability in their responsiveness. Is that correct?

Dr Clandinin: Yes, basically we find that the fish oil increases the LDL cholesterol in subjects who are high P/S consumers.

Dr Vega: Was this the case irrespective of the levels of triglycerides?

Dr Clandinin: Well, I think that one consistent thing was that in essentially all subjects, regardless of their P/S group, the triglyceride level was reduced by the fish oil. The degree of reduction was a little greater in the subjects on the low P/S treatment.

Dr Vega: This phenomenon seems to be quite similar to that of gemfibrozil in that you can have a slight increment in the LDL cholesterol by reducing the triglyceride. I wonder if that is a shift of cholesterol from the VLDL to LDL and what exactly this means?

Dr Clandinin: It is possible. I think that I would not get excited about the overall change in the LDL cholesterol levels in these control subjects because it is small. What precisely would happen in diabetic subjects might be another matter.

19

Lipoproteins, sex hormones and the gender difference in coronary heart disease

I.F. GODSLAND

Introduction

Between 35 and 44 years of age, age-standardized mortality from coronary heart disease may be as much as six-fold higher in men compared with women[1]. Men and women appear to have approximately equal *susceptibility* to risk factors for coronary heart disease. Therefore, the basis for the gender difference in coronary heart disease rates may be found in differences in *exposure* to risk factors[2-4]. Although this area remains surprisingly poorly researched, at least part of the gender difference in coronary heart disease rates may be accounted for by gender differences in lipoprotein risk factors[5].

Studies evaluating the safety and side-effects of synthetic gonadal steroids (such as oestrogens, androgens and anabolic steroids) have consistently demonstrated marked effects of these agents on serum lipids and lipoproteins[5]. An underlying pattern has emerged whereby synthetic steroids with oestrogenic activity induce a lipoprotein pattern consistent with reduced risk of coronary heart disease, whereas those with androgenic activity induce a pattern consistent with increased risk. It may not be appropriate to extrapolate effects of synthetic steroids to those of the equivalent endogenous hormones, and there are some inconsistencies in the overall picture. Nevertheless, evaluation of the effects of synthetic gonadal steroids on lipoprotein concentrations has lent support to the hypothesis that the lower incidence of coronary heart disease in women is due to the effects of endogenous sex hormones on serum lipoprotein risk factors for coronary heart disease. Furthermore, studies of the effects of gonadal steroids have highlighted the need for detailed evaluation of lipoprotein cholesterol fractions and subfractions, rather than measurement of serum total cholesterol alone. There may be substantial reciprocal changes in lipoprotein fractions and subfractions in response to gonadal steroids which are not reflected in changes in total cholesterol[6,7] (Figure 1).

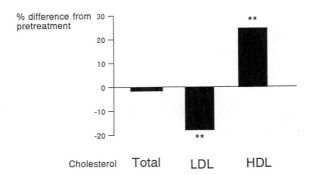

Figure 1 Percentage differences from pretreatment mean values for total, LDL and HDL cholesterol in 11 women receiving ethinyl oestradiol for 3 months or more. Adapted from Wynn *et al.*, *Clin. Endocrinol.*, **24**:183. Significant differences from pretreatment levels: ** $p < 0.01$

In the following review, gender differences in lipoprotein concentrations, primarily high density and low density lipoproteins (HDL and LDL, respectively) are summarized. The effects of exogenously administered gonadal steroids and sex hormones on serum lipoproteins are considered. Finally, the extent to which the gender differences in lipoprotein concentrations can be explained by the difference between the sexes in sex hormone levels is evaluated with regard to correlations between lipoprotein concentrations, sex hormone concentrations, and changes in gonadal status, such as puberty and the menopause.

Gender differences in lipid and lipoprotein concentrations

In societies in which coronary heart disease is considered to be a major health problem, and in which there is an appreciable gender difference in coronary heart disease rates, there are marked gender differences in serum lipid and lipoprotein concentrations[8–10]. The differences are consistent with the higher coronary heart disease rates in males. This is exemplified in data from the Lipid Research Clinics Prevalence Study Population (Table 1)[9]. For men and women aged 30–39 years, serum total cholesterol was 7% higher in men than in women, but underlying this difference were even greater differences in LDL and HDL cholesterol concentrations. LDL cholesterol was 12% higher in men and HDL cholesterol was 20% lower. The importance of these differences for coronary heart disease risk is illustrated by data from the Framingham Study, which show that when men and women are matched for HDL cholesterol

Table 1 Mean plasma total cholesterol (Chol), very low density lipoprotein (VLDL), low density lipoprotein (LDL) and high density lipoprotein (HDL) cholesterol (mg/dl) in white men and women in 11 North American populations

Gender	Ages	n	Chol	VLDL	LDL	HDL
M	20–29	371	173.4	16.2	112.4	44.9
F	20–29	513	175.9	13.4	107.7	55.0
M	30–39	775	196.7	22.6	129.7	44.5
F	30–39	637	184.1	13.7	115.3	55.5
M	40–49	712	209.0	25.0	139.3	44.8
F	40–49	648	201.9	16.1	127.3	58.6
M	50–59	601	214.0	24.5	143.8	45.6
F	50–59	508	222.9	18.9	142.0	62.1
M	60–69	236	218.5	19.3	148.1	51.3
F	60–69	212	237.6	17.6	158.8	61.3
M	70+	119	210.3	17.0	142.9	50.5
F	70+	127	224.8	16.2	148.9	60.1

Adapted from Rifkind, B.M. *et al. Lipids*, 1979; **14**: 105.

concentration the gender difference in coronary heart disease rates is no longer apparent[2,5].

The gender difference in HDL concentrations is due almost entirely to lower levels of the HDL_2 subfraction in men[11–13]. HDL_3 does not show such a marked difference between the sexes. These differences are clearly apparent in HDL_2 cholesterol concentration (Godsland *et al.*, unpublished observations). In age matched groups of men and women the gender difference in HDL cholesterol concentrations was almost entirely in the HDL_2 subfraction (Table 2).

A marked gender difference in VLDL cholesterol has also been observed, with men between 30 and 59 years of age having levels on average 50% higher than women in the same age range[9]. However, the status of triglyceride-rich lipoproteins as an independent risk factor for coronary heart disease is controversial[14]. For example, elevated triglyceride levels may not be associated with increased risk if HDL cholesterol levels are also high[15]. Furthermore, although gonadal steroids and sex hormones may affect VLDL levels, these associations are less well defined, and show a less consistent pattern with regard to gonadal steroid activity and gender differences, than do associations with HDL and LDL levels[5]. Therefore, in the following review, only HDL and LDL will be considered.

Table 2 HDL, HDL$_2$ and HDL$_3$ cholesterol concentrations (mg/dl) in healthy men and women from the UK, aged 20–60 years and less than 120% of ideal body weight[†]. Mean±SD

	n	Age	%IBW	HDL	HDL$_2$	HDL$_3$
Men	88	45.6±9.6	105.3±9.2	52.8±11.6	14.1±8.3	38.7±6.9
Women	77	48.1±8.1	105.1±6.7	63.2±12.0	22.4±9.0	40.8±6.5
		ns	ns	***	***	*

Significant differences between men and women: ns, non-significant; ***, $p < 0.001$; *, $p < 0.05$.
[†]Godsland, I.F. *et al.* Unpublished observations.

Effects on serum lipoproteins of gonadal steroid or sex hormone administration

Gonadal steroids with oestrogenic activity

Recognition that lipoprotein concentrations could be substantially affected by gonadal steroids dates back to the early work of Barr, Russ and Eder who described the characteristic increase in high density lipoprotein (HDL) cholesterol concentrations and decrease in low density lipoprotein (LDL) cholesterol concentrations seen in response to administration of ethinyl oestradiol[16]. This finding has been confirmed in a number of studies of orally administered oestrogens, not only ethinyl oestradiol, but also diethylstilboestrol, conjugated equine oestrogens (Premarin) and mestranol[17-19]. These effects have been mainly demonstrated in men and postmenopausal women. An increase in HDL cholesterol concentrations is also seen in premenopausal women[20], but the effects on LDL cholesterol are less marked, and this may be related to the relatively lower concentrations that are found in these women[21]. A reduction in LDL cholesterol and an increase in HDL cholesterol concentrations may also be seen when an alkylated oestrogen is administered by a non-oral route[22], suggesting that these effects are an intrinsic property of the steroid rather than a secondary effect on the liver of the high portal vein concentrations that result from oral administration (first-pass effect). The increase in HDL cholesterol in response to oestrogenic gonadal steroids appears to be primarily in the HDL$_2$ cholesterol subfraction[7,20,23].

Gonadal steroids with androgenic activity

Barr first reported that the orally administered, androgenic, 17-alkyl derivative, methyl testosterone could substantially raise total cholesterol and reduce cholesterol in the lipoprotein fraction corresponding to HDL[24]. It was subsequently confirmed that methyl testosterone could raise LDL cholesterol and lower HDL cholesterol in men and in pre- and postmenopausal women[17,25,26]. These changes were also seen with other orally administered steroids with androgenic activity, including other alkyl testosterone derivatives[27,28], the progestagens levonorgestrel and norethisterone acetate[29,30], the anabolic steroids stanozolol and oxandrolone[31,32] and the impeded androgen danazol[33]. When HDL subfractions were measured, it was primarily in the HDL_2 subfraction that the fall in HDL cholesterol occurred. The distinct effects on HDL_2 cholesterol of gonadal steroids with varying androgenic side effects is exemplified in our recent study in which the effects of seven different combined oral contraceptive formulations were compared[34]. These contained either levonorgestrel, norethindrone or desogestrel as progestagen, combined with a similar dose of ethinyl oestradiol in each formulation. The order of androgenicity of these progestagens is levonorgestrel > norethindrone > desogestrel. Levonorgestrel and norethindrone-containing oral contraceptives were each studied at three different progestagen doses. The percentage differences between mean values for HDL_2 cholesterol in each oral contraceptive group and a group of non-users are shown in Figure 2. The extent of the reduction in HDL_2 was proportional to the progestagen dose and was closely related to the degree of androgenicity.

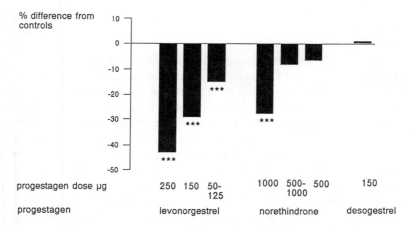

Figure 2 Percentage differences from non-user controls for HDL_2 cholesterol in groups of women taking combined oral contraceptives containing similar doses of ethinyl oestradiol combined with varying doses of the progestins levonorgestrel, norethindrone or desogestrel. Adapted from Godsland *et al.*, *N. Engl. J. Med.*, **323**:1375. Significant differences from controls: ***, $p < 0.001$

Orally administered alkylated androgens can have marked effects on the liver, associated with the hepatic first-pass effect, and it is possible that some of their effects on serum lipoprotein concentrations may be secondary to these hepatic effects[27].

17β-oestradiol

17β-oestradiol, administered orally, in micronized form or as oestradiol valerate, lowers LDL cholesterol and raises HDL cholesterol[35,36], principally in the HDL_2 subfraction[37]. However, when given parenterally, lipoprotein changes induced by oestradiol are more equivocal, and may depend on the route of administration. Administration of oestradiol as subdermal implants raises HDL cholesterol[38,39], whereas the predominant effect of transdermal administration appears to be to lower LDL cholesterol[40]. Intramuscular and percutaneous administration of oestradiol do not appear to affect LDL or HDL cholesterol[37,41,42]. Differences in potency may underly any discrepancies found between the effects of synthetic oestrogens and the natural hormones since, in experimental studies of the effects of oestrogens at the tissue level, ethinyl oestradiol has been shown to be approximately 100 times more potent than oestradiol[43].

Testosterone

Testosterone, administered by intramuscular injection as testosterone enanthate, generally lowers HDL cholesterol concentrations[44-48]. There is some evidence that LDL cholesterol can be raised by administration of testosterone[49,50], although most studies have found no effect or even a decrease.

The weight of evidence from studies of the effects on serum lipoproteins of exogenously administered gonadal steroids and sex hormones suggests that oestrogenic activity is associated with high levels of HDL cholesterol and low levels of LDL cholesterol, and androgenic activity is associated with the converse pattern. These associations are most apparent in studies of exogenously administered gonadal steroids. Changes with sex hormones are somewhat less well-defined, although generally consistent with the findings with gonadal steroids. Among studies of synthetic gonadal steroids there are, however, some striking inconsistencies. Higano *et al.* (1959) compared the effects of methyl testosterone and another anabolic testosterone derivative with markedly reduced androgenic activity. The latter compound caused the lipoprotein changes typical of methyl testosterone, but to a greater degree[51]. Wynn *et al.* (1986) studied the anti-androgen, cyproterone acetate[7]. As would be expected with an anti-androgen, LDL cholesterol concentrations fell on treatment. However, HDL_2 cholesterol concentrations also fell substantially. Thus there is some uncertainty whether the considerable amount of evidence from studies of exogenously administered gonadal steroids is relevant to the hypothesis that differences between men and women in sex hormone concentrations could contribute to differences in lipoprotein concentrations and the gender difference in coronary heart disease mortality.

Endogenous sex hormone levels and lipid and lipoprotein concentrations

If the gender difference in lipoprotein concentrations is a consequence of differences in sex hormone concentrations, it might be expected that plasma oestradiol concentrations would correlate positively with HDL and negatively with LDL concentrations. The converse relationships would be expected with plasma testosterone. Furthermore it would be expected that changing gonadal status would be associated with changes in lipoprotein concentrations. Thus, at puberty HDL concentrations would rise in girls and LDL concentrations would fall, the converse being the case in boys. During the menopause it would be expected that HDL concentrations in women would fall and LDL concentrations rise.

Correlations between plasma sex hormone concentrations and lipoproteins

Relationships between oestradiol and lipoprotein concentrations have been the subject of only very few studies. In premenopausal women either a weak positive[52] or no correlation[53] has been reported between total oestradiol and HDL cholesterol concentrations. In men free oestradiol has been found to correlate inversely with HDL cholesterol concentrations[54].

In a number of studies of the relationship between testosterone and lipoprotein concentrations in men, the most consistent finding has been a positive correlation between total testosterone and HDL cholesterol[5], and this is also seen with free testosterone[54,55]. There are no consistent findings regarding relationships between testosterone and LDL cholesterol concentrations.

Changes in lipoprotein concentrations at puberty

HDL cholesterol concentrations in males appear to fall during adolescence[56,57], whereas little change is seen in LDL cholesterol. No consistent changes are seen in females. The fall in HDL cholesterol concentrations in males correlates with sexual maturity[58,59], and a positive correlation between LDL cholesterol concentrations and maturity has been observed[59].

Changes in lipoprotein concentrations during the menopause

Although a number of studies have compared lipid and lipoprotein concentrations in pre- and postmenopausal women, there are very few that have not been subject to confounding effects that are independent of the menopause. Lipoprotein concentrations change with age, so any differences between pre- and postmenopausal women could be merely the result of ageing. On the other hand, if age-matched pre- and postmenopausal women are compared, then the groups may not be strictly comparable, since women in the postmenopausal group will have undergone the menopause at an earlier age than women in the premenopausal group. Furthermore, in the studies that have been carried out, menopausal status has rarely been adequately determined, or menopausal age taken into account.

Matthews *et al.* followed a cohort of women through the menopausal years and compared 65 women who underwent the menopause with age-matched women who remained premenopausal[60]. HDL cholesterol fell in the women who underwent the menopause. There was a rise in LDL cholesterol in women

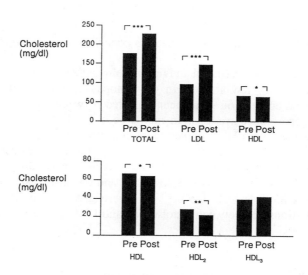

Figure 3 Total, LDL, HDL, HDL$_2$ and HDL$_3$ cholesterol concentrations in 395 premenopausal and 158 postmenopausal women. Adapted from: Stevenson *et al.* In Christiansen, C. and Overgaard, K. *Osteoporosis 1990*, pp. 1826. (Copenhagen: Osteopress ApS). Significant differences: *** $p < 0.001$, ** $p < 0.01$, ** $p < 0.05$

who remained premenopausal, but there was a greater rise in women who underwent the menopause. In our recent cross-sectional study of 553 healthy women, menopausal status was determined by measurement of gonadotropin levels, and age and body mass index were taken into account in the statistical analysis[61]. Postmenopausal women had higher LDL cholesterol and lower HDL cholesterol concentrations, and the difference in HDL cholesterol concentrations was entirely accounted for by a difference in HDL_2 cholesterol (Figure 3).

Discussion

Although changes in other lipids and lipoproteins have been reported in response to gonadal steroids and sex hormones, it is HDL and LDL that appear to be the most consistently affected. Despite some discrepancies, exogenously administered gonadal steroids, or sex hormones, with oestrogenic activity generally increase HDL cholesterol, and those with androgenic activity reduce HDL cholesterol. Converse changes are generally seen in LDL cholesterol, although they may be less clearly defined, particularly with administered sex hormones. Studies of gender differences in HDL and LDL are consistent with these observations. Changes in lipoprotein concentrations accompanying the menopause are also consistent, as are changes in males undergoing puberty. However, the expected changes in adolescent females are not seen, and in mature individuals the correlations seen between plasma sex hormone concentrations and lipoproteins are the inverse of what would be expected. A further qualification to observations supporting the hypothesis that differences in sex hormone concentrations are responsible for gender differences in lipoproteins is that these differences are not seen in men and women from non-Western, non-industrialized countries in which cardiovascular disease rates may be very low[5]. Furthermore, in studies of changes accompanying puberty in these societies, the fall in HDL cholesterol in males may be relatively small[62–64]. In the study of adolescent boys by Laskarzewski *et al*.[65] it was concluded that the fall in HDL cholesterol concentrations at puberty could be best accounted for by a combination of oestradiol and testosterone concentrations and adiposity, suggesting that factors other than sex hormone concentrations, for example, calorie intake, could contribute to the changes at puberty[65]. This is supported by the lack of effect of puberty seen in societies with a low cardiovascular disease incidence, and by the observation that among different ethnic groups in a Western-type society the fall in HDL at puberty is most apparent in white males[59].

In conclusion, gender differences in lipoprotein concentrations do appear to contribute to the gender difference in cardiovascular disease, and changes in endogenous sex hormone concentrations at puberty and the menopause may contribute to the gender difference in lipoprotein concentrations. However, an interaction with some other factor present in Western-type societies with a high incidence of cardiovascular disease must be invoked to account for the observed changes. Diet is a possibility, but this area remains virtually unexplored.

References

1. Uemura, K. and Pisa, Z. (1985). Recent trends in cardiovascular mortality in 27 industrialised countries. *World Hlth Stat. Q.*, **38**, 142–62
2. Gordon, T., Castelli, W., Hjortland, M., Kannel, W. and Dawber, T. (1977). High density lipoprotein as a protective factor against coronary heart disease. The Framingham study. *Am. J. Med.*, **62**, 707–14
3. Kannel, W. (1978). Hypertension, blood lipids and cigarette smoking as co-risk factors for coronary heart disease. *Ann. N.Y. Acad. Sci.*, **304**, 128
4. Friedman, G., Dales, L. and Ury, H. (1979). Mortality in middle aged smokers and non-smokers. *N. Engl. J. Med.*, **300**, 213–17
5. Godsland, I., Wynn, V., Crook, D. and Miller, N. (1987). Sex, plasma lipoproteins, and atherosclerosis: prevailing assumptions and outstanding questions. *Am. Heart J.*, **114**, 1467–503
6. Crook, D. (1989). Laboratory evaluation of lipid risk factors. *Int. Proc. J.*, **1**, 107–12
7. Wynn, V., Godsland, I., Seed, M. and Jacobs, H. (1986). Paradoxical effects of the antiandrogen, cyproterone acetate, on lipid and lipoprotein metabolism. *Clin. Endocrinol.*, **24**, 183–91
8. Carlson, L. and Ericsson, M. (1975). Quantitative and qualitative serum lipoprotein analysis. Part I. Studies in healthy men and women. *Atherosclerosis*, **21**, 417–33
9. Rifkind, B., Tamir, I., Heiss, G., Wallace, R. and Tyroler, H. (1979). Distribution of high density and other lipoproteins in selected LRC Prevalence Study populations. *Lipids*, **14**, 105–12
10. Wahl, P., Warnick, G., Albers, J. *et al.* (1981). Distribution of lipoprotein triglyceride and lipoprotein cholesterol in an adult population by age, sex and hormone use. *Atherosclerosis*, **39**, 111–24.
11. Barclay, M., Barclay, R. and Skipsi, V. (1967). High density lipoprotein concentrations in men and women. *Nature*, **200**, 362–3
12. Nichols, A. (1967). Human serum lipoproteins and their interrelationships. *Adv. Biol. Med. Phys.*, **11**, 109–58
13. Anderson, D., Nichols, A., Forte, T. and Lindgren, F. (1977). Particle distribution of human serum high density lipoproteins. *Biochim. Biophys. Acta*, **493**, 55–68
14. Avins, A., Haber, R. and Hulley, S. (1989). The status of hypertriglyceridemia as a risk factor for coronary heart disease. *Clin. Lab. Med.*, **9**, 153–68
15. Kannel, W. (1987). Metabolic risk factors for coronary heart disease in women: perspective from the Framingham Study. *Am. Heart J.*, **114**, 413–19
16. Barr, D., Russ, E. and Eder, H. (1952). Influence of estrogens on lipoproteins in atherosclerosis. *Trans. Assoc. Am. Physicians*, **65**, 102–11

17. Furman, R., Howard, R., Norcia, L. and Keaty, E. (1958). The influence of androgens, estrogens and related steroids on serum lipids and lipoproteins. *Am. J. Med.*, **24**, 80–97

18. Farish, E., Fletcher, C., Hart, D., Teo, C., Alazzawi, F. and Howie, C. (1986). The effects of conjugated equine estrogens with and without a cyclical progestagen on lipoproteins and HDL subfractions in postmenopausal women. *Acta Endocrinol.*, **113**, 123–7

19. Goldzieher, J., Chenault, C., de la Pena, A., Dozier, T. and Kraemer, D. (1978). Comparative studies of the ethinyl estrogens used in oral contraceptives. VII. Effects with and without progestational agents on ultracentrifugally fractionated plasma lipoproteins in humans, baboons and beagles. *Fertil. Steril.*, **30**, 522–33

20. Schaefer, E., Foster, D., Zech, L., Lindgren, F., Brewer Jr., H. and Levy, R. (1983). The effects of estrogen administration on plasma lipoprotein metabolism in premenopausal females. *Clin. Endocrinol. Metab.*, **57**, 262–7

21. Crook, D. and Seed, M. (1990). Endocrine control of plasma lipoprotein metabolism: effects of gonadal steroids. *Bailliere's Clin. Endocrinol. Metab.*, **4**, 851–75

22. Goebelsmann, U., Maschchak, C. and Mishell, D. (1985). Comparison of hepatic impact of oral and vaginal administration of ethinyl estradiol. *Am. J. Obstet. Gynecol.*, **151**, 868–77

23. Applebaum-Bowden, D., McLean, P., Steinmerz, A. *et al.* (1989). Lipoprotein, apolipoprotein, and lipolytic enzyme changes following estrogen administration in postmenopausal women. *J. Lipid Res.*, **30**, 1895–906

24. Barr, D. (1953). Some factors in the pathogenesis of atherosclerosis. *Circulation*, **8**, 641–54

25. Russ, E., Eder, H. and Barr, D. (1955). Influence of gonadal hormones on protein-lipid relationships in human plasma. *Am. J. Med.*, **19**, 4–24

26. Oliver, M. and Boyd, G. (1956). Endocrine aspects of coronary sclerosis. *Lancet*, **2**, 1273–6

27. Furman, R., Conrad, L. and Howard, R. (1954). A serum lipoprotein pattern characteristic of biliary obstruction with some comments on jaundice due to methyl testosterone. *Circulation*, **10**, 586

28. Furman, R., Howard, R., Smith, C. and Norcia, L. (1956). Comparison of the effects of oral methyltestosterone, 19-nortestosterone and 17-methyl-19-nortestosterone on serum lipids and lipoproteins. *J. Lab. Clin. Med.*, **48**, 808–9

29. Silfverstolpe, G., Gustafson, A., Samsioe, G. and Svanborg, A. (1979). Lipid metabolic studies in oophorectomized women. *Acta Obstet. Gynecol. Scand.* (Suppl.), **88**, 89–95

30. Tikkanen, M., Nikkilä, E., Kuusi, T. and Sipinen, S. (1981). Reduction of plasma high-density lipoprotein 2 cholesterol and increase of postheparin plasma hepatic lipase activity during progestin treatment. *Clin. Chim Acta*, **115**, 63–71

31. Taggart, H., Applebaum-Bowden, D., Haffner, S. *et al.* (1982). Reduction in high density lipoproteins by anabolic steroid (stanozolol) therapy for post-menopausal osteoporosis. *Metabolism*, **31**, 1147–52

32. Cheung, M., Albers, J. and Wahl, P. High density lipoproteins during hypolipidemic therapy: a comparative study of four drugs. *Atherosclerosis*, **35**, 215–28

33. Crook, D., Gardner, R., Worthington, M., Nolan, J., Stevenson, J. and Shaw, R. (1989). Zoladex versus danazol in the treatment of pelvic endometriosis: effects on plasma lipid risk factors. *Horm. Res.*, **32** (Suppl 1), 157–60

34. Godsland, I., Crook, D., Simpson, R. *et al.* (1990). The effects of different formulations of oral contraceptive agents on lipid and carbohydrate metabolism. *N. Engl. J. Med.*, **323**, 1375–81

35. Tikkanen, M., Nikkilä, E. and Vartiainen, E. (1978). Natural oestrogen as an effective treatment for type II hyperlipoproteinaemia in postmenopausal women. *Lancet*, **2**, 490–2

36. Enk, L., Crona, N., Samsioe, G. and Silfverstolpe, G. (1986). Dose and duration effects of estradiol valerate on serum and lipoprotein lipids. *Horm. Metab., Res.*, **18**, 551–4

37. Fahreus, L. and Wallentin, L. (1983). High density lipoprotein subfractions during oral and cutaneous administration of 17β-estradiol to menopausal women. *Clin. Endocrinol. Metab.*, **56**, 797–801

38. Farish, E., Fletcher, C., Hart, D., Al Azzawi, F., Abdalla, H. and Gray, C. (1984). The effects of hormone implants on serum lipoproteins and steroid hormones in bilaterally oophorectomised women. *Acta Endocrinol.*, **106**, 116–20

39. Crook, D., Montgomery, J., Godsland, I. *et al.* (1991). Lipid and carbohydrate metabolism in premenopausal women given subdermal estradiol pellets. *Horm. Metab. Res.*, **23**, 174–7

40. Crook, D., Cust, M., Gangar, K. *et al.* (1990). Transdermal administration of oestrogen/progestogen: effects on lipid risk markers. *Sixth International Congress on the Menopause: Abstracts 1990*; abstract 186

41. Buckman, M., Johnson, J., Ellis, H., Srivastava, L. and Peake, G. (1980). Differential lipemic and proteinemic response to oral ethinyl estradiol and parenteral estradiol cypionate. *Metabolism*, **29**, 803–5

42. DeLignieres, B., Basdevant, A., Thomas, G. *et al.* (1986). Biological effects of estradiol-17β in postmenopausal women: oral versus percutaneous administration. *J. Clin. Endocrinol. Metab.*, **62**, 536–41

43. Dickson, R. and Eisenfeld, A. (1981). 17-alpha ethinyl estradiol is more potent than estradiol in receptor interactions with isolated hepatic parenchymal cells. *Endocrinology*, **108**, 1511–18

44. Webb, O., Laskarzewski, P. and Glueck, C. (1984). Severe depression of high-density lipoprotein cholesterol levels in weight lifters and body builders by self-administered exogenous testosterone, and anabolic-androgenic steroids. *Metabolism*, **33**, 971–5

45. Hinkel, G., Hanefeld, M., Jaross, W., Leonhardt, W. and Trübsbach, A. (1985). Effects of high doses of oestrogens and androgens on lipoproteins: observations in the treatment of excessive growth with sexual hormones. *Exp. Clin. Endocrinol.*, **86**, 17–25

46. Kirkland, R., Keenan, B., Probstfield, J. *et al.* (1987). Decrease in plasma high-density lipoprotein cholesterol levels at puberty in boys with delayed adolescence. *J. Am. Med. Assoc.*, **257**, 502–7

47. Sorva, R., Kuusi, T., Taskinen, M-R., Perheentupa, J. and Nikkilä, E. (1988). Testosterone substitution increases the activity of lipoprotein lipase and hepatic lipase in hypogonadal males. *Atherosclerosis*, **69**, 191–7

48. Thompson, P., Cullinane, E., Sady, S. *et al.* (1989). Contrasting effects of testosterone and stanozolol on serum lipoprotein levels. *J. Am. Med. Assoc.*, **261**, 1165–8

49. ffrench-Constant, C., Spengel, F. and Thompson, G. (1985). Hyperlipidaemia and premature coronary artery disease associated with sex change in a female. *Postgrad. Med. J.*, **61**, 61–3
50. Jones, D., Higgins, B., Billet, J. *et al.* (1989). The effects of testosterone replacement on plasma lipids and apolipoproteins. *Eur. J. Clin. Invest.*, **19**, 438–41
51. Higano, N., Cohen, W. and Robinson, R. (1959). Effects of sex steroids on lipids. *Ann. N.Y. Acad. Sci.*, **72**, 970–9
52. Maserai, J., Armstrong, B., Skinner, M. *et al.* (1980). HDL-cholesterol and sex hormone status. *Lancet*, **1**, 208
53. Haffner, S., Katz, M., Stern, M. and Dunn, J. (1989). Association of decreased sex hormone binding globulin and cardiovascular risk factors. *Arteriosclerosis*, **9**, 136–43
54. Hamalainen, E., Adlercreutz, H., Enholm, C. and Puska, P. (1986). Relationships of serum lipoproteins and apoproteins to sex hormones and to the binding capacity of sex hormone binding globulin in healthy Finnish men. *Metabolism*, **35**, 535–41
55. Semmens, J., Rouse, I., Beilen, L. and Masarei, J. (1982). Sex hormone levels as determinants of HDL-cholesterol levels [abstract]. *Eur. J. Clin. Invest.*, **12**, Abstr. 39
56. Morrison, J., deGroot, I., Edward, B. *et al.* (1978). Lipid and lipoproteins in 967 schoolchildren age 6–17 years. *Pediatrics*, **62**, 990–5
57. Beaglehole, R., Trost, D., Tamir, I. *et al.* (1980). Plasma high-density lipoprotein cholesterol in children and young adults. The Lipid Research Clinics Program Prevalence Study. *Circulation*, **62** (Suppl. IV), 83–92
58. Orchard, T., Rodgers, M., Hedley, A. and Mitchell, J. (1980). Changes in blood lipids and blood pressure during adolescence. *Br. Med. J.*, **280**, 1563–7
59. Berenson, G., Srinivasan, S., Cresanta, J., Foster, T. and Weber, L. (1981). Dynamic changes in serum lipoproteins in children during adolescence and sexual maturation. *Am. J. Epidemiol.*, **113**, 157–70
60. Matthews, K., Meilahn, E., Kuller, L., Kelsey, S., Caggiula, A. and Wing, R. (1989). Menopause and risk factors for coronary heart disease. *N. Engl. J. Med.*, **321**, 641–6
61. Stevenson, J., Crook, D. and Godsland, I. (1990). Effects of age and menopause on lipid metabolism. In Christiansen, C. and Overgaard, K. (eds.) *Osteoporosis 1990*, pp. 1826–8. (Copenhagen: Osteopress ApS)
62. Walker, A. and Walker, B. (1978). High density lipoprotein cholesterol in African children and adults in a population free of coronary heart disease. *Br. Med. J.*, **2**, 1336–7
63. Miller, G. and Gilson, R. (1981). Similarity in males and females of HDL2 and HDL3 cholesterol concentration in a Caribbean rural community. *Atherosclerosis*, **40**, 75–80
64. Mendoza, S., Nucete, H., Zerpa, A. *et al.* (1980). Lipids and lipoproteins in 13–18 year old Venezuelan and American schoolchildren. *Atherosclerosis*, **37**, 219–29
65. Laskarzewski, P., Morrison, J., Gutai, J., Orchard, T., Khoury, P. and Glueck, C. (1983). High and low density lipoprotein cholesterol in adolescent boys: relationships with endogenous testosterone, estradiol and Quetelet index. *Metabolism*, **32**, 262–71

Discussion

Dr Parsons: Hormones that I did not see mentioned were prolactin and the hormones of pregnancy. For example, breast feeding raises plasma prolactin levels and what effect would this have on plasma lipoprotein cholesterol levels? I ask this question for a mother who was 3 days postpartum and breast feeding and she asked me when she should have her cholesterol rechecked as her cholesterol was 8 mmol/l in the 6th month of pregnancy.

Dr Godsland: There is normally quite a substantial rise in LDL cholesterol and apo B during pregnancy, which levels off during the last 2–3 months and returns to normal after the birth, so it is possible that the elevated cholesterol in this woman was a rather extreme example of this phenomenon. I do not know of any work on the effects of prolactin on LDL and cholesterol concentrations. With regard to the effects of pregnancy on other lipids and lipoproteins, there is a rise in HDL cholesterol that parallels the rise in LDL cholesterol and also a rise in serum triglycerides.

Dr Connor: With regard to the gender differences in CHD, there is a population in the United States, the Chicago blacks, in which the women seem to have an even higher rate of CHD than the men. These are menstruating women. In fact, they have about the highest rate in our country and I wonder if you have any explanation for that?

Dr Godsland: I have no explanation for the excessive rate. Certainly in American blacks there is some evidence for there being little difference in HDL cholesterol concentrations between men and women. The Bogulusa Heart Study studied paralleled groups of black and white children and did not see the kind of reduction in HDL cholesterol concentrations in the black children as they saw in the white children.

Dr Roncari: Let me comment on the previous point. Prolactin is interesting actually because it inhibits adipose tissue lipoprotein lipase and enhances mammary lipoprotein lipase. Triglycerides do rise and fuel is shunted from the periphery to the mammary gland where it is needed. So, actually there are some increases in VLDL and triglyceride.

Dr Godsland: On that subject, there is also mobilization of lower segment fat as opposed to central fat during lactation which is another confounding factor in these changes during pregnancy.

Dr Vega: If we could follow up on the question about the relationship between triglyceride and HDL a little bit, is there any increase in the triglyceride levels in postmenopausal women compared to premenopausal women? If there is an increase in the triglyceride, is there a reciprocal relationship between the triglyceride levels and HDL_2 subfraction?

Dr Godsland: In our own studies we have found increased triglyceride and reduced HDL_2 cholesterol concentrations in postmenopausal women and this was independent of age and body mass index. There are a number of conflicting reports in the literature regarding the effects of menopause on lipid and lipoprotein levels, possible reasons being the confounding effect of age on lipid metabolism and inaccuracies in the assignment of menopausal status.

Dr Parsons: Athletes persist in using anabolic steroids. Could you comment on the likelihood of an elevated LDL cholesterol and what work has been done on that?

Dr Godsland: A lot of work has been done on anabolic steroids and lipoprotein concentrations. The anabolic steroids are really considered under the androgenic steroid subhead and they are probably among the most potent elevators of LDL and reducers of HDL cholesterol. There are a few anecdotal accounts of premature coronary heart disease in anabolic steroid users but there has not been anything like a controlled trial; individual case reports are really all we have at the moment.

20
Children's health and the cholesterol/fat issue

R.B. GOLDBLOOM

Let me begin by professing my bias concerning this and other issues of disease prevention. After 15 years of working alongside people concerned with disease prevention, I have become deeply committed to the methodological principles elaborated and adopted by the Canadian Task Force on the Periodic Health Examination and the US Preventive Services Task Force. These principles require that in making recommendations for preventive health care, scientific evidence should take precedence over consensus and that the strength of that evidence be graded according to the quality of the studies on which it is based. When such a methodology is used to formulate recommendations there is little place for concepts that say, in effect: 'Well, it *probably* will do no harm and we think it *may* do some good'. Admittedly, the rigorous viewpoint of the Canadian and US Task Forces is not universally accepted. In 1984, Wynder and Berenson[1] editorialized in *Preventive Medicine* on 'Preventive Strategies for Reducing Hyperlipidaemias in Childhood'. They stated that a passive decision was ill-advised and that 'recommendations for action are needed *before* all the data are complete and success is guaranteed'. Among other recommendations, they advised that childrens' energy intake from fat be reduced to 25–30% of total calories and that routine school health exams be expanded to include periodic determination of blood lipids. Finally, they suggested (without presenting supportive evidence) that these and other measures would result in a major reduction in health care costs.

In discussing the paediatric aspects of the fat and cholesterol issues, we must draw a clear distinction between the management of individual ostensibly healthy patients in clinical encounters, management of those already identified to be at high risk, and recommendations directed broadside at the entire population. The situations have vastly different risk: benefit characteristics and cost implications. Our terms of reference must be very clear.

It is accepted that reduction of LDL-C levels in *adult men* (by whatever means) is associated with a reduction in coronary heart disease (CHD) morbidity (though a reduction in all-cause mortality has yet to be demonstrated and there have been worrisome increases in mortality due to other causes). It has also been demonstrated that serum lipid and lipoprotein levels have some tendency to track from childhood to adulthood – though, as we shall see, this tendency is not all that strong, and is of more statistical than clinical significance.

Let's consider the issue of serum cholesterol screening in unselected children. The first criterion for widespread adoption of *any* screening method to detect pre-symptomatic disease is that it must be demonstrated in well-designed, properly controlled trials that the screening method in question has a high level of sensitivity and specificity; second, that early detection improves outcome; and third, that in actual practice, detection by screening leads to treatment which has been demonstrated to do more good than harm. (The last two conditions are the ones most regularly forgotten or simply brushed aside). Have these criteria been met in the case of screening children for elevated serum cholesterol levels?

In 1990, Dennison and associates[2] published their analysis of serum cholesterol screening of 2857 children and adolescents in the Bogalusa Heart Study. Using age, race and sex-specific 95th percentile cut-offs, they found that only 44–50% of subjects with elevated LDL-C levels were detected. Using the 75th percentile as the cut-off they found an unacceptably high percentage of false positives (81–84%). They concluded that 'the poor test characteristics make serum total cholesterol measurement inefficient as a screening tool for detecting elevated levels of LDL-C in children and adolescents'.

In the Muscatine Study, Lauer and Clarke[3] reviewed over 2000 boys and girls examined and followed to ages 20–30 years. Among children with serum cholesterol levels over the 75th percentile on two occasions, 75% of girls and 50% of boys would not qualify for intervention by the National Cholesterol Education Program (NCEP) criteria. Using values over the 90th percentile on two occasions, 57% of girls and 30% of boys would still not qualify. A single childhood measurement produced a large number of false positives. These findings underline the maxim known to all paediatricians but often forgotten by others, that children are not simply miniature adults.

Results such as I have quoted are hardly calculated to inspire confidence in serum cholesterol screening in unselected children or child populations. When you superimpose the inescapable variables that are added to the equation when such a screening procedure is implemented widely e.g. nationally, involving multiple laboratories and innumerable physicians, the pre-existing errors are compounded and new ones added. Thus a survey of 71 cholesterol screening programs in 50 states and D.C. demonstrated frequent unsanitary conditions as well as poorly calibrated and poorly maintained equipment. In addition, most patients with serum cholesterol levels over 200 mg/dl were not told to see their doctor[4].

It is unsafe to assume that results achieved in a controlled experimental situation will be replicated in the hurly-burly of clinical practice or in public health applications. Within the last 2 months Lannon and Earp reported on the effects of screening children for high serum cholesterol in a middle-class, well-educated population in Chapel Hill, NC[5]. Of 440 children screened, 134 (30%) had levels above the recommended cut-point of 175 mg/dl (75th percentile). Parents were notified of the results and encouraged to comply with AAP guidelines. Only 64 children (48%) returned for follow-up. One-third of parents felt that 'confirmation of an elevated cholesterol would make the child worry too much'. Only 29 of 101 parents of children with high levels talked to a dietitian. If these results reflect the realities of experience with middle-class, well-educated families, what can we expect of less fortunate families in lower socio-economic groups whose children may be at above average risk?

Newman and colleagues[6] have proposed that three criteria must be met to justify serum cholesterol screening in childhood:

1. Measurement of blood cholesterol must allow identification of children at substantially increased risk of CHD.

2. Interventions to reduce the risk (of CHD) must be more effective when begun in childhood.

3. Cholesterol screening and intervention in childhood can be accomplished with little risk to the child.

Reviewing the evidence, they conclude that since these three criteria have not been met, and that since the benefits of cholesterol screening are unlikely to exceed the risks, children should not be screened for high cholesterol levels. Finally, the weak predictive power of serum cholesterol levels for coronary heart disease in individual subjects adds a further note of caution in considering widespread screening.

Cost issues in cholesterol screening

Shrinking monetary resources for health care require that the cost implications of *every* proposed preventive intervention be considered comprehensively and seriously before recommending or implementing public health policy. Such evaluations must never be limited to the health and financial burdens imposed by the target disease under scrutiny. As Louise Russell has pointed out[7] most preventive interventions represent add-on costs that exceed considerably the moneys saved by reductions in the mortality and morbidity of the target condition. In the case of screening for hypercholesterolaemia, Stephen Grover and associates[8] at McGill University recently estimated the cost of screening

335

all Canadians aged 30 years or more at between $432 million and $561 million for the first year. They questioned whether the potential benefits would offset such costs in an already overburdened health care system.

Needless to say, these views are not shared universally and there are those who continue to recommend universal serum cholesterol screening for children over 2 years of age.

What about the question of selective screening of children for hyperlipidaemia, based on pre-screening for a positive family history of premature coronary artery disease? Three recent studies have shown that, using a positive family history as the criterion, about 50% of children with high LDL levels will be missed. It can be argued, with some justification, that detecting even half of such children may be a worthwhile exercise, though we have little knowledge of the long-term benefits or undesirable side-effects of early detection and lifetime treatment of affected youngsters. Certainly such children need to be managed in well-supervised circumstances with careful ongoing evaluation of all aspects of possible benefit or harm.

The next issue is whether the diets of otherwise healthy, growing children should be modified and if so, by how much, so as to reduce the dietary intake of total fat, saturated fat and cholesterol. I can tell you at the outset that, following a lengthy review of the scientific evidence, the Canadian Task Force on the Periodic Health Examination concluded that for adult males aged 30–69 years there was *fair* evidence to include in the periodic health exam dietary advice on lowering intake of total fat to <30% of total calories and cholesterol to <300mg/day. At the same time, the Task Force concluded that there was *poor* evidence to support inclusion or exclusion of such advice for children, young men, elderly men and women of all ages.

The average North American diet is reported to have a fat content exceeding 40% of total calories and over 500 mg of cholesterol per day, though a recent study[9] of Texas schoolchildren showed an average total fat intake of 35.6% of total calories with 13.4% as saturated fat and 6.6% polyunsaturated. Seventeen percent consumed <30% of all calories from fat, while 34% consumed ≥38%. Thus, at least in this study, many children had intakes at or near currently recommended guidelines.

There is good evidence that blood lipids can be lowered by dietary manipulation in well-controlled settings, but the situation in free-living populations may be quite different. Further, the long-term safety of dietary changes currently recommended is unknown, especially where growing children are concerned.

Dr Fima Lifshitz[10] has documented significant growth retardation and/or delay of puberty in children, resulting from overzealous dietary control aimed at long-term prevention of coronary heart disease. In Manhasset, NY, he also found that 38% of high school students were currently dieting to lose weight and 72% had made serious efforts to diet in recent months. He expressed

concern that many individuals or groups who have made dietary recommendations for North Americans do not differentiate between adults and children,
since they recommend the same dietary pattern for everyone over the age of 2.
Predictably, some parents will decide that if some reduction in fat is good then
greater reduction will be even better.

The selection of a single figure, such as 30% of total calories as the
appropriate upper limit of intake for all children may end up doing more harm
than good, and suggests a level of precision that is not supported by adequate
scientific information. It does not take into account the well documented wide
variation in individual children's energy needs for growth, activity, learning
and development, or the potential economic impact of such dietary recommendations on poorer segments of our population. Children whose fat intake
is restricted have to make up the difference in their energy needs from complex
carbohydrate foods that tend to be filling. Also lean meat costs more than meat
with the usual fat content.

It may be much easier to *plan* a low fat diet that meets childrens' energy
requirements than to get them to eat it. The argument has been made, with
some logic, that if we are to change the dietary habits of the general population
the eating habits of the entire family, including the children, must be changed.
However, longitudinal studies designed to lower serum cholesterol in children
by dietary means have given conflicting results. Walter and colleagues[11]
studied 3388 children in 37 schools in the Bronx and Westchester County,
NY. Schools in both areas were randomly assigned to receive a teacher-
delivered curriculum that focused on diet, exercise and smoking, or to serve
as non-intervention controls. After 5 years, the net change in plasma levels of
total cholesterol (i.e. between treated and controls) was −1.7 mg/dl in Westchester County and −1.0 mg/dl in the Bronx. Although both trends were
favourable, only the change in Westchester County schools achieved statistical
significance. The program had no detectable effects on body mass, physical
fitness or blood pressure.

Plasma cholesterol fell somewhat in both intervention and non-intervention
groups, but even in the intervention groups the mean decline was only
−2.1 ± 1.0 mg/dl. The authors note that in the two other published school-
based studies (both from Europe) net mean reductions in plasma ranged from
only 2 to 4%, whereas substantial reductions in smoking were effected.
Although the authors seem to have taken some encouragement from the
Westchester/Bronx findings, the results can hardly be regarded as spectacular.
Dr Susan Harris, Director of the Human Nutrition Institute in Washington has
pointed out that in prescribing dietary guidelines for any national childhood
population, several practical issues must be taken into account[12]. First, if the
fat content of the diet is successfully reduced below its current level, families
will need to buy more food to maintain the same energy intake. Second, diets
that are promoted as 'nutritious' can be rather boring from a child's viewpoint.

Third, the emphasis on *fresh* fruit and vegetables may also do a disservice to the many families in our populations that have a low family income, since following this advice raises the cost of their food. Finally, there are serious concerns that any reduction of children's fat intake below 30% of total calories may carry a significant risk of deficiency in other nutrients and/or failure to meet children's energy requirments.

The recommendations proposed by various authoritative bodies for the population at large may also fail to allow for individual variations in nutritional requirements. Birch *et al*.[13] recently documented normal intakes varying from 1100 to 1800 kcal/day (4600–7530 kJ) in a group of pre-schoolers.

Even in adult patients with suspected or proven coronary heart disease, the observed rate of treatment is low. Cohen *et al*.[14] evaluated 95 patients admitted for chest pain and investigated with coronary angiography at Montefiore Medical Center. 1–2 years after the initial investigation only 17% of those with hypercholesterolaemia or low LDL-C were being actively treated with diet or drugs. The experience was similar in patients 1–2 years post-bypass. However the proportion under such treatment rose to 35% 2 years later.

Dr Neil Holtzman[15] of Johns Hopkins University in a recent commentary that bears the catchy title 'The Great God Cholesterol' discusses proposed paediatric interventions that are designed to prevent coronary artery disease. He rejects universal serum cholesterol screening for reasons presented earlier, pointing out that even among children whose elevated serum cholesterol levels will persist, the vast majority will never manifest coronary artery disease. He also expresses concern about telling children that if they do not adhere to a certain regimen they are at risk of dying, and quotes a study in which only 2% of children with elevated cholesterol levels who were given dietary advice actually maintained dietary change at follow-up.

In its 1986 statement on Dietary Fat and Cholesterol in Children, the American Academy of Pediatrics[16] reiterated its concern that any recommendations for dietary patterns more restrictive than 30–40% of total energy intake from fat should await demonstration that such restrictions would support adequate growth and development for children and adolescents. Based on reading the relevant literature, such evidence has yet to be presented, and there is some evidence of undesirable outcomes of over-zealous restriction. In my view, the Academy wisely suggested a range of intakes rather than a level which none should exceed. In doing so, they documented their respect for individuality and the glory of normal human variation – a respect that all of us should continue to emulate.

References

1. Wynder, E.L. and Berenson, G.S. (1984). Preventive strategies for reducing hyperlipidemias in childhood (Editorial). *Prev. Med.*, **13**, 327-9
2. Dennison, B.A. *et al.* (1990). Serum total cholesterol screening for the detection of elevated LDL in children and adolescents: The Bogalusa Heart Study. *Pediatrics*, **85**, 472-9
3. Lauer, R.M. and Clarke, W.R. (1990). Use of cholesterol measurements in childhood for the prediction of adult hypercholesterolemia. The Muscative Study. *J. Am. Med. Assoc.*, 3034-8
4. Loupe, D.E. (1989). Turning up the dirt in cholesterol screens. **136**, 359
5. Lannon, C.M. and Earp, J.A. (1991).Effects of screening children for high cholesterol. *Am. J. Dis. Child.*, **145**, 399 (abstr.)
6. Newman, T.B., Browner, W.S. and Hulley, S.B. (1990). The case against childhood cholesterol screening. *J. Am. Med. Assoc.*, **264**, 3039-43
7. Russell, L. (1986). *Is Prevention Better than Cure?* (Washington, DC: The Brookings Institution)
8. Grover, S.A., Coupal, L., Fahkry, R. and Suissa, S. (1991). Screening for hypercholesterolemia among Canadians: How much will it cost? *Can. Med. Assoc. J.*, **144**, 161-8
9. McPherson, R.S., Nichaman, M.Z., Kohl, H.W. *et al.* (1990). Intake and food sources of dietary fat among children in the woodlands, Texas. *Pediatrics*, **86**, 520-6
10. Lifshitz, F. and Moses, N. (1989). Growth failure. A complication of dietary treatment of hypercholesterolemia. *Am. J. Dis. Child.*, **143**, 537-42
11. Walter, H.J., Hofman, A., Vaughan, R.D. and Wynder, E.L. (1988). Modification of risk factors for coronary heart disease. *N. Engl. J. Med.*, **318**, 1093-100
12. Harris, S. Personal communication
13. Birch, L.L., Johnson, M.S., Andresen, G., Peters, J.C. and Schulte, M.C. (1991). The variability of young children's energy intake. *N. Engl. J. Med.*, **324**, 232-5
14. Cohen, M.V., Byrne, M.J., Levine, B., Gutowski, T. and Adelson, R. (1991). Low rate of treatment of hypercholesterolemia by cardiologists in patients with suspected and proven coronary heart disease. *Circulation*, **83**, 1294-304
15. Holtzman, N.A. (1991). The great god cholesterol. *Pediatrics*, **87**, 943-5
16. American Academy of Pediatrics. (1986). Committee on Nutrition. Prudent lifestyle for children: dietary fat and cholesterol. *Pediatrics*, **78**, 521-5

Discussion

Dr Parsons: There has been a great deal of difficulty in coming out with a positional statement in regard to the paediatric population and the Canadian Consensus Conference could not arrive at any. There are well-documented cases of familial hypercholesterolaemia. For example, one of my patients had his first infarct when he was 27. He had a cholesterol of 12 mmol/l and it is now down to 7.0 mmol/l on cholestyramine and lovostatin. His son is 13 and has a similar profile. What would you suggest to do in this case?

Dr Goldbloom: I think that these children do have to be treated and they have to be followed very closely. I think that they have to be supervised, not merely from the point of view of their lipids, but also from the viewpoint of their growth, maturation, and their general well-being and happiness. As I suggested earlier, we do not know for sure, at least in anything that I have read, that we are really capable of prolonging life in these children. Perhaps we can, and it is certainly worth trying. I wonder, from experience with other chronic diseases, such as diabetes in adolescence, how successful we are likely to be in persuading children to follow life long dietary regimens, even if they happen to be desirable. One of the paediatricians that I admire, the late Dr Harry Gordon, used to say that the doctor's mission is to relieve anxiety and that all our research, diagnostic efforts and treatment are nothing more than a means to that end. I still believe very much in this concept when dealing with individual patients. Treatment of these children cannot be turned into some sort of parlour trick, based simply on biochemical measurements. Certainly these children may not have a great future, but we must accept the fact that we are using somewhat experimental treatment on them and they may or may not accept it in the long term.

Dr Naylor: I have a question related to, to borrow a term, 'collateral damage' to children. We know that adults are treated and that adults under treatment are going to change their diets in a family way. We also know that, as a result of public health promotion, there are secular trends in diet in the whole population, in that many segments are showing dietary change. Do we have evidence from the paediatric community that shows deleterious effects when a child's mother or father change their diet or when the family changes its diet? Also, do we have similar data for population-wide trends?

Dr Goldbloom: I am not aware of any data other than what I mentioned. Since his original publication, I understand that Dr Lifshitz has detected many more in his growth clinic. A surprising number of children coming into that clinic because of delayed growth and delayed puberty have turned out to be the result of over-zealous attempts to provide a 'healthy' diet. These are the problems that can arise between prescribing a theoretically ideal regimen and its application in the field. Until one sees what happens in the general population, it is very difficult to prejudge effectiveness. It is also important to distinguish the effectiveness of exhortation versus that of regulation. Let me cite the analogy of accident prevention. Preaching to people about accident prevention has had a notoriously poor track record. When one looks at the success in accident prevention, whether it be seatbelts or preventing strangulation from babies sticking their heads through the bars of the crib or preventing accidental poisoning, every one of the real successes has been achieved by legislation or regulation. I think that possibly a modest lowering of fat intake through the marketplace is likely to have more success than exhortation of the entire population.

Dr Roncari: I agree with everything you said and I would like to re-emphasize that a lot of physical and emotional harm has been done by cholesterolphobia to children. However, in your answer to Dr Parsons, if we now have very effective means for treating these unusual cases, let's say of familial hypercholesterolaemia and, as you said yourself, they have a poor prognosis without treatment, I do not think it is different from having an insulin-dependent diabetic that requires insulin. Just as you would expect compliance of an insulin-dependent diabetic to insulin, I think one should expect compliance to these effective agents which we have now. But, I know these are unusual cases, 1 in 500 or so.

Dr Goldbloom: Yes I know, I agree that they should be treated. However, they have to be treated with an eye on the realities of life. This is a lifelong problem for these children, it carries for many families enormous costs and the child may reject the treatment at some point. This creates enormous problems. Whenever we put the burden of treatment on the victim, we often create problems while attempting to solve them. As far as treatment beginning in childhood is concerned, we still do not know if we are going to prolong the lives of those children, or if we do, by how much. It may seem to make sense to do it, but that is another story.

Dr Parsons: I would like to comment about when other structures have been put in place in children's lives. For example, the suicide incidence in teenagers increased when suicide prevention was taught in the schools. When driver education came to the schools the number of deaths went up from driving.

Dr Kubow: I would like to make some comments in support of Dr Goldbloom's position in terms of dietary recommendations for children. First of all in setting recommendations for 30% total fat and 10% saturated fat, if they are to be used on an individual basis for children, you would anticipate normal distribution of intakes. This would mean, for all individuals to meet the 30% total fat guidelines, that the distribution of total fat intake would go much below 30%. As well, in this bell-shaped curve of intakes that the population would have, you would see a significant proportion of children that would have intakes in the low 20s as a percentage of total fat.

There exist third world data showing that intakes of fat in the low 20s of total fat is associated with severe growth retardation in children. Beyond this, we also have to examine the issue of bioavailability of trace elements in low-fat diets which decrease mineral bioavailability by increasing the intake of cereal and plant proteins and fibres. This can occur even though the food composition tables may show similar intakes of trace elements on these types of diets. Rosalin Gibson at the University of Guelph has shown that diets with high plant protein content are associated with low hair zinc content and growth retardation in male children. So, I believe we have to consider the impact of mineral bioavailability when making recommendations of this nature for children.

Lastly, in terms of studies that are carried out to investigate fat intake in children, one has also to look at the dietary methodology that is being used. A recent publication in the *Journal of Nutrition* this year has shown that you need for male children about 277 days of daily food records in order to assess dietary cholesterol intake and 23 days of daily food records for assessing total fat intake accurately. You require such a large number of daily food records measuring fat intake in children because of the high variability of fat intake. I believe many of the studies in children have not looked properly at this in terms of assessing fat intake.

Dr Horlick: Dr Goldbloom, I just wanted to direct your attention to the recently published PDAY study*. This is a study of the pathological lesions of atherosclerosis in young adolescents who died accidentally, and in whom it was possible to obtain recent postmortem blood cholesterol. A rather nice correlation between the cholesterol levels and the degree of atherosclerosis both in the aorta and in the coronary arteries of these young people, who died accidentally, was demonstrated. This suggests again, that there is a link, and that perhaps we should address that link.

Dr Goldbloom: You have no argument from me on that.

---

* Relationship of atherosclerosis in young men to serum lipoprotein cholesterol concentrations and smoking. A preliminary report from the pathobiological determinants of atherosclerosis in youth (PDAY) research group. *J. Am. Med. Assoc.*, 1990, **264**, 3018

21
Coronary heart disease: prevention and treatment by nutritional change

S.L. CONNOR and W.E. CONNOR

Diet greatly affects many of the risk factors which cause coronary heart disease. In fact, nutrition itself must be listed as one of the major risk factors because of its tremendous modifying effects on the disease process, atherosclerosis. The most important risk factor in which diet plays the major role, both in causation and in treatment, is hyperlipidemia (See Figure 1).

Hyperlipidemia is important because it forms the basis for the excessive infiltration of lipid into the arterial intima with atherosclerosis an ultimate consequence. Stage 1 in the development of coronary heart disease is hyperlipidemia or, as depicted in the figure, hypercholesterolemia, but this could indicate any abnormality of the plasma lipids – lipoproteins including cholesterol, low density lipoprotein (LDL), very low density lipoprotein (VLDL), triglyceride, high density lipoprotein (HDL), and the remnants of chylomicrons and VLDL. If hyperlipidemia is not present, then atherosclerosis does not result. Should atherosclerosis be prevented, then stage 3, coronary heart disease, the clinical expression of this underlying and silent disorder, will not occur.

The cause of hyperlipidemia is clearcut for 1% or less of the population. Hyperlipidemia will result regardless of environmental factors because of genetic predisposition. Familial hypercholesterolemia is the classic example of genetic hyperlipidemia, but there are many others. For the other 99% of the population, dietary factors are crucial in the development of hyperlipidemia. Even dietary factors will affect the hyperlipidemia of genetically based disorders but, in most instances, will probably not make the situation completely normal. Pharmaceutical agents will be required, but these act synergistically with diet.

First published in Connor, S.L. and Connor, W.E. (1990). Coronary heart disease: prevention and treatment by nutritional change. In Carroll, K.K. (ed.), *Canadian Royal Society of Medicine Symposium*, pp. 33–72. (Montreal, Quebec: McGill-Queen's University Press). Reproduced by permission of McGill-Queen's University Press.

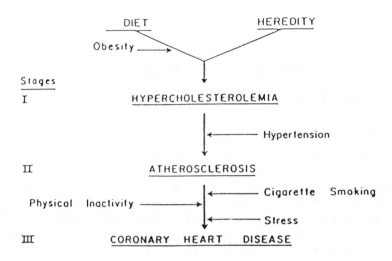

Figure 1 The stages and important factors in the development of coronary heart disease

The second risk factor affected by diet is thrombosis, a critical event in the evolution of the atherosclerotic plaque to complete coronary occlusion. Certain nutritional factors are thrombogenic, others are antithrombogenic. In both hyperlipidemia and thrombosis, the amount and kind of dietary fat are important.

A third risk factor, one obviously important and affected by nutrition, is obesity, which influences in turn hyperlipidemia, thrombosis and hypertension. Overweight may develop when another risk factor is abolished (i.e. cigarette smoking). Finally, the important risk factor, hypertension, is greatly affected by dietary electrolytes: sodium raises and potassium lowers blood pressure[1]. Fortunately, from the point of view of therapeutic simplicity, the same dietary lifestyle can be used to modify all four of these coronary risk factors: hyperlipidemia, thrombosis, obesity and hypertension.

The goals of this paper are 1) to review the precise roles that nutritional factors play in the causation of the atherosclerotic plaque, which is the underlying lesion of coronary heart disease (Figure 1), and 2) to delineate a practical approach to the dietary prevention and treatment of atherosclerosis. Attention will be given to the two components of the atherosclerotic plaque that lead to the development of overt coronary heart disease – namely, the lipid-rich, fibrous atheroma and the superimposed thrombotic lesion.

Dietary factors affect both the initiation and growth of the atherosclerotic plaque and the final thrombotic episode. The evidence about dietary factors and the genesis of atherosclerosis is best illustrated by the numerous experiments over the past 30 years carried out in subhuman primates. In these experiments dietary cholesterol and fat were the 'sine qua non' components necessary to produce hypercholesterolemia and atherosclerosis in many species of monkeys[2-4]. The atherosclerosis produced was severe and complicated, culminating in some monkeys in myocardial infarction, stroke and gangrene of an extremity[4]. These clinical features have reproduced the spectrum of the consequences of atherosclerotic disease in humans. In all of these experiments, diet exerted its effect on atherosclerosis by raising plasma lipid and lipoprotein concentrations.

The epidemiological evidence is likewise clearcut: populations consuming a low-cholesterol, low-fat diet have little coronary heart disease, whereas in populations of the Western world where the diet concentrates upon animal foods rich in cholesterol and saturated fat, the incidence of coronary heart disease is very high[5]. Japan is a classic example of a country with modern technology and a high living standard and yet a low incidence of coronary heart disease. The Japanese consume a low-cholesterol, low-fat diet and habitually have low plasma cholesterol levels. Here, again, the links between diet and clinical expression of coronary heart disease are the lifelong plasma cholesterol and LDL concentrations. In addition, populations with a low incidence of coronary heart disease and a low-fat dietary background also have a low incidence of clinical thrombosis.

The review of information on the vital role of plasma lipid and lipoprotein concentrations in the development of atherosclerosis raises a crucial question: Can dietary change lower elevated plasma lipid and lipoprotein concentrations in patients and in population subgroups of the Western world? The answer is an unequivocal yes. Experiments over the past 30 years have indicated which dietary components have an important effect upon plasma lipid and lipoprotein concentrations in humans. The major dietary factors to be considered include the following:

(1) Cholesterol
(2) Total fat
    Saturated fat
    Monounsaturated fat
    Polyunsaturated fat (omega-3 and omega-6)
(3) Carbohydrate, fibre, starch and sugars
(4) Protein
(5) Other nutrients (calories, alcohol, lecithin, vitamins and minerals)

Dietary cholesterol

Dietary cholesterol enters the body via the chylomicron pathway and is removed from the plasma by the liver as a component of chylomicron remnants. Only about 40% of ingested cholesterol is absorbed, the remaining 60% passing out in the stool. Dietary cholesterol is thus added to the cholesterol synthesized by the body, since feedback inhibition of cholesterol biosynthesis in the body only partially occurs in man even when a large amount of dietary cholesterol is ingested[6]. Because the ring structure of the sterol nucleus cannot be broken down by the tissues of the body as does occur for fat, protein and carbohydrate, it must be either excreted or stored. Thus, it is easy to see how the body or a particular tissue, i.e. a coronary artery, can become overloaded with cholesterol if there are limitations in cholesterol excretion from the body and from certain tissues. Cholesterol is excreted in the bile and ultimately in the stool, either as such or as bile acids synthesized in the liver from cholesterol. Both of these pathways of excretion are limited and, furthermore, the very efficient enterohepatic reabsorption and circulation returns much of what is excreted into the bile back into the body.

Dietary cholesterol does not directly enter into the formation of the lipoproteins synthesized in the liver, VLDL and LDL, since it is removed by the liver as a component of the chylomicron remnants. It can, however, profoundly affect the catabolism of LDL as mediated through the LDL receptor. Since dietary cholesterol ultimately contributes to the total amount of hepatic cell cholesterol, it can affect the biosynthesis of cholesterol and modify LDL receptor activity in the liver. In particular, an increase in hepatic cell cholesterol will decrease LDL receptor activity and, subsequently, cause an *increase* in the level of LDL cholesterol in the plasma[7-10]. Conversely, a drastic decrease in dietary cholesterol will increase the LDL receptor activity in the liver, enhance LDL removal and, hence, lower plasma LDL levels. Table 1 lists the effects of dietary cholesterol.

Over the past 30 years, some 26 separate metabolic experiments involving 196 human subjects and patients have shown decisive effects of dietary cholesterol upon plasma cholesterol and LDL levels[11-14]. Even patients with familial hypercholesterolemia respond greatly to dietary cholesterol. Table 2 shows that the plasma cholesterol level decreased 18% and 21% in two patients with FH (homozygotes) in response to the removal of cholesterol from the diet. This is similar to the mean plasma cholesterol increase of 17% that occurred when 1000 mg dietary cholesterol was added to a cholesterol-free diet in 25 subjects (11 normal, 7 with type II-a mild, 5 with II-a severe, and 9 with type IV hyperlipidemia)[15] (Figure 2).

Table 1 Effects of dietary cholesterol on LDL levels

---

1 Increased chylomicrons and remnants
2 Increased hepatic cell cholesterol
   Consequences:
   Decreased cholesterol biosynthesis
   Partial compensation in excretion of biliary cholesterol and bile acids to lessen
   hepatic cholesterol
   Decreased synthesis of LDL receptors
   Increased plasma LDL
3 Increased plasma LDL
   Consequence:
   Deposition of cholesterol into the arterial wall

Table 2 The effect of a cholesterol-free diet on the plasma cholesterol level in two patients with familial hypercholesterolemia (homozygotes)

| Diet | Plasma cholesterol (mg/dl) | |
	DL	DC
Cholesterol, 250 mg/day	737	786
Cholesterol-free	578	644
Change	–21 %	–18 %
Hyperalimentation	401	418

LDL increased very significantly in all groups, again showing indirectly the effects of dietary cholesterol upon the LDL receptor. These data further document the importance of dietary factors in hyperlipidemia of any phenotype or genotype. However, as pointed out years ago, the doubling or tripling of the amounts of dietary cholesterol will not necessarily increase the plasma levels if the initial amount of dietary cholesterol is already substantial, i.e. an increase to 950 mg per day from a previous intake of 475 mg per day[12]. Despite this earlier literature, such attempts are still being carried out and are highly touted as showing that dietary cholesterol has no effect on the plasma cholesterol levels. There is a review for those who wish to explore the subject more fully[16].

The effects upon the plasma cholesterol as the amount of dietary cholesterol is gradually increased may be depicted in Figure 3, and are supported by both animal and human experiments. With a baseline cholesterol-free diet, the amount of dietary cholesterol necessary to produce an increase in the plasma cholesterol concentration is termed 'the threshold amount'. Then, as the amount of dietary cholesterol is increased, the plasma cholesterol increases

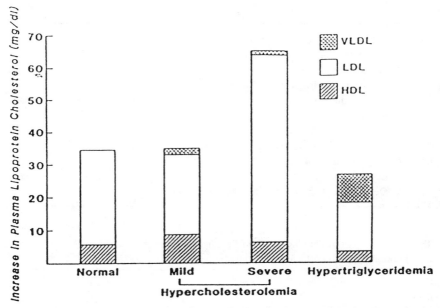

Figure 2 The effects of 1000 mg cholesterol diet on the content of cholesterol in the different lipoprotein (LP) fractions

likewise until the second important point on this curve is reached, which is termed 'the ceiling amount'. Further increases in dietary cholesterol do not lead to higher levels of the plasma cholesterol even if phenomenally high amounts may be fed. Each animal or human being probably has its own distinctive threshold and ceiling amounts. Generally speaking, however, and again based on the experimental literature, we would suggest that an average threshold amount for human beings would be 100 mg/day. An average ceiling amount of dietary cholesterol would be in the neighbourhood of 300–400 mg/day. Further experiments will be necessary to provide more precise information about the ceiling. Thus, a baseline dietary cholesterol intake of 500 mg/day from two eggs would, for most individuals, already exceed the ceiling. The addition of two more egg yolks for a total of 1000 mg/day would not then further increase the plasma cholesterol concentration. Yet, beginning with a baseline very low cholesterol diet under 100 mg/day and adding the equivalent of two egg yolks, or 426 mg, to this baseline amount would produce a striking change in plasma cholesterol concentrations, perhaps 60 mg/dl as shown in many experiments.

Recent dietary surveys indicate that the average American intake of dietary cholesterol is about 400 mg/day for women and 500 mg/day for men[17]. Decreasing these amounts of dietary cholesterol, as would take place in

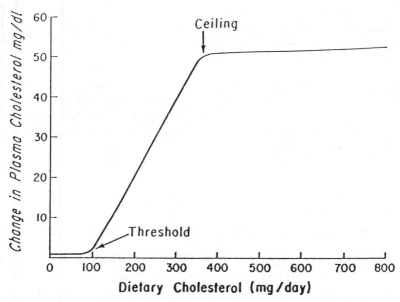

Figure 3 The effects upon the plasma cholesterol level of gradually increasing the amount of dietary cholesterol in human subjects whose background diet is very low in cholesterol content. See the text for discussion of the threshold and ceiling concepts

therapeutic and preventive diets to be amplified subsequently, would then have a profound effect on plasma cholesterol concentrations because operationally one would be on the descending limb of the curve as exemplified in Figure 3.

There has been recent discussion about the wide distribution of individual response to change in dietary cholesterol intake[18] although this finding is not new[11–13,18–22]. Further, variation in individual plasma cholesterol response occurs with other nutrients as well as with lipid-lowering drugs. Katan *et al.*[18] recently showed that 2% of their subjects had a negative or minimal response to dietary cholesterol feeding. Sixteen percent had responses less than half of the mean and 84% had a plasma cholesterol increase greater than half the mean. Therefore, the majority of people could be expected to respond significantly to a decrease in dietary cholesterol from 400–500 mg/day to 100 mg/day or less. Unfortunately, studies to date do not provide a way to predict who would have less than a 10% decrease and who would have greater than a 10% decrease in the plasma cholesterol level in response to maximal dietary changes. Studies are needed to provide a means by which one could correctly identify individuals with regard to plasma cholesterol response to decreases in dietary cholesterol and saturated fat intakes.

Also intriguing are the possible metabolic sequelae that could contribute to this individual variation in response, such as the LDL receptor which dietary cholesterol has been shown to down-regulate[8]. Mistry *et al.* suggested that individual differences in plasm lipid and lipoprotein response to dietary cholesterol appear to be related in part to differences in the capacity of peripheral cells to catabolize LDL and to down-regulate cholesterol synthesis[23]. Recent data indicate that the various apolipoprotein E alleles may be involved, with the E-2 isoform causing less binding to the LDL receptor[24] and the E-4 isoform possibly increasing VLDL catabolism independently of the LDL receptor[25].

Fat

The effects of dietary fats upon the plasma lipids and lipoproteins

The amount and kind of fat in the diet have a well-documented effect upon the plasma lipid concentrations[26,27]. The *total* amount of dietary fat is important in that the formation of chylomicrons in the intestinal mucosa and their subsequent circulation in the blood is directly proportional to the amount of fat which has been consumed in the diet. A fatty meal will result in the production of large numbers of chylomicrons and will impart the characteristic lactescent appearance to post-prandial plasma observed some three to five hours after meal consumption. A typical American diet with 110 gm of fat would produce 110 gm of chylomicron triglyceride per day. 'Remnant' production from chylomicrons is proportional to the number of chylomicrons synthesized. Chylomicron remnants are considered atherogenic particles[28]. Fat is important in cholesterol metabolism since cholesterol is absorbed in the presence of dietary fat and is transported in chylomicrons.

However, the most important effect of dietary fat upon the plasma cholesterol level relates to the *type* of fat. Fats may be divided into three major classes identified by saturation and unsaturation characteristics. Long-chain, *saturated fatty acids* have no double bonds, are not essential nutrients, and may be readily synthesized in the body from acetate. Dietary saturated fatty acids have a profound hyper-cholesterolemic effect, increase the concentrations of LDL and have thrombogenic implications[26,27]. All animal fats are highly saturated (30% or more of the fat is saturated) except for those which occur in fish and shellfish, these latter being, contrastingly, highly polyunsaturated. The molecular basis for the effects of dietary saturated fat on the plasma cholesterol level is now well understood and rests upon its influence on the LDL receptor activity of liver cells, as described by Brown and Goldstein[29]. Dietary saturated fat suppresses hepatic LDL receptor activity, decreases the removal of LDL from the blood and thus increases the concentration of LDL cholesterol in the blood[7]. Cholesterol augments the effect of saturated fat by further suppressing hepatic LDL receptor activity and raising the plasma LDL cholesterol level[8]. Conversely, a decrease in dietary cholesterol and saturated fat increases the LDL receptor activity of the liver cells, enhances the hepatic pickup of LDL cholesterol and lowers the concentration of LDL cholesterol in the blood[8]. Metabolic studies suggest that one can expect an average plasma cholesterol lowering of 10–20% by maximally decreasing dietary cholesterol and saturated fat intake.

Attention has been called to the fact that some saturated fats are not hypercholesterolemic (see Table 3). Medium-chain triglycerides (C8 and C10 saturated fatty acids) are handled metabolically more like carbohydrate and are transported to the liver via the portal vein blood rather than as chylomicrons. These fatty acids do not elevate the plasma cholesterol concentration. Stearic acid, an 18-carbon saturated fatty acid, likewise has a limited effect upon the plasma cholesterol concentration. This is because the body resists the accumulation of stearic acid and the liver converts excessive stearic acid from the diet into oleic acid, a monounsaturated fatty acid, by virtue of the action of a desaturase enzyme. Feeding animals large quantities of a fat such as cocoa butter containing a considerable percentage of its total fatty acids as stearic acid (33%) does not result in the deposition of stearic acid in the adipose tissue as would occur with mono- and polyunsaturated fat feeding[30]. This again is because of the action of the desaturase enzyme.

Table 3 Effects of saturated fatty acids upon plasma cholesterol levels

C8, C10	Medium chain	Neutral
C12	Lauric	Increase
C14, C16	Myristic, palmitic	Increase
C18	Stearic	Netural

The practical importance of these observations on certain saturated fatty acids is limited because they are not present to any appreciable extent in the diet. The equations developed for the prediction of plasma cholesterol change have been based upon the changes produced by a given fat, including its concentration of stearic acid. Thus, all of the information which has accumulated about the hypercholesterolemic and atherogenic properties of a given fat such as beef fat, butterfat, lard, palm oil, cocoa butter and coconut oil is completely valid. To be emphasized is the fact that palmitic acid, which is the most common saturated fatty acid found in our food supply, is intensely hypercholesterolemic. It has 16 carbons; myristic acid and lauric acid with 14 and 12 carbons respectively are likewise intensely hypercholesterolemic. It is these fatty acids which are present in dietary fats and which cause their unfortunate effects. Amounts of stearic acid in the American diet are not great compared with palmitic acid.

The second class of dietary fats consists of the characteristic *monounsaturated fatty acids* present in all animal and vegetable fats. For practical purposes, oleic acid, having one double bond at the omega-9 position, is the only significant dietary monounsaturated fatty acid. In general, the effects of dietary monounsaturated fatty acids have been 'neutral' in terms of their effects on the plasma cholesterol concentrations, neither raising nor lowering them[31]. However, reports that Mediterranean basin populations who consume olive oil in relatively large quantities have fewer heart attacks then people in this country has led to further investigations. Recent studies have shown that large amounts of monounsaturated fat, like polyunsaturated oils, lower plasma cholesterol and LDL levels when compared with saturated fat[32,33]. Furthermore, unlike polyunsaturated oils, monounsaturated fat did not lower the plasma HDL cholesterol level. However, distinct from omega-3 fatty acids from fish oil, monounsaturated fat does not decrease the plasma triglyceride concentrations[32,33]. Furthermore, monounsaturated fat has no known effect upon prostaglandin metabolism or upon platelet function. Omega-3 fatty acids are antithrombotic; monounsaturated fat has no such action.

There are several additional points to be made in regard to these recent studies: 1) The Mediterranean diet is also rich in fish, beans, fruit and vegetables, and is *low* in saturated fat and cholesterol. These could be the decisive factors which influence the lessened incidence of coronary disease and lower plasma cholesterol levels. 2) Olive oil is low in saturated fatty acids (which raise plasma cholesterol levels); this may be why the recent metabolic experiments have shown some cholesterol lowering from large amounts of monounsaturates in the diet. 3) Large amounts of any kind of fat should be avoided to lower the risk of other diseases such as colon or breast cancer and obesity. And all fats, after absorption, form large particles (remnants) which circulate in the blood and are atherogenic. One translation of the latest research on monounsaturated fats is to recommend that patients include them as part of a general lower-fat eating style – use olive oil in salad dressing and Italian dishes. Use peanut oil for special stir-fried dishes. Avocado is delicious but high in fat, so use as a garnish only.

Polyunsaturated fatty acids, the third class of fatty acids, are vital constituents of cellular membranes and serve as prostaglandin precursors[34]. Because they cannot be synthesized by the body and are only obtainable from dietary sources, they are 'essential' fatty acids. The two classes of polyunsaturated fatty acids are the omega-6 and omega-3 fatty acids (Figure 4). The most common examples of omega-6 fatty acids are linoleic acid, found in food, and arachidonic acid, 20 carbons in length with four double bonds, usually synthesized in the body from linoleic acid by the liver. Since the basic structure of omega-6 fatty acids cannot be synthesized by the body, up to 2–3% of total

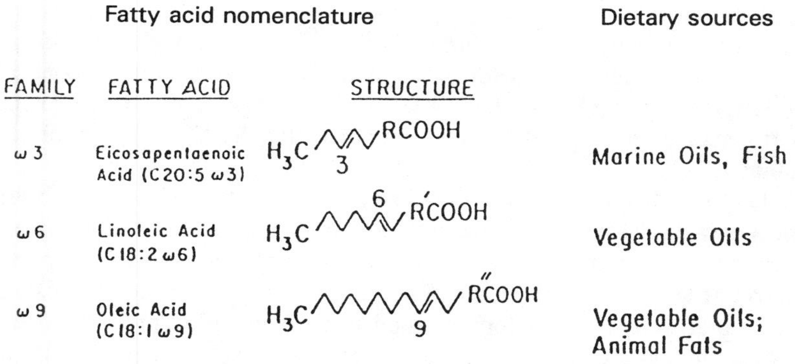

Figure 4 Fatty acids can be organized into families according to the position of the first double bond from the terminal methyl group. Typical fatty acids from three common families are shown in this figure. Omega-3 fatty acids all have three carbons between the methyl end and the first double bond. Besides eicosapentaenoic acid (C20:5), other common omega-3 fatty acids are linolenic acid (C18:3) and docosahexaenoic acid (C22:6). Linoleic acid (C18:2) and arachidonic acid (C20:4) are the most important omega-6 fatty acids, while oleic acid (C18:1) is the commonest fatty acid in the omega-9 family

energy in the diet must be supplied as linoleic acid to meet the requirements of the body for the omega-6 structure, i.e. an essential fatty acid.

Omega-3 fatty acids differ in the position of the first double bond counting from the methyl end of the molecule, this double bond being at the number 3 carbon. Omega-3 fatty acids are also an essential nutrient for human beings since the body is unable to synthesize this particular structure. Omega-6 and omega-3 fatty acids are not interconvertible. The dietary sources of omega-3 fatty acids are from plant foods – some, but not all, vegetable oils, and leafy vegetables (which are especially rich in omega-3 fatty acids) and, in particular, fish and shellfish. Linolenic acid, C18:3, is obtained from vegetable products. Eicosapentaenoic acid, C20:5, and docosahexaenoic acid, C22:6, are derived from fish, shellfish and phytoplankton (the plants of the ocean) and are highly concentrated in fish oils. Once either the omega-3 or omega-6 structure comes into the body as the 18 carbon linoleic or linolenic acid, the body can synthesize the longer chain and more highly polyunsaturated omega-6 or omega-3 fatty acids (20 and 22 carbons).

There are distinctly different functions in the body for omega-3 and omega-6 fatty acids. Both serve as substrate for the formation of different prostaglandins[34] and are rich in phospholipid membranes. Both omega-3 and omega-6 fatty acids are particularly concentrated in nervous tissue. Omega-3 fatty acids are rich in the retina, spermatozoa, the gonads, and many other organs. Omega-6 fatty acids are concentrated in the different plasma lipid

353

classes (cholesterol esters, phospholipids, etc.) and, in addition, are concerned with lipid transport.

Polyunsaturated fatty acids in large amounts, of either the omega-6 or omega-3 structure, depress plasma total and LDL cholesterol concentrations[22,31]. Omega-3 fatty acids have a second additional action in lowering plasma triglyceride concentrations and, in particular, VLDL, chylomicrons and remnants[35,36].

Already stressed is the wealth of evidence from experimental animals about the important and *sine qua non* necessity of dietary cholesterol and fat being present in the nutrition of animals to produce atherosclerosis. Several important studies in regard to fish oil containing omega-3 fatty acids have indicated much less atherosclerosis developing when fish oil was present in the diet. The species studied to date have been pigs[37] and rhesus monkeys[38]. Both coronary and aortic atherosclerosis have been greatly reduced by fish oil. This reduction in experimental atherosclerosis from omega-3 fatty acids is not necessarily explainable by changes in the plasma lipid–lipoprotein concentration. Since these were lowered only partially or not at all during the experimental atherosclerosis period, other mechanisms, possibly involving prostaglandins, must be postulated to explain the anti-atherogenic effects of fish oil. Table 4 lists possible effects of omega-3 fatty acids from fish oil upon coronary heart disease.

Table 4 Cardiovascular effects of omega-3 fatty acids

1 Hypolipidemic: decrease plasma lipids-lipoproteins, cholesterol, triglycerides, LDL, VLDL, chylomicrons and remnants.
2 Anti-thrombotic and vasodilatory: decrease platelet stickiness; increase bleeding time.
3 Lower blood pressure.

It is not known exactly how the evidence about omega-3 fatty acids should translate in eating behaviour. However, one study from the Netherlands showed that men who included fish in their diet twice a week had fewer deaths from heart disease[39]. Even very low-fat seafood contains an appreciable amount of omega-3 fatty acids. Eating a total of 12 oz. of a variety of fish and shellfish each week would provide 1000 to 5000 mg of omega-3 fatty acids, as well as protein, vitamins and minerals. The patient with hyperlipidemia could be expected to have only beneficial effects from following this dietary advice, especially if the fish replaced meat in the diet.

Most of the comparisons of the effects of saturated and polyunsaturated fat upon the plasma lipids have indicated that gram for gram, saturated fat is up to two times greater at raising plasma cholesterol than is polyunsaturated fat in depressing it[40,41]. Regression equations have been calculated to indicate the plasma cholesterol changes from dietary manipulations of saturated fat, polyunsaturated fat and cholesterol. These will be discussed later in the development of the cholesterol–saturated fat index of foods.

Many, but not all, of the currently marketed vegetable oils, shortenings, and margarines are only partially hydrogenated and thus retain the basic unsaturated characteristics of vegetable oils. The trend in industry is to produce margarines and shortenings with a minimum of the principal by-product of hydrogenation, elaidic acid, which is the trans isomer of oleic acid. This is desirable because in a recent study large amounts of trans fatty acid, 10% of calories providing about 33 g per day, significantly increased the plasma LDL and decreased the plasma HDL cholesterol levels[42]. In contrast the trans fatty acid availability in the United States is 8 g per person per day[43]. In that low amount, a significant LDL or HDL effect is doubtful. In the recommended 20% fat diet people would eat half as much fat. This alone would cut the amount of trans fatty acid in half to 4 g per day, an insignificant amount.

Coconut oil, cocoa butter (the fat of chocolate) and palm oil are common 'saturated' vegetable fats consumed in quantities; they have a hypercholesterolemic effect. The ratio of polyunsaturated to saturated fatty acids in a given fat or oil is termed the P/S value. Fats with a high P/S value of 2 and above, compared to 0.4 and less, are generally recognized as being hypocholesterolemic. The typical Western diet has a P/S value of 0.4. In the suggested low-fat, high-carbohydrate diet to prevent coronary disease, the P/S value is above 1.0.

Dietary fat and thrombosis

Table 5 lists possible dietary effects on thrombosis and platelet aggregation. These effects are based upon both experimental and epidemiological evidence. As may be appreciated, firm documentation in this arena may not always be possible and no clinical trials have been conducted to support the suggested relationships. However, both *in vitro* and *in vivo*, saturated fatty acids of a chain length C12 and above appear to be thrombogenic, activating the coagulation cascade and aggregating platelets[44-47]. Any circumstance which elevates the levels of free fatty acids in the plasma such as starvation, diabetic acidosis, myocardial infarction, or certain hormonal stimulation must be considered as having a thrombotic effect as well[48-52]. For example, in starvation, free fatty acids are released into the plasma from adipose tissue triglyceride. The mechanism of this effect may occur from a level of free fatty acids exceeding the two tight binding sites on the albumin molecule, the usual transport form of free fatty acids[53]. This, then, allows the free fatty acids to interact with various coagulation proteins and with platelets.

Table 5 Dietary factors affecting thrombosis and platelet function

---

1 Thrombotic factors
    Saturated fatty acids
    Free fatty acids
2 Anti-thrombotic factors
    Low-fat, high CHO diet
    Polyunsaturated fat
        omega-6 fatty acids (linoleic) from vegetable oils
        omega-3 fatty acids (eicosapentaenoic) from fish oil

Polyunsaturated fat, in general, has an antithrombotic effect. This effect is best documented by dietary studies in human beings[34] and by the epidemiological evidence in the Greenland Eskimos who have a low incidence of thrombotic disease[54]. They consume fish and seal, both rich in the omega-3 fatty acids, eicosapentaenoic and docosahexaenoic fatty acids[55]. The feeding of fish and fish oil to humans or their presence in a natural diet not only has a hypolipidemic effect but also increases the bleeding time and reduces platelet aggregation[56,57]. On the other hand, the ingestion of a low-fat diet high in carbohydrate and fibre is associated with a low incidence of thrombosis in certain population groups, such as the Ugandans[58-60]. These populations ingest a low-fat diet and consume most of their fat in the form of polyunsaturated fatty acids with a very low intake of saturated fat.

Accordingly, an antithrombotic diet for human beings would be low in total fat and saturated fat and might contain fish. It should also be a high-carbohydrate, high-fibre diet. High circulating levels of the plasma-free fatty acids should also be avoided. This is particularly important in obese patients with vascular disease who are given low calorie diets. Such diets should avoid ketosis, which would be an indication that plasma-free fatty acid concentrations are greatly increased. They should contain sufficient calories in general, about 700–1000 kcalories/day, in which the chief sources of calories would be carbohydrate and protein.

Carbohydrate

If the total fat content of an anti-coronary diet is reduced from the current American intake of 40% to 20% of the total calories and if protein is to be kept constant, the difference in caloric intake between a high-fat diet and a low-fat diet must be made up by increasing the carbohydrate content of the diet. As already indicated, both the epidemiological evidence and experimental studies buttress this basic concept, since populations ingesting a high-carbohydrate diet, usually from complex carbohydrates, have a low incidence of coronary disease and other thrombotic conditions.

Over 25 years ago it was demonstrated that a sudden increase in the amount of dietary carbohydrate in Americans accustomed to a high-fat diet would increase the plasma triglyceride concentration rather dramatically[61]. However, after many weeks, adaptation occurs, and the hypertriglyceridemia regresses[62,63]. We regard this situation as metabolically normal, since it is a universal occurrence in Americans given a high-carbohydrate diet. It is analogous to the hyperglycemia which results in individuals who have previously been consuming a reduced number of calories or a low-carbohydrate diet and are given a glucose load. In order to obtain a valid glucose tolerance curve, an individual must eat a diet reasonably high in carbohydrate for at least three days before the test.

High-carbohydrate diets have been used in diabetic patients over a long period of time without impairment of glucose tolerance and without the occurrence of hypertriglyceridemia[62]. Since any lasting dietary change is adopted gradually, as will be emphasized in the behavioural modification approach taken to educate patients about dietary change, it is highly unlikely that any patient with coronary disease asked to follow the low-cholesterol, low-fat, high-carbohydrate diet would develop hypertriglyceridemia. There would be ample time for adaptation as he passed through the three or more phases of this dietary approach.

We recently increased the dietary carbohydrate intake gradually from 45% kcal to 65% kcal over a 28-day period in eight mildly hypertriglyceridemic subjects. There was a significant lowering of the mean plasma cholesterol level from 232 to 198 mg/dl, –15% ($p < 0.0001$), whereas the mean plasma triglyceride did not change significantly, 213 mg/dl to 230 mg/dl[64].

Studies in rats have indicated that sucrose and fructose have a hypertriglyceridemic effect in contrast to starch or glucose[65]. The evidence in human beings that even very large amounts of sucrose (over 50% of the total calories) produce hyperlipidemia is not completely convincing. However, even if large quantities of sucrose have a mild hypertriglyceridemic and perhaps also a hypercholesterolemic effect, this does not bear particularly upon the dietary design of the anti-coronary diet as envisioned. In the low-fat, high-carbohydrate diet the vast majority of the carbohydrate is in the form of cereals and legumes, not sucrose. Americans commonly consume about 20% of the total calories as sucrose or about half of their carbohydrate intake. In the dietary changes being suggested, sucrose would fall to 10–15% of the total calories, and so any effect from sucrose would be diminished rather than accentuated by the dietary change.

Fibre

Dietary fibre is a broad nondescript term which includes several carbohydrates thought to be indigestible by the human gut. These include cellulose, hemicelluloses, lignin, pectin and beta glucans. Dietary fibre is only found in plants and is commonly present in unprocessed cereals, legumes, vegetables and fruits. In ruminant animals, dietary fibre is completely digested by the microbial flora of the rumen, so that fibre provides a major source of energy for these animals. In man, however, dietary fibre contributes little to the caloric content of the diet, promotes satiety through its bulk, and affects colonic function greatly. A high-fibre diet produces larger stools and a more rapid intestinal transit, factors which may prevent certain diseases of the colon (i.e. diverticulitis, colon cancer). A high-fibre diet increases the emptying time of the stomach, thereby promoting slower absorption of nutrients, especially glucose.

Fibre experiments date back at least 30 years[66,67]. Fibre added to semisynthetic diets fed to rats has usually had a plasma cholesterol lowering effect. In humans, fibre fed predominantly in the insoluble form was not hypocholesterolemic[68]. A study in which large amounts of soluble fibre (17 g/2000 kcal) from oat bran and beans were fed to people produced a 20% lowering of the plasma total and LDL cholesterol levels[69]. Other studies have produced similar results[70,71]. Rich sources of soluble fibre include fruits, pectin being a soluble fibre, oats and other cereals, legumes and vegetables. One way soluble fibre acts is to bind bile acids in the gut, prevent their reabsorption and thus lower cholesterol levels much like the bile acid-binding resins like cholestyramine.

A high-fibre diet is integral to the dietary concepts for the treatment of hyperlipidemia. The consumption of more foods from vegetable sources will automatically mean a higher consumption of both total and soluble fibre.

Protein

The dietary treatment of hyperlipidemia involves, in general, a shift from the consumption of protein derived from animal sources, such as meat and dairy products, to the consumption of more protein from plants. The nutritional adequacy of such protein shifts is assured, because mixtures of vegetable proteins, plus the provision of ample low-fat animal protein sources, provide abundantly for essential amino acid requirements. Ranges of protein intake from 25 to 150 g have been tested over the years for effects upon blood lipids and have been found to have no effect within amounts commonly consumed by Americans. However, experiments in animals have suggested that an animal protein such as casein (from milk) is definitely hypercholesterolemic and that

358

a vegetable protein such as soy protein has the opposite effect. There have been few definitive experiments in humans to test the hypocholesterolemic effect of vegetable proteins vis à vis animal proteins. As might be expected, it is difficult to control all the variables, including the cholesterol and fat content. However, there are suggestions that the consumption of vegetable protein may have some hypocholesterolemic action. Thus, it may be postulated that a shift in protein intake to include more vegetable protein carries no harm and may confer some benefit to the hyperlipidemic individual.

Calories

Excessive caloric intake and adiposity can contribute also to both hypertriglyceridemia and hypercholesterolemia by stimulating the liver to overproduce VLDL. The plasma triglyceride and VLDL concentrations of hypertriglyceridemic patients greatly improve after weight reduction and are increased by the hypercaloric state[72-74]. There is little direct evidence, however, that the LDL receptor and plasma cholesterol and LDL concentrations are directly affected by caloric excess. Nonetheless, it is known that obese individuals have a total body cholesterol production which is higher than in individuals of normal weight. Weight reduction and fasting, which involve a decrease in the consumption of cholesterol and saturated fat from the diet, could certainly upregulate the LDL receptor and could be expected to improve LDL levels in patients with familial hypercholesterolemia. It is, therefore, reasonable to advise caloric control and the avoidance of obesity in the dietary management of hyperlipidemia. The role of increased physical activity is most important in weight control.

Alcohol

Results from large population studies have shown that people who report consuming alcohol have a lower incidence of coronary heart disease than people who do not drink[75,76]. These studies, while indicating trends in large populations, need to be reinforced by the much stronger evidence provided by controlled experiments in which other factors that influence the plasma HDL cholesterol level such as body weight, smoking, exercise habits and diet are accounted for. Many such studies testing the effect of alcohol consumption on HDL cholesterol levels have been conducted. These studies have shown significant increases in HDL cholesterol after alcohol consumption ranging from an equivalent of two beers to seven beers per day over three to six weeks compared to a similar abstention period. The type of alcohol given (beer, wine, spirits) did not appear to influence results. Alcohol appears to increase the HDL$_3$ component of HDL which is less related to protection against coronary heart disease[77]. It is HDL$_2$, affected by exercise but not alcohol, which is more protective[78]. Because of these results, and since the increased levels of HDL have been linked to lower rates of atherosclerosis, some drinkers have been tempted to drink more, claiming that alcohol is 'good for the heart'. Should alcohol consumption be encouraged to protect against coronary heart disease?

Specific recommendations are not easy to make, because the effects of alcohol consumption are complex, affecting other components of the plasma in addition to HDL cholesterol. Most of the metabolic studies have involved people with plasma cholesterol values below 190 mg/dl, and these results may not translate directly to patients with hyperlipidemia. The effects of alcohol on the levels of HDL$_2$ (linked to reduced coronary disease) and HDL$_3$ (no relationship to coronary disease) are controversial. Alcohol is packed with calories. There are about 290 kcalories in two 12-ounce beers or two 6-ounce glasses of wine. On the average, up to 8% of calories consumed by adult Americans come from alcohol. This may be one of the reasons why so many people who drink heavily are overweight and have alcohol-related problems. Theoretically, the amount of alcohol it would take to increase a person's HDL cholesterol from below 30 to above 40 mg/dl is five to six drinks per day. Other consequences of alcohol consumption – admittedly when excessive – include cirrhosis of the liver, certain cancers, gastritis, mental deterioration, neuropathies and, of course, the personal and social ravages of chronic alcoholism.

We do not think that alcohol should be part of a daily diet, rather – for those who enjoy an occasional drink – we suggest a limit of one to two drinks on any given day and up to four to five drinks per week. The inclusion of alcohol in the diet to increase HDL cholesterol levels is not recommended.

Lecithin

This phospholipid derived from soybeans is commonly sold in health food stores and is widely publicized as a popular remedy for hypercholesterolemia. Aside from its high content of linoleic acid, the consumption of lecithin has little or no effect upon lipid metabolism. Contrary to popular belief, lecithin is not absorbed as such from the digestive tract but is hydrolyzed into its constituent fatty acids and choline. Choline is a lipotrophic substance which was tested in the treatment of hypercholesterolemia 30 years ago and found to be of no value[79]. The plasma phospholipid levels have not been affected by the addition of lecithin to the diet; the circulating plasma phospholipids are largely synthesized by the liver. Parenthetically, high levels of plasma phospholipids are found in patients with familial hypercholesterolemia.

Minerals and vitamins

Under the assumption that the minimum daily requirements have been met in the diet, there is no information to indicate that additional vitamins and minerals above and beyond the content of a nutritionally adequate diet will have any effect upon the plasma lipid concentrations. This comment applies equally to vitamin C[80] and vitamin E[81], both enthusiastically consumed by the public without there being any proof of benefit. On the contrary, massive doses of vitamin A may produce liver damage[82]. The sole exception is niacin, a B-vitamin used in massive doses for the treatment of hyperlipidemia.

Design of a dietary approach for treating and preventing coronary heart disease

In view of the evidence about dietary factors, hyperlipidemia, thrombosis and coronary heart disease, it should now be possible to indicate the features of an appropriate and effective preventive diet against coronary heart disease in patients with hyperlipidemia and for the public at large. In general terms, such a diet, from what has already been indicated in this chapter, should be hypolipidemic and antithrombotic. It should be nutritionally adequate and meet the necessary nutritional requirements during childhood and adult life. This feature is essential because the dietary approach is less likely to succeed unless it is familial. Coronary heart disease occurs in families. Many in the family who have not yet developed overt symptomatology of coronary heart disease are undoubtedly at risk for subsequent coronary heart disease. Another criterion of the dietary approach is that it should be no more costly than the current Western diet. Finally, its use should be facilitated and supported by recipes and menu plans to make it possible for interested patients and their families to incorporate the proposed dietary changes into their lifestyle after a suitable educational and training period. The dietary approach presented here, i.e. the low-fat, high-carbohydrate diet, is intended to produce a maximal lowering of plasma total and LDL cholesterol concentrations, to reduce excess body weight when this is present, and to respond to all of the evidence concerning antithrombotic dietary factors. This diet can be used to treat the many different types of hyperlipidemia. No longer is it necessary to have a different diet for each phenotype of hyperlipidemia. The same diet with slight modification can be used for any type of hyperlipidemia. This single diet concept has been delineated in detail elsewhere[83,84].

The cholesterol-saturated fat index (CSI) of foods[85]

The major plasma cholesterol elevating effects of a given food reside in its cholesterol and saturated fat content. To help understand the contribution of these two factors in a single food item and to compare one food with another, we have computed a cholesterol-saturated fat index (CSI) for selected foods (Figure 5 and Table 6). This index was based on a modification of the regression equation used earlier to calculate the cholesterol index of foods[86]. Since the objective of the low-fat, high-carbohydrate diet is to maintain, but not to increase, the current intake of polyunsaturated fat, we chose not to include the polyunsaturated fat component of the equation in assessing an individual food item. The cholesterol index of foods was thus modified and is called the cholesterol-saturated fat index (CSI): CSI = (1.01 × gm saturated fat) + (0.05× mg cholesterol), where the amounts of saturated fat and cholesterol in a given amount of a food item are entered into this equation.

In this context it is particularly instructive to compare the CSI of fish versus moderately fat beef. A 100 gm portion of cooked fish contains 66 mg of cholesterol and 0.20 gm of saturated fat. This contrasts to a 96 mg cholesterol content and 8.1 gm of saturated fat of 20% fat beef. The CSI for 100 gm (3.5 oz) fish is 4, while that of beef is 13. The caloric value of these two portions also differs greatly (91 for fish and 286 for beef). The CSI of cooked chicken and turkey (without the skin) is also preferable to beef and other red meats. Again, the total fat content is quite a bit lower and the saturated fat per 100 gm is 1.3, with the cholesterol 87 mg. The CSI of poultry is 6. Table 6 lists the CSI for various foods.

Shellfish have low CSIs because their saturated fat content is extremely low, despite the fact that their cholesterol or total sterol content is 2.5 to 3 times higher than fish, poultry or red meat. This means that, when considering both cholesterol and saturated fat, shellfish have a CSI of 6, very much like poultry, and are a better choice than even the leanest red meats. Salmon also has a low CSI and is preferred to meat.

The low-fat, high-carbohydrate diet

The relationship between nutrients and coronary heart disease presents both responsibility and opportunity. The challenge is to define dietary objectives in specific and very practical terms relating to shopping, food preparation and eating[87]. One of the first low-cholesterol, low-fat cookbooks was produced by Dobbin *et al.* in 1957[88]. Our own such diet plan and cookbook is called *The New American Diet*[87]. The first objective of all low-fat diets must be to reduce cholesterol consumption from 500 to less than 100 mg per day. This requires keeping egg yolk consumption to a minimum since 45% of dietary cholesterol

Table 6 The cholesterol-saturated fat index (CSI) and kilocalorie content of selected foods

	CSI	kcalories
Fish, poultry, red meat (3^1/2 ounces or 100 grams cooked)		
Whitefish-snapper, perch, sole, cod, halibut, etc.	4	91
Salmon	5	149
Shellfish (shrimp, crab, lobster)	6	104
Poultry, no skin	6	171
Beef, pork and lamb:		
10 per cent fat (ground sirloin, flank steak)	9	214
15 per cent fat (ground round)	10	258
20 per cent fat (ground chuck, pot roasts)	13	286
30 per cent fat (ground beef, pork, and lamb, steaks, ribs, pork and lamb chops, roasts)	18	381
Cheeses (3^1/2 ounces or 100 grams)		
Low-fat cottage cheese, tofu (bean curd), pot cheese	1	98
Cottage cheese, Lite-line, Lite'n Lively, part-skim ricotta, reduced calories Laughing Cow	6	139
Imitation Mozzarella, Cheezola, Min Chol (Swedish low fat), Hickory Farm Lyte, Saffola American*	6	317
Olympia Low Fat, Green River, Keil Kase (lower fat cheddars), part-skim mozzarella, Neufchatel (lower fat cream cheese), Skim American	12	256
Cheddar, Roquefort, Swiss, Brie, jack, American, cream cheese, Velveeta, cheese spreads (jars), and most other cheeses	26	386
Eggs		
Whites (three)	0	32
Egg substitute (equivalent to two eggs)	1	98
Whole (two)	25	158
Fats (^{1}/4 cup or 4 tablespoons)		
Peanut butter	6	380
Mayonnaise	8	404
Most vegetable oils	6	491
Soft vegetable margarines	8	420
Soft shortenings	13	464
Bacon grease	20	464
Butter	36	409
Coconut oil, palm oil	38	491
Frozen desserts (1 cup)		
Water ices	0	245
Sherbet or frozen yogurt	2	290
Ice milk	6	214
Ice cream, 10% fat	13	272
Rich ice cream, 16% fat	18	349
Specialty ice cream, 22% fat	34	768

Continued

Table 6 (continued)

	CSI	kcalories
Milk products (1 cup)		
Skim milk (0.1% fat), or skim milk yogurt	<1	88
1% milk, buttermilk	2	115
2% milk or plain low-fat yogurt	5	144
Whole milk (3.5% fat) or whole milk yogurt	10	159
Liquid non-dairy creamers: soy bean oil	4	326
Liquid non-dairy creamers: coconut oil	23	326
Sour cream	39	468
Imitation sour cream (IMO)	43	499

*Cheeses made with skim milk and vegetable oils.

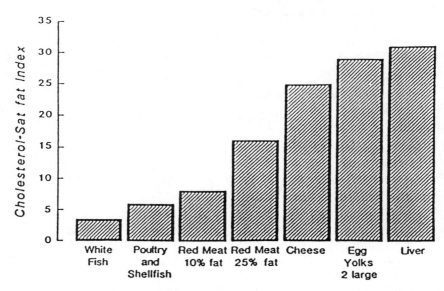

Figure 5 The cholesterol-saturated fat index (CSI) of $3^1/2$ oz. of fish, poultry, shellfish, meat, cheese, egg yolk, and liver. The CSI for poultry is the average CSI for cooked light and dark chicken without skin. The CSI for shellfish is the average CSI of cooked crab, lobster, shrimp, clams, oysters and scallops. The CSI for cheese is the average CSI of cheddar, Swiss and processed cheese

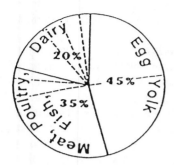

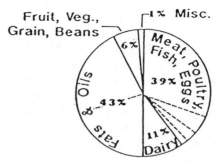

Figure 6 The sources of dietary cholesterol for people in the United States. Forty-five percent of the dietary cholesterol is derived from egg yolk, with half of that being from visible eggs (1–2 eggs per week) and half from eggs used in food preparation (the broken line in the egg yolk segment). Twenty-eight percent of the cholesterol is from red meats, poultry (4%), and fish (2%). Twenty percent is from dairy products: 8% from milk, 5% from cheese, 4% from butter, and 2% from ice cream

Figure 7 The sources of dietary fat for people in the United States. Thirty percent of the dietary fat is derived from red meats, poultry (5%), eggs (3%), and fish (1%), as per the broken lines dividing that segment of the circle. Eleven percent is from dairy products. Forty-three percent is directly from fats and oils, 21.5% being from visible fat (spreads and dressings) and 21.5% from fat used in cooking and baking. Six percent is from fruits, vegetables, grains, and beans, and 1% is from miscellaneous sources

comes from egg yolk, with approximately half from visible eggs and half from eggs incorporated into foods (Figure 6)[89]. Meat and poultry and fish are limited as well as the use of lower-fat dairy products.

The second objective is to reduce fat intake by one-half, from 40 to 20% of calories. This can be done by avoiding fried foods, reducing the fat used in baked goods by one-third and using low-fat dairy products. Added fat should be limited to three teaspoons per day for women and children and five teaspoons per day for teenagers and men. Peanut butter should be used as part of a meal and not as a snack, and nuts used sparingly as condiments.

Another objective is to decrease the current saturated fat intake by two-thirds, from 14 to 5–6% of calories. This requires eating red meat or cheese no more than twice a week, using lower-fat cheeses (20% fat or less), avoiding products containing coconut and palm oil, limiting ice cream and chocolate to once a month and using soft margarines and oils sparingly.

When people are advised to decrease the amount of fat in their diets, they usually think only of visible fat and are surprised to learn that fat added at the table represents only 22% of their fat intake (Figure 7)[89]. Decreasing dietary fat would be very difficult without knowing that 78% is invisible, with the majority coming from red meat, cheese, ice cream and other dairy products, and fat used in food preparation.

If dietary fat is reduced from 40 to 20% of calories and protein kept constant at 15% of calories to maintain weight, carbohydrate intake must be increased from 45 to 65% of total calories. What this means practically is that at least two complex carbohydrate-containing foods should be eaten at each meal. For example, eating toast *and* cereal for breakfast, a sandwich (two slices of bread) or bean soup and low-fat crackers at lunch, and 1–2 cups of rice, pasta, potatoes, corn, etc. *with* bread at dinner, in addition to selecting complex carbohydrate snacks such as popcorn or low-fat crackers and low-fat cookies. This is a significant change, as most Americans currently limit carbohydrate foods to no more than *one* per meal. To reach the increased carbohydrate objective, the patient must also eat three to five cups of legumes per week and two to four cups of vegetables per day. While research supports the value of a high-carbohydrate diet, many people are reluctant to adopt it because 'starchy' foods are falsely associated with gaining weight and are viewed as the food of the poor. Another objective is to eat three to five pieces of fruit per day with a concomitant decrease in refined sugar intake from 20% of calories to 10%. This means that sweets (pop *or* candy *or* desserts) must be limited to no more than one serving per day.

The phases of the low-fat, high-carbohydrate diet

Even well-motivated patients do not make abrupt changes in their dietary habits that are maintained over time. It will take many months and even years to make permanent changes in food consumption patterns. Therefore, we suggest that the recommended changes be approached in a gradual manner, with each phase introducing more changes toward the low-fat, high-carbohydrate diet pattern[84,87,91]. The manner in which patients are guided through these phases can be individualized. An example of three phases is summarized in Table 7.

Phase I The aim of Phase I is to decrease the consumption of foods high in cholesterol and saturated fat (Table 6). This can be accomplished by deleting egg yolk, butterfat, lard, and organ meats from the diet and by using substitute products when possible: soft margarine for butter, vegetable oils and shortening for lard, skim milk for whole milk, and egg whites for whole eggs. Many alternative foods can replace foods that contain large amounts of cholesterol and saturated fat. Increasing numbers of new products low in cholesterol and saturated fat are now marketed: low-fat cheeses, egg substitutes, soy meats, and frozen yogurt are a few examples.

366

Table 7 Summary of the three phrases of the low-fat, high-carbohydrate diet

Phase I: Substitutions	This is accomplished by: avoiding egg yolks, butterfat, lard and organ meats (liver, heart, brains, kidney, gizzards); substituting soft margarine for butter; substituting vegetable oils and shortening for lard; substituting skim milk and skim milk products for whole milk and whole milk products; substituting egg whites for whole eggs;	trimming fat off meat and skin from chicken choosing commercial food products lower in cholesterol and fat (low-fat cheeses, egg substitutes, soy meat substitutes, frozen yogurt, etc.) modifying favourite recipes by using less fat or sugar and vegetable oils instead of butter or lard;
Phase II: New recipes	This step involves: reducing amounts of meat and cheese eaten and replacing them with chicken and fish; eating meat, chicken or fish only once a day; cutting down on fat; as spreads, in salads, cooking and baking;	eating more grains, beans, fruit and vegetables; when eating out, make low-fat, low-cholesterol choices; finding new recipes to replace those which cannot be altered
Phase III: A new way of eating	The final phase means: eating meat, cheese, poultry and fish as 'condiments' to other foods, rather than as main courses; eating more beans and grain products as protein sources; using no more than 2–4 teaspoons of fat per day as spreads, salad dressings, or in cooking and baking	drinking 4–6 glasses of water per day; keeping extra meat, shellfish, regular cheese, chocolate, candy, coconut, and richer home-baked or commercially prepared food for special occasions (once a month or less enjoying a wide variety of new food and repertoire of totally new and savory recipes).

Many recipes currently in use can easily be altered. For example, most recipes, including baked items, can be made without egg yolks. Usually $1\frac{1}{2}$ to 2 egg whites can be used successfully in place of one whole egg in making cakes, cookies, custards, potato salad and many other products without changing their quality.

Phase II The goal of Phase II is a reduction of meat and cheese consumption with a gradual transition from the Western ideal of up to a pound of meat a day to no more than 6–8 ounces per day (Table 7). The use of lean, well-trimmed meat will help to decrease greatly the amount of saturated fat. Fatter meats such as lunch meats, bacon, sausage, wieners, spareribs and others should be saved for very special occasions. Meat or cheese should be used no more than *once* a day. One significant point is the change in the composition of the traditional sandwich. Meat and cheese are not necessarily essential parts of a sandwich, nor is a sandwich always necessary for lunch. In addition, less fat and cheese should be used. Broiling, baking, steaming or braising should be the methods of cooking instead of frying. Fewer foods should be used which contain a lot of fat. Only cheeses with part or all skim milk (20% fat or less) should be selected for daily cooking. Cheeses made from whole milk should be used sparingly, one ounce of cheese being substituted for three ounces of lean meat.

At this point, new recipes will be needed to replace the recipes which cannot be altered to meet these new requirements. Recipes centered about meat or high-fat dairy products (cream cheese, butter, sour cream, cheese) can be replaced with recipes that use larger amounts of grains, legumes, vegetables and fruits. Furthermore, because of the world-wide concern for the conservation of natural resources and the use of economical foods as well as the current interest in gourmet cooking and exotic foods, a large number of new recipes can be found in current cookbooks, magazines and newspapers. Many of these stress the use of non-animal food products.

Many other cultures have developed delicious meals which are low in cholesterol and in fat. A wide variety of spices and different products and foods from the cuisines of other countries can be used. Oriental dishes emphasize fresh vegetables and rice products; Mexican dishes make use of tortillas, peppers and beans. The Mediterranean countries (Greece, Italy and Spain) incorporate pastas and vegetable sauces. The cuisine of the Middle Eastern countries employs a variety of wheat products and legume dishes.

Phase III In Phase III the final goals of the low-fat, high-carbohydrate diet are attained. The cholesterol content of the diet is reduced to 100 mg per day and the saturated fat lowered to 5 or 6% of the total calories. These changes mean that consumption of meat and cheese, in particular, must be reduced. For most patients this will present a considerable challenge. We take an historical approach to the consumption of meat. Man has always eaten meat. What he had not done is to eat meat every day, let alone several times a day. Even today, *daily* meat consumption is only possible for the affluent minority of the world's population. It is not to our advantage, from the standpoints of either health or the wise use of resources, to consume large amounts of meat every day.

We propose, therefore, in Phase III, that meat, fish and poultry be used as 'condiments' rather than 'aliments'. With this philosophy, no longer will the meat dish occupy the centre of the table. Instead, meat in smaller quantities will spice up vegetable–rice–cereal–legume based dishes, much as in Oriental, Indian and Mediterranean cookery. The use of low-fat, low-cholesterol cheeses is also an important component of Phase III.

The total of meat, shellfish (shrimp, crab, lobster) and poultry should average three to four ounces per day. Poultry and especially fish should be stressed instead of meat because of their lower saturated fat content. In lieu of meat or poultry, fish and molluscs (clams, oysters, scallops) may be included in the diet in amounts up to six ounces per day because of the omega-3 fatty acids.

By this time, new recipes will be emphasizing whole grains and legumes. In Phase II of the low-fat, high-carbohydrate diet, lunch, the smaller meal of the day, was changed by using beans, grains and low-fat animal products in place of meat. In Phase III the larger meal of the day becomes very different. A large variety of new flavours and spices will be introduced. An example of entrées for dinner over a week include lean beef or pork for 1–2 days, poultry for 2–3 days, fish for 2–3 days, and meatless for 1–2 days. During Phase III, the transition from the current Western diet to the low-fat, high-carbohydrate diet will have been completed (Table 7). Sample menus for one week are provided in Table 8.

Special occasions: eating away from home, and entertainment Many restaurants serve a variety of the foods recommended in Phase III of the low-fat, high-carbohydrate diet. Oriental, Italian, Mexican and Middle Eastern restaurants all have tasty foods to choose from. In the inevitable situation where the food choices are minimal, such as at parties or when eating in friends' homes, one can concentrate upon the salad, vegetable, fruit and cereal foods and take small amounts of the animal foods to be used as condiments. Guests entertained at home can be introduced to a new way of eating which they will discover to be attractive, tasty and healthful. Obviously, meeting the goals for Phase III is very difficult when eating out of the home. Therefore, one needs to eat meals at home which are as low-fat as possible to meet the goals. Then, by being selective about the frequency of eating out and by making choices, one can afford to have special occasions or feasts which include extra meat, cheese, chocolate and coconut.

Chemical and nutrient content The chemical composition of the Western diet and the three phases of the low-fat, high-carbohydrate diet are given in Figure 8. The Western diet contains approximately 500 mg cholesterol per day. This is decreased in Phase I to 350 mg, in Phase II to 200 mg, and in Phase III to 100 mg per day. The fat content decreases from 40% of calories

Table 8 Low fat, high carbohydrate sample menus

Day 1	Day 2	Day 3	Day 4	Day 5	Day 6	Day 7
Cantaloupe Raisin bran cereal Skim milk English muffin with jam	Orange juice Whole wheat pancakes topped with unsweetened applesauce	Plain low-fat yogurt with banana, cereal Bran muffins*	Berries Shredded wheat Skim milk Whole grain toast	Grapefruit half Potatoes (hashbrowned with small amount of oil in non-stick pan) Whole grain toast with marmalade	Blueberries Hot whole grain cereal Skim milk English muffin	Fresh melon German oven pancakes*
Tuna sandwich (water-packed tuna mixed with tangy dressing* or fat-free mayonnaise) Carrot sticks Fresh fruit	Chili bean salad* in whole wheat pocket bread Tomato soup (Campbell's low-sodium) Fresh fruit Graham crackers	Lentil soup* Low-fat crackers Laughing Cow reduced calories cheese Fresh fruit	Bean burritos Lettuce and sliced tomato Fresh fruit	Salad bar (greens topped with kidney beans, tomato, radishes, garbanzo beans, and cucumbers) Low-calorie commercial or Western dressing* Bagel Fruit	Peanut butter and jelly sandwich Vegetable sticks (carrot, celery, etc) Fresh orange Whole wheat fig bar	Minestrone soup Wheat berry rolls Low-fat cottage cheese Fresh fruit
Bean lasagna* Tossed salad with Western dressing* French bread Fresh berries	Cashew chicken* Steamed rice Fresh pineapple slices Wheat berry rolls Hot fudge pudding cake*	Easy tuna noodle casserole* Steamed broccoli Confetti Appleslaw* Wheat rolls Strawberry ice*	Pizza rice casserole* Green peas Green salad with low-calorie dressing Sourdough rolls Gingersnaps	Baked herbed fish* Baked potato with mock sour cream* Steamed zucchini Waldorf salad* Caraway puffs*	Corn chips* with bean dip* Creamy enchiladas* Meatless Spanish rice Shredded lettuce and tomato Fresh fruit	Spaghetti with marinara sauce* Tossed salad with low-calorie dressing Steamed green beans seasoned with lemon and pepper, French bread, Fresh fruit

*Recipes from ref. 87

370

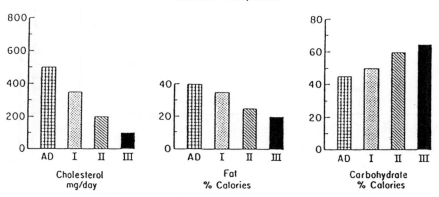

Phases of the "Alternative American Diet"
Chemical Composition

*Saturated fat not to exceed 6% total calories

Figure 8 The cholesterol, fat, and carbohydrate content of the Western diet (AD) and the phases of the low fat, high carbohydrate diet (I, II, III)

in the Western diet to 35% in Phase I, to 25% in Phase II, and to 20% in Phase III, with special consideration given to the decrease of saturated fat. In order to have sufficient calories to meet body needs we propose a gradual increase in carbohydrate, with emphasis on the use of the fibre-containing complex carbohydrates found in whole grains, cereal products and legumes. The increase in carbohydrate content to 65% in Phase III increases the bulk of the diet considerably, a feature which induces satiety sooner per unit of calories and helps to promote weight loss. The dietary fibre content of the low-fat, high-carbohydrate diet increases from 10 to 12 g per day to 35 to 50 g per day. Increasing the complex carbohydrate as fruits, vegetables, grains and beans will ensure that 30% of the fibre intake is soluble fibre (11–15 g). Even though the total carbohydrate is increased, the refined sugar content is actually decreased, from 20 to 10% of calories, and a greater emphasis is placed on eating more fruit.

Using the low-fat, high-carbohydrate diet for patients who are also hypertensive or diabetic A persistent problem in the dietary treatment of disease has been the use of a separate and individual diet for each disease. A good example would be the hyperlipidemic patient who also has high blood pressure and has been advised to follow a low-sodium, high-potassium diet. Such a diet is completely compatible with the low-fat, high-carbohydrate diet, which has incorporated into its design a phased approach to a low-sodium and high-potassium intake[83,84,87]. Should caloric reduction be required to treat obesity, the low-fat, high-carbohydrate diet in reduced calories can be utilized. This diet has also been used in the treatment of diabetic patients[62]. The high

Table 9 Predicted plasma cholesterol lowering from the three phases of the low fat, high carbohydrate diet

	Total Fat*	Saturated Fat*	Polyun-saturated Fat*	P/S	Cholesterol (mg/day)	Predicted total change in plasma cholesterol from Western diet to each phase (per cent)	Predicted change in plasma cholesterol from phase to phase (per cent)
Western diet	40	15	6	0.4	500		
Low fat, high carbohydrate diet							
Phase 1	35	14	9	0.6	350	−6	−6
Phase II	25	8	8	1.0	200	−13	−7
Phase III	20	5	8	1.3	100	−19	−6

*per cent of the total calories
calculated per the formula of Hegsted, McGandy, Myers, and Stare[40]

Chol = 2.16 S − 1.65 P + 6.77 C − 0.53

Where Chol = the change in plasma cholesterol in mg/dl

S = the change in saturated fat as per cent of total calories

P = the change in polyunsaturated fat as per cent of total calories

C = the change in dietary cholesterol intake in decigrams/day

The baseline diet from which changes have been made is the Western diet.

intakes of complex carbohydrate and fibre are in keeping with the latest trends in diabetic diets.

Predicted plasma cholesterol lowering from the three phases of the low-fat, high-carbohydrate diet As has been emphasized, both dietary cholesterol and saturated fat elevate plasma cholesterol levels, whereas polyunsaturated fat has a mild depressing effect. By steps, the cholesterol and saturated fat of each phase of the low-fat, high-carbohydrate diet are progressively reduced, with Phase III providing for the lowest intakes. According to calculations derived from Hegsted and co-workers[40], one would expect a 6 to 7% decrease, on the average, in the plasma total and LDL cholesterol level for each dietary phase (Table 9). If a patient were to reach Phase III goals there would be, on the average, an 18 to 21% lowering of the plasma cholesterol level. Approximately one-half of the plasma cholesterol lowering would result from decreasing dietary cholesterol intake from 500 to 100 mg/day and one-half of the lowering would result from decreasing saturated fat intake from 14 to 5% of calories.

For example, a patient with a plasma cholesterol level of 300 mg/dl when consuming the typical Western diet would have a plasma cholesterol level of 237 to 246 mg/dl if Phase III goals were to be achieved. Then a small dose of one of the hypocholesterolemic drugs would be used to decrease the plasma cholesterol further to below 200 mg/dl.

The scenario just described represents a mean plasma cholesterol response to dietary change. Based on the data from Katan *et al.*[18], one would estimate that 75 to 85% of people who achieved maximal dietary changes would have a plasma cholesterol decrease of 9% or greater and 50% of those people would have an 18% or greater reduction in the plasma cholesterol level. Extrapolation from the Lipid Research Clinics Primary Prevention Trial results, which showed a 2% reduction in risk for coronary disease for every 1% reduction in plasma cholesterol[92], one might then expect that 50% of individuals maximally reducing their plasma cholesterol level by diet would decrease their coronary risk by 36% and 75 to 85% of individuals having such reductions would decrease their coronary risk by 18%.

Summary and conclusions

The dietary treatment and prevention of the atherosclerotic lesions underlying coronary heart disease have a logical and well-established rationale which has been developed over the past three decades. The low-fat, high-carbohydrate diet for these purposes is designed to prevent and treat hyperlipidemia and to have an antithrombotic action. The proposed low-cholesterol, low-fat diet is safe, inexpensive, and can become habitual through the process of gradual change, practice and patience. It offers a practical means of dealing with some of the key risk factors in coronary heart disease, especially hyperlipidemia. Furthermore, the same dietary philosophy may be applied to hyperlipidemias of differing severity, of different etiologies and of different lipoprotein types.

This dietary approach may be used with therapeutic benefit at any stage in the development of coronary heart disease. Atherosclerosis is inevitably progressive but focal. The same coronary artery may have occlusive lesions in one location and in neighbouring locations only beginning lesions. Likewise, in other coronaries the lesions may be minimal, severe or variable. Thus, the complete therapy of coronary heart disease must concentrate upon the removal or alleviation of those factors causing plaques to worsen and upon enhancing those factors promoting regression of atherosclerosis.

The primary prevention of coronary heart disease is clearly the ultimate goal to deal most effectively with the current epidemic of coronary heart disease. The dietary changes suggested for the coronary patient are completely safe and are prudent measures to be followed by any population (i.e., Western) at serious risk for coronary disease. These nutritional changes should be instituted early in life when they will have the greatest impact. This is a familial disease and its control and treatment can best be approached on a family basis.

The primary prevention of coronary heart disease is dependent upon the prevention of diet-induced hyperlipidemia.

Acknowledgements

Permission has been granted by the publishers to reproduce material from references[83-85].

References

1. Intersalt Cooperative Research Group. (1988). Intersalt: an international study of electrolyte excretion and blood pressure. Results for 24 hour urinary sodium and potassium excretion. *Br. Med. J.*, **297**, 319–28
2. Armstrong, M.L., Warner, E.D. and Connor, W.E. (1970). Regression of coronary atheromatosis in Rhesus monkeys. *Circ. Res.*, **27**, 59–67
3. Armstrong, M.L., Connor, W.E. and Warner, E.D. (1967). Xanthomatosis in Rhesus monkeys fed a hypercholesterolemic diet. *Arch. Pathol.*, **84**, 226–37
4. Taylor, C.B., Cox, G.E., Counts, M. *et al.* (1959). Fatal myocardial infarction in Rhesus monkeys with diet-induced hypercholesterolemia. *Circulation*, **20**, 975. (Abstract)
5. Connor, W.E. and Connor, S.L. (1972). The key role of nutritional factors in the prevention of coronary heart disease. *Prev. Med.*, **1**, 49–83
6. Lin, D.S. and Connor, W.E. (1981). The long-term effects of dietary cholesterol upon the plasma lipids, lipoproteins, cholesterol absorption, and the sterol balance in man: the demonstration of feedback inhibition of cholesterol biosynthesis and increased bile acid excretion. *J. Lipid Res.*, **21**, 1042–52
7. Spady, D.K. and Dietschy, J.M. (1985). Dietary saturated triacylglycerols suppress hepatic low density lipoprotein receptor activity in the hamster. *Proc. Natl. Acad. Sci. USA*, **82**, 4526–30
8. Spady, D.K. and Dietschy, J.M. (1988). Interaction of dietary cholesterol and triglycerides in the regulation of hepatic low density lipoprotein transport in the hamster. *J. Clin. Invest.*, **81**, 300–9
9. Kovanen, P.T., Brown, M.S., Basu, S.K., Bilheimer, D.W. and Goldstein, J.L. (1981). Saturation and suppression of hepatic lipoprotein receptors: a mechanism for the hypercholesterolemia of cholesterol-fed rabbits. *Proc. Natl. Acad. Sci. USA*, **78**, 1396–400
10. Mahley, R.W., Hui, D.Y., Innerarity, T.L. and Weisgraber, K.H. (1981). Two independent lipoprotein receptors on hepatic membranes of dog, swine and man. *J. Clin. Invest.*, **68**, 1197–206
11. Beveridge, J.M.R., Connell, W.F., Mayer, G.A. and Haust, H.L. (1960). The response of man to dietary cholesterol. *J. Nutr.*, **71**, 61–5
12. Connor, W.E., Hodges, R.E. and Bleiler, R.E. (1961). The serum lipids in men receiving high cholesterol and cholesterol-free diets. *J. Clin. Invest.*, **40**, 894–900

13. Connor, W.E., Stone, D.B. and Hodges, R.E. (1964). The interrelated effects of dietary cholesterol and fat upon the human serum lipid levels. *J. Clin. Invest.*, **43**, 1691–6

14. Steiner, A., Howard, E.J. and Akgun, S. (1962). Importance of dietary cholesterol in man. *J. Am. Med. Assoc.*, **181**, 186–90

15. Connor, W.E. and Connor, S.L. (1986). Dietary cholesterol and fat and the prevention of coronary heart disease: risks and benefits of nutritional change. In Hallgren, B. *et al.* (eds.) *Diet and Prevention of Coronary Heart Disease and Cancer*, pp. 113–47. (New York: Raven Press)

16. Roberts, S.L., McMurry, M. and Connor, W.E. (1981). Does egg feeding (i.e. dietary cholesterol) affect plasma cholesterol levels in humans? The results of a double-blind study. *Am. J. Clin. Nutr.*, **34**, 2092–9

17. Gordon, T., Fisher, M., Ernst, N. and Rifkind, B.M. (1982). Relation of diet to LDL cholesterol, VLDL cholesterol and plasma total cholesterol and triglycerides in white adults. *Arteriosclerosis*, **2**, 502–12

18. Katan, M.B., Beynen, A.C., De Vries, J.H.M. and Nobels, A. (1986). Existence of consistent hypo- and hyperresponders to dietary cholesterol in man. *Am. J. Epidemiol.*, **123**, 221–34

19. Connor, W.E., Rohwedder, J.J. and Hoak, J.C. (1963). The production of hypercholesterolemia and atherosclerosis by a diet rich in shellfish. *J. Nutr.*, **79**, 443–50

20. Flaim, E., Ferreri, L.F., Thye, F.W., Hill, J.E. and Ritchey, S.F. (1981). Plasma lipid and lipoprotein cholesterol concentrations in adult males consuming normal and high cholesterol diets under controlled conditions. *Am. J. Clin. Nutr.*, **34**, 1103–8

21. Connor, W.E., Hodges, R.E. and Bleiler, R.E. (1961). The effect of dietary cholesterol upon the serum lipids in man. *J. Lab. Clin. Med.*, **57**, 331–42

22. Connor, W.E., Witiak, D.T., Stone, D.B. and Armstrong, M.L. (1969). Cholesterol balance and fecal neutral steroid and bile acid excretion in normal men fed dietary fats of different fatty acid composition. *J. Clin. Invest.*, **48**, 1363–75

23. Mistry, P., Miller, N.E., Laker, M., Hazzard, W.R. and Lewis, B. (1981). Individual variations in the effect of dietary cholesterol on plasma lipoproteins and cellular cholesterol homeostasis in man. *J. Clin. Invest.*, **67**, 493–502

24. Mahley, R.W., Innerarity, T., Rall, S.C. *et al.* (1984). Plasma lipoproteins: apolipoprotein structure and function. *J. Lipid. Res.*, **25**, 1277–94

25. Gregg, R.E. and Brewer, H.B. Jr. (1986). The role of apolipoprotein E in modulating the metabolism of apolipoprotein B-48 and apolipoprotein B-100 containing lipoproteins in humans. In Angel, A. and Frohlich, J. (eds.) Lipoprotein deficiency syndromes. *Adv. Exp. Med. Biol.*, **201**, 289–98

26. Ahrens, E.H., Hirsch, J. and Insull, W. (1957). The influence of dietary fats on serum lipid levels in man. *Lancet*, **1**, 943–53

27. Keys, A., Anderson, J.T. and Grande, F. (1957). Serum cholesterol response to dietary fat. *Lancet*, **1**, 787

28. Zilversmit, D.B. (1979). Atherogenesis: a postprandial phenomenon. *Circulation*, **60**, 473–85

29. Brown, M.S. and Goldstein, J.L. (1986). A receptor-mediated pathway for cholesterol homeostasis. *Science*, **232**, 34–47

30. Lin, D.S., Spenler, C.W. and Connor, W.E. The effects of different dietary fatty acids upon the fatty acid composition of adipose tissue: saturated, monounsaturated and n-3 and n-6 polyunsaturated fatty acids. Unpublished observations

31. Becker, N., Illingworth, D.R., Alaupovic, P., Connor, W.E. and Sundberg, E.E. (1983). Effects of saturated, monounsaturated, and omega-6 polyunsaturated fatty acids on plasma lipids, lipoproteins and apoproteins in humans. *Am. J. Clin. Nutr.*, **37**, 355–60

32. Grundy, S.M. (1986). Comparison of monounsaturated fatty acids and carbohydrates for lowering plasma cholesterol. *N. Engl. J. Med.*, **314**, 745–8

33. Mattson, F.H. and Grundy, S.M. (1985). Comparison of effects of dietary saturated, monounsaturated and polyunsaturated fatty acids on plasma lipids and lipoproteins in men. *J. Lipid Res.*, **26**, 194–202

34. Goodnight, S.H. Jr., Harris, W.S., Connor, W.E. and Illingworth, D.R. (1982). Polyunsaturated fatty acids, hyperlipidemia and thrombosis. *Arteriosclerosis*, **2**, 87–113

35. Harris, W.S. and Connor, W.E. (1980). The effects of salmon oil upon plasma lipids, lipoprotein and triglyceride clearance. *Trans. Assoc. Am. Physicians*, **93**, 148–55

36. Harris, W.S., Connor, W.E., Alam, N. and Illingworth, D.R. (1988). The reduction of postprandial triglyceridemia in humans by dietary n-3 fatty acids. *J. Lipid Res.*, **29**, 1451–60

37. Weiner, B.H., Ockene, I.S., Levine, P.H. *et al.* (1986). Inhibition of atherosclerosis by cod liver oil in a hyperlipidemic swine model. *N. Engl. J. Med.*, **315**, 841–6

38. Davis, H.R., Bridenstine, R.T., Vesselinovitch, D. and Wissler, R.W. (1987). Fish oil inhibits development of atherosclerosis in Rhesus monkeys. *Arteriosclerosis*, **7**, 441–9

39. Kromhout, D., Bosschieter, E.B. and Coulander, CdeL. (1985). The inverse relation between fish consumption and 20-year mortality from coronary heart disease. *N. Engl. J. Med.*, **312**, 1205–9

40. Hegsted, D.M., McGandy, R.B., Myers, M.L. and Stare, F.J. (1965). Quantitative effects of dietary fat on serum cholesterol in man. *Am. J. Clin. Nutr.*, **17**, 281–95

41. Keys, A., Anderson, J.T. and Grande, F. (1957). Prediction of serum-cholesterol responses of man to changes in fats in the diet. *Lancet*, **2**, 959–66

42. Mensink, R.P. and Katan, M.B. (1990). Effect of dietary trans fatty acids on high-density and low-density lipoprotein cholesterol levels in healthy subjects. *N. Engl. J. Med.*, **323**, 439–45

43. Hunter, J.E. and Applewhite, T.H. (1991). Reassessment of *trans* fatty acid availability in the US diet. *Am. J. Clin. Nutr.*, **54**, 363–9

44. Haslam, R.J. (1964). Role of adenosine diphosphate in the aggregation of human blood-platelets by thrombin and by fatty acids. *Nature*, **202**, 765–8

45. Hoak, J.C., Warner, E.D. and Connor, W.E. (1967). Platelets, fatty acids and thrombosis. *Circ. Res.*, **20**, 11–17

46. Mahadevan, V., Singh, M.H. and Lundberg, W.O. (1966). Effects of saturated and unsaturated fatty acids on blood platelet aggregation in vitro. *Proc. Soc. Exp. Biol. Med.*, **121**, 82–5

47. Renaud, S., Kinlough, R.L. and Mustard, J.F. (1970). Relationship between platelet aggregation and the thrombotic tendency in rats fed hyperlipemic diets. *Lab. Invest.*, **22**, 339–43

48. Beckett, A.G. and Lewis, J.G. (1960). Mobilization and utilization of body fat as an aetiological factor in occlusive vascular disease in diabetes mellitus. *Lancet*, **2**, 14–18

49. Fredrickson, D.S. and Gordon, R.S. Jr. (1958). Transport of fatty acids. *Physiol. Rev.*, **38**, 585–630

50. Gjesdal, K. (1976). Platelet function and plasma free fatty acids during acute myocardial infarction and severe angina pectoris. *Scand. J. Haematol.*, **17**, 205–12

51. Gjesdal, K., Nordoy, A., Wang, H., Berntsen, H. and Mjos, O.D. (1976). Effects of fasting on plasma and platelet-free fatty acids and platelet function in healthy males. *Thromb. Haemost.*, **36**, 325–33

52. Kurien, V.A. and Oliver, M.F. (1966). Serum free fatty acids after myocardial infarction and cerebral vascular occlusion. *Lancet*, **1**, 122–7

53. Connor, W.E., Hoak, J.C. and Warner, E.D. (1969). Plasma free fatty acids, hypercoagulability and thrombosis. In Sherry, S., Brinkhous, K.M., Genton, E.D. and Stengle, J.M. (eds.) *Thrombosis*, pp. 355–73. (Washington, DC: Natl. Acad. Sci.)

54. Bang, H.O. and Dyerberg, J. (1980). Lipid metabolism and ischemic heart disease in Greenland Eskimos. In Draper, H.H. (ed.) *Advanced Nutrition Research*, vol. 3, pp. 1–22. (New York: Plenum Press)

55. Bang, H.O., Dyerberg, J. and Hjorne, N. (1973). The composition of food consumed by Greenlandic Eskimos. *Acta Med. Scand.*, **200**, 69–73

56. Dyerberg, J. and Bang, H.O. (1979). Hemostatic function and platelet polyunsaturated fatty acids in Eskimos. *Lancet*, **2**, 433–5

57. Goodnight, S.H. Jr., Harris, W.S. and Connor, W.E. (1981). The effects of dietary omega-3 fatty acids upon platelet composition and function in man: a prospective, controlled study. *Blood*, **58**, 880–5

58. Burkitt, D.P. (1972). Varicose veins, deep vein thrombosis, and hemorrhoids. *Br. Med. J.*, **2**, 556–61

59. Davies, J.N.P. (1948). Pathology of central African natives. IX Cardiovascular diseases. *East African Med. J.*, **25**, 454–67

60. Latto, C. (1981). Hemorrhoids, diverticular disease and deep vein thrombosis. In: Trowell, H.C. and Burkitt, D.P. (eds.) *Western Diseases: Their Emergence and Prevention*, pp. 421–4. (Cambridge, Ma: Harvard University Press)

61. Ahrens, E.H., Hirsch, J., Oette, K., Farquhar, J.W. and Stein, Y. (1961). Carbohydrate-induced and fat-induced lipemia. *Trans. Assoc. Am. Physicians*, **74**, 134–46

62. Stone, D.B. and Connor, W.E. (1963). The prolonged effects of a low cholesterol, high carbohydrate diet upon the serum lipids in diabetic patients. *Diabetes*, **12**, 127–32

63. Weinsier, R.L., Seeman, A., Herrera, M.G., Assul, J-P., Soeldner, J.S. and Gleason, R.G. (1974). High and low carbohydrate diets in diabetes: study of effects on diabetic control, insulin secretion and blood lipids. *Ann. Intern. Med.*, **80**, 332–41

64. Ullmann, D., Connor, W.E., Hatcher, L.F., Connor, S.L. and Flavell, D.P. (1991). Will a high-carbohydrate low-fat diet lower plasma lipids and lipoproteins without producing hypertriglyceridemia? *Arteriosclerosis and Thrombosis*, **11**, 1059–67

65. Nikkila, E.A. and Ojala, K. (1965). Induction of hypertriglyceridemia by fructose in the rat. *Life Sci.*, **4**, 937–43

66. Keys, A., Grande, F. and Anderson, J.T. (1961). Fiber and pectin in the diet and serum cholesterol concentration in man. *Proc. Soc. Exp. Biol. Med.*, **106**, 555–8

67. Grande, F., Anderson, J.T. and Keys, A. (1965). Effect of carbohydrates of leguminous seeds, wheat and potatoes on serum cholesterol concentration in man. *J. Nutr.*, **86**, 313–17

68. Raymond, T.L., Connor, W.E., Lin, D.S., Warner, S., Fry, M.M. and Connor, S.L. (1971). The interaction of dietary fibers and cholesterol upon the plasma lipids and lipoproteins, the sterol balance, and bowel function in human subjects. *J. Clin. Invest.*, **60**, 1429–37

69. Anderson, J.W., Story, L., Sieling, B., Chen, W.J.L., Petro, M.S. and Story, J. (1984). Hypocholesterolemic effects of oat-bran or bean intake for hypercholesterolemic men. *Am. J. Clin. Nutr.*, **40**, 1146–55

70. Kay, R.M. and Truswell, A.S. (1977). Effect of citrus pectin on blood lipids and fecal steroid excretion in man. *Am. J. Clin. Nutr.*, **30**, 171–5

71. McLean Ross, A.H., Eastwood, M.A., Anderson, J.R. and Anderson, D.M.W. (1983). A study of the effects of dietary gum arabic in humans. *Am. J. Clin. Nutr.*, **37**, 368–75

72. Galbraith, W.B., Connor, W.E. and Stone, D.B. (1966). Weight loss and serum lipid changes in obese subjects given low-calorie diets of varied cholesterol content. *Ann. Intern. Med.*, **64**, 268–75

73. Olefsky, J., Reaven, G.M. and Farquhar, J.W. (1974). Effects of weight reduction on obesity. *J. Clin. Invest.*, **53**, 64–76

74. Schwartz, R.S. and Brunzell, J.D. (1981). Increase of adipose tissue lipoprotein lipase activity with weight loss. *J. Clin. Invest.*, **67**, 1425–30

75. Castelli, W.P., Gordon, T., Hjortland, M.C. *et al.* (1977). Alcohol and blood lipids. *Lancet*, **2**, 153–5

76. St Leger, A.S., Cochrance, A.L. and Moore, F. (1979). Factors associated with cardiac mortality in developed countries with particular reference to the consumption of wine. *Lancet*, **1**, 1017–20

77. Haskell, W.L., Camargo, C., Williams, P.T. *et al.* (1984). The effect of cessation and resumption of moderate alcohol intake on serum high-density-lipoprotein subfractions. *N. Engl. J. Med.*, **310**, 805–10

78. Wood, P.D., Haskell, W.L., Blair, S.N. *et al.* (1983). Increased exercise level and plasma lipoprotein concentrations: a one-year randomized, controlled study in sedentary middle-aged men. *Metabolism*, **32**, 31–9

79. Katz, L.N., Stamler, J. and Pick, R. (1958). *Nutrition and Atherosclerosis*, p. 98. (Philadelphia: Lea and Febiger)

80. Peterson, V.E., Crapo, P.A., Weininger, J. *et al.* (1975). Quantification of plasma cholesterol and triglyceride levels in hypercholesterolemic subjects receiving ascorbic acid supplements. *Am. J. Clin. Nutr.*, **28**, 584–7

81. Beveridge, J.M.R., Connell, W.F. and Mayer, G.A. (1957). The nature of the substances in dietary fat affecting the level of plasma cholesterol in humans. *Can. J. Biochem. Physiol.*, **35**, 257–70

82. Muenter, M.D., Perry, H.O. and Jurgen, L. (1971). Chronic vitamin A intoxication in adults. *Am. J. Med.*, **50**, 129–36

83. Connor, W.E. and Connor, S.L. (1982). The dietary treatment of hyperlipidemia: rationale, technique and efficacy. In Havel, R.J. (ed.) Lipid Disorders. *Med. Clin. N. Am.*, **66**, 485–518

84. Connor, W.E. and Connor, S.L. (1985). The dietary prevention and treatment of coronary heart disease. In Connor, W.E. and Bristow, J.D. (eds.) *Coronary Heart Disease: Prevention, Complications and Treatment*, pp. 43–64. (Philadelphia: Lippincott)

85. Connor, S.L., Artaud-Wild, S.M., Classick-Kohn, C.J. *et al.* (1986). The cholesterol saturated fat index: an indication of the hypercholesterolemic and atherogenic potential of food. *Lancet*, **1**, 1229–32

86. Zilversmit, D.B. (1979). Cholesterol index of foods. *J. Am. Dietet. Assoc.*, **74**, 562–5

87. Connor, S.L. and Connor, W.E. (1986). *The New American Diet*. (New York: Simon & Schuster)

88. Dobbin, L.V., Gofman, H.F., Jones, L. *et al.* (1957). *The Low Fat, Low Cholesterol Diet*. (New York: Doubleday)

89. Brewster, L. and Jacobson, M.F. (1978). *The Changing American Diet*. (Washington, DC: Center for Science in the Public Interest)

90. Welsh, S.O. and Marston, R.M. (1982). Review of trends in food use in the United States, 1909 to 1980. *J. Am. Dietet. Assoc.*, **81**, 120–5

91. Connor, W.E., Connor, S.L., Fry, M.M. and Warner, S. (1976). *The Alternative Diet Book*. (Iowa City: University of Iowa Press)

92. Lipid research clinics programs: the lipid research clinics coronary primary prevention trial results: I. Reduction in incidence of coronary heart disease. (1984). *J. Am. Med. Assoc.*, **251**, 351–64

Discussion

Dr Wood: I would like to know what is the mean life expectancy of the Tarahumara Indians. Secondly, what was the composition of the fat compared to the United States in the study where you had the 25 humans?

Dr Connor: Let me answer the second part of your question first. In regard to the composition of the fat, there was a P/S ratio of about one, so this is a little less saturated than the typical American intake. But certainly this was not a highly polyunsaturated fat diet. The fats used in that experiment were a combination of peanut oil, cocoa butter and a little safflower oil.

The life expectancy of all people living like the Tarahumara Indians with no sanitation, with a high prevalence of infectious disease, living in caves or log cabins in which there is a lot of smoke, fire in the centre of the building coming out through an opening, is not very great. There are old Tarahumaras and we were able to find them. The Tarahumaras have the typical life expectancy that was present in the United States at the time of the revolutionary war, which was in the neighbourhood of 35 years. With sanitation and adequate nutrition I think their life expectancy would be pretty good. A comparable population, which was alluded to yesterday, would be the Japanese population, which in preaffluent Japan, were consuming a diet which was chemically not too different from the Tarahumara diet. So, if the Tarahumara Indians were able to obtain enough to eat and their sanitation problems were solved, I think they would probably have a good life expectancy. Mind you, I am not advocating that we return to the diet or the lifestyle of the Tarahumara Indians, which none of us would find very satisfying.

Dr Horlick: You told us what we might expect from maximal diet modification, what might we expect for instance, by implementing the National Cholesterol Education Program (NCEP) guidelines?

Dr Connor: I think that we do not know for sure, but one could make some sort of prediction. I think we will have a dietary change somewhat similar to what we obtained in our family heart study in Portland, Oregon. Our family heart study went on for over 5 years in over 800 healthy people, including children. During this time we had many births in this young adult population. I think we saw approximately a 4% plasma cholesterol level change totally. I think the guidelines will produce something in this neighbourhood over a certain period of time. However, I think the changes will occur more rapidly now because industry and agriculture are providing low-fat products which will make a lower fat way of eating much easier. I think these changes will occur much easier than in our family heart study which we started in the late 1970s.

Dr Grover: Your data are interesting and point out one of the potential complications of diet and that is that it looks like HDL cholesterol follows the same general direction as total cholesterol. In other words, if the total cholesterol comes down 20%, HDL comes down 20% as well. If we extrapolate from both the Framingham data and studies like the Helsinki Heart Study, one would predict that lowering of HDL cholesterol would have a negative impact or an inverse effect on CHD. In other words, if you lower total serum cholesterol you lower your risk, but if you lower HDL cholesterol, you increase the risk by the same amount. Could you comment on that please?

Dr Connor: I think that is a possibility, but unlikely because LDL cholesterol also falls. We have to appreciate that there are no trials in which HDL alone has been increased or lowered. I believe that the favourable result of the Helsinki Heart Trial has been misinterpreted as an HDL effect. Actually, the main effect was on VLDL and total triglyceride and was the result of the agent, gemfibrozil. I think that this is really what happened, rather than the not too great HDL changes. However, the publicity concerning this study has focused on HDL. There really is not a precise answer to your question but I think cholesterol lowering diets will, in general, lower HDL but the upshot is that, LDL is going to be lowered further. As far as we know in experimental animals, it is LDL that produces atherosclerosis and not low HDL concentrations. Populations with both low LDL and HDL levels (i.e. the Tarahumara Indians) do not develop coronary heart disease.

Dr Goldbloom: I wonder, in the experiments you quoted earlier in your talk of the high- and low-fat diet in monkeys, did you observe any behavioural change in the animals when they were undergoing the low-fat diet?

Dr Connor: No, of course one has to appreciate that the diet of the monkey in the wild is very low in fat and these monkeys had been maintained on low-fat Purina monkey chow ever since we encountered them, so that we really continued their low-fat diet. We did not observe any behavioural changes.

Dr Goldbloom: What about on the high-fat intake? Did they become less aggressive or more aggressive?

Dr Connor: Caged Rhesus monkeys are aggressive at all times, regardless of diet.

Dr Isles: How does the CSI of a Mediterranean diet and the low coronary mortality of the French, Italians and Greeks fit into your scheme of things?

Dr Connor: I would say it fits in beautifully because their diet would be a low CSI diet. We have to appreciate the fact that the Mediterranean diet was low in cholesterol and saturated fat even though it had a good deal of olive oil in it. Even in Crete where the olive oil consumption was 40% of the total calories, the CSI was relatively low. I showed you the data on olive oil, which has a relatively low CSI. However, those countries are changing their diets as Ancel Keys' seven country data are illustrating. What is happening is that they are consuming less olive oil and having more butter and more dairy products and more meat, so that the CSI is increasing and also the propensity to develop coronary heart disease.

Dr Naylor: I was struck that you drew a comparison between your aboriginal population and potential life expectancy in Japan. Would it not be true that in Japan the intake of fish would be an important confounder in terms of ω-3 fatty acids and that the analogy might not be all that convincing if you consider that as a confounder?

The second point that I would like to make is that you alluded to the Hegsted equations and modifications thereof. As I understand it, those equations were developed in metabolic ward studies using diets extremely high in polyunsaturates which probably, in light of their effects on HDL, would not be regarded as desirable today. Could you comment on how the Hegsted equations, or modifications, might lead to overestimates of the dietary effects to be obtained with the step one and step two diets of the American Heart Association?

Dr Connor: I accept your modification of the Japanese diet as having more fish, certainly it does. The Tarahumara Indians liked fish also, although they did not have it has often as the Japanese. What I had wanted to illustrate by referring to the Japanese was that, until recently, they represented a population which consumed a low-fat diet, not much higher than the Tarahumara diet. I did not mean to imply that their diets were identical.

The Hegsted equations were based on literally dozens and dozens of metabolic ward experiments. In these studies, not only was polyunsaturated fat used, but various combinations of saturated and monounsaturated fat. Monounsaturated fats were taken out of the equations because they appeared to be relatively neutral compared to saturated and polyunsaturated fat. We have found that the predictive value from using these equations in our metabolic experiments, that were done later than those of Keys and Hegsted, fit the equations fairly well.

Dr Skrabanek: If you believe what you say, would you stick to your convictions and recommend the Tarahumara diet for people with high risk of heart disease? Second, would you expect, again if you believe what you say, that these people would not die of heart disease and also would not die of something else instead? A simple and interesting experiment would be to give the Tarahumara population, or half of them, enough to eat and to improve their sanitation. Then you would wait and see if this really improves their life expectancy beyond that of the American population. I think that there is no relevance for the rest of the affluent world to use examples of Tarahumara Indians or Masai or Eskimo except to show that the human species is wonderfully adaptable. Humans can survive on a 75% carbohydrate diet or, in the case of Masai, on a diet consisting of 50% fat, but to extrapolate this to people in the Western world with relatively high life expectancy simply does not follow.

Dr Connor: I think that depends on the point of view. I would stress that the World Health Organization has made as a major health effort the prevention of CHD in these developing populations. Obviously, the cost of health care for coronary patients in the two billion Chinese, should they move to a high-fat diet, would be astronomical. If these developing populations adopt the Western way of life, including their diet, it is estimated by all who look at the situation that CHD is going to become very common in those countries, a very costly problem and a significant cause of death and disability as it is in our own society. What we have not mentioned in our discussions thus far is the high cost of CHD from the point of view of health care delivery and the high cost in terms of suffering and morbidity that our population currently has. It would seem that any approach to health care must address these problems. To think that coronary heart disease will go away without decisive public health measures is merely wishful thinking.

Dr Skrabanek: You said that the diet is so protective of heart disease, so why not recommend this diet to the population at high risk? I know you said that you would not recommend this diet to the general population because it is not palatable but if you are really desperate to help those with heart disease, why would you not recommend this kind of diet then?

Dr Connor: The Tarahumara diet is ideal for Tarahumaras but would not be appropriate for all populations. Americans simply will not eat that kind of a diet. You made the suggestion that humans are infinitely adaptable and I think that is partly true but, I do not think that we are adaptable enough to eat it even with the best motivation. We lost weight on the diet and were more than glad to see a bowl of corn flakes on the way home to the United States. The Tarahumara diet is too bulky and monotonous. It is too coarse a diet. I would not recommend that diet. However, I would recommend a consideration of a lower fat diet, not as low as 12%, I think that is probably not necessary, but in the 20–25% range with a cholesterol intake of around 100 mg per day. I think that is a reasonable approach. In such a diet, we could use the kinds of foods as I illustrated from those recipes that we are already accustomed to. So, it is not a very drastic change in our way of life but it might be a change that would ultimately foster a much lower coronary attack rate.

Dr Parsons: Which part of the Tarahumara diet did you have trouble with, the corn or the beans? I ask this specifically because we are into another component here which is fibre, and did that play a role in the diet?

Dr Connor: The beans produced enough gas to keep some of us awake at night. That certainly is a socially undesirable quality of beans. If one is going to eat a lot of beans, they should be gradually introduced. Some people will be more susceptible to the bean effects than others. I think the bulk of the diet, eight tortillas, high in fibre, is too much. One tortilla is fine but eight at a sitting cannot be consumed with relish by a 'westernized' stomach!

22
The relationship between serum cholesterol and the incidence of type-specific stroke in Honolulu Japanese men

K. YANO and D.M. REED

Although the association of serum total cholesterol with coronary heart disease is well established, its relationship to stroke is less clear. In Japan, where stroke is more common than coronary heart disease, ecological and prospective epidemiological studies indicated an inverse association of serum cholesterol with stroke, especially cerebral haemorrhage[1-5]. In the United States and Europe, most studies demonstrated no significant relationship between serum cholesterol and total stroke or cerebral infarct, while little attention has been paid to cerebral haemorrhage because of its relative scarcity[6-10]. Recently, however, Iso and his associates have reported on the basis of 6 years follow-up of 350 977 American men who participated in the Multiple Risk Factor Intervention Trial (MRFIT) screening examination that the mortality from intracranial haemorrhage was three times higher in men with serum cholesterol levels below 4.14 mmol/l (160 mg/dl) than those with higher cholesterol levels, and that this inverse association was confined to hypertensive men with diastolic blood pressure 90 mmHg or higher[11].

In earlier reports from the Honolulu Heart Program based on 6 and 10 years follow-up of approximately 8000 Japanese-American men in Hawaii, it was demonstrated that there was a significant inverse association of serum cholesterol with haemorrhagic stroke after controlling for age and other risk factors, while no significant relationship was found between serum cholesterol and thromboembolic stroke[12,13]. We present here results of our recent investigation on the relationship between baseline serum cholesterol levels and the incidence of type-specific stroke based on the expanding data of 20 years follow-up.

Methods

Study population

The Honolulu Heart Program is a prospective epidemiological investigation of coronary heart disease and stroke among men of Japanese ancestry who were born between 1900 and 1919 and were living on Oahu Island, Hawaii in 1965. Of the 11 136 eligible men identified through World War II Selective Service Registration files and located by updated information, 8006 participated in the initial examination during 1965–1968. Their ages at the entry examination ranged from 45 to 68. Repeat examinations were carried out 2 and 6 years later, with response rates of 95% and 90%, respectively. Also, the entire cohort has been followed for the development of coronary heart disease and stroke by a comprehensive morbidity and mortality surveillance based on hospital records and death certificates. Details of procedures for recruitment, examination, and surveillance are described elsewhere[14–17].

Case ascertainment

The ascertainment of incident stroke cases was made by a study neurologist who reviewed all hospital records with discharge diagnosis of definite or suspected stroke. The diagnosis of type-specific stroke was made on the basis of characteristic neurological symptoms and signs, lumbar puncture, the findings of neuroimaging such as nuclear brain scan, CT scan and arteriography, surgical intervention, and autopsy findings. The diagnostic certainty was also evaluated, and each stroke event was classified into definite, probable, possible, or doubtful by the specified criteria. Details of procedures for the diagnosis of stroke are given elsewhere[12].

In this report we included only definite or probable cases identified as the first event of incident stroke during the follow-up after the initial examination through December 1986. The length of follow-up was 18–21 years with an average of 19 years and 9 months. Less than 2% of the cohort were lost to follow-up, and virtually all definite or probable cases of stroke were hospitalized.

Risk factor measurement

At the initial examination, blood pressure was determined three times in the sitting position using a mercury sphygmomanometer. The average of three readings was used for the diagnosis of hypertension according to the WHO criteria. Body mass index, as an indicator of obesity, was determined by weight (kg)/height (m)^2. Serum total cholesterol, glucose and uric acid were determined using an Autoanalyzer on venous blood specimens 1 h after ingestion of 50 g glucose. Information on family history, past medical history, cigarette smoking, alcohol consumption, diet and physical activity have been obtained by an interview. Details of these procedures are given elsewhere[15].

Statistical analysis

In order to examine the relationship between baseline levels of serum cholesterol and the risk of type-specific stroke, age-adjusted incidence rates (per 1000 person-years) of stroke were calculated by the indirect method for seven subgroups of serum cholesterol ranging from below 4.14 mmol/l (160 mg/dl) to over 6.72 mmol/l (260 mg/dl), divided by an equal interval of 0.517 mmol/l (20 mg/dl). The association between serum cholesterol (as a continuous variable) and the incidence of stroke was tested using the Cox proportional hazards model[18], with age as a covariate. The statistical significance of the association was judged by Z value (beta/standard error). Also, a quadratic term of serum cholesterol was included in the model to examine whether a significant non-linear component (U-shaped or J-shaped curve) did exist in the relationship.

Furthermore, separate analyses were performed for hypertensive men and normotensive men to examine the possibility that the association of serum cholesterol with stroke was restricted to hypertensive men. As a statistical test for the significance of the interaction of serum cholesterol and hypertension, the product of these two variables was added in the Cox regression model.

Finally, in order to summarize the relationship between serum cholesterol and each type of stroke, the interquintile (highest/lowest) relative risk and the 95% confidence interval were estimated using the Cox regression model on the basis of the regression coefficient and the difference in mean serum cholesterol values between the highest and the lowest quintile groups, after adjusting first for age alone, and then for age and other risk factors including hypertension (0,1), diabetes (0,1), body mass index (kg/m^2), cigarette smoking (cigarettes/day), and alcohol consumption (oz/month).

Results

During 20 years of follow-up of 7850 men who were free of stroke and had cholesterol determinations at the initial examination, a total of 523 cases were identified as having the first event of definite or probable stroke. These include 38 cases of subarachnoid haemorrhage (SAH), 78 intracerebral haemorrhage (ICH), 355 thromboembolic stroke (TE), and 52 unspecified type.

Table 1 presents clinical characteristics of each stroke type excluding the unspecified type. The mean age at diagnosis was youngest for SAH and oldest for TE. The case fatality ratio, defined as the proportion of stroke cases who died within one month after the onset, was highest for SAH (58%), followed by ICH (49%), and lowest for TE (13%). The diagnosis was confirmed by autopsy or surgery in 43% of SAH, 27% of ICH, and only 3% of TE. The CT scan became available in 1975 and has been commonly used since 1978. This modern technology confirmed the diagnosis in 56% of ICH, 32% of TE, and only 8% of SAH. The diagnosis was confirmed by arteriography in 21%

Table 1 Clinical characteristics of type-specific stroke

Clinical characteristics	Subarachnoid haemorrhage ($n=38$)	Intracerebral haemorrhage ($n=78$)	Thromboembolic stroke ($n=355$)
Mean age at diagnosis	63.4	67.5	68.2
Case fatality ratio (%)*	58	49	13
Diagnosis confirmed by:			
Autopsy (%)	32	19	3
Surgery (%)	11	8	0
CT Scan(%)	8	56	32
Arteriography (%)	21	9	8

*Case fatality ratio was based on deaths within 1 month of the onset of stroke.

Table 2 Age-adjusted means of selected variables at baseline examination for type-specific stroke cases and non-stroke subjects

Baseline variable	Subarachnoid haemorrhage ($n=38$)	Intracerebral haemorrhage ($n=78$)	Thromboembolic stroke ($n=355$)	Non-stroke subjects ($n=7327$)
Systolic blood pressure (mmHg)	146*	147*	144*	133
Diastolic blood pressure (mmHg)	88*	92*	86*	82
Body mass index (kg/m^2)	24.6	24.1	24.4	23.8
Serum cholesterol (mg/dl)	207	208*	223*	218
Serum glucose (mg/dl)	160	165	180*	160
Cigarettes/day	17*	13	15*	10
Alcohol consumption (oz/month)	22*	27*	15	14

*These values are significantly different ($p < 0.05$) from those for the non-stroke group.

388

of SAH, 9% of ICH, and 8% of TE. These figures are not mutually exclusive, and the diagnosis was made solely by neurological symptoms and signs (including lumbar puncture findings) in 42% of SAH, 21% of ICH, and 53% of TE.

Table 2 shows age-adjusted means of selected variables measured at the initial examination for type-specific stroke cases and non-stroke subjects. As compared with the non-stroke group, all groups of stroke had significantly higher blood pressure. Serum cholesterol was significantly lower in ICH and significantly higher in TE. It was lowest in SAH, but the difference was not statistically significant. Body mass index and 1-h post-load serum glucose were significantly higher only in TE. The number of cigarettes smoked per day was greater in all stroke groups than the non-stroke group, but the difference was significant only in SAH and TE. Usual alcohol consumption (oz/month) was significantly greater in SAH and ICH.

Figure 1 shows distributions of the baseline serum cholesterol levels for hypertensive men and normotensive men, separately. The distribution curves in both groups were quite similar and slightly skewed to the high side. Therefore, raw values of serum cholesterol rather than logarithmic transformations were used in all analyses. The overall average serum cholesterol level was 5.64 mmol/l (218 mg/dl), and only 366 men (4.7%) had serum cholesterol less than 4.14 mmol/l (160 mg/dl).

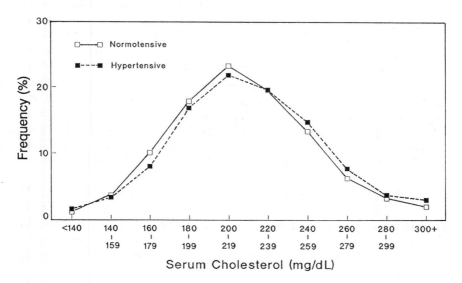

Figure 1 Distribution of baseline serum cholesterol levels by hypertension status. Normotensives: average blood pressure < systolic 140 and diastolic 90. Hypertensives: average blood pressure ≥ 140 systolic, or diastolic 90

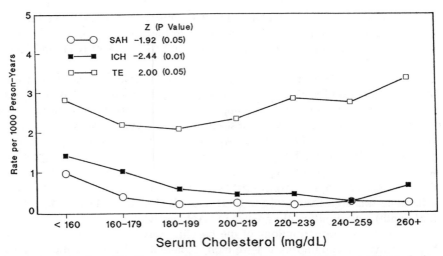

Figure 2 Age-adjusted incidence rates (per 1000 person-years) of type-specific stroke by baseline serum cholesterol level. SAH: subarachnoid haemorrhage, ICH: intracerebral haemorrhage, TE: thromboembolic stroke, Z: regression coefficient/standard error of coefficient

Figure 2 presents age-adjusted incidence rates (per 1000 person-years) of type-specific stroke by the baseline level of serum cholesterol divided into seven subgroups with an interval of 0.517 mmol/l (20 mg/dl). In both SAH and ICH the highest rate was noted for the lowest category of serum cholesterol (< 4.14 mmol/l or 160 mg/dl). In SAH the rate declined substantially (from 1.00 to 0.21) between the lowest and the third lowest groups of serum cholesterol, and thereafter stayed nearly flat. In ICH the rate declined progressively (from 1.41 to 0.44) with increasing serum cholesterol level up to 5.69 mmol/l (220 mg/dl) and turned slightly upward in the highest category of cholesterol (6.72 mmol/l, or 260 mg/dl). In TE the rate declined (from 2.82 to 2.19) between the lowest and the third lowest groups of serum cholesterol, and thereafter it showed an upward trend with increasing cholesterol levels, and reached the highest rate (3.37) in the highest cholesterol group. As indicated by Z statistic, the inverse association of serum cholesterol with SAH was borderline significant ($p=0.054$), the inverse association with ICH was significant ($p=0.014$), while the direct association with TE was weakly significant ($p=0.045$). There was no evidence for significant non-linear component in any of these curves tested by quadratic terms.

The next three figures show age-adjusted incidence rates of type-specific stroke by baseline serum cholesterol level for 3232 hypertensive men and 4618 normotensive men, separately. The analyses were carried out using three different criteria for hypertension: (1) men with systolic blood pressure (SBP)

≥ 140 or diastolic blood pressure (DBP) ≥ 90, or on antihypertensive medication; (2) men with SBP ≥ 140 regardless of DBP or medication; and (3) men with DBP ≥ 90 regardless of SBP or medication. Very similar patterns of the relationship between serum cholesterol and each type of stroke were demonstrated in all three criteria. Therefore, only the results using the first criterion are presented here, since it is the most comprehensive criterion for hypertension.

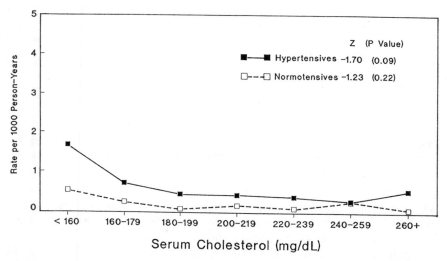

Figure 3 Age-adjusted incidence rates (per 1000 person-years) of subarachnoid haemorrhage by baseline serum cholesterol level among hypertensives and normotensives. See footnotes of Figures 1 and 2

Figure 3 shows that in both hypertensives and normotensives there was a trend of decline in age-adjusted rate of SAH between the lowest and the third lowest categories of serum cholesterol, but thereafter no consistent trend was noted. As indicated by Z statistic, the inverse association was not statistically significant in either hypertensives or normotensives. However, the rate of SAH was higher among hypertensives than among normotensives in all but one category of serum cholesterol.

Figure 4 demonstrates that in hypertensives there was a substantial decline in age-adjusted rate of ICH between the lowest and the second lowest categories of serum cholesterol (from 2.49 to 0.94), but thereafter no consistent trend was noted. In normotensives the rate of ICH was relatively high in the two lowest categories of serum cholesterol, followed by a substantial decline between the second and the third lowest categories (from 1.09 to 0.13) and a nearly flat trend thereafter. As indicated by Z statistic, the inverse association

391

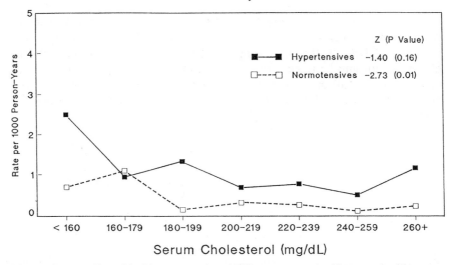

Figure 4 Age-adjusted incidence rates (per 1000 person-years) of intracerebral haemorrhage by baseline serum cholesterol level among hypertensives and normotensives. See footnotes of Figures 1 and 2.

was statistically significant only in normotensives. Similar to SAH, the rate of ICH was substantially higher among hypertensives than among normotensives in all but one category of serum cholesterol.

Figure 5 shows that in hypertensives there was a nearly flat trend in age-adjusted rate of TE except for a drop between the lowest and the second lowest categories of serum cholesterol. In normotensives the trend appeared to show a J-shaped curve, with the highest rate of TE in the highest level of serum cholesterol. As indicated by Z statistic, there was a statistically significant direct association of serum cholesterol with TE among normotensives, but no significant relationship among hypertensives. There was no evidence of significant non-linear component in these trends when quadratic terms of serum cholesterol were included in the model. The rate of TE was consistently higher among hypertensives than among normotensives at every level of cholesterol.

Thus, the associations of serum cholesterol with type-specific stroke (inversely with ICH and directly with TE) were statistically significant only among normotensives. However, a formal statistical test did not indicate evidence for a significant interaction of serum cholesterol and hypertension.

Table 3 presents the interquintile relative risk (highest/lowest) of type-specific stroke and the 95% confidence interval by the baseline level of serum cholesterol. After adjustment for age alone, the risks of both SAH and ICH were less than half in the highest quintile of serum cholesterol as compared

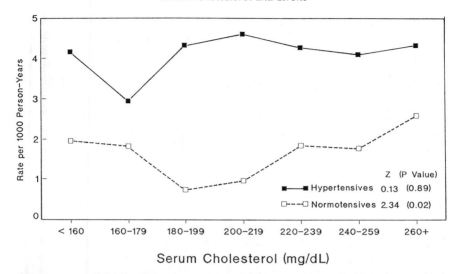

Figure 5 Age-adjusted incidence rates (per 1000 person-years) of thromboembolic stroke by baseline serum cholesterol level among hypertensives and normotensives. See footnotes of Figures 1 and 2

Table 3 Interquintile relative risk (highest/lowest) of type-specific stroke by baseline serum cholesterol

Stroke type	Adjustment	Relative risk[†]	95% confidence interval
Subarachnoid	Age alone	0.40	0.16–1.02
haemorrhage	Age and risk factors*	0.45	0.16–1.14
Intracerebral	Age alone	0.44	0.23–0.85
haemorrhage	Age and risk factors*	0.46	0.24–0.88
Thromboembolic	Age alone	1.33	1.01–1.77
stroke	Age and risk factors*	1.26	0.94–1.65

*Risk factors included hypertension (0,1), diabetes (0,1), body mass index (kg/m^2), cigarettes/day, alcohol consumption (oz/month).
†Relative risks were estimated, using the proportional hazards model, on the basis of regression coefficients for serum cholesterol and interquintile differences (highest-lowest) in mean serum cholesterol values (2.72 mmol/l, or 105 mg/dl).

with the lowest quintile, where the interquintile difference in mean cholesterol was 2.72 mmol/l (105 mg/dl). On the other hand, the risk of TE increased one-third in the highest quintile of serum cholesterol, as compared with the lowest quintile. As indicated by the 95% confidence interval, the reduced risk of SAH was not statistically significant, while the reduced risk of ICH and the increased risk of TE were both significant. However, after further adjustment for age and other risk factors including hypertension, diabetes, body mass index, cigarette smoking, and alcohol consumption, only the reduced risk of ICH (relative risk: 0.46) remained significant.

Discussion

In the present study relating serum cholesterol to the risk of type-specific stroke among Japanese-American men, we found a statistically significant association of serum cholesterol only with ICH (inversely) after controlling for age and other possible confounders. This inverse association was noted only below the level of 5.17 mmol/l (200 mg/dl), with the highest rate of ICH in men with serum cholesterol less than 4.14 mmol/l (160 mg/dl). When separate analyses were done for hypertensives and normotensives, the inverse association of serum cholesterol with ICH was observed in both groups, but the association was statistically significant only among normotensives. There was no statistical evidence for the interaction of serum cholesterol and blood pressure.

The inverse association of serum cholesterol with ICH noted in the present study is in accord with the findings reported by other studies in Japan[1-5] and by the MRFIT Study in the United States[11]. In contrast to the present study, however, the inverse association was restricted to hypertensive men in the MRFIT Study. Although there are some differences in the endpoint (mortality vs. incidence) definition of hypertension and covariates used for adjustment between the two studies, this discrepancy appears to be mainly due to different methods of calculating the relative risk. In the present study as shown in Figure 4, if the relative risk was calculated using the lowest serum cholesterol level <4.14 mmol/l (160 mg/dl) as the reference group, instead of the interquintile (highest/lowest) comparison, the inverse association of serum cholesterol with ICH would be significant among hypertensives, but not among normotensives. Thus, the results would be similar in both the present study and the MRFIT Study. Also, in one Japanese study[4], the inverse association of serum cholesterol with cerebral haemorrhage was noted in both hypertensive and normotensive men. It may need further studies to determine whether the inverse association of serum cholesterol with ICH exists only at very low levels, such as <4.14 mmol/l (160 mg/dl), or whether it is linear within the normal range below 5.17 mmol/l (200 mg/dl), and whether the inverse association is restricted to hypertensive men.

The biological mechanism of the inverse association of low serum cholesterol with ICH is still not well understood. There are, however, several plausible explanations based on pathological and experimental investigations, as well as epidemiological observations.

Cholesterol is an important component of the cell membrane and is essential in maintaining the normal cellular function of the vascular endothelium. Some evidence suggests that very low serum cholesterol plays a role in the pathogenesis of ICH through its adverse effects upon osmotic fragility of the cell membrane which may lead to the development of arterionecrosis in small intracerebral arteries[19,20]. In spontaneously hypertensive rats, feeding with high cholesterol diet prevented the development of ICH[21].

Low serum cholesterol may also be a manifestation of inadequate nutrition, especially if there is a low intake of animal protein and fat. It is known that farmers in northern Japan, where ICH is prevalent, have very low serum cholesterol and eat little animal food[3]. Furthermore, in a study of trends for coronary heart disease and stroke and their risk factors in Japan[5], it was found that the decline in the incidence of stroke between 1963 and 1983 in rural communities of north-east Japan paralleled an increase in the intake of animal protein and fat, as well as in the average level of serum cholesterol, during the same period.

Also, in a comparative epidemiological study of stroke in Japan and Hawaii[22], it was found that the incidence of stroke (both haemorrhagic and non-haemorrhagic) was three times as high in Japan as in Japanese-American men in Hawaii, despite nearly equal levels of average blood pressure. The intake of animal protein and fat and the average level of serum cholesterol were substantially higher in Hawaii than in Japan.

These findings appear to suggest that very low serum cholesterol, which might reflect poor nutrition with inadequate intake of animal food, could enhance the vulnerability of small intracerebral arteries and lead to the development of ICH, especially in the presence of hypertension. However, low serum cholesterol might be merely a marker for a disease or constitution characterized by blood vessel fragility which enhances the susceptibility to ICH.

Even assuming a causal relation between low serum cholesterol levels and ICH, its public health implications would depend upon characteristics of populations in terms of the relative frequency of ICH and the distribution of serum cholesterol levels. In the United States and other Western countries, where the average level of serum cholesterol and the prevalence of coronary heart disease are high, haemorrhagic stroke occurs much less commonly than thromboembolic stroke[7]. As indicated in the MRFIT Study[11], only a small fraction of the population has very low serum cholesterol levels, and the relative frequency of ICH is low. In these countries, therefore, the public health impact of the inverse association of serum cholesterol with ICH would not be serious. On the other hand, in Japan and Asian countries where the average level of serum cholesterol is low, and the frequency of stroke is high with haemorrhagic stroke accounting for more than one-third of all strokes[23,24], an appropriate public health goal appears to be the maintenance of optimal levels of serum cholesterol (4.65–5.17 mmol/l, or 180–200 mg/dl) which would not increase the risk of either stroke (haemorrhagic and non-haemorrhagic) or coronary heart disease.

References

1. Shibuya, R., Kimura, N., Isomura, K. *et al.* (1975). Ecological aspects of nutritional status as limiting factors of life expectancy of Japanese. Ecological background for CVA and CHD in Japan. In Ashina, K. and Shigiya, R. (eds.) *Physiological Adaptability and Nutritional Status of the Japanese*, pp. 127–65. (Tokyo: University of Tokyo Press)
2. Ueshima, H., Iida, M., Shimamoto, T. *et al.* (1980). Multivariate analysis of risk factors for stroke. Eight-year follow-up study of farming villages in Akita, Japan. *Prev. Med.*, **9**, 722–40
3. Tanaka, H., Ueda, Y., Hayashi, M. *et al.* (1982). Risk factors for cerebral hemorrhage and cerebral infarction in a Japanese rural community. *Stroke*, **13**, 62–73
4. Lin, C.H., Shimizu, Y., Kato, H. *et al.* (1984). Cerebrovascular diseases in a fixed population of Hiroshima and Nagasaki, with special reference to relationship between type and risk factors. *Stroke*, **4**, 653–60
5. Shimamoto, T., Komachi, Y., Inada, H. *et al.* (1989). Trends for coronary heart disease and stroke and their risk factors in Japan. *Circulation*, **79**, 503–15
6. Kannel, W.B. (1971). Current status of the epidemiology of brain infarction associated with occlusive arterial disease. *Stroke*, **4**, 295–318
7. Ostfeld, A.M. (1980). A review of stroke epidemiology. *Epidemiol. Rev.*, **2**, 136–52
8. Dyken, M.L., Wolf, P.A., Barnett, H.J.M. *et al.* (1984). Risk factors in stroke. A statement for physicians by the subcommittee on risk factors and stroke of the stroke council. *Stroke*, **15**, 1105–11
9. Welin, L., Svardsudd, K., Wilhelmsen, L. *et al.* (1987). Analysis of risk factors for stroke in a cohort of men born in 1913. *N. Engl. J. Med.*, **317**, 521–6
10. Harmsen, P., Rosengren, A., Tsipogianni, A. *et al.* (1990). Risk factors for stroke in middle-aged men in Göteborg, Sweden. *Stroke*, **21**, 223–9
11. Iso, H., Jacobs, D.R. Jr, Wentworth, D. *et al.* (1989). Serum cholesterol levels and six-year mortality from stroke in 350,977 men screened for the Multiple Risk Factor Intervention Trial. *N. Engl. J. Med.*, **320**, 904–10
12. Kagan, A., Popper, J.S. and Rhoads, G.G. (1980). Factors related to stroke incidence in Hawaii Japanese men. The Honolulu Heart Study. *Stroke*, **11**, 14–21

13. Kagan, A., Popper, J.S., Rhoads G.G. *et al.* (1985). Dietary and other risk factors for stroke in Hawaiian Japanese men. *Stroke,* **16** 390-6

14. Worth, R.M., Kato, H., Rhoads, G.G. *et al.* (1975). Epidemiologic studies of coronary heart disease and stroke in Japanese men living in Japan, Hawaii and California: mortality. *Am. J. Epidemiol.,* **102,** 481-90

15. Belsky, J.L., Kagan, A., Syme, S.L. (1971). Epidemiologic studies of coronary heart disease and stroke in Japanese men living in Japan, Hawaii and California. Research plan. *Atomic Bomb Casualty Commission Technical Report,* pp. 12-71

16. Kagan, A., Harris, B.R., Winkelstein, W. Jr *et al.* (1974). Epidemiologic studies of coronary heart disease and stroke in Japanese men living in Japan, Hawaii and California: demographic, physical, dietary and biochemical characteristics. *J. Chronic Dis.,* **27,** 345-64

17. Rhoads, G.G., Kagan, A. and Yano, K. (1975). Usefulness of community surveillance for the ascertainment of coronary heart disease. *Int. J. Epidemiol.,* **4,** 275-70

18. Cox, D.R. (1972). Regression models and life tables (with discussion). *J. R. Stat. Soc.,* **34** (Series B), 187-220

19. Oneda, G., Yoshida, Y., Suzuki, K. *et al.* (1978). Smooth muscle cells in the development of plasmatic arterionecrosis, arteriosclerosis, and arterial contraction. *Blood Vessels,* **15,** 148-56

20. Konishi, M., Terao, A., Doi, M. *et al.* (1982). Osmotic resistance and cholesterol content of the erythrocyte membrane in cerebral hemorrhage (in Japanese). *Igaku no Ayumi,* **120,** 30-2

21. Yamori, Y., Horie, K., Ohtaka, M. *et al.* (1976). Effects of hypercholesterolemic diet on the incidence of cerebrovascular and myocardial lesions in spontaneously hypertensive rats (SHR). *Clin. Exp. Pharmacol. Physiol.* (Suppl. 3), 205-8

22. Takeya, Y., Popper, J.S., Shimizu, Y. *et al.* (1984). Epidemiologic studies of coronary heart disease and stroke in Japanese men living in Japan, Hawaii and California: incidence of stroke in Japan and Hawaii. *Stroke,* **15,** 15-23

23. Tanaka, H., Ueda, Y., Date, C. *et al.* (1981). Incidence of stroke in Shibata, Japan: 1976-1978. *Stroke,* **12,** 460-6

24. Komachi, Y., Tanaka, H., Shimamoto, T. *et al.* (1984). A collaborative study of stroke incidence in Japan: 1975-1979. *Stroke,* **15,** 28-36

Discussion

Dr Goldbloom: I was just wondering if you have any information about the dietary intake of these groups? The reason why I am asking this question is because, as I listened to this discussion of the increased incidence of haemorrhagic stroke, I was reminded of a report that came out about a year ago. This study involved a group of children who were being given fish oil capsules. Subsequently, they developed haemorrhagic manifestations, mostly in the form of nose bleeds but quite severe haemorrhagic manifestations, such that the fish oil had to be stopped.

Dr Yano: In our study, there was not a significant difference in the dietary intake between the stroke and non-stroke groups, although the former group tended to eat less protein and fat. In particular, the fish consumption did not show any significant differences. Also, there was no significant relationship between fish consumption and either the serum cholesterol level or the stroke incidence. I might add that there was a study conducted in Japan which indicated that in residents of a fishing village, the average intake of fish was much higher than in residents of a farming village. The blood level of ω-3 fatty acids was also higher in the fishing village than in the farming village. Also, the platelet function was lower in the fishing village compared to the farming village. However, between these two villages, there was no statistically significant difference in either CHD or stroke mortality.

Dr Dietschy: I have two minor methodological questions. Obviously, this is now pretty much classic work, but I wonder if there is some possible misclassification of the haemorrhagic vs. the non-haemorrhagic strokes, given the lack of availability of objective measures. Some of your 'p' values are pretty marginal, especially given multiple comparisons and so on. Did you leave out the clinically diagnosed strokes and clinical assignations from the model and remodel, going only with those strokes that were confirmed as to aetiology by CAT scan or autopsy or other means?

Dr Yano: Yes, there certainly is the possibility of misclassification especially between haemorrhagic and non-haemorrhagic stroke. However, our diagnosis was made not only on the clinical symptoms and signs but on all available diagnostic tests, including CAT scan, surgery and autopsy findings. So, I think that the diagnosis of the different types of stroke was fairly reliable, although I cannot assure it with certainty.

Dr Dietschy: I would just like to press this point a tiny bit, even though I do not think it is all that important. Since there were overlapping numbers within each of the groups for the classification of stroke, and that the one under intracranial haemorrhage added up to 93, and that there was overlap within it, surely there must have been a certain proportion of the patients who were diagnosed without reference to CAT scan, autopsy or other definitive measures? Was the analysis repeated by backing those patients out of the model? I am saying that there are some whose classification might be ambiguous and therefore should be excluded from the model if they were not confirmed by CAT scan or autopsy. We have seen this with the thrombolysis trials, where the assignation of events is highly controversial in ISIS3 because of the issue of CAT scan or autopsy confirmation and the misclassification that occurs with clinical and other measures.

Dr Yano: Yes, I think it would be worthwhile to re-analyze the data, using only definite cases with objective evidence for the diagnosis.

23
Dyslipidaemias and the primary prevention of coronary heart disease: reflections on some unresolved policy issues

C.D. NAYLOR

Guidelines for the prevention of coronary heart disease [CHD] through clinical modification of lipid profiles have been promulgated in Europe[1], Britain[2-7], North America[8-13], and even as far afield as South Africa[14]. These guidelines vary among and within countries in several respects, including target populations for case-finding, tests for initial screening and follow-up, threshold values leading to further testing and treatment, and the place of other risk factors in treatment decisions. The evidence available to the various expert panels, consensus bodies, and task forces has been similar. Differing policies therefore reflect divergent interpretations of evidence, as well as the priorities and values of the experts and their sponsors. This report reviews several unresolved issues that have lent themselves to differences of expert opinion in the lipid and cholesterol field.

Prognostic misclassification: beyond the serum cholesterol

In all proposed programmes of clinical prevention, the accuracy and precision of laboratory measures is a concern, particularly with the anticipated application of lipid testing to large populations using local laboratories. Repetition of any abnormal values is mandatory in light of the intraindividual variation in cholesterol levels. Given the distribution of cholesterol values in most industrialized populations, the lower the cut-point for individualized intervention and follow-up, the greater will be the proportion of persons misclassified categorically for any level of laboratory imprecision or bias. However, even were superb laboratories available to all practitioners, the underlying issue is the prognostic worth of the measurement itself.

Molecular biologists and epidemiologists alike would probably agree that the total serum cholesterol [TC] is a mediocre marker for risk of CHD.

Imagine, for example, that a new diagnostic assay is introduced in an enzymology laboratory. A group of normals is tested and their range of values compared to those known to have the disease of interest. The ideal results would see two quite distinct curves, with little overlap. Conversely, Figure 1, drawn from the Framingham study[15], shows the distribution of TC values for men who did and did not develop CHD over a 16-year follow-up period starting from middle-age. The overlap is striking.

Comparison of these two curves creates a situation analogous to measures of sensitivity and specificity, wherein prevalence or incidence are divorced from the equation. More clinically-useful measures assess positive and negative predictive value of TC and thereby show the real burden of misclassification. Figure 2, a transformation of Figure 1, helps in that regard (Ref. 11, pp. 1045–6). It shows first, that about seven times as many men did **not** have coronary events, as compared to those who did. One also sees clearly that there is no discrete cut-point beyond which all or even most persons develop CHD. Instead, there are trade-offs in the ratio of 'true positives' to 'false positives': the proportion of subjects labelled and treated, who would not have developed CHD in the next 16 years, rises as one lowers the threshold value for 'normal' serum TC.

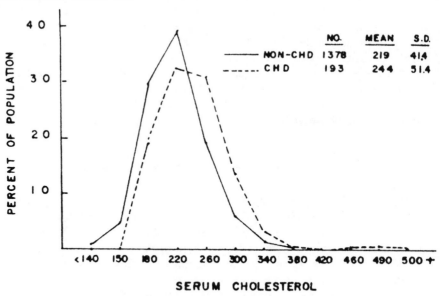

Figure 1 Distribution of serum cholesterol levels (mg/dl) in men aged 30–49 years at entry, who did and did not subsequently develop coronary heart disease in 16 years (Framingham study). Source: ref. 15

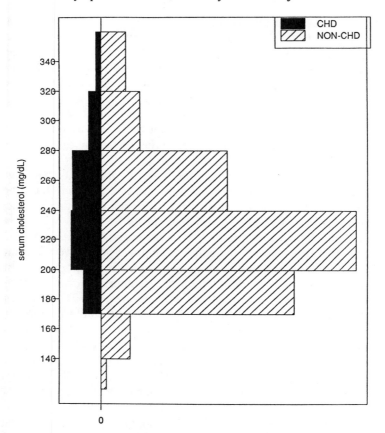

Figure 2 This figure is reconstructed by interpolation from Framingham data (see Figure 1). Males initially free of CHD were entered between ages 30 and 49 years, and followed for 16 years. The proportions who did and did not develop symptomatic CHD are shown for varying initial TC levels. This illustrates the 16-year burden of treatment relative to potential yield at various proposed TC cutpoints, and also sheds light on the 'prevention paradox' (see text). Source: ref. 11, p. 1046

If anything, this example may overstate the predictive value of TC on several scores: (i) the annual hazard rates are much higher among middle-aged males than younger adults of either sex, and same-aged females; (ii) the 16-year cumulative incidence of CHD is therefore higher; and (iii) while the rising incidence of CHD with age should improve the predictive value of TC among the elderly, some studies suggest that this factor is counterbalanced by a weakening of the risk relationship between TC and CHD.

Figure 2 also illustrates how the poor clinical predictive value of TC relates to the so-called prevention paradox[16,17]. If one treats only those with very high TC levels, there are so few persons affected that little impact is made on the total burden of CHD in society. If one lowers the cut-point for active treatment, the ratio of false positives to true positives rises to such an extent that individualized intervention bears small marginal returns and large numbers of persons who will not develop premature CHD are treated for every one who stands to benefit (Ref. 11, pp. 1046–9).

Such poor predictive performance is not sufprising. Not only are there many other potent risk factors for CHD, but more importantly, the serum cholesterol cannot adequately reflect the myriad metabolic disturbances that appear to feed the atherosclerotic process.

Attempted redress for the prognostic poverty of the TC has involved incorporating other lipid measures and non-lipid risk factors into testing and treatment plans. For example, under the National Cholesterol Education Program in the USA [NCEP][12], all adults are to be tested, with a low TC cut-point demarcating abnormality on initial screening (5.2 mmol/l), and other lipid markers measured thereafter to improve predictive performance. Non-lipid risk factors are used to guide both the need for more sophisticated lipid tests, and the aggressivity of treatment. Another approach is not to rely on TC as the sole screen, but use other lipid measures with TC at the first test step. This stance is understandable, given the poor predictive performance of TC alone. The role of triglycerides as an independent risk factor remains moot (Ref. 11, pp. 1041–2), but modest improvements in predictive value with measurement of high-density lipoprotein cholesterol [HDL] have been documented for some subgroups of patients (Ref. 11, pp. 1042–3). The most important of these subgroups is the elderly. Unfortunately, algorithms for more generous use of HDL seem to increase rather than decrease the numbers of persons labelled and treated[18], indirectly supporting the concept that the incremental predictive value of HDL is oversold. A simplified interpretation is that HDL improves our ability to predict CHD, particularly at the lower ranges of TC. However, as a predictor – alone or in combination with TC – it has the same inherent limitations as the parent cholesterol measure, albeit inverted as befits its risk relationship with CHD. If we put the threshold for abnormal HDL too low, we miss the bulk of persons with CHD. If we raise it, we then label many persons as having abnormally low HDL who have low CHD event rates. Furthermore, since a 'lowish' HDL may co-exist with relatively normal TC, we end up adding more persons to the pool for follow-up and treatment.

An alternative approach suggested in some policy statements[6,8,9,11] is the use of non-lipid risk factors to help target initial testing. The definite drawback to this approach is the weak clustering of dyslipidaemia with other CHD risk factors, and negative family history in at least 20% of patients with inherited dyslipidaemias, so that many patients with isolated lipid abnormalities will be missed. The rationale is that for elevations of TC without other non-lipid risk factors, the absolute short- and intermediate-term risk of CHD is unquestionably low.

There is no obvious way out of this prognostic quagmire, particularly when one also considers the limited published evidence on the range of predictive interactions between the subfractions of TC and non-lipid risk factors. The standard measures – TC, HDL, low density lipoprotein cholesterol [LDL] and triglycerides – alone, or in combination, are inadequate in telling clinicians which asymptomatic patients will actually develop CHD in the near future. On the other hand, evidence for some of the promising newer markers is incomplete. The most exciting markers are Lp(a) and ApoB. Lp(a) has the advantage of showing sharp gradients in measured values between persons with and without CHD, but such case-control comparisons aside, there is limited prospective evidence[19-22]. Apo B is readily measured, almost certainly reduces misclassification of CHD risk as compared to TC, and has been used as a pivotal measure in one positive RCT[22-26]. However, as with Lp(a), the risk relationships have been defined largely from case-control comparisons, and the RCT in question involved predominantly persons with pre-existing CHD. One could nonetheless argue for switching to newer markers before all the evidence is in, if only because the older markers have such poor performance. In any event, it is probable that the newer markers will reduce prognostic misclassification, enhance the efficiency of any detection programme, and permit greater agreement on both testing strategies and cutpoints for individualized follow-up.

All-cause mortality: clinical and public policy concerns

All-cause mortality benefits have not been demonstrable in any of the single factor lipid trials, individually or in combination, in the context of primary prevention. Muldoon *et al.*[27] have aggregated data from six primary prevention trials that randomized 24 847 men and treated them primarily with diet (Los Angeles VA study, Minnesota Coronary Survey) or drugs (Helsinki Heart Study, Lipid Research Clinics Coronary Primary Prevention Trial, Colestipol–Upjohn Trial, and World Health Organization Study). The mean duration of follow-up was 4.8 years. Total mortality was unchanged (odds ratio 1.07, 95% Cl: 0.94 to 1.21), even after excluding the WHO study wherein clofibrate was associated with excess all-cause mortality. There was, as expected, a clear trend to reduction in CHD mortality (odds ratio 0.85, 95% Cl: 0.69 to 1.05). However, this was counterbalanced by increases in non-CHD causes of death. The most notable was 'deaths from other causes', typically violent causes (suicides, accidents, and homicides), with an odds ratio of 1.76, 95% Cl, 1.19 to 2.58.

Other meta-analyses of the primary prevention trials, including multiple risk factor interventions, have failed to show any all-cause mortality benefit[28-35]. Indeed, if one aggregates all the primary and secondary prevention trials, the net effect is a non-significant increase in all-cause mortality, with narrowing of confidence intervals such that the likelihood of benefit is small[28]. Inadequate statistical power is thereby ruled out as the best explanation for the lack of benefit. Instead, there are three important caveats.

First, could this simply be a statistical fluke, as suggested by MacMahon and Peto[29,30] and Yusuf *et al.*[32,36]? Yusuf *et al.*[36], in particular, have argued that a causal connection between cholesterol lowering and non-CHD deaths is unlikely given: (a) little epidemiological, experimental, or mechanistic evidence to support a claim of excess in non-CHD disease; (b) no relationship between the intensity of lowering the level of cholesterol and excess non-CHD deaths; and (c) no increase in specific causes of death, other than hepatobiliary diseases with the fibric acid derivatives. However, on the latter point, one cannot ignore the above-noted excess in 'other' causes of death demonstrable on meta-analysis of the primary prevention trials[27]. The excess mortality from various non-CHD causes recurs in trial after trial of both primary and secondary prevention[37], and there is also observational evidence from cohort studies linking low cholesterol to increased risks of both cancer and haemorrhagic stroke (see below). In sum, it seems unlikely that cholesterol-lowering is devoid of biological side-effects.

Second, is the problem one of duration of follow-up? Observational data show that, upon comparing asymptomatic middle-aged persons with relatively normal lipid profiles to those with dyslipidaemias, a decade must elapse before any all-cause mortality differences emerge[38]. On the other hand, all-cause mortality benefit attributed to static differences between two groups may not justify assumptions about the effects of dynamic changes within one of those groups at higher risk (Ref. 11, pp. 1061–2). Furthermore, modelling by our group has not shown a relationship between duration of single-factor trials and extent of all-cause mortality reduction. It is encouraging that the MRFIT follow-up data at 10.5 years indicate a significant 7.7% reduction in all-cause mortality[39]. But whether this is due to lipid modifications, or to the changes in other risk factors, remains unknown*.

Third, is the problem one of extent of cholesterol lowering? This is not implausible, particularly if one considers that there may be a combined

---

* Caution is also needed since the multiple risk factor trials have not been consistent in their results. An Oslo trial included very high risk males (TC 7.5–9.8 mmol/l, 80% smokers) and showed all-cause mortality benefit from dietary and anti-smoking interventions, while a Helsinki study of men with one or more CHD risk factors showed no benefit, even for coronary events, and total mortality was slightly higher in treated subjects, albeit not statistically significant.

deficiency in both extent of cholesterol lowering and duration of follow-up. On the basis of his meta-analysis, Holme has suggested that a sustained 8–9% reduction in cholesterol is required before all-cause mortality benefits are likely[28]. This unproven hypothesis must nonetheless be viewed with caution on two scores. First, it is generated from a combination of primary and secondary prevention data, and the latter overstate the likelihood of all-cause mortality benefit from intervention in asymptomatic subjects. Second, long-term (e.g. 23-year follow-up) cohort studies among males suggest that hypertension and smoking are much more important than cholesterol in predicting all-cause mortality[40]. Thus, we should not make unduly optimistic assumptions about the extent of benefit to be expected even with more effective lipid-lowering interventions.

Controversy about cholesterol-lowering, primary prevention of CHD, and all-cause mortality is likely to continue until new trials of more powerful cholesterol-lowering interventions and/or longer-term follow-up of earlier trials are completed. At present, as suggested elsewhere (ref. 11, p. 1063), the significant increase in non-CHD deaths could be attributed to one or more of the following causes: (i) chance alone, i.e. a type 1 error, which seems most unlikely; (ii) true adverse effects of treatment with diet or drugs, albeit with protean biological manifestations; or (iii) some as yet unexplained emergence of competing risks when CHD mortality is reduced for the middle-aged males who represent the majority of trial subjects to date. The latter, however, is also unlikely, given that certain non-CHD causes of death seem to predominate. In sum, while the trial evidence leads to the conclusion that cholesterol-lowering does reduce CHD mortality, and thereby experimentally validates the basic cholesterol-CHD hypothesis, there is legitimate concern about the lack of reduction in all-cause mortality in primary prevention trials.

What, then, of a population strategy, i.e. attempts to promote community-wide changes in diet that would lead to reduction in the average population TC? Various authors have warned of the pitfalls in attempting to control CHD by population-wide interventions[35,41,42]. The Toronto Working Group on Cholesterol Policy drew more optimistic conclusions about public health promotion[11], but we were remiss in not taking fuller account of the potential impact of excess all-cause mortality in association with low cholesterol. Many prospective studies have now shown J-shaped curves, with excess cause-specific or total mortality at low TC levels[43-56]. From an all-cause mortality standpoint, the optimal TC level could well lie somewhere between 4.9 and 5.3 mmol/l. An excess in haemorrhagic stroke is a particularly recurrent finding in association with low cholesterol and its increased incidence obviously cannot be attributed to some pre-clinical disease state[47-49]. In contrast, while cancer has also been frequently associated with low cholesterol, there has been much debate about cause and effect, with some studies suggesting that the lowering of cholesterol may itself be a result of undetected cancer, and others not[49-55].

Parenthetically, excess non-CHD risks with low cholesterol tempt one to draw parallels with the above-noted increases found in randomized trials of cholesterol-lowering. However, it is probably unreasonable to indict cholesterol-lowering treatment for individuals in the highest quintile of TC on the basis of phenomena affecting persons in the lowest cholesterol quintile in observational studies. Few persons treated for high TC are likely to lower their values into the range where excess all-cause mortality has been observed, and the balance of risks and benefits is further tipped by the excess CHD risk faced by those with high TC. Nonetheless, there is a biological parallel that is difficult to ignore.

Where concerns arise are with the effects of a community-wide cholesterol-lowering strategy on those who already have normal cholesterol. In particular, if deaths from all-causes are increased in those with low TC, could dietary change actually increase the risk of death among persons who already have normal values[56]? A possible rejoinder is that many persons with normal or low TC are unlikely to be affected. These persons could be in one of two protected subgroups. The first will be those who follow a prudent diet already, and who are unlikely to change further in response to community-wide health promotion pressures. The second are those who do eat higher than desired levels of saturated fats, but who are genetically able to moderate dietary influences, so that a more healthy diet may conversely have limited impact. If these optimistic speculations are false, and if many persons are pulled into lower TC ranges, what risks will be incurred? The short answer is that no one knows, although Frank and Reed[56] have produced preliminary and disquieting answers that suggest no net all-cause mortality benefit whatsoever even under assumptions that bias their model against non-CHD risks.

The issue is especially vexing since it adds another dimension to the prevention paradox. Recall that even though a majority of CHD events actually occur among those with 'normal' TC or modest elevations, the individual risks of CHD among such persons tend to be either low, or if not, conditioned by risk factors other than lipids. Hence, as stated above, individualized lipid intervention is difficult to justify for such persons, and a community health strategy promoting general dietary change has been advocated by various authors as the most practical approach[7,11,16,17,57-59]. Yet this same untargetted policy could lead those with low-normal TC to reduce their TC into the range where an excess in all-cause mortality has been demonstrated.

In conclusion, we currently have inadequate trial or observational evidence to rule in all-cause mortality benefit from application of a medical strategy to lower cholesterol among persons with high levels, and inadequate observational or trial evidence to rule out all-cause mortality harm from a community-wide strategy of dietary change that could reduce cholesterol among those who already have normal or low levels. Pronouncements from experts who claim to be marshalling 'The Cholesterol Facts' have yet to make these observations go away[60].

The trial evidence: limits of design and populations

Community-wide health promotion strategies are difficult to test in a randomized context (ref. 11, pp. 1060–1,1087–9) but clinical interventions are more amenable to trial-based evaluation. One can accordingly ask: what experimental evidence should ideally be available before adoption of a clinical programme or medical strategy for detection and management of dyslipidaemias? An idealized answer would be: randomized controlled trial evidence derived in the community, proving that the programme has an all-cause mortality impact, with acceptable side-effects and morbidity benefits such that overall quality-adjusted life years or healthy life-year equivalents are increased, and at an incremental cost per life-year gained that is comparable to other funded programmes and interventions.

While trial after trial has been mounted to prove the 'lipid hypothesis', or show regression of coronary atherosclerosis in subjects with known CHD, no study has realistically assessed the impact of a screening or case-finding programme as it might be mounted in the community. The latter is crucial because innumerable points of slippage occur that render the generalizability of the very design of the trials questionable, independent of concerns about the populations enrolled.

Most of the extant single-factor trials start at the referral centre spout, not at the primary care funnel. They are sited in academic hospitals and clinics, take for granted that superb laboratory facilities will be generally available, and that numerous nurses and dietitians will be available to enforce compliance. They use selected populations of volunteers with high lipid levels, usually middle-aged males, and take no account of persons at lower risk who would be tested and treated in aggressive programmes, and for whom the risk-benefit ratio may be less favourable.

Furthermore, the follow-up in all trials has been inadequate in both length and focus. The focus on CHD events, both fatal and non-fatal, has actually been used in rather innovative ways to rationalize the failure of primary prevention trials to show all-cause mortality benefits. One rationalization is that the focus on mortality is misplaced because cholesterol-lowering also has morbidity-reducing effects through reducing CHD events and complications. This ignores all other causes of morbidity, including those associated with the excess non-CHD mortality that has been demonstrated repeatedly in clinical trials. The second argument is a corollary, namely, that ethically, the trials cannot be extended long enough to show all-cause mortality benefits because significant differences in CHD events emerge much earlier. This is based on a slippery moral calculus, whereby the outcomes of interest to the trialists are all that should matter to patients and society. Some overall quality of life measure is absolutely necessary to capture, on the positive side, morbidity reductions from reduced CHD events, and on the negative side, the impact of other diseases as either inevitable background morbidity limiting the quality-of-life impact of CHD reductions or actually induced by treatment. Other negative quality-of-life outcomes to be captured are psychological labelling effects[61-64], the inconvenience and cost of continuing medical care, the usual drug side-effects (gastrointestinal distress, rashes, and so on), and the loss of habitual gustatory pleasures consequent upon dietary therapy.

Indeed, the ideal trial would actually set out two case-finding programmes, e.g. one aggressive, and another more conservative. The organizers would recruit individual family physicians, or group practices, allocating the practitioners or practices randomly to one level of intervention or another. The function of trials nurses would be to review the protocols with the participating primary care MDs and their office staff, not to enforce protocol compliance on the part of the patients since such enforced compliance would unduly exaggerate the impact of treatment. In this 'effectiveness' or 'programme' trial, there would be no special laboratories, only the usual laboratories and quality control measures of the region. Perhaps resources for dietary therapy might be bolstered, simply to avoid unfair restraint on the potential success of the trial. But the army of trained dietitians that figures in some trials would not be in the field. There would be guidelines for family physicians to refer the patient on for endocrinological opinions. Whether the referral occurred would be up to the family doctor – again as occurs in real life – and once a patient was referred, the specialist physician or endocrinologist would be free to follow his/her own preferred protocol, as again will be the case in the 'real world'. This clinical freedom, incidentally, is a positive feature of such a trial: conventional trials could underestimate effectiveness of interventions because they do not allow patients to change drugs or dosages if metabolic responses do not occur (ref. 11, p. 1062).

Some thought would also have to be given to the extent of background community health promotion in such a trial. In the past, claims have been advanced that risk factor modification trials failed because rapid community changes in risk factors narrowed the gap between control and intervention arms[65]. This confounder made it all but impossible to determine the true effectiveness of the North Karelia[66-68] community health promotion experiment. Overall changes in diet and life-style might similarly narrow the gap between a conservative and aggressive screening and treatment programme. (Indeed, the same potential effect of community-wide behavioural changes led the Toronto Working Group[11] to endorse a conservative approach to clinical intervention against hypercholesterolaemia, combined with a strong public health campaign against CHD risk factors generally.)

In such an outcomes-oriented trial, patients would need to be followed for about 10 years. The outcomes might include only three basic measures: date of death; cause of death; and regular measurements of health status (and/or quality-of-life) using a battery of indices. There should also be costing of the two protocols, using a randomly drawn sub-sample of patients. The costing should include elements from the perspective of both a third-party payer, and society at large (i.e. costs for medical services as well as indirect costs from time off work, and so on.)

We are far removed from having this type of evidence. Lack of evidence cannot, of course, paralyse policy-making; action in the face of uncertainty is a hallmark of clinical practice. But an awareness of deficiencies in evidence might at least encourage a more prudent approach to the clinical cholesterol crusade than has been evident in America and Europe thus far.

Lastly, as implied above, there are definite concerns about the extent to which the results of primary prevention trials to date can be generalized to other, lower-risk groups, particularly females. Short-term effort–yield ratios even with groups of very high risk males indicate that between 1000 and 2000 patient-years of drug treatment are required per CHD death prevented (Ref. 11, p. 1062). Longer-term treatment may enhance the efficiency of drug therapy, and generate disproportionate benefits that reduce these effort–yield ratios. However, when one extrapolates to lower risk groups, most of whom would not merit drug therapy, the effort–yield ratios rise to the point where one must question the prudence of cholesterol-lowering for such persons in a clinical context as opposed to a population-based strategy which would promote community-wide dietary change.

Informed consent or unformed dissent? Patient perceptions and preferences in treatment policies

As noted above, it is almost paradoxical that a recurrent argument in favour of aggressive detection and management of dyslipidaemias is the effect of lipid-lowering on non-fatal coronary events. The overall decrease in non-fatal coronary events is encouraging. But since none of the trials was designed to demonstrate changes in non-coronary morbidity, and these outcomes were neither uniformly sought nor reported, the tally remains seriously imbalanced[37]. This, again, is why it is vital to perform overall quality-of-life measurements in the context of lipid-lowering trials.

Until those data are acquired experimentally, one can logically ask: at what level do psychological labelling effects, drug side-effects or unhappiness stemming from dietary change lead to shifts away from aggressive treatment and towards more conservative strategies? Krahn and co-workers from our group have assessed this issue using a three-state (health, CHD, and death) Markov model[69]. Two sets of guidelines were compared: an aggressive programme (roughly based on the NCEP) and a much more conservative programme (analogous to a draft proposal from the Canadian Task Force on the Periodic Health Examination). The guidelines were applied to a theoretical cohort of middle-aged men, constructed to parallel the subjects in the Lipid Research Clinics Coronary Primary Prevention trial[70,71] [LRC-CPPT], but under an assumption that the TC levels had the distribution of an age/sex matched general population. Table 1 shows the proportions of men that would receive treatment in this model.

Table 1 Aggressive versus conservative testing and treatment programme: impact on a theoretical cohort of middle-aged males

	Aggressive	*Conservative*
No therapy	45.6%	81.3%
Diet alone	36.7%	6.9%
Diet and drugs	17.7%	11.8%

Source: ref. 69.

Quality-adjusted life expectancy was calculated based on each of these programmes. The baseline disutility of diet was assumed to be 0.02 and of drugs to be 0.02. The disutility of CHD was set at 0.20, so that once any non-fatal CHD event was incurred, quality-adjusted life-expectancy of all affected subjects was penalized under an assumption of impaired health status. As per the LRC-CPPT[70,71] and other sources, diet was assumed to reduce TC by 4.9%, while drugs were to reduce TC by 13.4%.

Assumptions that might have favoured the more aggressive programme were built into the model. For example, there was long-term follow-up, and the state transition probabilities were calculated using bivariate (age and cholesterol) proportional hazards and logistic regression functions derived primarily from the Framingham study. In other words, all-cause mortality benefits were assumed on the basis of between-subjects observational data, contrary trial evidence about within-subject effects notwithstanding. Use of a population of middle-aged males would also exaggerate the benefits from an aggressive programme such as the NCEP.

The conservative programme was slightly favoured in most scenarios, and the result was robust under a wide range of assumptions and sensitivity analyses. *Ceteris paribus*, the aggressive programme was favoured only when the dietary disutility term was reduced below 0.0014. Holding treatment disutilities constant, the aggressive programme could also be favoured if several other variables were shifted simultaneously (e.g. improve TC-lowering effectiveness of drugs and dietary intervention and/or raise mortality associated with any myocardial infarction and/or increase the disutility of CHD). Among the interesting findings was that adaptation to a low-fat diet, with time-related decrease in the disutility of dietary change, could be a potent force in mitigating the negative impact of any cholesterol-lowering programme.

One concern in this model is that survival differences for either programme versus no programme whatsoever were small (about 0.25 years on average after 20 years of follow-up!). This suggests, in part, the relatively minor effect that any cholesterol-lowering programme would have on the longevity of populations. But it also may reflect the tendency of any cyclical model (in this case, a 7.4 year cycle based on the LRC-CPPT) to underestimate longevity differences. On the other hand, so many biases in favour of treatment were built into the model that such concerns may be irrelevant.

The main lessons, in any case, are three. First, at an aggregate level, these findings constitute a warning against unduly aggressive cholesterol-lowering programmes in the clinical context. Unless we are sure that drugs and diets are very well-tolerated, and that patients are not psychologically harmed by disease-equivalent labels such as 'dyslipidaemia' or 'high cholesterol', a prudent approach seems warranted. Second, at an individual clinical level, the findings underscore the need to determine just how patients perceive the process of treatment. It should be recalled here that the concept of 'average' disutilities is almost a contradiction in terms. We should pay close attention to our patient's preferences and anxieties before pressing hypolipidaemic drugs or aggressive dietary therapy on them. Third, from a policy-making standpoint, it is frankly staggering that we were unable to find any literature in 1990 that rigorously addressed the disutility of drug and dietary therapy for hypercholesterolaemia. Some patients may well feel better on diet; others may find the medicalization of their food intake to be a nightmare. Some may adapt quickly; others may find that their low-fat diet is a constant struggle against implicit familial and community pressures. This is an area that urgently demands research.

Three inter-related areas of patients' preferences and perceptions also remain unexplored, but are particularly germane to the field of preventive policy. These are: (a) the accuracy of patients' perceptions of their CHD risk, before they agree to long-term treatment; (b) the framing effects of various methods whereby risks and benefits are presented to patients; and (c) the time-preferences of patients.

We suspect that patients diagnosed with dyslipidaemia develop an exaggerated perception of personal CHD risk, along with undue expectations of how much difference treatment makes to that risk. Furthermore, all preventive

413

programmes involve investments: patients suffer the inconvenience and side-effects of treatment now, and over many years, in hopes of averting some unpleasant future event. If patients are not aware of when that event is likely to occur, their implicit consent to treatment may be based on shaky foundations since most of us have strong time preferences. Ask, for example, whether a person wants, say, $100 now, or $100 a year from now: the answer is a foregone conclusion. To assess strength of time preference, one can carry on with a trade-off task, e.g. if the choice is for $100 now, the questioner increases the deferred amount to $110, to $120, and so on, until the subject chooses to wait. Similar exercises can be performed with health-related expectations[72], but no work has been done in the field of hypercholesterolaemia, even though most primary prevention benefits are deferred. Our group is now gearing up to initiate such studies. Our particular concern is that patients may have grossly exaggerated perceptions of their coronary risk per unit time, and that the propensity to accept aggressive treatment is actually contingent on a misperception of both when benefit is likely to occur, and how much benefit is likely. That is, the patient perceives that he/she has, say, an 80% risk of having an MI in the next 5 years, and that the risk is cut to 20% by taking hypolipidaemic therapy. How would the patient's attitudes change if the risk was much lower in the short-term, and rose only with advancing age? In such a circumstance, even dramatic benefits might look less attractive. Brett has reviewed some of these issues in the general context of risk factor modification[73], and emphasized the role of framing effects in obtaining consent to treatment with lipid-lowering drugs[74]. For instance, patients could be expected to respond differently if told that treatment with a hypolipidaemic drug will reduce their (relative) risk of CHD by 25%, as opposed to information that a cumulative and absolute reduction of 0.5% in fatal CHD events is projected over their next 10 years of drug therapy. Alternatively, one might frame efforts and yields, e.g. based on the Helsinki Heart Study[75], a middle-aged man on gemfibrozil faces an average of 350 patient-years of treatment per CHD event prevented, or a 1 in 70 chance of avoiding some fatal or non-fatal CHD event after 5 years of treatment. One could also turn to the LRC-CPPT[70,71], and advise patients that on average, 10.3 metric tonnes of cholestyramine were consumed per CHD death prevented (ref. 11, p. 1062)!

In sum, as practitioners and researchers, we need to explore patients' treatment preferences and perceptions, and their responses to various ways of framing treatment data. Research is especially important to determine just how individualized dietary therapy affects the quality of patients' lives. There is truly an ethical imperative to study the process by which patients give consent to these long-term therapies, since so little is known about this area.

Misguided guidelines? The practitioners' dilemma

The simple dissemination of guidelines has seldom done much to guide clinical practice[76]. While lack of awareness of the content of guidelines is one barrier to compliance, even a knowledgeable and well-motivated family physician might have trouble deciding which guidelines to follow for detection and management of dyslipidaemias in North America or England. For example, in Canada, there have been separate and slightly divergent pronouncements from the Canadian Consensus Conference on Cholesterol[9], the Toronto Working Group on Cholesterol Policy[11], the Canadian Task Force on the Periodic Health Examination[10], and the Canadian Lipoprotein Society[8]. In Britain, Leitch[77] has neatly summarized the still-larger number of different recommendations that a GP may encounter. In sum, no 'meta-consensus' has emerged about clinical policies for dyslipidaemias in Canada and the UK.

Let us say, however, that a practitioner does decide on a given set of guidelines. There is no assurance that the guidelines will be comprehensive and clear. For example, the Canadian Task Force on the Periodic Health Examination was a pioneer in attempting to rank evidence on preventive policies according to the methodological rigour of the studies pertaining to a given issue. The Task Force also adopted a grading system for its recommendations about including a manoeuvre in the periodic health examination, viz. A = good evidence for inclusion, B = fair evidence for inclusion, C = poor evidence for inclusion, but recommendations may be made on other grounds, D = fair evidence for exclusion, and E = good evidence for exclusion. The Task Force has published scores of recommendations, but has yet to assess the impact of this rather vague grading system on practitioners' perceptions and practices.

Assuming that a set of guidelines is chosen and is clearly written, can they actually be implemented? Unfortunately, even conservative guidelines may be virtually impossible for a conscientious GP to implement for the following reasons. First, somewhere between 50% and 100% of all adults would have to be tested under various guidelines, and then retested every 5 years. Follow-up tests will have to be performed on all subjects above a given cut-point. This means call-backs to the office or telephone time to persuade patients to return to the laboratory. Furthermore, a tracking system is needed to ensure that the GP looks over results for all patients so tested; otherwise, the lab slips will disappear into patient files. Second, the proportion of patients who are to receive individualized counselling and formal dietary therapy, with or without drug intervention, varies according to the cut-points used in the guidelines but could easily include scores of adults in any given family practice. In Canada, there is a shortage of dietitians, and most GPs lack the training and any reasonable financial incentives to become personally involved in ongoing dietary counselling. Each patient consigned to individualized follow-up is also a source of ongoing appointments, and a certain amount of laboratory testing. It is not inconceivable that 10% of adults in a practice could end up on lipid-lowering drugs under aggressive guidelines such as those of the NCEP[12]. Since many GPs already run busy practices, it is hard to imagine how they will cope with such a programme[78]. These practical considerations, coupled with uncertain patient compliance, support Browner's observation that the actual yield from many preventive programmes is likely to be much less than enthusiasts would have us believe[79].

Even if we assume that the practitioner is willing and able to follow a given set of guidelines, one might also ask whether the guidelines are internally consistent. We have analysed the recommendations of the Adult Treatment Panel of the NCEP in that latter regard[80]. The NCEP has three grades of treatment intensity: dietary advice, formal dietary therapy, and drug therapy. Intensity of treatment depends on a given patient's lipid values and other risk factors. Because of uncertainty about patients' attitudes to long-term treatment, we chose to model an intermediate-term follow-up period, and therefore used the multiple logistic regression equation from the Framingham study to derive predicted 8-year cumulative risks for any CHD event according to different age–sex groupings[81]. TC values were chosen in light of the NCEP cut-points for TC and LDL. Additional risk factors – hypertension, glucose intolerance, and smoking – were considered in combination for each of these values.

Women and men in younger age groups who would be candidates for drug treatment because of lipid values alone were usually at low levels of risk compared to those with much lower TC values and other risk factors. Furthermore, in every age grouping, women with high TC (>6.9 mmol/l) and two other risk factors were in the drug treatment category, but had 8-year CHD risks that were often much lower than males with one other risk factor and lower TC levels who would be candidates for dietary advice or dietary therapy respectively. Table 2 shows some of the discrepancies within a given age bracket, while Table 3 summarizes the highest and lowest 8-year risk within any given category of treatment intensity. Data in Table 3 are broken down by age brackets; moving down the columns, the discrepancies are revealed to be much greater when age is allowed to vary as well.

Perhaps the most important lesson is that no practitioner can adequately estimate CHD risk in the context of multiple risk factors, especially given the changing event rates across age groupings. Add to this the need to estimate the *reduction* in risk from modifying one or more risk factors, so that the most efficient (and least disruptive) strategy can be devised for a given patient, and the problem with virtually all extant guidelines becomes apparent. The more complex they become on paper, the harder they will be for a practitioner to follow in a busy office. But the more simplistic guidelines will also be characterized by glaring internal inconsistencies, and could lead to over-emphasis on some risk factors relative to others.

Table 2 Eight year risk of developing any CHD manifestation, starting from age 45 years, per 100 000 population

Risk profile	*Serum cholesterol* (mg/dl)			
	185 Rx	*220 Rx*	*265 Rx*	*300 Rx*
Female	1 010 A	1 344 A	1 937 D	2 570 R
Male	2 420 A	3 450 A	5 406 D	7 609 R
Female + smoking				
+ glucose intol.	1 473 A	1 958 D	2 814 R	3 722 R
Male + glucose intol.	3 030 A	4 309 D	6 719 R	9 403 R
Male + smoking	3 703 A	5 251 D	8 143 R	11 327 R
Female + SBP 165 mmHg				
+ smoking	1 523 A	2 024 D	2 908 R	3 845 R
Female + SBP 165 mmHg				
+ glucose intol.	3 137 A	4 142 D	5 897 R	7 720 R
Male + SBP 165 mmHg	4 046 A	5 729 D	8 859 R	12 286 R
Male + SBP 165 mmHg				
+ smoking	6 139 A	8 613 D	13 101 R	17 848 R

A = General dietary advice; D = Formal dietary therapy; R = Drug treatment in addition to diet. Source: ref. 80.

Table 3 Lowest and highest 8-year risks of developing CHD, per 100 000 population

Age	8-year risk	*Diet advice*		*Diet therapy*		*Drug therapy*	
		Male	*Female*	*Male*	*Female*	*Male*	*Female*
35	Lowest	675	230	1 387	487	2 590	770
	Highest	1 762	727	2 859	1 047	8 371	2 402
45	Lowest	2 420	1 010	4 309	1 937	6 719	2 570
	Highest	6 139	3 137	8 613	4 142	17 848	7 720
55	Lowest	5 486	2 756	8 471	4 370	11 130	5 331
	Highest	13 276	8 250	16 229	9 975	24 906	15 156
65	Lowest	8 023	4 713	9 984	6 227	10 969	7 023
	Highest	18 706	13 561	20 357	15 144	24 529	19 329

Source: ref. 80.

The best solution may be to use specially-programmed hand-held calculating devices (or software programs for office computers) that allow physicians and nurse-practitioners to assess the individual risk profile of patients and most efficient strategies for reducing their CHD risk. Such a programme could also provide some sense to the patient of what he or she could expect in the way of gains with various strategies, and thereby abet the process of bringing the patient's perceptions and preferences into play. While this sounds cumbersome, the alternative is to consign individuals to lifetime therapy in an inappropriate fashion.

Secondary versus primary prevention: the baby in the bathwater[82]?

For virtually all diseases, the conventional wisdom in epidemiology and public health policy is that primary prevention is valued over secondary prevention. The logic is compelling: keeping persons healthy is better than treating those who are sick, and the condition may no longer be reversible if one waits. Certainly in Canada, the debate about cholesterol has thus far focused on primary prevention. Yet even as controversy continues about primary prevention, too little has been said of secondary prevention. The following points are noteworthy:

(1) CHD event rates (fatal or non-fatal myocardial infarction [MI] or reinfarction) are strikingly higher once a person has angina or has had an MI. For example, Pekkanen *et al.* report from an LRC Prevalence Study that the 10-year risk of death from cardiovascular disease rose from 3.8% to 19.6% with rising TC levels among men with known CHD, while the risk for men free of CHD at baseline rose from 1.7% to 4.9%[83]. The relative risks are, of course, different. But what is most notable is the divergence in absolute differences in event rates: 15.8% excess risk versus only 3.2%. This heralds a tremendous potential increase in the efficiency of treatment when dealing with secondary prevention.

(2) Trial evidence clearly supports the merits of lipid-altering intervention, thereby reducing theoretical concerns about lack of reversibility in the presence of established disease. Setting aside the various quantitative coronary angiography studies (which rest on surrogate measures rather than clinical events), overviews of clinical endpoints in the secondary prevention trials confirm that the aggregate relative reduction in events is similar to that found in the primary prevention trials[28,84]. Moreover, because there are about four times as many fatal and non-fatal infarcts (as compared to asymptomatic populations), the absolute yield in CHD events averted is greater for any relative risk reduction.

(3) The extent of all-cause mortality benefits from lipid-altering in primary CHD prevention remains uncertain for reasons summarized above. Of note, in secondary prevention trials there is a similar pattern to primary

prevention trials, with recurring increases in non-CHD causes of death. However, once afflicted with clinically-manifest CHD, a given individual is sufficiently likely to die of CHD that all-cause mortality benefits also are much more likely to accrue over time. Support for this concept comes from two trials of secondary prevention – the Coronary Drug Project[85-87] and the Stockholm Ischemic Heart Disease Study[88]. Both have demonstrated a significant all-cause mortality benefit, albeit only after long-term follow-up. While this benefit has not been confirmed for all the secondary prevention trials when aggregated through meta-analysis, there is at least a trend towards all-cause mortality benefit[84]. No such trends have been demonstrated in the single-factor primary prevention trials.

(4) Arguments about the predictive value of various lipid markers become largely irrelevant. Whatever the lipid profile, it is atherosclerotic in the context of that individual. Smoking cessation is arguably the single most critical step, where applicable. But logic dictates that dietary intervention at minimum is also warranted for the majority of these patients.

(5) Issues of 'labelling' and 'medicalization', pertinent to individualized primary preventive manoeuvres, are only weakly applicable. After all, one is dealing with a person who is ill, and who has already been legitimately labelled as having a disease. Patients' risk perceptions bear study in the context of secondary prevention, just as they do for those who have never had a coronary event. However, we hypothesize that many such persons will have particularly pressing fears of recurrent CHD events, and that they may feel psychologically empowered by taking personal steps that could reduce their subsequent risk of CHD events.

(6) Economic efficiency should be substantially superior to primary preventive manoeuvres, both because of the higher baseline event rates, and because of the assured costs of downstream treatment in all affected individuals. As argued elsewhere, it is crucial to recall that clinical efficiency and cost-effectiveness are both contingent on differences in absolute event rates between treated and untreated patients (ref. 11, p. 1093). A recent cost-effectiveness analysis by Goldman *et al.*[89] supports the view that lipid-lowering drugs are an economically efficient intervention in almost all patients with *established CHD*, whereas our review of drug therapy for *primary prevention* suggested competitive cost-effectiveness ratios were likely only for patients in selected high-risk subgroups (ref. 11, pp. 1093–101).

In sum, it is arguable that this patient population should not be viewed in the same light as persons subjected to primary clinical prevention. While debate about primary preventive programmes continues in an attempt to resolve many issues (including some reviewed in this essay), more attention should be paid to those who primary prevention has failed – our patients with established CHD.

Acknowledgements

Almost all the foregoing material draws on collaborative work with a number of Toronto colleagues who should share the credit but none of the blame for errors. They are: Drs John W. Frank, Antoni Basinski, Michael M. Rachlis, Murray D. Krahn, Hilary Llewellyn-Thomas and Warren McIsaac.

Supported in part by a Career Scientist Award to the author from the Ontario Ministry of Health.

References

1. Study group, European Atherosclerosis Society. (1987). Strategies for the prevention of coronary heart disease. *Eur. Heart J.*, **8**, 77–88
2. Consensus statement: blood cholesterol measurement in the prevention of coronary heart disease. (1989). *Lancet*, **2**, 115–16
3. Report of the British Cardiac Society Working Group on Coronary Disease Prevention. London: British Cardiac Society, 1987
4. British Cardiac Society Working Group on Coronary Prevention. (1987). *Br. Heart J.*, **57**, 188–9
5. Shepherd, J., Betteridge, D.J., Durrington, D. *et al.* (1987). Strategies for reducing coronary heart disease and desirable limits for blood lipid concentrations: guidelines of the British Hyperlipidaemia Association. *Br. Med. J.*, **295**, 1245–6
6. Smith, W.C.S., Kenicer, M.B., Maryon Davis, A., Evans, A.E. and Yarnell, J. (1989). Blood cholesterol: is population screening warranted in the UK? *Lancet*, **1**, 372–3
7. Risk assessment: its role in the prevention of coronary heart disease. (1987). Recommendations of the scientific and medical advisory committee of the Coronary Prevention Group. *Br. Med. J.*, **295**, 1246
8. Canadian Lipoprotein Conference ad hoc committee on guidelines for dyslipoproteinemia. (1990). Guidelines for the detection of high-risk lipoprotein profiles and the treatment of dyslipoproteinemias. *Can. Med. Assoc. J.*, **142**, 1371–82
9. The Canadian Consensus Conference on Cholesterol: Final Report. (1988). *Can. Med. Assoc. J.*, **139** (Suppl.), 1–8
10. Logan, A. (1988). The conclusions of the Canadian Task Force on the Periodic Health Examination. Paper 10: Presentations from the Canadian Consensus Conference on Cholesterol, March 9–10, 1988. [Mimeographed proceedings]

11. Toronto Working Group on Cholesterol Policy: Naylor, C.D., Basinski, A., Frank, J.W. and Rachlis M.M. (1990). Asymptomatic hypercholesterolemia: a clinical policy review. *J. Clin. Epidemiol.*, **43**, 1021–122

12. The Expert Panel. Report of the National Cholesterol Education Program Expert Panel on Detection, Evaluation, and Treatment of High Blood Cholesterol in Adults. (1988). *Arch. Intern. Med.*, **148**, 36–69

13. Garber, A.M., Sox, H.C. Jr, and Littenberg, B. (1989). Screening asymptomatic adults for cardiac risk factors: the serum cholesterol level. *Ann. Intern. Med.*, **110**, 622–39

14. Roussow, J.E., Steyn, K., Berger, G.M.B. *et al.* (1988). Action limits for serum total cholesterol. A statement for the medical profession by an ad hoc committee of the Heart Foundation of Southern Africa. *S. Afr. Med. J.*, **73**, 693–700

15. Kannel, W.B., Castelli, W.P. and Gordon, T. (1979). Cholesterol in the prediction of atherosclerotic disease. New perspectives based on the Framingham Study. *Ann. Intern. Med.*, **90**, 1985–91

16. Rose, G. (1985). Sick individuals and sick populations. *Int. J. Epidemiol.*, **14**, 32–8

17. Rose, G. (1981). Strategy for prevention: lessons from cardiovascular disease. *Br. Med. J.*, **282**, 1847–51

18. Glueck, C.J., Sanghvi, V.R., Laemmle, P. *et al.* (1989). Misclassification of coronary heart disease risk by HDL cholesterol in subjects with desirable total cholesterol. *Clin. Res.*, **37**, 937A

19. Utterman, G. (1989). The mysteries of Lp(a). *Science*, **246**, 904–10

20. Acanu, A.M. and Fless, G.M. (1990). Lipoprotein (a): heterogeneity and biological significance. *J. Clin. Invest.*, **85**, 1709–15

21. Breckenridge, W.C. (1990). Lipoprotein (a): genetic marker for atherosclerosis? *Can. Med. Assoc. J.*, **143**, 115

22. Durrington, P.N., Ishola, M., Hunt, L., Arrol, S. and Bhatnagar, D. (1988). Apolipoproteins (a), Al, and B and parental history in men with early onset ischaemic heart disease. *Lancet*, **1**, 1070-3

23. Barbir, M., Wile, D., Trayner, I., Aber, V.R. and Thompson, G.R. (1988). High prevalence of hypertriglyceridemia and apolipoprotein abnormalities in coronary artery disease. *Br. Heart J.*, **60**, 397–403

24. Sniderman, A.D. (1988). Apolipoprotein B and apolipoprotein Al as predictors of coronary artery disease. *Can. J. Cardiol.*, **4** (Suppl. A), 24-30A

25. Sniderman, A.D. and Silberberg, J. (1990). Is it time to measure apolipoprotein B? *Arteriosclerosis*, **10**, 665–7

26. Brown, G., Alberts, J.J., Fisher, L.D. *et al.* (1990). Regression of coronary artery disease as a result of intensive lipid lowering therapy in men with high levels of apolipoprotein B. *N. Engl. J. Med.*, **323**, 1289–98

27. Muldoon, M.F., Manuck, S.B. and Matthews, K.A. (1990). Lowering cholesterol concentrations and mortality: a quantitative review of primary prevention trials. *Br. Med. J.*, **301**, 309–14

28. Holme, I. (1990). An analysis of randomized trials evaluating the effect of cholesterol reduction on total mortality and coronary heart disease incidence. *Circulation*, **82**, 1916–24

29. MacMahon, S. and Peto, R. (1988). Randomized trials of cholesterol reduction in the context of observational epidemiology. Paper presented to the Canadian Consensus Conference on Cholesterol. Ottawa, March 9–11, 1988
30. MacMahon, S., Peto, R., Collins, R. and Yusuf, S. (1988). Randomized trials of cholesterol reduction in the context of observational epidemiology. First National Cholesterol Conference 1988, Arlington, Va. Program Book, p. 42 (abstract)
31. Yusuf, S. and Furberg C.D. (1987). Single factor trials: Control through lifestyle changes. In Olsson, A.G. *et al.* (eds.) *Atherosclerosis*, pp. 389–92. (New York: Churchill Livingstone)
32. Yusuf, S. and Cutler, J. (1987). Single factor trials: Drug studies. In Olsson, A.G. *et al.* (eds.) *Atherosclerosis*, pp. 393–8. (New York: Churchill Livingstone)
33. Furberg, C.D. and Cutler, J. (1987). Multiple factor intervention: Controlled trials. In Olsson, A.G. *et al.* (eds.) *Atherosclerosis*, pp. 399–401. (New York: Churchill Livingstone)
34. Yusuf, S., Wittes, J. and Friedman, L. (1988). Overview of results of randomized clinical trials in heart disease. II. Unstable angina, heart failure, primary prevention with aspirin, and risk factor modification. *J. Am. Med. Assoc.*, **260**, 2259–63
35. McCormick, J. and Skrabanek, P. (1988). Coronary heart disease is not preventable by population interventions. *Lancet*, **2**, 839–41
36. Yusuf, S., Wittes, J. and Friedman, L. (1989). Randomized clinical trials in heart disease. *J. Am. Med. Assoc.*, **261**, 2953–4
37. Basinski, A., Naylor, C.D., Frank, J.W. and Rachlis, M.M. (1989). Randomized clinical trials in heart disease. *J. Am. Med. Assoc.*, **261**, 2952–3
38. Anderson, K.M., Castelli, W.P. and Levy, D. (1987). Cholesterol and Mortality. 30 Years of follow-up from the Framingham Study. *J. Am. Med. Assoc.*, **257**, 2176–80
39. Multiple Risk Factor Intervention Trial Research Group. (1990). Mortality rates after 10.5 years for participants in the multiple risk factor intervention trial: findings related to *a priori* hypotheses of the trial. *J. Am. Med. Assoc.*, **268**, 1795–801
40. Goldbourt, U. and Yaari, S. (1990). Cholesterol and coronary heart disease mortality: a 23-year follow-up study of 9902 men in Israel. *Arteriosclerosis*, **10**, 512–19
41. Oliver, M.F. (1984). Coronary risk factors: should we not forget about mass control? *World Health Forum*, **5**, 5–8
42. Oliver, M.F. (1981). Serum cholesterol – the knave of hearts and the joker. *Lancet*, **2**, 1090–5
43. Forette, B., Tortrat, D. and Wolmark, Y. (1989). Cholesterol as a risk factor for mortality in elderly women. *Lancet*, **1**, 868–70
44. Kagan, A., McGee, D.L., Yano, K. *et al.* (1981). Serum cholesterol and mortality in a Japanese–American population. *Am. J. Epidemiol.*, **114**, 11–20
45. Peterson, B., Trell, E. and Sterby, N.H. (1981). Low cholesterol levels as risk factor for non-coronary death in middle-aged men. *J. Am. Med. Assoc.*, **245**, 2056–7
46. Salmond, C.E., Beaglehole, R. and Prior, I.A. (1985). Are low cholesterol values associated with excess mortality? *Br. Med. J.*, **290**, 422–4

47. Iso, H., Jacobs, D.R., Wentworth, D. *et al.* (1989). Serum cholesterol levels and six-year mortality from stroke in 350,977 men screened for the Multiple Risk Factor Intervention Trial. *N. Engl. J. Med.*, **320**, 904–10

48. Yano, K., Reed, D.M. and Maclean, C.J. (1989). Serum cholesterol and hemorrhagic stroke in the Honolulu Heart Program. *Stroke*, **20**, 1460–5

49. Reed, D.R., Yano, K. and Kagan, A. (1986). Lipids and lipoproteins as predictors of coronary heart disease, stroke and cancer in the Honolulu Heart Program. *Am. J. Med.*, **80**, 871–8

50. Yaari, S., Goldbourt, U., Even-Aohar, S. *et al.* (1981). Associations of serum high density lipoprotein and total cholesterol with total cardiovascular and cancer mortality in a 7-year prospective study of 10,000 men. *Lancet*, **1**, 1011–15

51. Isles, C.G., Hole, D.J., Gillis, C.R. *et al.* (1989). Plasma cholesterol, coronary heart disease, and cancer in the Renfrew and Paisley survey. *Br. Med. J.*, **298**, 920–4

52. Sherwin, R.W., Wentworth, D.N., Cutler, J.A. *et al.* (1987). Serum cholesterol and cancer mortality in 361,662 men screened for the multiple risk factor intervention trial. *J. Am. Med. Assoc.*, **257**, 943–8

53. Tornberg, S.A., Holm, L-E., Carstensen, J.M. and Eklund, G.A. (1989). Cancer incidence and cancer mortality in relation to serum cholesterol. *J. Natl. Cancer Inst.*, **81**, 1917–21

54. Wingard, D.L., Criqui, M.H., Holdbrook, M.J. *et al.* (1984). Plasma cholesterol and cancer morbidity and mortality in an adult community. *J. Chronic Dis.*, **37**, 401–6

55. Cowan, L.D., O'Connell, D.L., Criqui, M.H., Barrett-Connor, E., Bush, T. and Wallace, R.B. (1990). Cancer mortality and lipid and lipoprotein levels: the lipid research clinics program mortality follow-up study. *Am. J. Epidemiol.*, **131**, 468

56. Frank, J.W. and Reed, D.M. (1990). Will lowering mean population levels of serum cholesterol affect total mortality? Evidence from the Honolulu Heart Program. Abstract of presentation to the Annual Meeting of the American Epidemiological Society, Baltimore, March 23, 1990

57. Beaglehole, R., Jackson, R. and Stewart, A. (1988). Diet, serum cholesterol and the prevention of coronary heart disease in New Zealand. *N.Z. Med. J.*, **101**, 415–18

58. McNeil, J.J. (1988). Cholesterol: action or caution? *Med. J. Aust.*, **148**, 1–3

59. Kottke, T.E., Gatewood, L.C., Wu, S-C. and Park, H.-A. (1988). Preventing heart disease: is treating the high risk sufficient? *J. Clin. Epidemiol.*, **41**, 1083–93

60. Gotto, A.M., LaRosa, J.C., Hunninghake, D. *et al.* (1990). The cholesterol facts: a summary of the evidence relating dietary fats, serum cholesterol, and coronary heart disease. *Circulation*, **81**, 1721–33

61. Haynes, R.B., Sackett, D.L., Taylor, D.W. *et al.* (1978). Increased absenteeism from work after detection and labelling of hypertensive patients. *N. Engl. J. Med.*, **299**, 741–4

62. Sackett, D.L., Macdonald, L., Haynes, R.B. *et al.* (1983). Labelling of hypertensive patients. *N. Engl. J. Med.*, **309**, 1253

63. Lefebvre, R.C., Hursey, K.G. and Carleton, R.A. (1988). Labeling of participants in high blood pressure screening programs. Implications for blood cholesterol screenings. *Arch. Intern. Med.*, **148**, 1993–7

64. Forrow, L., Calkins, D., Allshouse, K. and Delbanco, T. (1989). Effects of cholesterol screening on health perceptions. *Clin. Res.*, **37**, 818A
65. Wilhelmsen, L., Berglund, G., Elmfeldt, D. *et al.* (1986). The multifactor primary prevention trial in Goteborg, Sweden. *Eur. Heart J.*, **7**, 279–88 (See the Commentary by G.A. Rose)
66. Puska, P., Nissinen, A., Tuomilehto, J. *et al.* (1985). The community-based strategy to prevent coronary heart disease: conclusions from the ten years of the North Karelia Project. Annu. Rev. Publ. Hlth., **6**, 147–93
67. Puska, P. (1987). Multiple factor intervention: Community studies. In Olsson, A.G. *et al.* (eds.) *Atherosclerosis*, pp. 403–8. (New York: Churchill Livingstone)
68. Salonen, J.T. (1987). Did the North Karelia Project reduce coronary mortality? (Letter) *Lancet*, **2**, 269
69. Krahn, M.D., Naylor, C.D., Basinski, A. and Detsky, A.S. (1991). A comparison of an aggressive (U.S.) and a less aggressive (Canadian) policy for cholesterol screening and treatment. *Ann. Intern. Med.*, **115**, 248–55
70. Lipid Research Clinics Program. The Lipid Research Clinics coronary primary prevention trial results. I. Reduction in incidence of coronary heart disease. *J. Am. Med. Assoc.*, **251**, 351–64
71. Lipid Research Clinics Program. (1984). The Lipid Research Clinics Coronary Primary Prevention Trial Results. II. The relation in the reduction in incidence of coronary heart disease to cholesterol lowering. *J. Am. Med. Assoc.*, **251**, 365–74
72. McNeil, B.J., Pauker, S.G., Sox, H.C. Jr. and Tversky, A. (1982). On the elicitation of preferences for alternative therapies. *N. Engl. J. Med.*, **306**, 1259–62
73. Brett, A.S. (1984). Ethical issues in risk factor intervention. *Am. J. Med.*, **76**, 557–61
74. Brett, A.S. (1989). Treating hypercholesterolemia: how should practicing physicians interpret the published data for patients? *N. Engl. J. Med.*, **321**, 676–80
75. Frick, M.H., Elo, O., Haapa, K. *et al.* (1987). Helsinki heart study: primary prevention trial with gemfibrozil in middle-aged men with dyslipidemia. *N. Engl. J. Med.*, **317**, 1237–45
76. Lomas, J., Anderson, G.M., Domnick-Pierre, K., Vayda, E., Enkin, M.W. and Hannah, W.J. (1989). Do practice guidelines guide practice? The effect of a consensus statement on the practice of physicians. *N. Engl. J. Med.*, **321**, 1306–11
77. Leitch, D. (1989). Who should have their cholesterol concentration measured? What experts in the United Kingdom suggest. *Br. Med. J.*, **298**, 1615–16
78. McElroy, J.R. (1990). Detecting and treating dyslipoproteinemias. *Can. Med. Assoc. J.*, **142**, 607–8
79. Browner, W.S. (1986). Estimating the impact of risk factor modification programs. *Am. J. Epidemiol.*, **123**, 143–53
80. Mclsaac, W., Naylor, C.D. and Basinski, A. (1991). Mismatch of treatment intensity and coronary risk under the National Cholesterol Education Program guidelines. *J. Gen. Intern. Med.* (in press)
81. McGee, D. (1973). *The Probability of Developing Certain Cardiovascular Diseases in Eight Years at Specified Values of some Characteristics.* (Framingham section 28). US-DHEW Publication no. 74-618
82. Naylor, C.D. (1991). Secondary vs primary prevention: if at first you don't succeed. *Can. Lipidol. Rev.*, **1**, 7

83. Pekkanen, J., Linn, S., Heiss, G. *et al.* (1990). Ten-year mortality from cardio-vascular disease in relation to cholesterol level among men with and without pre-existing cardiovascular disease. *N. Engl. J. Med.*, **322**, 1700–7
84. Roussow, J.E., Lewis, B. and Rifkind, B.M. (1990). The value of lowering cholesterol after myocardial infarction. *N. Engl. J. Med.*, **323**, 1112–19
85. Coronary Drug Project Research Group. (1973). The Coronary Drug Project: design, methods, and baseline results. *Circulation*, **47** (Suppl. 1), 1-179
86. Coronary Drug Project Research Group. (1975). Clofibrate and niacin in coronary heart disease. *J. Am. Med. Assoc.*, **231**, 360–81
87. Canner, P.L., Berge, K.G., Wenger, N.K., Stamler, J., Friedman, L., Prineas, R.J. *et al.* (1985). Fifteen year mortality in the Coronary Drug Project patients: Long-term benefit with niacin. *J. Am. Coll. Cardiol.*, **8**, 1245–55
88. Carlson, L.A. and Rosenhamer, G. (1988). Reduction of mortality in the Stockholm ischaemic heart disease secondary prevention study by combined treatment with clofibrate and nicotinic acid. *Acta Med. Scand.*, **223**, 405–18
89. Goldman, L., Weinstein, M.C., Goldman, P.A. and Williams, L.W. (1991). Cost-effectiveness of HMG-CoA reductase inhibition for primary and secondary prevention of coronary heart disease. *J. Am. Med. Assoc.*, **265**, 1145–51

Discussion

Dr Horlick: I have a couple of questions. Why are you not concerned about a risk ratio of 4? In most conditions a risk ratio of 4 would ring great alarm bells in the heads of epidemiologists.

Dr Naylor: There are a few things that need to be said. The first is that traditionally epidemiology and particularly population epidemiology has focused on relative risk. However, when you come down to the individual patient level, what matters is not relative risk but the absolute risk differences. Although the relative risk is impressive at 4, it is like the relative risk I incurred in the last 2 weeks by making four airplane flights. It is greater than someone who flew once, but in absolute terms it is a small risk and I am still going to take it. When we compare those small absolute risks to those that occur with multiple risk factors, you are looking at very different gradients. The relative risk gradient is probably quite small when you have two risk factors and go from low to high cholesterol, but the difference in absolute risk is quite astonishing. So, my instinct is to focus on the absolute risk rather than the relative risk and to worry less about many of those individuals who are sitting at 6.8 or 7 who we might not pick up. If we do pick them up, we should be very wary of how aggressively we treat them.

Dr Horlick: The second question I would like to ask is how did you arrive at the dysutility of diet? I am really somewhat amazed that you have the same dysutility figures for diet and for drugs.

Dr Naylor: We arrived at that partly by formal measures in anti-hypertensive drug studies and also by talking to some of our medical colleagues and to dieticians. We were also influenced, perhaps unduly, by some work that Toni Basinski had done. This was qualitative research, talking to families of individuals who were placed on dietary therapy, and we were struck by the extent to which dietary modification actually became a battleground within some families. From this we had a clear sense that there are some individuals who have virtually no dysutility from dietary change, who are happy with their diet and are compliant. They may actually have a tiny positive utility. They may feel virtuous and empowered by getting rid of all that high-fat stuff. Unfortunately we are missing, and I think this is particularly true in the lower socioeconomic classes, a large number of individuals who might have quite profound effects. Our major message is not to say that dietary therapy is out and it is a terrible thing. Rather, we would like the side-effects of dietary therapy to be considered. Very often we think of diet as benign, but let us start looking at it and studying it more carefully.

426

Dr Holub: With respect to diet and the prevention of heart disease, we have to be open to the consideration of risk factors for heart disease in addition to the blood lipid profile before writing off a dietary appreciation. A recent paper by Trip *et al.* in the *New England Journal of Medicine* (1990, **322**, 1549–54) showed the very great importance of platelet aggregability in terms of the risk of a second myocardial infarct in men who had their first. This brings me to a consideration of the work by Burr *et al.* (*Lancet*, 1989, **2**, 757–61) who showed that just by advising men, following their first myocardial infarct, to eat fish three times a week, which did not lower their blood cholesterol, it reduced their second-year mortality from heart disease and all causes by 29%. So, I think the diet consideration has to encompass a wide range of risk factors for cardiovascular disease.

Dr Naylor: I certainly agree with that. I did not have time to get into the whole issue of secondary prevention. Sometimes in the interpretation of the data, primary and secondary prevention are rolled together and I have problems with that. There is a biological rationale there, but epidemiologically, across middle aged males particularly, the baseline event rate in the secondary prevention setting is four times as high as in the primary prevention setting. This is true even in relatively high risk middle-aged males. If you start treating those individuals who have established coronary disease, it is not surprising that you are going to show more of a trend to all-cause mortality benefit because those individuals are likely to die of their coronary disease, as already established. Labelling issues can be thrown aside; they are already labelled. I am much less concerned about the dysutility of dietary therapy there because many of those individuals are going to feel helpless. They have had their first infarct; doing something that they can control may make them feel empowered about their illness. This may be especially so when they are being bombarded with multiple drugs. So, if we are talking about the post-infarct population, the secondary prevention population, I am quite happy to be more aggressive. But, with primary prevention I still think there are concerns about where we are going and about how aggressive we have been.

Dr Roncari: How about children, could you comment further upon your concerns or recommendations regarding the paediatric age group?

Dr Naylor: I certainly could not improve further on Dr Goldbloom's comments except to make one comment. Although we look at the heterozygous familial hypercholesterolaemias, we may be talking about one in 500 persons. Those individuals who get infarcts in their twenties are a tiny minority. There is part of me that says, yes, atherosclerosis may be starting then, but let us deal with it by a prudent diet on a population-wide basis and leave childhood alone. Let children enjoy their ice cream and everything else, and let's start the consent process when they are at least old enough to take account of some of this information in an adult way. At our house we follow a low-fat diet. I do not eat a lot of red meat; I am quite careful about that, except when I go out and treat myself. In our house we have two types of ice cream. There are the sorbets and the low-fat ice cream for my wife and myself and the high-fat ice cream for my children. Invariably we put both tubs on the table, the children eat the high-fat ice cream, and we eat our low-fat ice cream. Then my wife and I look longingly into their tubs and by the end of the meal we have been dipping into theirs as well. If you have been raised on a high-fat diet, a lot of the low-fat products simply taste abysmal and you only get your kicks eating something a little bit richer. I am in that camp!

Dr Roncari: I would like to register my major concern about public recommendations involving children because of the increasing evidence of the impairment of development and maturation with restriction of fat. Of course treatment is indicated in those who have specific dyslipidaemias, but otherwise I have major concerns about public health recommendations involving children. There is increasing evidence that there is a multiplicity of lipid factors which are essential for appropriate development of the visual and higher cerebral systems.

Dr Naylor: I suppose we are dealing with the possibility of a generation of kids who will have no insulation of their neurons.

Dr Connor: I thought it would be of interest to give you the data from our family heart study on the effect in mood in 800 people who followed a lower fat way of eating, and not a drastic change. Affect, or mood, actually improved. For example, in the opinion of our consulting psychologist, they were less likely to slay their brothers or take their own lives. So, I think that when people feel that they are taking control of their lives, as you indicated, they may feel better about themselves if they feel they are going in the right direction. We have in our population what we call 'fat attacks'. In addition to feeling better after a low-fat diet, you avoid these 'fat attacks' which people, who are accustomed to a low-fat diet, develop on the spree that they may have at a time of celebration.

Dr Naylor: That may well be a pretty exceptional situation and it is encouraging. However, consider a small town in Ontario where a solo general practitioner is operating with the hospital dietitian and badgering his or her patients about apple pie as well as lobsters and oysters. I am not so sure that we are going to get the same happy group of patients that you may be able to generate in your clinic. But, point well taken, I just think that we need to look more at that issue.

Dr Goldbloom: I would just like to make a brief comment to underline a couple of things that Dr Naylor has said. I agree that it is important that the undertaker should always have a difficult time getting the smile off your face, in other words, the quality of life is very important. The other comment I would like to make is really an expansion of something I alluded to previously. I think that we need to be very cognizant of the four quantum leaps that exist between the laboratory, the clinical trial, individual patient application and public health application.

I get to see a fair number of obese youngsters, particularly teenagers, and, as far as we can tell from both the scientific and clinical evidence, the vast majority are obese as a result of genetic abnormalities that are incompletely understood. Yet, the main form of treatment that is usually prescribed for them is diet. This occurs despite the fact that clinical trials indicate that dietary treatment of obese children is notoriously ineffective except in very tightly controlled circumstances and over the very short term. I make it a point to ask these youngsters what mealtime is like for them and, let me assure you, it is a horror. The adults sit around the table and watch disapprovingly every bite that enters the child's mouth. The children dread mealtime and they are fighting a condition which is largely genetically determined and over which they have no control. I suspect that in the issue of CHD we have only begun to tap the genetic pool in terms of recognizing a few specific genetic atherogenic entities. I also suspect that the next decade will bring to light several more and will allow us to treat people more as individuals and less as a common herd.

Dr Godsland: The point that has been raised during the last couple of days is that the 35-year-old women with a cholesterol of 250 mg/dl is apparently not at increased risk of a myocardial infarct as compared to her 35-year-old male equivalent. At this age it is not a problem for her, but women do go on to become 45, 55, and 65 years of age. As of yet we do not know that the diet she has been exposed to at 35 will not have any long term implications for disease at a later date. Do you think that is a fair comment?

Dr Naylor: I think that is a fair comment and I think this ties in a number of issues here. The first is stability of cholesterol measures over time and the tendency for women who have a cholesterol reading of 250 mg/dl at age 35 to acquire much higher readings by the time they are 55 years of age. You are also dealing with whether or not your recommendations on an individual testing basis include differential testing by age. Many of us are pretty comfortable ignoring the 35-year-old woman with no other risk factors, but some of us are starting to get less comfortable about ignoring the same woman when she is 45 or 50. If she has no other risk factors, certainly I could live with not testing her. If there is one other risk factor and she is postmenopausal

429

I could probably live with testing her and looking at her cholesterol at that point. I think the bottom line is that the absolute event rates are sufficiently low during the first 10 or 15 years of that woman's period post age 35 that being aggressive is very hard to justify. Her event rates scoot up postmenopausally. If we believe the clinical trials we can make a difference to those events within a few years. Starting treatment at age 50 may not be that terrible as opposed to subjecting her to 15 years of treatment between the ages of 35 and 50.

Dr Godsland: You showed a slide in which there was the statement that measures which confirm large benefit on the community do not benefit the individual. Taken on its own, that statement does not make much sense to me because the community is obviously made up of individuals who represent the benefit there is to the community.

Dr Naylor: You are taking a direct quote from the slide so let me return to the prose that I hope accompanied the slide. When we look back at Geoffrey Rose's statement about the prevention paradox in the setting of coronary disease, what I hoped to underscore was the notion as follows. First, if you treat those with cholesterols of 350 mg/dl or 330 mg/dl plus or minus other risk factors, the risk–benefit ratio and efficiency is more impressive. If you drop down to treating individuals who have lower cholesterols, a medical framework is inefficient and if you advocate community-wide dietary change, it is also inefficient. Compliance may be low and variable and those individuals may have very tiny increases in average life expectancy. If my cholesterol is 220 mg/dl and I change my diet, as I did some years ago, my potential benefit is pretty small on average. If you were to ask me to quantify my benefits and to decide whether my dietary change was worth it, who knows where I, or many people would come down. The benefits on average are tiny, yet aggregated across the whole population they can make a major difference to population health status. I think that is the kernel of the prevention paradox, both in medical treatment and at a population-wide level.

24
Canadian Consensus Conference on Cholesterol (CCCC)

L. HORLICK

The CCCC[1] was held in March of 1988. It was the fourth conference of its kind, having been preceded by the British[2], American[3] and European[4] Consensus conferences. The objective was to provide a distinctly Canadian viewpoint on coronary heart disease (CHD) prevention based on frequency and distribution of risk factors and the burden of CHD in Canada and to develop a policy on prevention. The policy aspects were to include the priority of a population or high-risk approach, and the appropriate screening of the population. In addition we hoped to build on distinctive Canadian contributions to the knowledge of lipoproteins and to design a system which would fit with our universal health system.

The format followed very closely that of the American Consensus organized by NHLBI. The Panel consisted of a family practitioner, a layman (barrister), two clinical biochemists, two nutritionists and two epidemiologists. The chairman was a cardiologist with a long-standing interest in lipid metabolism. The Panel considered the evidence linking cholesterol and coronary heart disease (CHD) which was presented by a group of experts, and was also asked to consider a series of questions prepared by the organizing committee. After the evidence had been presented to them by the experts, the Panel withdrew to formulate their conclusions. During the next 16 hours, the panellists discussed the issues and were able to reach a consensus, which was modified somewhat by the feedback received at the reporting session and subsequently.

In preparing its recommendations, the Panel was strongly influenced by the data available from the Nova Scotia Heart Health Study[5] which had been completed shortly before the Consensus Conference. This was the first major epidemiological survey of risk factors carried out in Canada, and the forerunner of what has become a national programme. It showed that 39% of males and 31% of females aged 35–64 had blood cholesterol levels above 220 mg/dl. It also showed that only 29% of the population aged 17–74, both sexes, was free of the three cardinal risk factors (hypercholesterolaemia, hypertension, smoking). Although we only had the data from Nova Scotia at the time, we

431

assumed that similar data would be forthcoming from the other Provincial surveys, and we have since been proved right. It was the Nova Scotia data that led us to make our most important decision, namely to opt for a population-based strategy for control of hypercholesterolaemia. In this respect we differed from the American Consensus[3] which initially opted for a high-risk case-finding strategy.

It was clear to us that only a total population approach could hope to remedy the situation and reduce the risk. It was based on health promotion strategies for the entire population, and included action on all the risk factors rather than on cholesterol alone. It would require the collective involvement of health service personnel at all levels of government. We have therefore made important recommendations concerning dietary changes for the entire population, food products, and a new population goal for total cholesterol. We recommended a reduction in total fat and saturated fat in the Canadian diet, to 30% and less than 10% respectively, and this has since been incorporated in the new Nutrition Recommendations for Canada[6]. We also recommended that the agriculture and food industries be encouraged to maintain and continue efforts to produce foods low in total fat, saturated fat and cholesterol. Restaurants, fast-food outlets, industrial and school cafeterias were encouraged to offer such foods. We recommended strongly that consumers should have better, more explicit food information/labelling in order to facilitate healthy food choices. We also recommended as a feasible long-term goal a mean population serum cholesterol of 190 mg/dl, a level considered attainable through public health measures and commensurate with a low incidence of CHD.

We did not ignore the problem of the high-risk individuals in our society. However we gave it a lower priority than the population approach. The Panel made recommendations for screening which were aimed at individuals known to be at risk, but reserved universal screening for a time when resources would permit. It recommended the lipid parameters to be screened, and then made some basic recommendations for intervention. Thus we advocated the determination of total cholesterol, triglyceride, HDL cholesterol and LDL cholesterol in the fasting state as the basic screen. In this respect we differed from the NCEP recommendations which used non-fasting cholesterol as the basic screen. New evidence has emerged in the last few years which indicates the importance of triglycerides and HDL as discriminating factors for CHD and lends support to our initial decision to include these tests in the screen. Screening was reserved for individuals with known CHD or a strong family history of CHD and/or hyperlipidaemia occurring before age 60, or for those with other risk factors such as hypertension, smoking, diabetes, renal failure and obesity. The emphasis in treatment was on the dietary intervention, and we gave only very general advice about drug treatment. Simplified cut-off points were used stratified into two age classes, but not by sex. For men and women over age 30 a cholesterol level under 5.2 mmol/l (200 mg/dl) was regarded as acceptable and should be re-checked in 5 years. Individuals in the range 5.2-6.2 mmol/l (200–240 mg/dl) should have dietary education provided, while those in this range but with LDL cholesterol levels above 3.4 mmol/l (130 mg/dl) or HDL cholesterol levels below 0.9 mmol/l (35 mg/dl) required intensive dietary therapy. Cholesterol levels above 6.2 mmol/l (240 mg/dl), which were resistant to intensive dietary therapy might require pharmacological measures (Table 1).

Table 1 CCCC recommendations

1 – SCREENING	Individuals with CHD	
	Family history of hyperlipidaemia or CHD < 60	
	Hypertension, diabetes, renal failure,	
	obesity, (smoking).	
	As part of periodic health examination for	
	all adults (as circumstances permit).	
2 – INTERVENTION	Males and females > age 30	
	Total cholesterol	
	5.2–6.2 mmol/l	**Dietary advice**
	and LDLC > 3.4, or	
	HDLC < 0.9 or Trig > 2.3	**Dietary instruction**
	> 6.2 mmol/l	and hypolipidaemic drugs after minimum 6 months of intensive diet.
	Males and females age 18–29	
	Total cholesterol	
	4.6–5.7 mmol/l	Dietary advice
	and LDLC > 3.0, or	
	HDLC < 0.9 or Trig > 2.3	**Dietary instruction**
	> 5.7 mmol/l	and hypolipidaemic drugs after minimum 6 months of intensive diet

Like the other consensuses we were concerned that there be an accurate diagnosis, and a rigorous 6-month trial of diet before drug therapy was undertaken. We felt that the decision as to when to initiate drug therapy should be made by the physician taking into account his knowledge of all the factors concerning the individual involved. We stressed the importance of acting on all risk factors rather than on cholesterol alone.

A vigorous high-risk approach will have important cost implications for the health-care system, and will create major problems for physicians, dietitians, and laboratory services. The Panel recognized that dietary counselling was probably the weakest link in the chain, and that we needed many more dietitians and nutritionists in order to cope with the more than one-third of our adult population with cholesterol levels in the range of moderate and high risk. We will need to upgrade our laboratory services to ensure that accurate and reproducible measurements can be made.

Since the CCCC recommendations were made there have been a number of promising developments in Canada. We have almost completed the risk-factor surveys which will give us the best national risk-factor inventory anywhere in the world, and enable us to plan preventive and therapeutic programmes for the different regions of Canada. A number of pilot programmes supported by the provinces and NHW are being planned, and some are already under way in Nova Scotia. A prime target will be that part of the population in the lower socio-economic bracket which has the highest incidence of disease, and which is not being reached by current programmes.

Table 2 The Canadian Lipoprotein Conference guidelines

		CHD risk		
Age	*Normal*	*Borderline*	*High*	*Very high*
Plasma total cholesterol final screen (mmol/l)				
≤19	<4.0	>4.0	>4.5	>5.0
20–29	<4.5	>4.5	>5.0	>6.0
30–39	<5.0	>5.0	>5.5	>6.5
≥40	<5.5	>5.5	>6.0	>7.0
Plasma LDL-C (mmol/l)				
≤19	<2.5	>2.5	>2.8	>3.2
20–29	<3.0	>3.0	>3.5	>4.0
30–39	<3.5	>3.5	>4.0	>4.5
≥40	<4.0	>4.0	>4.5	>5.0
Retest	5 yrs	<6 mo	<2 mo	<2 mo
Intensive		if CHD risk		
diet R		factors +	yes	yes
Retest		6–12 mo	6 mo	<6 mo
Drug R			CHD+	
			TC or LDLC	
			remain high or very high	

We have new national dietary recommendations for Canada which limit fat intake to 30% of calories and urge reduction of saturated fat and cholesterol[6]. The CCCC recommendations have been widely circulated and have had a major influence on Canadian physicians. Unfortunately we did not provide precise cut-off points for drug therapy, and this has sparked controversy and confusion[7]. This issue has since been addressed by the Canadian Lipoprotein Conference[8] and they have come up with cut-off points which are somewhat more conservative than those of the National Cholesterol Education Expert Panel[9] (Table 2), but not as conservative as those suggested by the Toronto Working Group on Cholesterol Policy[7] (Table 3). The CCCC Panel placed top priority on the population approach realizing that its success would in the end greatly reduce the number of individuals who might require expensive drug treatment. We must not allow ourselves to be distracted by this controversy over cut-off points for the high-risk individual from the objective of reducing risk for the population as a whole.

Table 3 Toronto Working Group recommendations

	Total cholesterol (mmol/l)		
	<6.2	6.2–6.9	>6.9
Repeat cholesterol	—	+	+
Fractionate	—	+/–	+
Modify other RFs	+	+	+
Dietary advice	—	+	+
Dietary therapy	—	+ if male with one RF/or female two RFs	+

LDL cholesterol (mmol/l)	
4.9–5.5	>5.5
Drug treatment	
+/– Intensify diet and RF reduction	+
If no improvement after 6 months diet therapy	If no improvement after 3 months dietary therapy
and unmodified RFs remain	

References

1. Canadian Consensus Conference on Cholesterol; final report. *Can. Med. Assoc. J.*, **139**, 1–8, 1988
2. Report of the British Cardiac Society Working Group on Coronary Disease Prevention. London, British Cardiac Society, 1987
3. Consensus Conference: Lowering blood cholesterol to prevent heart disease. *J. Am. Med. Assoc.*, **253**, 2080–6, 1985
4. Study Group. European Atherosclerosis Society. (1987). Strategies for the prevention of coronary heart disease. *Eur. Heart J.*, **8**, 77–88
5. Report of the Nova Scotia Heart Health Study (1986). Nova Scotia Department of Health and Department of National Health and Welfare (Canada)
6. Nutrition Recommendations. A Call for Action. National Health and Welfare Canada. Report of the Scientific Review Committee and the Communications/Implementation Committee, 1989
7. Detection and Management of Asymptomatic Hypercholesterolemia. A Policy Document by the Toronto Working Group on Cholesterol Policy. Prepared for the Task Force on the Use and Provision of Medical Services. Ontario Ministry of Health, 1989
8. Guidelines for the detection of high-risk lipoprotein profiles and the treatment of dyslipoproteinemias. The Canadian Lipoprotein Conference ad hoc committee on guidelines for dyslipoproteinemia. *Can. Med. Assoc. J.*, **142**, 1371–81, 1990
9. Report of the National Cholesterol Education Program Expert Panel on Detection, Evaluation and Treatment of High Blood Cholesterol in Adults. *Arch. Intern. Med.*, **148**, 36–39, 1988

Discussion

Dr Gold: In the initial slide you showed us the first recommendation, a general address of all risk factors. I do not think that there is anyone in the room who would disagree that tobacco consumption is the number one controllable parameter as concerns CHD. The control of blood pressure is certainly another major area but of all of the risk factors, why did the Consensus Conference choose to address the lipid problem only, when smoking and blood pressure control, I think, would have gotten you a consensus in the first 30 seconds of the meeting? Certainly these two parameters have not yet gained universal societal acceptance. On the other hand, the recommendations concerning lipid intake and serum cholesterol appear to have opened a Pandora's Box vis-à-vis recommendations, interpretations of recommendations and media transmission to the population of these recommendations before all of the evidence is in.

Dr Horlick: Well, we had to start somewhere. The evidence for cholesterol seemed strong and we decided to focus in on this but, as I pointed out before, we never lost sight of the fact that there are other risk factors which are important as well.

Dr Gold: Then why not just say, as a definite recommendation, that cigarette smoking should be eliminated in the Canadian population?

Dr Horlick: I do not disagree with you at all, perhaps it was a mistake not to say that.

Dr Skrabanek: As you mentioned that this was meant to be a contribution to the health of the Canadian people, I wonder if you would at least consider the possibility that this could be the contribution to ill health in the Canadian people. I say this because all interventions, particularly intervention in healthy people, carries some kind of risk. If the benefit is small, then even a small risk would overweigh the benefit. You, for example, recommend intense counselling for someone who has a cholesterol of 240 mg/dl. As you did not have any age limit on this I take it that this could even apply for a 70-year-old woman. If such a woman would have 6 months of intense counselling, do you not think that it would have some effect on her psychological well-being? How can you say that a cholesterol more than 220 mg/dl is a risk factor, for young or old, for women? I think that if you issue this kind of recommendation, surely there must be some kind of ethical obligation to provide people with the full information that is available and to inform the public that there is no evidence from control trials that this kind of intervention reduces mortality.

These people are not going to live any longer and I think the public should be entitled to that kind of information as well.

Dr Horlick: First of all I disagree with you on several points. There is evidence to suggest that there is a continuing relationship between cholesterol and morbidity and mortality from CHD into old age. These data come from the 30-year Framingham study. There are also a number of other small studies that confirm these data in older people. I think there is a benefit to everyone in the population by knowing about these relationships.

The second part is that physicians are not idiots. You are assuming that they are going to act the same way with a 30-year-old male as they would with an 80-year-old female – they are not. We gave them some credit for having good sense and having the ability to apply the guidelines in a sensible way and, I think that in fact, that is what they are doing. Intervention has both its upside and its downside, there is no question about that. I think that there is enough evidence to suggest that the upside of intervention, particularly in a problem that affects so many people and that costs the Canadian taxpayer somewhere in the range of five billion dollars a year, is worth doing.

Dr Gold: You give your colleagues too much credit, Dr Horlick.

Dr Grover: I think the Canadian Consensus on Cholesterol was a fairly moderate document in a number of ways. I agree with you that first and foremost it was aimed at identifying the role of cholesterol in the development of atherosclerosis and bringing to the attention of the Canadian public that this was a potential problem. I think it was also moderate in terms of the use of pharmacological agents which a number of other consensus conferences were much more aggressive about.

However, I have two major problems with the document. Firstly, it really does not discriminate in terms of cut-off points across age and sex. As you have shown with data here, and as I and others have shown, based on these recommendations, we are basically identifying the vast majority of elderly women as being at risk when everything we know from Framingham and epidemiologic data suggests that this is the group that is going to benefit the least. We have to remind ourselves that, if you have reached the age of 65 and have never had a chest pain, you have already demonstrated that you are fairly tolerant of whatever cholesterol level and constellation of risk factors you have. So, my first concern is that we have to tease out older individuals from these recommendations.

The other thing you did not really touch on was recommendations for children. I thought that this was a good thing, however, it has not prevented others in our society from doing so. These people have used the recommendations as a jumping-off point and now we are talking about following a specific diet for everybody over the age of two. I am not an expert in paediatrics but I am a parent and it absolutely frightens me when I see my kids playing in the basement, pretending they are at McDonalds and they are serving each other low-cholesterol french fries or something. How did my kids ever get worried about such issues? All I am getting at, and the recommendations originally said this, was that they represent a starting point and that we need to come back and make them better. I really believe that it is time to get back and to make them better.

Dr Horlick: In response to your comments, I think that they are well taken. In regard to your first point, I agree that it would have been better if we had been able to break this down by age ranges. However, in the interest of simplicity, and the fact that people do not remember large streams of numbers, we opted for this. I showed the Canadian Lipoprotein Conference Recommendations where there is a long stream of numbers and I am perfectly certain that if you talked to any practicing physician, he or she could not give you the numbers. However, they can remember simple numbers and I agree, you pay a price for that.

With respect to your second point, of course we did say in the consensus document that we could not reach consensus about children. We felt that as far as children were concerned, we did not advocate any major dietary changes for healthy children. However, children who were known to be dyslipidaemic, needed to be treated and I think that is a sensible recommendation. We cannot be held responsible for the irresponsible interpretation of our data by others.

Sheila Murphy: Do you have any information on the socioeconomic breakdown of who is dying from heart disease?

Dr Horlick: I do not have that data here but National Health and Welfare Canada has a lot of data on the socioeconomic breakdown for CHD and for all other diseases as well. We are currently analyzing the Saskatchewan Heart Health Study data for that and I can tell you, without quoting numbers, that there is definitely a concentration of increased risk in the lower socioeconomic stratum. This is clearly an area that we are not reaching.

General Discussion

PAUL BRADLEY ADDIS
University of Minnesota
St. Paul, Minnesota, USA

I do not believe that the conference has changed my views but it has been an exceptional experience. I started at sea level, went to the top and came back down to sea level. The trip has been informative but has not changed my viewpoint – namely, that the lipid hypothesis is rather weak. That is not to say that it is totally fallacious but it is a weak hypothesis. I think that an extreme adherence to the hypothesis has necessarily excluded other promising avenues of research on coronary artery disease (CAD) including fish oils, lipid oxidation products and platelets. David Naylor's comments about the need to look at other types of markers of CAD that might be more accurate than serum cholesterol are another example of an area that should be investigated. Numerous criticisms may be raised about the research cited to support the lipid hypothesis but I will mention only a few: (1) the short period of time used; (2) the lack of concern about cholesterol oxidation products in cholesterol-feeding studies; (3) the extrapolation to free-living people from those in metabolic wards; and (4) lack of control or inappropriate fatty acid compositions in cholesterol-feeding studies. As Stan Kubow pointed out, the work of Eddington of Oxford University is seminal in pointing out the fact that even responders could be reclassified as nonresponders if the experimental protocol is carried out for a total of 8 weeks rather than for shorter time periods and appropriate diets are fed. Another comment has to do with the relative importance of HDL and LDL. William Connor told us that saturated fat, while it raised LDL, also raised HDL, but that this increase in HDL was not a benefit or 'was not important'. Other speakers told us that HDL is important. I think we have to decide, is it important or is it not? I don't think we can have it both ways. There needs to be consistency in the message we are sending out to the public. We must be willing to admit when 'our hypothesis' is not supported by experimental results. A final comment is that I am very interested in using the techniques we have developed in the area of quantification of lipid oxidation products in combination with the abilities of the people in this room. Joint activities such as cooperative research ventures and cooperative attempts to obtain research funding will be welcomed by our research group at the University of Minnesota.

KEAVEN ANDERSON
Centocor
Malvern, PA, USA

I would like to make a few comments about mortality and also about some age, sex issues.

There are various 'rules of thumb' that I use to help guide me when thinking about certain problems. One of these is that if you eliminated coronary heart disease, you would expect to increase average life span by a maximum of 2 years. Certainly, the later in life you wait to prevent heart disease by altering its underlying causes, the less you expect to increase population life-expectancy. In any case, using mortality, or life-expectancy, as your endpoint, you are not giving yourself much of a chance for gain.

In the Framingham cohort, if you start with a relatively healthy population aged 30–50 and follow that population for 30 years, there is a striking relationship between cholesterol measured at that 'young' age and subsequent mortality. I believe that Dr Grover's models combine multiple shorter term follow-ups to estimate long-term associations between cholesterol and mortality. In general, that 'joining together' weakens the long-term relationship between cholesterol and mortality.

Running clinical trials concerning the treatment of coronary heart disease to study mortality is often not appropriate. By the time you would be able to show differences in mortality, you would have had such big differences in morbidity that it would have been unethical to continue the trials.

I have a few comments about lipids in the elderly. I was interested in Louis Horlick's remark about wanting a simple measure that you could use across all age groups – and using that in defence of calling, say, a 60 or 70-year-old woman with a 250 mg/dl cholesterol at high risk. If you look exclusively at that group in the Framingham Study, the single measure you would want would be HDL cholesterol. If you divide people by tertiles of HDL with the cut points coming about 45 and 55 mg/dl, the high risk group would have about a 20% CHD incidence over the course of 12 years, whereas the low risk group would have about a 5% incidence. Thus lipid measurements can still be quite useful in stratifying a population into high and low risk groups even among elderly women. The reason I and others at Framingham promote the total to HDL cholesterol ratio is that it stratifies risk well across all sex and age-groups from age 30 to over age 70.

Both the Whitehall and Framingham studies suggest that over the long-term, cholesterol is still a risk factor in the elderly. In particular, a recent analysis of the Whitehall study was nicely done. They found that the further in time a cholesterol measurement was taken before a follow-up period, the stronger it was related to CHD incidence in that period. On the other hand, you do not see strong associations with cholesterol measured at an elderly age and subsequent disease. An exception to this is the Honolulu Study where the biggest differences in absolute risk associated with cholesterol come in elderly men.

In Framingham, we recently measured carotid artery stenosis. The measurements of cholesterol that were most strongly associated with stenosis measurement were those taken 30 years prior!

There are a couple of plausible explanations for why we do not always see associates of cholesterol with coronary heart disease in the elderly. One is that there might be a harvesting effect going on and that those sensitive to cholesterol have gotten heart disease before they become elderly. In Honolulu, where CHD prevalence was lower at 'old' age, incidence was associated with cholesterol. A second possibility, which is difficult to study statistically, is that a fall in cholesterol, weight, vital capacity, or blood pressure is predictive of subsequent mortality. Thus, a low cholesterol group in an elderly population may be a mixture of low risk individuals who always had low cholesterol and high risk individuals who have only recently achieved a low cholesterol. In such a case, one would not expect to find much of an association between cholesterol and subsequent CHD incidence.

PIERRE BUDOWSKI
The Hebrew University of Jerusalem
Revohot, Israel

One of my concerns has to do with the widespread use – and abuse – of the P/S ratio in the context of nutrition and CHD. 'P' stands for polyunsaturated fatty acids, but for all practical purposes it means linoleic acid. However, there is a second PUFA family, the n-3 fatty acids, whose main representative in our diet is α-linolenic acid and whose effects are different from those of linoleic acid. It is therefore wrong to lump the two fatty acid families together under the heading 'P'. My second concern is about extremely unbalanced PUFA intakes: this may be either an excessive linoleic acid consumption (a trend that has been observed in our dietary habits) or a dietary excess of n-3 fatty acids, as demonstrated by Hugh Sinclair, who consumed during 100 days an Eskimo diet of seal, fish and crustaceans with unpleasant results. We must find out what the desirable PUFA balance ought to be. Undoubtedly, more fish in our diet would help to redress what appears to be a PUFA imbalance favoring linoleic acid. Perhaps we should also think of ways to increase the consumption of α-linolenic acid: new food products have already appeared, such as ground linseed and linseed bread, which have excellent organoleptic properties. We may expect to see more such developments in the future.

M.T. (TOM) CLANDININ
University of Alberta
Edmonton, Alberta, Canada

I agree with Phil Yeagle in that the public awareness aspect of science is very important, and that these days it is very important that scientists talk about what they do so that the public will continue to support science and indeed begin to understand science better. I have been impressed with some of the epidemiological stories I have heard and I suspect that the 35 people in the room here would have 35 different stories, all of which are not really right or wrong but are interesting views of how the perspective of this disease evolves. From my own perspective, I am not entirely convinced by the epidemiology because I like to see mechanisms and, therefore, I do not like to base general dietary advice just on the epidemiology without clear mechanisms. I think as a reflection on the topics that we have covered and not covered, there are several areas with which I am a little uncomfortable. We have not really discussed the role of platelets in this whole disease process and I think we need to pay more attention to the developmental aspects of lipoprotein metabolism. This is not necessarily with the view of making dietary changes in young children, it is more with the perspective that there may be some earlier markers that we are missing because we are not really looking at that period of time. We have heard from the pathologists that this is a process that begins in the fetus and thus there is a period of development that we have not looked at in terms of how the disease evolves. One of the other areas that has been ignored is the aspect of lipoprotein phospholipids and fatty acid metabolism. This is an area we need to cover in some way. I am also concerned that we do not know enough or have not found other dynamic measures for the regulation of cholesterol synthesis. I think some of these sorts of approaches might be fairly revealing to look at how the individual responds to diet to sort out why we have responders and nonresponders. I think, too, that we have traditionally viewed the gastrointestinal tract as passing on the composition of much of what we eat in different ways and not doing too much with it. We need to take a little more careful look at the gut because I think it is doing a lot more than just that. The ability to respond or not respond may be related to what the gut is doing. In terms of our public health approach, I have some concerns about the recommendations, partly because we have been involved for some years now in assessing dietary intakes in fairly well educated people that are health conscious, and who volunteer for various kinds of studies. Even in those subjects who are well informed, it is very difficult to find subjects that have low saturated fat intakes and have high polyunsaturated fat intakes, even though they think that they should do so. This tells me that people are relatively ineffective at translating recommendations into some sort of action that they can take at the level of foods. As a nutritionist, one of the things that you cope with is that everybody who eats is an expert in nutrition and they have certain preconceived ideas. We have sort of bamboozled the public with recommendations, but the consumer still does not know how to translate low cholesterol or specific types of fatty acid into foods. The public has been encouraged to label foods as good or bad and I think that understanding does not reflect the most appropriate form of communication.

WILLIAM E. CONNOR
Oregon Health Sciences University
Portland, Oregon, USA

This has been a most interesting conference because of the diversity of opinions. I think both wit and perspective are enhanced if there is wit and controversy rather than patting each other on the back and saying, 'We know it all so let's go home'. I would like to comment on a couple of issues but, in particular, to emphasize that, while there seems to be unanimity about cigarette smoking, I deduce very few markers for those who smoke who will develop lung cancer, coronary disease and cancer of the bladder and larynx. I happen to be in a family in which there are a large number of smokers and they continue to smoke regardless of the evidence that has been given by numerous Surgeon General reports. They say, 'How do I know that I am the one who is going to develop lung cancer, do you have any information?' and obviously, I do not. I think we have to be sceptical in all areas and not just necessarily assume that we should quit smoking and not respond to similar bits of evidence in which there may be better markers about dietary fat. I am not advocating smoking mind you, but the tobacco lobby does have that point well in hand and they have continued to shout about it. We have to be careful about using the same scientific scrutiny about all aspects of health when we focus upon dietary fats and cholesterol.

I would emphasize the vessel wall. We have two factors in coronary disease. We have the blood factors and we have the vessel wall itself. We know very little about why some people with high LDLs will develop coronary disease and others do not. I have a number of elderly patients with familial hypercholesterolaemia and indeed, we are collecting such examples, both women and men, who lived past 70 and even into the 80s with this supposedly lethal disease. Why are these people spared? We do not know a lot about the vessel wall and, in particular, the factors that contribute to thrombosis. The critical event which causes myocardial infarction is thrombotic. Atherosclerosis is the underlying disease, but the event rate is thrombotic. I suspect that women are spared from coronary disease because they are less susceptible to thrombosis, particularly in the premenopausal years, for reasons that are not completely understood. White showed a long time ago in Minneapolis that the amount of atherosclerotic disease in both sexes was basically parallel with age. Women had as much atherosclerosis as men but they did not have as many coronary events. So, we need to think about the factors in the diet and in the lifestyle that leads to thrombosis. Obviously, physical inactivity is a major contributor to causing thrombosis.

Children. The big issue here is that we do not know completely the proper nutrition for infants. We have, as the head paediatrician at the Johns Hopkins Hospital has said, 100 years of experimenting with infant formulas, but still do not know the correct infant formula. Many of us are very concerned about the ω-6–ω-3 balance and imbalance in current infant formulas. I think that we need to know a lot more about what is the proper nutrition for children. We do not have the answer yet, so changing the diet of children is a moot point. We need to find out what the best diet is for children and a lot of experiments have to be done to ascertain that.

Basically, I am an optimist in regard to the coronary epidemic – Sir William Osler said in 1920, in one of his editions of the *Textbook of Medicine* (of course, he was a Canadian) that, 'angina pectoris is a rare disease in hospitals'. He stated that one would see, in the large city hospitals of North America, one or two cases of angina pectoris a year, so I think we have had a disease become epidemic since the 1920s but is now an epidemic which is waning. I think that is a cause for optimism. Coronary heart disease is waning because of declining risk factors in our Western populations (dietary change to low fat and cholesterol, cessation of smoking, less hypertension, etc.).

MICHELINE DE BELDER
Montreal Heart Institute
Montréal, Québec, Canada

I am the chief dietician at the Montreal Heart Institute, so I need practical and safe information on prevention.

I came here to get answers but I am leaving with more questions.

For me, low fat diet, as proposed by the Canadian Consensus Conference on Cholesterol, is well adapted to the first-step diet for people at risk for heart disease. I have no problems teaching this diet to these patients, but when it concerns whole populations, including infants and children, it is more difficult to transpose this on an individual basis. For example, parents who are eating only 'light' foods because of concerns about heart disease may also feed this diet to their children.

Eating patterns are usually habitual, so any modification of diet composition through manipulation of fatty acids, additives, etc. will greatly alter overall nutritional intake.

The second point is that 'light' foods or vegetable fats are not seen by people as being bad or that they should be limited. So people eat as much as they want, thinking these foods are free of any bad effects. Ultimately, nutrient consumption can be different but the total fat intake will not necessarily be lower. In 'light' foods, fiber content is higher, some minerals are less abundant, fatty acids are in new proportions, and 'new' fatty acids are introduced ..... What will the result be in the next generation?

JOHN M. DIETSCHY
University of Texas
Dallas, Texas, USA

I do not want to deal with public policy matters, but I would like to comment on something that David Naylor said. When a patient presents with a complication of atherosclerotic disease, there are really at least three components involved. First, there is the problem of LDL cholesterol levels and how these levels are associated with the development of atherosclerosis. The principles involved in the regulation of LDL levels are now fairly well understood. Second, there is also the problem of atheroma formation. Presumably, if one had a large number of individuals with the same LDL-cholesterol level, there presumably would be genetic variation in the rate at which each of these individuals went ahead to develop atherosclerosis. Third, there is also the problem of genetic variation in clotting. Clearly, for any level of atheroma formation, there may be differences among different individuals in terms of when vascular occlusion occurs secondary to clotting. Thus, there are at least three major processes involved in the development of overt clinical atherosclerotic disease and each of these is subject to genetic variation. It seems unlikely, therefore, that any single marker will necessarily identify the patients who are at risk. Nevertheless, the close association between LDL-cholesterol levels and atherosclerosis and the availability of very potent new forms of therapy make it very reasonable to attack this particular aspect of the problem at this time.

IAN F. GODSLAND
Wynn Institute for Metabolic Research
London, United Kingdom

I work for two old hands in the cholesterol game. One is Professor Victor Wynn who, 20 years ago, was severely criticized for wasting resources by measuring cholesterol in middle-aged men, with the intention of identifying and modifying their risk of coronary heart disease. The other is Professor Michael Oliver, who some of you may know as a moderating voice in calls for mass screening and population modification of cholesterol levels. So I came into this meeting with my views fairly evenly balanced on either side of the debate. I have come out cautiously in favour of intervention, and the metabolic and cell biology data that we have seen have been mainly responsible for that. Studies exemplified by the work of John Dietschy leave me in little doubt that modification of dietary fat intake can modify circulating cholesterol levels. From the results reported by Martijn Katan, it is evident that such diet-induced changes can be difficult to detect in the population as a whole, but it does seem possible, given sufficiently careful experimental design. Against these arguments in favour of dietary intervention and cholesterol-lowering, I think we should be paying more attention to the possible effects of low cholesterol concentrations. I certainly take Martijn Katan's point that societies with low cholesterol clearly do not have cancer or suicide epidemics. But I think there is a difference between having a low cholesterol and having one's cholesterol lowered. I wonder if we, in so-called Western societies, are to some extent cholesterol junkies, and, if our supply is cut, our physiology goes rather crazy. Among other issues that I think could be given more attention, there is the parallelism between changes in HDL and LDL cholesterol in response to diet, and the evident importance of lipid oxidation products in this whole area. On balance, however, I think it would be unfortunate if consideration of these issues was to detract from the positive steps towards modifying coronary heart disease rates that are under way at the moment. Whilst this evidence is not conclusive, there does seem to be enough of it to justify taking practical measures towards lowering cholesterol in the population as a whole.

RICHARD B. GOLDBLOOM
Dalhousie University
Halifax, Nova Scotia

I do not know if any ideas have changed a great deal as a result of this conference, but that is probably a function of age and perhaps because my serum cholesterol is not very subject to change at this stage. However, the experience reminded me that, as one sage put it ... 'Good research does not necessarily give the answers but it certainly sharpens the questions'. Many questions have been sharpened over the last 2 days and that has been a tremendous help to me as an interested bystander.

I mentioned yesterday that I was disturbed by the current TV commercial depicting three toddlers discussing the Surgeon General's report on cholesterol. I am equally disturbed by the TV news pictures of youngsters starving elsewhere in the world. The contrast places in stark focus what an extraordinary luxury it is to be able to sit around a table in this opulent hotel and talk about a health problem which affects, for the most part, the elderly in our society, who already live twice as long as most people in the world. I do think that we have to maintain a balanced perspective. The other concern I have after listening to the presentations is how we interpret risk both to the public and to the individual patient. In paediatric practice, when we see a child born with congenital anomalies, it may be determined that there is a 5% chance of recurrence in subsequent children, and most parents want to know the recurrence risk. Physicians fall into two groups: some focus on the 5% risk of recurrence and others focus on the 95% risk of normalcy. The mathematics are the same but the impact can be very different. This is an important aspect of balance in the perception of risk. I frankly worry when I see risk factor charts for coronary disease. Not so much in the mathematics but in how it is applied. What are people going to be told by their doctors? Most doctors and patients like binary decisions: do it or don't do it. They are not interested in various gradations of options or risk. From an emotional point of view, we have to ask ourselves, are we doing more good than harm by the clinical application of this kind of information.

Another issue which was not discussed very much here was the question of cost and cost benefit. These must be considered not only in relation to the target disease but to all health outcomes. Not everything can be measured in dollars. In a country like Canada where the health care system is entirely publicly funded, we must weigh the cost of intervening in a preventive or therapeutic form for cardiovascular disease against other issues such as mammography, programs to detect cervical cancer, etc. Thus, we may be approaching the point where we will have to compare disparate options in order to make public policy decisions. The science of cost effectiveness analysis is in its infancy. I attended a presentation last year by David Eddy in the United States, who used a computer model to compare the costs of various interventions to prevent cardiovascular disease. Though I do not recall the exact figures, the cost of various models of screening and intervention at different ages ran to billions of dollars. Where resources are limited, we cannot ignore such realities.

Another striking omission from our deliberations was the applicability of the information we discussed to the highest risk in our society, i.e. the poor. In inner cities, where a young, black American man may have a one in four chance of dying by violence before the age of 35, it is going to be very difficult to interest that young man or his family in the serum cholesterol issue. During the Vietnam war, someone studied the future thinking of the Vietnamese and showed that they were virtually incapable of thinking beyond the next 24 hours because their whole focus of survival was through that time period. In the same way, for many poor people in our society, the world ends about five blocks from home and life can only be planned perhaps 6 months ahead. Therefore, even if we had the indisputable answers, the selling job would be (understandably) very difficult among the groups at highest risk in our society. Ours is a very middle-class approach to the problem.

Finally, I think we must be very selective in clinical practice about how we interpret information like this to individual patients. Too often, we inadvertently blame the victim. A couple of years ago I attended a nutrition conference at the University of Western Ontario and someone quoted a study of the eating habits of dieticians. It showed that their eating habits were no different than those of the rest of the population. So often we ask patients to do things that we are incapable of doing ourselves. When we do so, we inadvertently blame the victim; an act which runs exactly counter to the physician's ultimate mission to the patient, which is to relieve anxiety.

STEVEN A. GROVER
McGill University
Montréal, Québec, Canada

There has been some excellent science presented at this conference during the past few days. The data presented demonstrate how good scientific research has helped us to arrive at this point in the diet/coronary heart disease debate. Perhaps more importantly, the questions generated by these data show us where we must go in our future work. I would hope that this conference has underscored that there is still a lot to be learned, with many questions to be answered. With hard work and a little luck, the outstanding issues will be resolved and the cholesterol debate will truly become a consensus. Until that time, I believe that our dietary guidelines to the population-at-large should be every bit as prudent at the diets we are recommending.

K.C. HAYES
Brandeis University
Waltham, MS, USA

In terms of where I come from and where I have been, my approach to the conference was from the perspective of atherogenesis, as an investigator interested in nutritional aspects of the mechanism and pathology involved.

450

Based on observations of arterial lesions in monkeys during manipulations with dietary fat and cholesterol, I have come to think of atherogenesis as having two major components: (1) cholesterolaemia and, (2) a thrombogenic component, both interacting with the vessel wall. At the same time, it is apparent by studying different species that the genetic component is very important. Some species are very susceptible, others quite resistant to the atherosclerotic process under the same nutritional challenge. The primary influence of diet is its effect on the lipoprotein profile. Having said this, one of the missing components in this conference was any discussion of the mechanisms contributing to atherogenesis. The epidemiology of dietary fat and cholesterol intake is useful in that it tells us which hypotheses to pursue, but epidemiology cannot prove anything nor establish a mechanism.

Mechanistic studies have demonstrated that increasing apo B or apo E-rich lipoproteins in any species will induce atherosclerosis if their concentrations are high enough for a sufficient length of time, providing the thrombogenic component of the host is also activated. Thus cholesterolemia and thrombosis (platelet aggregation) are the two major contributors to atherosclerosis.

In this conference we did not talk much about the thrombogenic component and platelet aggregation, but it is now well established that once this cascade begins at the arterial intima, a myriad of cytokines and inflammatory responses are generated in the arterial wall that can be modulated by the environment, the diet being one aspect of the environment.

Having said that, what do we tell the public? That becomes a difficult task because the detailed facts are extremely complicated from a public health point of view. Nor do we completely understand all the facts or we would not be sitting here now. Based on the clear evidence, we should provide general information to the public with the proviso that individual requirements and risks vary considerably. Atherogenesis is unfortunately an individual problem, based on one's genetic background interaction with lifestyle and environmental factors. If we can educate the public in a general sense to the overall aspect of the problem and more precisely educate our physicians and clinical nutritionists or dieticians, who are interacting one on one with the public, to identify the high-risk people and work with them, we should make steady progress.

From my point of view, the public health policy of the past 20 years has been beneficial, i.e. lower the fat intake to about 30% of calories. Try and lower saturates the most and if fat is added, polyunsaturates are preferred because it is important that the person with hyperlipidemia maintain at least 5% energy from polyunsaturated fat. That level of polyunsaturates is what the average American consumes now. Thus, our recommendations should not change until the more complicated, more sophisticated aspects of the issue are sorted out. We still do not know everything about which fatty acid is doing what. But the basic overview is quite apparent, and we should continue to disseminate this information as best we can.

BRUCE J. HOLUB
University of Guelph
Guelph, Ontario, Canada

First, I would like to say that I appreciate the invitation to be here. Overall, I believe that the 1990 Nutrition Recommendations (Health and Welfare Canada) are extremely prudent and practical for the general population. These recommendations included the choice of low-fat dairy products as part of Canada's Guidelines for Healthy Eating. I think there are some limitations in the Nutrition Recommendations that need tightening but I am sure that this will come with time. The recommendations, while advising a lowered intake of total fat and saturated fat, which is very appropriate, did not adequately address the issue of the '*trans*' fatty acids. Because of the excellent work of Dr Martijn Katan, who is present at this meeting, and some of the work done previously, we are concerned with the potential for the '*trans*' to elevate plasma LDL-cholesterol levels while lowering the HDL. A 1979 expert committee meeting in Canada to deal with the topic of '*trans*' fatty acids, recommended that the food manufacturers in Canada should be encouraged to significantly control the increase in '*trans*' fatty acid appearance in the Canadian food supply. For reasons which one can only speculate on, these recommendations did not become properly instituted. I do think that leaving the '*trans*' fatty acid issue out of food regulations and nutrition recommendations has serious limitations. So, I would like to think that future recommendations would indicate that we control our intake of total fat, saturated fat, plus '*trans*' fatty acids. I think we need better food labelling regulations in Canada and also in the United States to deal with this issue. We currently have allowance for 'cholesterol-free' labelling on processed foods and it is well known that such labelling can help promote the market shares of a commodity. In a few cases, this may be appropriate, but for many products it is potentially misleading to the health-conscious consumer, since most of these products never contained cholesterol to begin with. Also, for cholesterol-free labelling in Canada, the product must not only be cholesterol-free, or have a minor amount of cholesterol, but must also have a minimal amount of saturated fat. Consequently, many of the cholesterol-free products that we have analyzed in our laboratory are very high in fat because fat levels are not covered in the regulation. Secondly, they are often very high in '*trans*' fatty acids, sometimes having two or three times the level of '*trans*' as compared to the saturates. Thus, the extensive use of hydrogenated vegetable oils containing '*trans*' are not covered by the regulation. Our regulatory

452

agencies should provide for the listing of saturates plus *'trans'* on labels rather than only declaring the saturates. This would also provide a fairer representation across the commodity groups. The inclusion in the regulations and in food labelling of saturates plus *'trans'* would also educate the public regarding the impact that *'trans'* fatty acids may have on blood lipids which can approach that of saturated fats in terms of overall risk. I think the balance of polyunsaturates such as n-6 to n-3 (ω-3) fatty acids is also very important. We have an n-6 polyunsaturate to n-3 polyunsaturate ratio in the diet which is about 11 to 1 in North America. Recent Canadian recommendations have indicated that the ratio (n-6 over n-3) should be brought down to as low as four, but somewhere in the region of the 4–10 range; I think this is a very appropriate recommendation. We will have to wrestle with time as to the relative nutritional equivalency of linolenic acid (ω-3) versus docosahexaenoic acid (ω-3), DHA, the latter being the essential one for biological function (brain and retina) and the former being a precursor of DHA in the body. The big question is: what is the convertibility and therefore the equivalency of dietary linolenic versus DHA? In this regard, is one part of dietary DHA equal to 6–30 parts of dietary linolenic acid? This needs to be resolved as we hopefully get into food labelling in the future, where we recognize n-3 as well as n-6 fatty acids as essential nutritionally. Also, the nutritional impact of the n-6 fatty acids as dietary linoleic acid (plant plus animal foods) versus arachidonic acid (animal foods) needs resolution since the former is also a precursor of the latter. Arachidonic acid forms thromboxane A_2, a potentiator of blood platelet aggregation.

Finally, I would like to conclude and concur with my colleagues on the importance of dietary effects on thrombogenicity and platelet reactivity in assessing the risk of cardiovascular disease. I think this is a key area for future research and we need some very aggressive and extensive studies, at least equal to what has been done on dietary effects, on blood cholesterol and lipoprotein levels. This work, directed towards the dietary management of blood platelet reactivity and the thrombogenic risk, is critical if we are really going to further reduce our excessive death rates due to heart disease and, hopefully, approach the much lower levels which exist in Japan and some other countries.

LOUIS HORLICK
University of Saskatchewan
Saskatoon, Saskatchewan, Canada

There is no substitute for good science. Many of the disagreements which emerged in this meeting, such as the potential benefits of pharmacologic and dietary intervention in hypercholesterolemia in women and the elderly, are the result of incomplete information, and cannot be resolved until more information becomes available. Unfortunately, because of the high costs of carrying out the necessary studies and the deteriorating economic situation, it is unlikely that they will ever be done. The Canadian Consensus Conference on Cholesterol considered the best available information and proposed what I consider to be a reasonable approach involving both a population and high-risk strategy for preventing and ameliorating the effects of the risk factors for ischemic heart disease. The CCCC recommendations are not carved in stone; as new, or better information becomes available those recommendations will have to be changed.

During the past few years we have seen an enormous increase in knowledge of the genetic bases of the dyslipidemias. In the future, we may be able to identify some individuals at risk and concentrate our efforts on them. However, in the vast majority of individuals at risk, the process is multifactorial and represents an interaction between genes and environment. Intervention aimed at changing an unhealthy environment and unhealthy human behaviour must continue to be one of our main goals. Human behaviour can be changed; we need only attend to what has been happening with smoking behaviour. Changing from a high-fat, cholesterol-rich diet is no more 'dysfunctional' than stopping smoking. The diet consumed by our population is an anomaly in a world where fewer calories and very low fat intake are the rule, and are associated with better health, as in Japan.

Atherosclerosis is a cumulative process and proceeds in fits and starts throughout our lifetime. It proceeds more slowly initially in women, but they catch up following the menopause. Intervention should begin in youth in men and women and be a lifelong process. Current interventions will probably have only a modest effect, but when multiplied by the very large numbers at risk, the results will be very rewarding.

CHRISTOPHER G. ISLES
Dumfries and Galloway Infirmary
Dumfries, Scotland

I have enjoyed this conference enormously and feel that the standard of contributions has been extremely high. I was also delighted to see that what started out as a rather bad tempered affair became rather more good humoured as time has gone on. There are three points that I would like to make: first, a few words on the use of national mortality data which were dismissed rather uncharitably by William Stehbens. The advantages to epidemiologists are the large number of endpoints, but, on the other hand, there are legitimate concerns about the accuracy of death certification.

In my view, the critical point in favour of national mortality data is that they are unlikely to be subject to systematic bias. Moreover, overdiagnosis of coronary death by death certificate will tend to weaken rather than strengthen any association between cholesterol and heart disease, which means that, if you can still observe that association, it is more rather than less likely to be real. So there, if you like, is a defence of epidemiology from a clinician.

The second point is that I often think the best lessons to be learned are from the pieces of a jigsaw which do not fit easily into the puzzle. For me, France is one such awkwardly fitting piece. I am not sure that Dr Connor was correct when he said the CSI (cholesterol saturated fat index) of French food was low and I feel that this is an area which merits further research. The French, incidentally, seem more relevant to me than primitive Indians because if the answer does turn out to be dietary, then it would be considerably easier to adopt a Mediterranean diet than to eat eight tortillas a day.

My final thought is that people who hold extreme views at either end of the spectrum might be wiser to hold their counsel until after the results of the Statin trials are available. I say this not just for their own sakes but also because the views of the extremists make the best headlines and are, therefore, most likely to confuse our public.

This advice also goes for the American Heart Association, who presumably are going to have to throw the whole process of cholesterol lowering into reverse if the Statin trials do not show the expected benefits. For the time being, therefore, it seems safer to sit on the fence.

MARTIJN B. KATAN
Wageningen Agricultural University
Wageningen, The Netherlands

A number of presentations have dealt with the implications of the cholesterol issue for society. I thought they were excellently balanced in discussing the pros and cons and they agreed with my own feelings on the subject. On the one hand, it is undeniable that there is a causal relation between high levels of LDL cholesterol and coronary heart disease and that levels of LDL cholesterol can be changed by dietary manipulation. I think we would be doing a disservice to the dairy farmers of Canada, who sponsored this meeting, by saying that cholesterol is bosh and that the issue will fade away. It will not go away if only because we here are just one out of a 100 or so expert conferences sifting through the data and they all, more or less, come up with the same conclusion. On the other hand, I was glad to hear stressed the problems that we have in bringing this conclusion to the public. Cholesterol is not like a polio virus where you give a simple vaccination and eliminate totally, a terrible disease which strikes people in their youth. Coronary heart disease is a disease that largely strikes in the later phase of life and even if you prevent it, you are often going to get some other disease not too much later. So, we need some nuances and subtleties in what we are going to tell people and that needs to be tailored to their own risk. I think the whole diet/cholesterol/heart disease issue is very much an issue of cost and benefit. We should try to explain to people what the benefit is, but we should also monitor the costs, not just in terms of dollars but also in terms of what David Naylor has termed 'disutility'. I was delighted to see his presentation and I am going to look forward to seeing it in the *Annals* because I think we very much need to try and estimate how much people have to pay in terms of discomfort or unhappiness in order to lower their cholesterol by diet or by drugs. I am not sure that being a coronary patient is only ten times as bad as being on a cholesterol-lowering diet. I think it is much worse. In fact, I myself am quite happy eating more fruits, seafood and olive oil, and less butter and sausage, and I believe such a diet could be quite tolerable to all those people who are now trying to lower their cholesterol worldwide.

STAN KUBOW
MacDonald Campus of McGill University
Ste-Anne-de-Bellevue, Québec, Canada

First, I would like to urge researchers to take a closer look at the essential fatty acid content of the so-called atherogenic diets used in animal studies. These diets are typically deficient in essential fatty acids which can confound interpretation of these studies. I would also like to echo Dr Addis's comments that the addition of cholesterol to semi-purified diets may actually induce high levels of cholesterol oxidation products, which in turn could cause changes in cholesterol metabolism. Also, dietary additions of unsaturated oils, if not carefully monitored, could induce the formation of lipid peroxidation products and they need to be carefully controlled.

I would like to reiterate that the role of primary dietary intervention in cardiovascular disease is inconclusive, since well-controlled dietary trials have only recently begun to be carried out. For example, the double-blinded, randomized primary intervention trial of the Minnesota Coronary Survey, which looked at the effects of diet alone, did not see a change in the incidence of cardiovascular disease between the treatment group receiving a diet with a high P/S ratio of 1.6 versus the control group consuming a diet with a low P/S ratio of 0.3. I would also like to second Dr Budowski's comments that diets with a high P/S ratio may pose some risk. The recent secondary intervention trials of the Blakenhorn Cholesterol Lowering Intervention

Study showed that higher intakes of polyunsaturated fatty acids were associated with an increase in coronary lesion growth in coronary bypass patients.

The workshop has only peripherally examined the potential role of free radical biology in cardiovascular disease. There is increasing evidence, however, that free radical mechanisms do play a role in cardiovascular disease. There are suggestions by Gey in Switzerland and Duthie in England, that the antioxidant content of the diet may be of prime importance in terms of cardiovascular disease. With regard to this, it is worth noting that epidemiological studies have tended to see much stronger negative correlations between cereal, plant fibre and fruit intake with cardiovascular disease than the positive correlations that have been observed between cardiovascular disease incidence and saturated fat intake. In that light, it may be that the high antioxidant content found in fruits and vegetables is playing a key protective role. In this respect, I would like to mention France, whose population has a high saturated fat intake but which also has a low cardiovascular disease incidence. Interestingly, the French population has a very high intake of fruits and vegetables which may be exerting a protective influence. The Mediterranean populations which have a low cardiovascular incidence also consume a very high fat diet of 40%, although it is mostly monounsaturated. Hence, although a low fat diet may have some potential health benefits, I do not feel that this diet is necessarily the best diet in terms of the North American context. We are seeing an increased intake of fruits, vegetables and fish in North America and this may turn out to be a much more efficacious factor than changes in dietary fat *per se*. Dietary recommendations towards a more French- or Mediterranean-style diet may allow for a much more palatable and acceptable diet for Western tastes than the more extreme high-fibre, low-fat diet that is currently recommended. I would also like to emphasize the potential importance of n-3 fatty acids which need to be considered in terms of thrombotic lesions. In North America, n-3 fatty acid intake has decreased since the turn of the century. This has correlated much better with the increased incidence in cardiovascular disease since the 1900s than linoleic acid intake which has dramatically increased in the past century due to the development of vegetable oil processing techniques.

HÉLÈNE LAURENDEAU
Professional dietician
Montréal, Québec, Canada

I really enjoyed the conference and my comment will be one of a dietician with a background in epidemiology working with the media in communications. Although there are a lot of questions which still need to be answered we still have to work with real people in the meantime and give them our best advice. I think I am more and more convinced that the important focus is to eat a balanced, varied diet and to enjoy it. By 'variety' we mean what you eat and by 'moderation' we mean how much you eat. For this, no calculator should be needed. I am also very concerned about the fact that people do not eat to stay healthy any longer but they eat not to be sick. Because of this we see the appearance at market, of all kinds of 'imitation' food which Bruce Holub and Micheline de Belder mentioned are made with food additives and hydrogenated oils. I was once in a supermarket and someone asked me if there was any food I could suggest that contained 'good' cholesterol. I think there is something terribly wrong there and we need to work in that area.

Secondly, we need more environmental interventions to address this whole issue of health promotion with the industry, with the point of purchase, grocery stores, restaurants, cafeterias and workplaces, to reach the people in their areas. There is a need for government labelling – good labelling, because we have to remember that there are no good or bad foods, just good or bad diets.

SHEILA MURPHY
Professional dietician
Montréal, Québec, Canada

I am a dietician with a background in sociology. I work, not with individuals, but as a nutrition educator using the mass media, mostly radio and television. There are a few points I would like to make. One is that I was not aware, until coming to this meeting, that a risk factor was the cause of disease. I have been hearing the two terms used interchangeably during the course of this meeting and have come to the conclusion that they must be one and the same.

Second, I agree with Richard Goldbloom: there seems to be little or no consideration given to the effect of the socioeconomic or poverty factor on the incidence, on the treatment and on the education efforts concerning heart disease.

My third point is, in disagreement with some previous speakers, that I think we have been causing harm with the kinds of nutrition recommendations, including those from the Cholesterol Consensus Conference, that have been going out to the public. This belief stems from my own personal experience and from my recent reading. In a recent Gallup Poll, paid for by the American Dietetic Association, women were asked what steps they were taking to improve their health: 53% said that they had stopped eating red meat and 36% said that they had stopped using dairy products. I wonder what kinds of problems we are creating when an article published in the *New*

England Journal of Medicine states that the average American has insufficient intakes of vitamins B6, C, E and folic acid and that recommended intakes of calcium, iron, magnesium and zinc are also not being met. And all of this is happening with a sufficient, or even excessive, calorie intake!

We see the same thing in Canada. Louise Lambert-Lagace, a fellow Quebec dietician, in her book *The Nutrition Challenge for Women* says that one in five women has no iron reserves and one in ten is anaemic, the diets of many adolescents have only half the required calcium, and our calcium intake gets worse as we grow older.

The diets of many women lack sufficient magnesium and vitamin B6 and some women on meatless diets do not get enough protein.

I think that nutrition recommendations concerning cholesterol are to blame for this in the sense that they are contributing to the difficulty normal people seem to be having when it comes to choosing and eating a balanced diet. People think cholesterol is a killer and they think that all medical experts agree. From being here and listening to you, I know that there is no agreement, but the rest of the world does not know it! I think it is in the long run that the real harm will show up. The negative effects of today's nutrient deficiencies will be clear 20–30 years from now.

CYRIL NAIR
Statistics Canada
Ottawa, Ontario, Canada

Thank you for inviting me to this conference on Fats and Cholesterol. The experience has been most instructive, enlightening and revealing to me. After having listened to all the speakers, I must conclude that the views from both sides of the debate are very convincing and that dialogues of this nature are necessary to get a better understanding of the issue.

In Canada, the mortality rates for most forms of cardiovascular disease (CVD) have been declining and have done so since the late 1960s, with the declining trend intact even today. To what have we attributed these declines? Unfortunately, the simple answer to this is still quite equivocal as CVD incidence varies by age, sex, region, socioeconomic status as it does with risk factors. Nevertheless, data from the various health surveys in Canada have all shown that the change in cholesterol levels in the population over time has not been that significant. Dr Horlick presented data from the Nova Scotia Heart Study and indicated that the cholesterol levels in Nova Scotia were similar to those in Saskatchewan, as were some of the other risk factors, yet there are significant differences in the mortality rates between the two provinces and we have been unable to explain this divergence.

It is well documented that the single most important risk factor for cardiovascular disease is smoking. Yet, public opinion surveys reveal that most people associate smoking with cancer and not heart disease. The perception that smoking is not directly associated with the risk of developing CVD is well established, particularly with the young, a perception that needs to be changed.

On the other hand, most people seem to be more aware of the effects of cholesterol on heart disease than of smoking on heart disease.

MAHAMED NAVAB
UCLA School of Medicine
Los Angeles, California, USA

I learned a great deal in this meeting. Some of my views were affected by the talks by Doctors Katan, Grover and Naylor. I was reminded of important facts such as the need for better markers other than plasma cholesterol levels. I also believe that coronary heart disease, cancer and other major killers, which are affected by fat and cholesterol, are multifactorial diseases. They are affected genetically and environmentally. We see tremendous variability even among the inbred strains of experimental animals in response. On the other hand, we do see the beneficial effects of lowering fats and cholesterol in our diet. We do need more good science and more collaboration with the social science experts. Comparing the late 1960s Western diet and lifestyles compared to now, I think a lot of good has been done to the general public and I think that abuse and creation of public panic and hysteria should be opposed, and the adverse effects of intervention should not be overlooked. Finally, in recommending guidelines, one has to remember that attention to cultural differences is crucial. Guidelines for one particular country and population may not necessarily be suitable for another.

C. DAVID NAYLOR
Sunnybrook Health Science Centre
Toronto, Ontario, Canada

Consensus is a difficult thing because it implies unanimity of opinion. If the evidence were iron-clad, we would not have to debate anything; there would be unanimity anyway. Consensus on some levels is the death of science. You need a paradigm within which you do science, which is partly consensual. But the real progress in science comes when there is debate and disagreement and when the anomalies – the bits of evidence that do not fit the paradigm – are highlighted and become the focus for further activity. I think the organizers here are to be congratulated by not forcing a consensus. I think I must say that harm has been done to science in the last few years, by the forced consensus on the cholesterol issue.

With respect to the patient's stake in the debate, I really think that all of us in the health policy field have failed to look carefully enough at the process of consent of individual patients and their ability to assimilate and use information in the doctor–patient and dietician–patient encounter. Public input is also needed in terms of policy formulation. It is not enough to have a token lawyer on the Canadian Consensus Conference panel, and it is certainly inadequate to get four pointy-headed epidemiologists together in the Toronto Working Group and promulgate recommendations. We need ways to involve the lay public in an informed fashion in the decisions that we make about public health strategies that affect all of them, about regulations regarding labelling and content of foodstuffs and about clinical recommendations that are to be translated into practice across the country.

Keaven Anderson has raised the point that extending the follow-up of clinical trials may cause ethical problems. This is because cardiovascular morbidity endpoints in treatment groups diverge from controls faster than mortality endpoints. I would simply point out that none of the trials that have addressed cholesterol lowering have been designed to assess non-cardiovascular morbidity. No one has counted the number of days in hospital from gallbladder disease in fibric acid trials. Before we say that longer trials are not possible because of ethical concerns, I think we need to think about all-cause morbidity, rather than cardiovascular morbidity, as our endpoint.

On health care costs, I am struck by the fact that Japan has one of the lowest per capita cost profiles of any industrialized nation, and yet has the longest life expectancy. It appears there is something that can be done in terms of life expectancy by shifting national diets. However, genetic factors are an important confounder. And, even if we assume that we can obtain some life expectancy prolongation with a national dietary strategy, the differences are small. None of the industrialized nations has a radically longer life expectancy than any other, so I think we have to be realistic about what is to be gained.

Finally, on the issue of quality of life, there is a huge body of research in social science, psychology and medicine dealing with quality of life and happiness indices. In some of that research, good health is indeed a prerequisite to happiness or good quality of life. However, I am struck by the fact that most of us are well most of the time and, as Richard Goldbloom said, we are really very privileged. For that reason, any strategy that medicalizes the population and changes the way we perceive ourselves has to be looked at sceptically. I also look at the funds we may put into such programs, as compared to better education for our children, parks and playgrounds, and health outreach programs for the socioeconomically disadvantaged who have a disproportionate burden of illness of all kinds. I think we need to think critically about the potential benefits of these primary prevention programs before we go too far down the road.

HOWARD PARSONS
University of Calgary
Calgary, Alberta, Canada

This workshop has been a very interesting experience. The diverse nature of the group has been one of the major strengths of this conference. Many have reviewed their own work and suggested future studies. The lipid hypothesis has been scrutinized and in my view is still viable.

Multiple studies have shown that populations with elevated cholesterols are at greater risk for coronary vascular disease (CVD). Lowering of elevated plasma cholesterol levels has led to a decreased incidence of CVD and, in several studies, regression of atherosclerotic plaques. I agree with Dr Louis Horlick when he states there has been good science and we need more good science.

Before coming to this conference I had no major disagreement with the recommendations of the Canadian Consensus Conference on Cholesterol. Thirty percent of calories from fat, with 10% polyunsaturated, monounsaturated and saturated, does not create undue hardship. I suggest this recommendation is valid until we see more research to disprove it. One of the difficulties is that men and women are lumped together under the same recommendations due to a lack of data on women. Only with more data from women should these recommendations be changed. In addition, as outlined earlier, there are multiple-risk factors for atherosclerosis and all should be considered.

Of specific interest to me are children, as I am a paediatrician. Instructions for dietary intervention in children need to be done with prudence in order to prevent the occurrence of malnutrition because of an overzealous parent. In addition with more research (as pointed out by Dr Vega) we will better define our population in terms of those with and without genetic defects. Aggressive management of children should at present be limited to those with known genetic abnormalities. It is the responsibility of the medical community to identify those that require diet and pharmaceutical intervention.

I look forward to the time when such a diverse group can reach a consensus. Sharing of ideas, such as this group has done, will enhance such a consensus as areas of research needs are better defined.

DANIEL A.K. RONCARI
University of Toronto
Toronto, Ontario, Canada

This has indeed been an enriching meeting, bringing together constructively complementary disciplines. The following include some notable points that were addressed at this workshop: some persons are clearly at risk – e.g., those with familial hypercholesterolaemia who obviously require prompt and efficacious therapy. However, there is concern about blanket recommendations to the public at large. In particular, we are concerned about generic recommendations to children (Shiela Murphy, Richard Goldbloom, Micheline Ste. Marie), and similarly, the introduction of nutritional deficiencies. The brain, along with the visual system, contains an abundant and complex set of lipids. These, or their precursors, may be unduly restricted by certain diets resulting in potential, possibly subtle, problems, particularly during development. Cholesterol is an essential, ubiquitous constituent of mammalian and many other living cells. Thus, cholesterolphobia has to be eliminated by proper public education; populations must not be medicalized. There should be greater emphasis on quality of life.

Before concluding, we should congratulate the participants for coming up with some common sense and some common ground, and with direction for the future.

EMIL SKAMENE
McGill University
Montréal, Québec, Canada

The important thing I have learned at this conference is that the best way to prevent atherosclerosis and coronary heart disease is to choose your parents wisely. I would like to share with you my impressions as to where I see the research in this area going. I am impressed by how much men look like mice and I will use the patterns of response of the set of 30 recombinant inbred mouse strains to a high-fat diet as a concept (Figure 1). We were feeding mice of these different genotypes a very high-fat diet and we measured the phenotype of the magnitude of atherosclerotic plaque developing in the sinus valve area of ascending aorta. About half of all the strains on the left-hand side of the figure had no lesions at all. These happen to be the strains which did not become hyperlipidemic on a high-cholesterol diet. If you translate this conceptually to human populations, we are exposing, by our 'low-fat' dietary recommendations, at least half of the population to a diet which may not be enjoyable, and for no good reason. These individuals are genetic hyporesponders. Let us now look at the other half of mouse strains which do respond to this high-fat, high-cholesterol diet by the development of dys-

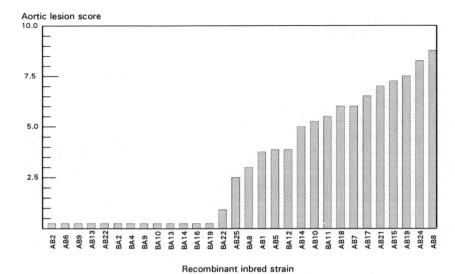

Figure 1 Phenotype of aortic plaque formation (aortic lesion score) in 30 recombinant inbred mouse strains derived from susceptible C57B6/J (B) and resistant A/J (A) progenitors. All mice were fed high cholesterol diet for 20 weeks. (from *Clinical Investigative Medicine*, **12**, 121, 1989, with permission)

lipidemia. The majority of them develop minimal lesions: aortic score is less than 5, which would just mean fat infiltration and a few foam cells, etc. Only a very few strains develop histopathological lesions characteristic of the atherosclerotic plaque. With regard to humans, in that half of the population who are hyperresponders, there is the question of how to reconstruct this situation which is clearly genetic and only genetic in nature. One way to do this would be to identify a chromosomal location of the regulatory genes in mice. This is quite possible. We could then apply a strategy of the mouse/human genomic homology. An alternative would be to search through the human genome for allelic markers which are linked to a defined phenotype of atherosclerosis. This is the challenge to this group: I could devise a human genetic study if I knew what it is that I look for as an 'intermediate phenotype'. Perhaps we should say that in the absence of a non-invasive diagnosis of atherosclerotic heart disease, we should start by looking at families with atherosclerosis, and start collecting DNA from them for storage. Alternatively, we can start looking at some intermediate phenotypes, such as lipid levels, etc. and attempt linkage analysis in families. With the advance in human genetics and genome mapping, we might be able to start providing some of the genetic markers of susceptibility which Louis Horlick was talking about, and the task may not be eventually as difficult as it seems to be at the moment.

PETR SKRABANEK
University of Dublin
Dublin, Ireland

I liked the fact that the chairman used the term 'hypothesis' when referring to lipid hypothesis, because if it is a hypothesis, we really talk about ways of testing it, although at times it seems it is a dogma. When you oppose a dogma, you become a heretic: if you question a hypothesis, it is just a legitimate scientific exercise. But, if it is a hypothesis, we should not marshal selectively all evidence in its favour, in an attempt to verify it, as advocates of a hypothesis do all the time. We should remember, as Wittgenstein said, that if you want to find the truth of a statement published in a newspaper, you would not get any wiser by buying another copy of the newspaper. You have to devise the most severe ways of falsifying the hypothesis. Only when it withstands severe tests, do you become more comfortable that it approaches the truth. The question is really: is this lipid hypothesis testable, i.e. is it formulated in a testable way?

Secondly, the talk about national diet, national cholesterol, national lifestyle, etc. has a very ominous ring. Who is the patient? – the nation is not a patient, and who is the doctor? – some kind of 'Big Brother' trying to introduce the tyranny of uniformity? Everyone should eat less than 30% fat? Everyone's cholesterol should be below 200, 190, 180 .....? People are not chickens on a chicken farm. And where do these recommendations come from? Based on what evidence? The consensus method, used in these cases, was compared by Richard Feynman to the search for the length of the Chinese Emperor's nose – the problem being that no one was allowed to see his august face. So how do you establish it? You go around the country and you ask the experts on the length of the Emperor's nose what they *think* it might be. Then you average it and *presto*, you have the estimate. It is likely to be accurate since many experts chipped in. That is exactly how the 'optimum' cholesterol for the whole nation has been determined.

The last point is that intervention in healthy people is not necessarily a good thing. Any kind of medicalization of life is potentially harmful, and health promotion may be damaging to one's health.

One thing I have learned from this conference is that the lipid hypothesis is even more complicated than I suspected. We should remember what H.L. Mencken said about quick fixes – every complex problem has a solution which is simple, direct, plausible – and wrong.

WILLIAM E. STEHBENS
Wellington School of Medicine
Newton, Wellington, New Zealand

This conference was very worthwhile for me because it provided the opportunity to debate the lipid hypothesis. At present there is a need for further scientific debate of this hypothesis and the entire cholesterol issue in a scientific journal, but in much more detail than has been possible at this conference. Like others I have learned something, and I too am concerned with the need for good science and scientific thinking, but I do not believe that all of what I have heard is good science. Many of the statements made at the meeting do not stand up to critical analysis. There is much loose talk about the lipid hypothesis, particularly in relation to coronary heart disease and by extrapolation to atherosclerosis. I am interested in the etiology of atherosclerosis and the pathogenesis of its complications, but the lipid hypothesis is not really a theory of the etiology of atherosclerosis. In reality, it is a theory for the infiltration of lipid into the blood vessel wall. It does not explain either the pathogenesis of intimal thickening that precedes lipid accumulation or the complications such as aneurysms, ulcerations, intimal tears, etc. The need for thrombogenic studies has been stressed, but it must be remembered that the thrombus is only secondary to the underlying lesion, i.e. the intimal tear.

At this conference, repeated extrapolations have been made from risk factors of coronary heart disease occurring mostly in the 6th decade and beyond to the etiology of atherosclerosis which commences in infancy, if not *in utero*. Such extrapolations are invalid. Risk factor has been used synonymously with cause and the etiology of atherosclerosis is thereby argued to be multifactorial. Petr Skrabanek and James McCormick, his colleague, have both indicated that the multifactorial concept is but a euphemism for ignorance and I agree. The stance is similar to the approach that predated the introduction to Koch's Postulates for causation of pathogenic bacteria. Unfortunately, consensus opinion seems to be moving towards such primitive philosophy of disease causation once more.

Such fundamental problems indicate that detailed analysis of absolutely every aspect of coronary heart disease epidemiology is essential. The pathology of atherosclerosis is a case in point, because the pathology of hypercholesterolemia and of the cholesterol-fed animal has been misrepresented. Discussion of the use of the word 'cause' and whether it should be used synonymously with 'risk factor' is indicated. Currently, some epidemiologists consider socioeconomic factors to be of equal or even greater importance than is the tubercle bacillus in the etiology of tuberculosis or the smallpox virus in smallpox. This is the philosophy and standard of logic that

466

underlies much of the coronary heart disease epidemiology, but not of modern day medical science and clinical management.

No good clinical scientist would treat all patients with subarachnoid hemorrhage in exactly the same manner because hemorrhage has many causes. Yet at this conference CHD is used as if it was one disorder, even though it is a non-specific condition complicating many diseases including familial hypercholesterolemia. Both the etiology and the pathogenesis of coronary heart disease in familial hypercholesterolemia are quite different from those in atherosclerosis. This is true of Type 3 hyperlipoproteinemia, and other dyslipidemias may also cause fat storage in blood vessels. Such factors indicate the need to exclude from consideration these diseases which confound the results and lead to selection bias for hypercholesterolemia. Lumping all cases of CHD together results in soup epidemiology.

It has been noted in animal experiments that there are hyperresponders and hyporesponders and this probably holds true for humans in regard to dietary lipid and even to hemodynamic stress. It adds emphasis to the need to investigate in more detail the individual metabolic disorders of lipids and to differentiate between such subjects and normolipidemic individuals.

Risk factors are only statistical associations with endpoint disease and are not causal in any sense. Yet we repeatedly heard reference to the etiology of atherosclerosis by extrapolation, an association that is scientifically invalid, and it is essential to realize that the causality is assumed and not proven. Such imprecise use of English results in misrepresentation and bad science.

In experimental atherogenesis there is a need to comply with specific criteria before any experimental model can be classified as atherosclerosis. We repeatedly heard reference to the cholesterol-fed animal in which the vascular lesions are dissimilar to atherosclerosis and devoid of the complications. Because the lesions contain lipid, the model is still assumed to be atherosclerosis. Surely it is a matter of logic that deductions from one disease are of little applicability to another when they are unrelated; having different pathology and a different pathogenesis negates applicability.

There are serious inconsistencies in the lipid hypothesis. Smith and others have drawn attention to many of them. The greatest inconsistency, quite apparent to everyone, is the fact that surgeons are regularly producing atherosclerosis in the human by producing an atrioventricular shunt for renal dialysis and also when producing a coronary venous bypass graft. Severe, accelerated atherosclerosis develops in the veins made use of, yet if those veins had been left intact, like other veins elsewhere in the individuals' bodies, the veins would have developed only minimal change during the rest of their life-long use. It is not cholesterol, nor any other circulating humoral agent, that is responsible but the stresses associated with the altered blood flow. Why has this inconsistency been totally ignored? It is a matter of logic that if there is one unexplained inconsistency in an hypothesis then the hypothesis fails and one must then review the premises on which the theory is based. Such inconsistencies stress the need for scientific review of CHD epidemiology and the lipid hypothesis.

I am also concerned that, today, one speaker suggested that 'anyone with extreme views should shut up'. My views are no doubt regarded in this light and the inference to be drawn is that my voice should be stifled. A working committee of the WHO also suggested similar muzzling and recommended government legislation to prevent people from objecting or interfering with the institution of changes in national diets. This reeks of Lysenkoism and the Inquisition and should be of great concern to the scientific community. People can have different views but the majority is certainly not always correct and, historically, has often been made an ass. Unless people are given freedom and the opportunity to debate the scientific aspects of the role of cholesterol and lipids in atherosclerosis in great detail, it will only increase the time before the problems of atherosclerosis, the most common underlying cause of CHD and stroke, are solved.

MICHELINE STE. MARIE
Dalhousie University
Halifax, Nova Scotia, Canada

I will try to limit remarks to what I know. I am not a scientist, I am a paediatric gastroenterologist and most of my interests lie in the clinical practice of paediatric gastroenterology and the teaching of paediatrics to medical students and residents. As a woman, I am glad to see that we have finally been taken to heart by people in this entire process.

I have learned at this conference that I am a mouse, a pigeon and a monkey to which I object strongly. I have never really liked being compared to an animal, although I suspect we come from the monkey that does no evil.

I have learned from John Dietschy, whom I admire very much, that the gut is indeed the starting point of this whole thing. I have always believed this. I think the gut has been forgotten as a primary organ of modulation and needs to be looked at in greater detail. I am concerned that this problem is a problem of an affluent society and that the follies committed by adults will have repercussions in children. I think this has been the story of our affluent society over the past 100 years. Children have suffered from the passive effects of smoke, for example. People have a way of dealing with life and including children into their follies which frightens me. There is a problem with the diet in North America and it is a problem of an affluent society. You have access to a lot of food, you can eat whatever you want and you overindulge. There is a need to decrease the amount of fat in the diet of the general population but I think that as far as children are concerned I would like to interject a word of caution. I have seen a lot of things being introduced as universal panaceas in infant nutrition that have had some deleterious consequences and have had to be abandoned.

The next unfortunate event I see happening is the disappearance of the most important infant food, breast milk. The infant formula companies are one step away from advertising infant formulas as being cholesterol-free. The physicians have lost the battle in the United States for advertising of infant formulas to the public and we will lose it in Canada in the next few years. I am really concerned that this hypothesis will be advertised with great exaggeration because of this.

My second concern is that the dietary changes referred to in this conference have also been described for an affluent society. We have talked about fresh fruits, vegetables, fish, etc. In Canada and in the Maritimes, where you would expect fish to be cheap, it is cheaper to buy a pound of beef than fish. It is definitely cheaper to buy a pound of beef than spinach or cauliflower.

Recommendations translated by us, the affluent members of this society (for practical purposes), may not be applicable to a population that is getting poorer, and this includes a large number of children. I would like to see other foodstuffs that could be taken as alternatives in the food chain, but in order to do that they have to be a popular choice; unfortunately the poor may well want to imitate the rich, i.e. when the rich decide not to breast feed, the poor may decide not to breast feed. It is a collective responsibility to be practical if you want to effect changes in the entire population.

I do not like percentages; I do not think that percentages should be introduced to the general public. It is true the well-intentioned and well-educated could interpret these appropriately, but other people do things to the extreme. We should strive not to tell them what to take away from their diet but what to add or how to achieve a better nutritional status.

I would also like to raise a point, as others have, in regard to the artificiality of our own diet: we may be changing one disease for another by moving into a very artificial diet that the human body has not been used to.

HIROTSUGU UESHIMA
Shiga University Medical School
Shiga, Japan

I say that chronic disease is induced by multiple causes, and results from many epidemiological and pathological studies have proved the cholesterol and coronary heart disease hypothesis. I, however, think of this statement as more of a theory. Past epidemiological studies have proved that the higher the cholesterol level, the higher the incidence and mortality of IHD, even in Japanese people.

Our country is lowest in CHD, but the Japanese are not exceptional people. Dr Yano showed that if I eat more fat, I will suffer from CHD. Although there is perhaps some kind of genetic factor involved, lifestyle and diet are also very important determinants of the disease. For example, the main risk factor for stroke is hypertension. Hypertension is not only a risk factor, it is also a cause. In Japan we decreased the mortality from stroke by 60% for men aged 60–69, and the blood pressure change was very small, only 15 mmHg or so. Thus, the risk factor was greatly affected even though the average blood pressure change was very small. When thinking about the differences in cholesterol levels among populations, the difference is not so large. Yet, cholesterol level is very important because it is a risk factor and there are variations in the mortality rate among countries. If we try to get populations to shift the risk factor distribution down to ideal levels, we may see very significant results. Therefore, the population strategy is very important. In order for population strategies to be effective, however, nutrition recommendations and lifestyle changes have to be implemented.

GLORIA LENA VEGA
University of Texas
Dallas, Texas, USA

Epidemiological studies have shown that high levels of plasma cholesterol and LDL cholesterol are a risk factor for coronary heart disease (CHD) and reduction of LDL cholesterol by hypolipidemic drugs reduces risk of mortality and morbidity from CHD.

Levels of plasma LDL cholesterol normally rise with age in both men and women, and persistent intake of dietary fat and cholesterol can increase further the levels of plasma cholesterol by about 25 mg/dl. Some saturated fats, but not all, have a cholesterol-raising effect. They may contribute to an increase of about 19 mg/dl, whereas dietary cholesterol may cause a rise of about 6 mg/dl. This implies that a reduced intake of saturated fat and cholesterol can cause a significant lowering of plasma cholesterol. A number of studies showed that aging and dietary fat seemingly cause down-regulation of LDL receptors, and this mechanism may be reversed in part by reduced intake of dietary fat.

Some genetic factors also have been identified as cholesterol-raising such as a defective gene for LDL receptors, or apolipoprotein B-100. The severity of the hypercholesterolemia in subjects heterozygote for either of these defects is quite varied and it has been postulated that other factors may counteract the effects of these monogenic defects. Hopefully, in the near

470

future, we shall have a better understanding of the genetic basis of susceptibility to hypercholesterolemia.

KENNETH F. WALKER
The Toronto Hospital
Toronto, Ontario, Canada

William Shakespeare made an apt remark about 500 years ago. He wrote 'Such as we are made of, such we be'. I leave this conference confirmed in the belief that to circumvent coronary disease it helps if you choose your parents very, very carefully! It is my opinion that genetics play a major role in the causation of atherosclerosis and heart disease as they do in many other medical problems. Since we cannot change genetics, my advice to patients and readers of my medical column remains the same, namely to follow a balanced lifestyle. Unfortunately, too many people today are the architects of their own misfortune. I see young people still smoking and everywhere rampant obesity in our society. Yes, I see more joggers than in former years. But on my way to work I daily witness 95% of workers standing immobile on an escalator rather than walking up 25 stairs. And these same people will be sitting at a desk for the rest of the day.

For years my syndicated medical column has defended the dairy industry against attack that it has caused an avalanche of coronary disease. I have pointed out that 'blaming farmers, hens and cows for this problem is like accusing the iceberg for sinking the Titanic'. It was a foolish captain that sank this great ship and similarly irresponsible people who often set the stage for heart disease. As the immortal bard wrote, 'The fault dear Brutus is not in our stars, but in ourselves'. Or as Pogo remarked, 'We have identified the enemy and the enemy is us'.

My worry is that we have now created 'cholesterolphobia', a national disease which doctors will treat with cholesterol-lowering drugs. I agree there may be sound indications for this medication in a select group of patients. But the vast majority of patients, in an already overmedicated society, do not require these drugs. And already studies are showing that their use will prove J.B. Molière right when he wrote in 1673 that, 'Nearly all men die of their medication and not their disease'.

The workshop has been a fascinating experience for me as I have heard international authorities debate the role of cholesterol in the causation of atherosclerosis and heart disease. And as I listened, I wondered if we are shooting at the wrong target. I have little doubt that cholesterol plays a role in cardiovascular problems. But it is my opinion that other factors such as hypertension causing injury to vessel walls may eventually prove to be more significant in causing atherosclerosis than increased blood cholesterol. I believe there is a reasonable possibility that we may find that it is a single abnormality that triggers atherosclerosis. But it is the sum total of many other factors such as genetics, obesity, smoking, diabetes, hypertension, increased blood fibrinogen, sticky platelets and lack of exercise that sets the stage for a coronary attack.

I thank you for the privilege of allowing me as a medical journalist to attend this absorbing meeting.

RANDALL WOOD
Texas A & M University
College Station, Texas, USA

I have to agree with William Connor that diversity and controversy are more important than a mutual admiration society. This meeting has helped me. I am in the process of writing two papers about dietary fats in humans. I think, hopefully, I will be more objective in my interpretation of my data after attending this meeting. I have a feeling that some of our differences and opinions are due to what we think the public policy should be. I have no objections to those who have high levels of serum lipids altering their diet and getting the treatment they need, but I do have concerns about making recommendations for the whole population. In my opinion, some 60–75% of the population are not affected adversely by most dietary fats and should not be misled to believing that they can avoid coronary heart disease by changing their diets. The common response heard is that 'recommendations will not hurt those even if it does not help them'. I would contend that this is one of the strongest endorsements for snake oil tonics and elixirs. We do not know that the dietary recommendations will not hurt or will not be harmful to some individuals. We do know that a lot of the recommendations have a negative bearing on some industries and that this should be taken into account. I recommend treatment for those who have high serum cholesterol levels but I do not think we should be making recommendations for the public at large until it is clear what the outcome will be. I think the public is confused about many items. For instance, most individuals do not know how to lower their fat to 30%. They simply are not equipped to compute that information and, further, I do not know how they determine that they have a 10/10/10 percentage of saturated, monounsaturated and polyunsaturated fat calories unless they are scientists. I personally do not know how that ratio came into being. There is certainly no scientific basis for it. Someone said it came from the McGovern conference but I cannot verify that.

KATSUHIKO YANO
The Honolulu Heart Program
Honolulu, Hawaii, USA

It is important and useful for epidemiologists and basic science researchers to meet together and exchange views on prevention of coronary heart disease and atherosclerotic diseases.

My comment is that we need more studies to search for optimal levels of serum cholesterol for populations or subgroups of populations with different cholesterol levels and disease patterns. Also, I would like to add that recent trends of dramatic decline in stroke mortality in Japan and yet no appreciable increases in coronary heart disease might be related to concurrent increase in fat intake. However, the average intake is still not enough to reach the current level of the United States.

PHILIP L. YEAGLE
State University of New York
Buffalo, New York, USA

My comments for this discussion come from the limited role I have had as an educator to the lay population. I believe that, as practicing scientists, we have an obligation to society as a whole to attempt to communicate the science that we are doing in as clear a fashion as possible. That has been my personal goal. In pursuing this goal, I have had contact with a number of lay, non-scientist populations. From this experience, I would share the following with you. One is that I am not sure that we can over-educate. I think that we underestimate the ability of much of the population to assimilate and understand in English what we are doing as researchers. We can dare to be a little more sophisticated in our attempts at communication. As a result, I think it is possible, if one is careful to be clear, to present some of the complications, some of the caveats, some of the positive indications and some of the contraindications to approaches to medical issues, based on medical science. In that regard, public education has really still not received enough sophistication and emphasis, and I think that it can stand the detail that is necessary to explain some of the issues that we have discussed here.

Let me now address two specific issues. One has to do with the elderly population. The elderly are the only population that I have found to express any sense of over-concern with respect to cholesterol. It may be necessary to communicate to the elderly in a diplomatic and gentle fashion that problems of long-term disease need to be addressed early in the disease process. Much of the benefit found from control of serum cholesterol accrues from early and life-long attention to the problem. The epidemiological studies and clinical intervention studies do not offer much support for starting rigorous cholesterol control in a 75-year-old woman. When you go into the public forum, you do get a lot of feedback from that particular population. Therefore, I would agree with that area of concern expressed in this conference.

However, for virtually every other area of the population, the education effort at this point does not seem to have super-saturated the market. I think there is a lot of benefit yet to be achieved from people knowing and understanding their cholesterol status. They are then in a position to exercise some personal judgement about it.

The other area that I would suggest needs further education and research is the status of post-bypass surgery. I have been impressed with the CLASS study that reported on the benefit from aggressive intervention for cholesterol control on the longevity of the grafts. There are still many cardiologists who do not offer effective education to their patients on the benefits of cholesterol control for graft lifetime. Therefore, I think there is still much education and research to be done in that area.

Abstracts –
English and French

Abstracts (English)

1

An updated coronary risk profile – a statement for health professionals

Keaven M. Anderson, PhD

Research and Development Division
Centocor, Inc.
Malvern, PA, USA
(Formerly with the National Heart, Lung, and Blood Institute, Framingham, MA)

Coronary heart disease (CHD) remains the most frequent cause of death in much of the world, and often kills without prior warning. We present a simple worksheet which stratifies over a large range predicted probabilities of developing CHD in previously disease-free individuals. This is based on an equation which updates previous Framingham Heart Study publications. The focus here is on the role of lipoprotein profiles in risk prediction. Factors considered include total cholesterol (T-C), high density lipoprotein cholesterol (HDL-C), age, gender, systolic blood pressure (SBP), cigarette smoking, diabetes, and left ventricular hypertrophy as measured by electrocardiogram (ECGLVH). The equation is based on the original and offspring Framingham cohorts. Baseline measurements were made in 1968–75 from 5573 men and women aged 30–74 years and CHD incidence times over the following 12 years. The population was free of CHD at baseline. Risk levels associated with a given lipid profile vary greatly according to the presence or absence of other risk factors. As an example, consider a 55-year-old man who smokes, has a T-C of 250 mg/dl, SBP of 130 mmHg, HDL-C of 35 mg/dl, no diabetes, and no ECGLVH. This man has a predicted 10-year CHD risk of 27%. A similar individual with an HDL-C of 60 mg/dl has a 16% risk. However, also eliminating smoking from the profile and find a T-C of 180 mg/dl suggests a risk of 6%. Model selection and its implications will be discussed. For instance, with HDL-C in the model, total cholesterol effects appear to be independent of age and sex. The worksheet emphasizes that there are multiple, additive precursors of CHD, and suggests that a CHD risk factor profile should be evaluated and treated as a whole rather than considering individual risk factors in isolation.

2

Cardiovascular disease prevention through dietary change

Steven A. Grover, MD, MPA, FRCP(C)

Director, Centre for Cardiovascular Risk Assessment
Montreal General Hospital
Assistant Professor
Departments of Medicine, Epidemiology and Biostatistics
McGill University
Montréal, Québec, Canada

Cardiovascular disease (CVD) remains the most common cause of death among Canadians despite recent advances in its diagnosis and treatment. There is no question that CVD can be prevented in certain individuals. The question is how much modification is required for how much prevention? We must determine these 'orders of magnitude' to understand the potential efficacy of dietary change for the average Canadian.

To address many of these questions, we have developed a computer model to predict the changes in life-expectancy and morbidity associated with risk factor modification. The coronary heart disease (CHD) primary prevention model calculates the annual probability of dying from CHD or other causes and the annual risk of specific CHD events for an individual free of CHD at entry into the model.

Our computer model suggests that some individuals may benefit from dietary change if they are at 'high risk' due to a high serum cholesterol and/or the presence of other CHD factors. On the other hand, the average change in life expectancy for many groups of Canadians may be less than 1 month as these individuals are already at 'low risk' for CHD.

We conclude that the risks, benefits, and costs of dietary modification must be better understood before devising a national strategy. Only then can a scientifically sound and economically feasible program be implemented.

3

Coronary risk factors today: a view from Scotland

Christopher G. Isles

Consulting Physician
Department of Medicine
Dumfries and Galloway Royal Infirmary
Dumfries, Scotland

Objective – To examine the relationships between coronary risk and coronary disease among an urban population of women in the West of Scotland.

Design – Longitudinal health study of a general population relating plasma cholesterol, cigarette smoking, diastolic blood pressure, obesity, and social class, to coronary mortality after 15 years of follow-up. Comparison was made with similar data in men.

Subjects – 15 399 adults aged 45 to 64 years, including 8262 women screened between 1972 and 1976 in Renfrew and Paisley, and followed until the end of 1989.

Main Outcome Measure – The analysis was based on 490 CHD deaths in women and 878 CHD deaths in men.

Results – Renfrew and Paisley women were more likely to have high cholesterol, to belong to social class 4 + 5, and less likely to smoke than men. The distribution of blood pressure and body mass index was similar in the two sexes. The relative risk (91% CI) of cholesterol for coronary death was the same in women (1.56 [1.28, 1.90]) and men (1.49 [1.26, 1.77]) but absolute risk was less in women. Thus women in the top quintile for cholesterol had lower coronary mortality (6.1 deaths per thousand patient years) than men in the bottom quintile (6.8 deaths per thousand patient years). Trends showing similar relative risk but lower absolute mortality in women were present for smoking, diastolic blood pressure, and social class. There was no relation between obesity and coronary death after adjusting for other risks. Age-specific CHD mortality was always less in women, even in those aged 60–64 years initially, for whom adjusted CHD rates were only half those of men of similar age.

Conclusions – These results suggest that some other factor or factors lowers CHD risk in women, and it follows, therefore, that the potential for reducing CHD death by stopping smoking, lowering blood pressure and cholesterol, is less in women than in men. Until the results of cholesterol lowering trials in women are available, decisions on lipid lowering therapy will have to be based on estimates of risk rather than of proven benefit. If it is accepted that such judgements should be determined by absolute and not relative risk, then the Renfrew and Paisley Survey suggests the threshold for the use of cholesterol lowering drugs in the primary prevention of coronary disease should be between 1 and 2 mmol/l higher in women than in men.

4

Effect of cholesterol-lowering treatment on coronary heart disease morbidity and mortality: the evidence from trials, and beyond

Martijn B. Katan, PhD

Professor of Human Nutrition
Department of Human Nutrition
Wageningen Agricultural University
Wageningen, The Netherlands

Evidence from controlled clinical trials shows convincingly that reducing serum cholesterol levels by diet or drug treatment reduces the incidence of coronary heart disease. On a population basis, the most important effect of cholesterol lowering might be postponement of the first symptoms of disease rather than postponement of death, because most cardiac deaths occur at an advanced age. No enhanced cancer mortality is seen either in populations with low serum cholesterol levels or in patients who, through a genetic defect, have a low-density-lipoprotein cholesterol of zero. This makes it unlikely that cholesterol-lowering treatment as such promotes cancer. Still, specific side effects and toxicity of drugs need careful scrutiny, and diet remains the treatment of choice for mild hypercholesterolaemia.

5

Trends in fat and cholesterol intake, serum cholesterol levels and cardiovascular disease in Japan

Hirotsugu Ueshima, MD

Head and Professor
Department of Health Science
Shiga University of Medical Science
Shiga, Japan

Mortality rates in Japan, compared with those of America and Europe, are higher for stroke and lower for ischaemic heart disease (IHD). Both mortality rates for stroke and IHD, have declined since 1965 and 1970, respectively.

Epidemiological follow-up studies in Japan have demonstrated that a major risk factor for stroke is hypertension. There is also a hypothesis that appropriate fat and animal protein intake may prevent stroke. On the other hand, many epidemiological studies in industrialized countries have revealed that major coronary risk factors are hypertension, hypercholesterolaemia and smoking. These risk factors may be applicable to Japanese people from findings of Japanese-Americans and some Japanese follow-up studies.

The age and sex-adjusted stroke mortality rate has declined by 64.9% during 1960–1985 and by 49.7% during 1975–1985, while IHD mortality increased up to 1975, and subsequently declined. During the period of 1975–1985, IHD mortality has declined by 32.6%. Fat consumption in Japan has increased more than twofold during the last 25 years. However, it remains about half the level of consumption of American and European people. Furthermore, the ratio of polyunsaturated and saturated fat consumption remains over 1.0 and is higher than the value of 0.5 for Americans and Europeans. Cholesterol intake has increased up to 1972 and then levelled off. Japanese people also eat more fish, shellfish, dishes which are cooked with vegetable oil, such as 'tempura', and less beef and dairy products compared to other industrialized countries.

The increasing trends in fat consumption and the Keys' lipid factor in Japan have slowed recently. These Japanese dietary habits reflect the blood cholesterol level. There may be still 15–20 mg/dl difference in the total cholesterol level between Japanese and Americans, although it becomes less year by year.

In conclusion, the traditional Japanese diet characterized by a low fat intake and a high P/S ratio, and favourable trends in salt and animal protein consumption may contribute to the decline of stroke mortality during the last 25 years and IHD mortality during the last 15 years.

6

The heart disease crusade – cui bono?

Petr Skrabanek, PhD

Senior Lecturer
Department of Community Health
Trinity College
University of Dublin
Dublin, Ireland

Attempts to manipulate 'natural cholesterol' by changes in 'national diet', as recommended by various groups of experts, are absurd expressions of the wish to eliminate coronary heart disease (CHD) as a cause of death. The folly is twofold. First, CHD is a disease of old age, with a mean age at CHD death of 75 years. Not dying of CHD would mean dying of cancer, stroke or Alzheimer's dementia. Secondly, the link between cholesterol and CHD is hypothetical, weak, and non-causal.

The cholesterol-CHD hypothesis rests on a number of weak or unproved links. The relationship between dietary cholesterol and blood cholesterol has not been demonstrated in many large studies, including the Framingham Study. Many studies showed that blood cholesterol does not correlate with the extent of coronary atheromatous lesions. There is no clear correlation between coronary atherosclerosis and CHD. Cholesterol is neither necessary nor sufficient cause of CHD; therefore, cholesterol is only a risk marker. It is a very weak risk marker: the cholesterol attributable risk to CHD is only about 10%. The official consensus that there is no safe threshold for cholesterol is absurd, as it implies that zero cholesterol would be optimal.

The acid test of the diet-heart hypothesis is population-intervention experiment. There are two kinds of evidence available: modification of high cholesterol as a single risk factor, and multiple risk factor intervention. In either case, randomised, controlled trials failed to show significant benefit for the intervention groups (McCormick and Skrabanek, 1988). The failure was encountered regardless whether the study population was in the low-risk or in the high-risk category.

If multiple risk factor intervention has been useless, it is less surprising that the concentration on a single risk factor (high cholesterol) was useless too.

Additional negative evidence comes from community-based trials, such as the Framingham Study and the Northern Karelia project. In Framingham, despite favourable modification of the major risk factors for CHD between 1953 and 1983, the incidence and mortality of CHD in middle-aged men during the same period *increased* (D'Agostino *et al.*, 1989). In Northern Karelia, community-based intervention had no effect on the underlying trend in CHD mortality (McCormick and Skrabanek, 1988).

As to the value of dietary intervention, numerous dietary trials failed to show any benefit to treated population. In the Minnesota Coronary Survey trial (Frantz *et al.*, 1989), 4500 men and 4500 women in mental institutions were randomly allocated to low saturated-fat diet and to normal hospital diet. Despite the fact that the mean cholesterol in the low-fat diet group was reduced by 15%, at 5-year follow up there were ten deaths more from CHD and 21 deaths more from all causes in this group.

It is a fascinating sociological phenomenon that the cholesterol consensus experts, in face of this massive, negative evidence for the value of population intervention as the means of preventing CHD, have come up with recommendations based on their wishful thinking and their dogmatic beliefs. They are guilty of unethical behaviour since they are imposing expensive and potentially dangerous interventions on healthy populations, while concealing from them that reducing cholesterol does not reduce mortality (Oliver, 1988).

References

D'Agostino, R., Kannel, W.B., Belanger, A.J. and Sytkowski, P.A. (1989). Trends in CHD and risk factors at age 55–64 in the Framingham study. *Int. J. Epidemiol.*, **3** (Suppl. 1), S67–S72

Frantz, I.D., Dawson, E.A., Ashman, P.L., Gatewood, L.C., Bartsch, G.E., Kuba, K. and Brewer, E.R. (1989). Test of effect of lipid lowering by diet on cardiovascular risk. *Arteriosclerosis*, **9**, 129–35

McCormick, J. and Skrabanek, P. (1988). Coronary heart disease is not preventable by population interventions. *Lancet*, **2**, 839–41

Oliver, M.F. (1988). Reducing cholesterol does not reduce mortality. *J. Am. Coll. Cardiol.*, **12**, 814–17

7

The role of blood flow in atherogenesis and the dietary cholesterol–fat hypothesis

William E. Stehbens, MD, DPhil

Professor of Pathology
Wellington School of Medicine
Wellington Hospital
Newtown, Wellington, New Zealand

Atherosclerosis is a degenerative disease of blood vessels affecting all humans and many lower species. It varies in severity from individual to individual and from vascular bed to vascular bed. The complications (intimal tears, ulcerations, mural thrombosis, tortuosity, aneurysms) can be explained on the basis of an acquired mural weakness. This and the predilection for arterial forks, junctions, and curvatures led to the haemodynamically-induced fatigue hypothesis which provides a plausible explanation for the complications. However, haemodynamics has been generally regarded merely as a localizing factor in atherosclerosis but without dietary manipulation, accelerated atherosclerosis can be induced by surgically altering the blood flow in sheep and rabbits and in man in coronary venous by-pass grafts and in the veins of therapeutic arteriovenous shunts for renal dialysis. These observations argue strongly against the dietary fat/cholesterol (lipid) hypothesis of atherogenesis which is only a theory of fat accumulation in the vessel wall and does not explain the pathogenesis or the complications.

The lipid hypothesis has dominated research in atherosclerosis for more than forty years despite misrepresentation of the vascular pathology of the cholesterol-fed animal and of familial hypercholesterolaemia. The pathogenesis of myocardial ischaemia associated with lipid storage in these conditions differs from that caused by atherosclerosis and there are other irreconcilable differences. The absence of pathological and experimental support negates the value of epidemiological studies of atherosclerosis. As well, there are major flaws and inconsistencies in the epidemiological evidence for the aetiology of atherosclerosis, including (1) misuse of cause and risk factor; (2) misuse of CHD as an inappropriate, non-pathognomonic surrogate monitor of severe atherosclerosis; (3) invalid extrapolations from CHD risk factors to the aetiology of atherosclerosis; (4) the maldiagnostic rate of $\pm 30\%$ for CHD; (5) selection bias in clinical trials by virtue of age and inclusion of familial hypercholesterolaemia; (6) the use of invalid national mortality rates and dietary data, and; (7) ecological factors. Currently there is no scientific evidence proving that dietary fat/cholesterol or elevated blood cholesterol levels can cause atherosclerosis. Until it is possible to assess the severity of atherosclerosis accurately, clinical epidemiological studies concerned with atherosclerosis will be of limited value.

8
Cellular and lipoprotein interactions in early atherogenesis

Mahamed Navab, PhD and Alan M. Fogelman

Associate Research Cardiologist
Division of Cardiology
School of Medicine
University of California at Los Angeles
Los Angeles, California, USA

Accumulating evidence suggests that oxidized lipoproteins may play a critical role in the development of atherosclerosis. These lipoproteins have been observed in atherosclerotic plaques in human and in experimental animals. Additionally, the development of lesions in cholesterol-fed or Watanabe rabbits can be diminished by treatment with antioxidants. Low density lipoprotein (LDL) has been demonstrated to undergo modification by the cells of the artery wall and by monocyte-macrophages in culture in the *absence* of serum. The modification of LDL in the vessel wall, however, must occur in the presence of plasma antioxidants such as α-tocopherol and β-carotene. We have used a multilayer co-culture of human aortic EC and SMC and studied the modification of native LDL in the presence of serum. We have found that incubation of LDL with artery wall cells results in a significant induction of monocyte chemotactic protein 1 (MCP-1) mRNA and protein, and in a marked increase in monocyte adhesion to and transmigration across the endothelial monolayer in the co-culture. High density lipoprotein (HDL) and antioxidants prevent these LDL induced effects. Based on the recent work from our laboratory and those of others, we propose a model for foam cell formation in the artery wall: In the lesion prone sites, plasma LDL enters the largely acellular subendothelial space (SES) where it is retained in microenvironments secluded from plasma antioxidants. LDL lipid is oxidatively modified giving rise to a minimally oxidized LDL, MM-LDL. Once formed MM-LDL stimulates the overlaying endothelium to produce an adhesion molecule(s) for blood monocytes, 'M-ELAM' and to secrete MCP-1 and M-CSF. These molecular events lead to the following cellular events: monocyte attachment to the EC; MCP-1 induced monocyte migration into the SES of the artery wall and M-CSF induced differentiation of monocytes into macrophages. Macrophage products such as reactive oxygen species, malondialdehyde, can then further modify MM-LDL to a highly modified (oxidized) form which is then recognized by the macrophage scavenger receptor leading to cholesterol ester accumulation and foam cell formation. If HDL is present in sufficient concentrations, the formation of biologically active MM-LDL is prevented and the inflammatory reaction may be blocked.

9

Animal models for studying the pathogenesis of atherosclerosis

J. Stewart-Phillips, J. Lough and <u>Emil Skamene</u>, MD, PhD, FRCP(C), FACP

McGill Centre for the Study of Host Resistance and the
Montreal General Hospital Research Institute
Montréal, Québec, Canada

In man, atherosclerosis is a slow, progressive disorder which develops over many years. In order to study its pathogenesis, a number of animal models have been developed, the best known of which include non-human primates, rabbits and pigeons. The choice of model rests largely on familiarity, availability and existence of previous data relevant to the parameter under investigation.

One of the important ways in which the pathogenesis of atherosclerosis can be studied is by establishing the genetic factors which determine susceptibility and resistance to the disease. To this end, the mouse has proved to be an invaluable model. A wide variety of genetically-characterized inbred strains of mice are readily available for studies of this nature. Moreover, there are many similarities between the lipoproteins and apoproteins of mice and those of humans, which are altered by high fat/high cholesterol feeding. Susceptible mice develop aortic lesions similar to human atherosclerotic plaques. Furthermore, the mouse had by far the most extensive gene-linkage map of any mammal and the discovery of many marker genes has facilitated the mapping of new genes.

In our laboratory, we have used mice derived from the susceptible C57BL/6J strain and resistant A/J strain to identify genetically-determined differences in both serum lipoproteins and macrophage activities which may contribute to the pathogenesis of diet-induced atherosclerosis. We have concluded that the difference in susceptibility exhibited by these two mouse strains is polygenic but that one gene, designated Ath-3, which apparently determines serum HDL levels, may exert a major effect. We have tentatively mapped this gene to mouse chromosome 7. We have also concluded that a genetically-determined difference in macrophage chemotactic activity between A/J and C57BL/6J mice contributes to the difference in their susceptibility to diet-induced atherosclerosis.

10
Obesity and associated apolipoprotein abnormalities: relation to coronary heart disease

Daniel A.K. Roncari, MD, PhD, FACP, FRCPC

Physician-in-Chief
Sunnybrook Health Science Centre
Professor of Medicine
University of Toronto
Toronto, Ontario, Canada

Obesity both triggers the development and aggravates a variety of lipopro-tein-apolipoprotein abnormalities. These confer increasing atherogenicity upon the individual. The aggravating influence is in obese subjects with specific genetic susceptibility to dyslipoproteinaemia, who then develop the more pronounced abnormalities. Hepatic production of very-low-density lipoproteins (VLDL) is augmented in obesity, particularly when the body weight is increasing or when the corpulence is maintained. The heterogeneous VLDL are atherogenic, to a greater extent particles that are denser because of higher apoB/cholesterol ester ratios. VLDL, in turn, are precursors of even more atherogenic lipoproteins, intermediate-density lipoproteins (IDL) and low-density lipoproteins (LDL). The augmented flux of free fatty acids from adipose tissue to liver promotes VLDL synthesis. Moreover, specific hepatic cholesterol esters influence significantly apoB production. ApoB is an essential constituent of the developing VLDL particles, which eventually are converted to LDL, whose exclusive apolipoprotein is apoB. Relatedly, dietary intake of lauric, myristic, and palmitic acids elevate plasma LDL-cholesterol, stearic acid is neutral, while oleic (under some conditions also neutral), linoleic, and (n-3) fatty acids decrease LDL-cholesterol levels. Particularly in obese individuals, especially those with abdominal expansion, IDL containing isoforms E-2 and E-4 are associated with dyslipidaemias, E-2 with increased plasma VLDL-triglycerides and decreased high-density lipoprotein-cholesterol (HDL-C), while E-4 with elevated plasma LDL-cho-lesterol, LDL-apoB, and triglycerides. IDL are more atherogenic than VLDL. Upon stripping of much of the remaining triglycerides from IDL by lipoprotein lipase (the activity of lipoprotein lipase, whose essential activator is apolipoprotein C-II, is augmented in obesity, promoting progression of the adiposity), with concurrent transfer of apoE and other constituents to different lipoproteins, low-density lipoproteins are formed. These highly atherogenic particles contain apoB-100 as the exclusive apolipoprotein and are enriched in cholesterol esters. In obesity, there is augmented flux of the atherogenic VLDL, IDL, and LDL, along with their apolipoproteins. Thus, even in the absence of elevated plasma levels, their excessive turnover imposes a substantial risk for coronary heart disease. Denser VLDL produce, via IDL, low-density lipoproteins with higher apoB/cholesterol ester ratios. The extreme situation is expressed by the syndrome of hyperapobetalipoproteinaemia, described by A. Sniderman *et al.* This is a highly atherogenic state, even when plasma cholesterol and triglycerides are within normal limits. Denser VLDL and LDL particles, as found in hyperapobetalipoproteinaemia, occur frequently in the setting of familial combined hyperlipidaemia, which has variable expression in different family members. While lipoprotein-apolipoprotein abnormalities occur generally in obesity, abdominal obesity is particularly characterized by augmented levels of VLDL-triglyceride and LDL-apoB (the influence of apoE isoforms has already been indicated), as well as HDL abnormalities, as follows. In both abdominal and diffuse obesity, the HDL species containing apoA-1 are decreased, partly because of increased disposal in adipose tissue, and in abdominal obesity, increased hepatic triglyceride lipase activity. Increased clearance is particularly prominent in abdominal depots. While much has yet to be learned about lipoprotein (a), its level is relatively decreased in obese subjects and it rises upon weight loss. In fact, in both children and adults, all the described abnormalities improve with effective dietary and exercise measures, although the ultimate degree of benefit is dictated by genetic factors. While the liver is a major site of apolipoprotein, lipid, and lipoprotein production and metabolism, adipose tissue modulates these hepatic functions. In obesity, adipose tissue contributes significantly to the pathogenesis of abnormal lipoprotein – apolipoprotein production and clearance, both through its influence on the liver, and through its action on lipoproteins (e.g. through adipose cell lipoprotein lipase). The numerous cellular and molecular abnormalities of adipose cells facilitating the development, progression, and recurrence of obesity will be reviewed in the context of the emergence of an increasingly atherogenic apolipoprotein – lipoprotein profile and metabolism.

11
Modulation of membrane function by cholesterol

Philip L. Yeagle, PhD

Department of Biochemistry
University at Buffalo School of Medicine
State University of New York
Buffalo, New York, USA

Cholesterol is an essential component of mammalian (and other cell) membranes. Mammalian cells cannot grow, mitose, or differentiate in the absence of cholesterol. Parallel behaviour can be found in other organisms, such as yeast, in which the required sterol is ergosterol. These cellular functions have been shown to require at a minimum a small level of a structurally specific sterol; i.e., other sterols cannot substitute for this specific sterol requirement. For example, ergosterol cannot substitute for cholesterol in mammalian cells and cholesterol cannot substitute for ergosterol in yeast cells. Much has been learned about the structural effects of cholesterol on lipid bilayers at high cholesterol content. Yet what role specific sterols play in the normal functioning of a cell has remained a mystery.

Recent data have led to the development of a comprehensive hypothesis to explain the essential role of cholesterol in mammalian cells. At low membrane levels, cholesterol stimulates the activity of membrane enzymes that are crucial to cellular function by a structurally specific, direct sterol-protein interaction. At high membrane levels, cholesterol modulates membrane protein activity by alteration of the bulk properties of the lipid bilayer of the cell membrane. This effect has been expressed as a change in the 'free volume' within the bilayer which affects the ability of a membrane protein to undergo the conformational transitions required for function.

Available data will be reviewed in the context of this hypothesis. Examples of these data that will be discussed are given in the following. Experiments under the conditions of sterol auxotrophy in mycoplasma and yeast revealed the structurally specific sterol requirement (Dahl and Dahl, 1988). Studies on Na^+-K^+-ATPase activity in plasma membranes from mammalian cells showed the structurally specific requirement for cholesterol to support pump activity, a membrane enzyme crucial to cellular function (Yeagle *et al.*, 1988). The inhibition by cholesterol at high membrane levels of Na^+-K^+-ATPase (Giraud *et al.*, 1981; Yeagle, 1983) and the photoreceptor rhodopsin (Boesze-Battaglia and Albert, 1990; Straume and Litman, 1988) showed that alteration of bulk properties of the membrane by cholesterol inhibited membrane function.

References

Boesze-Battaglia, K. and Albert, A. (1990). *J. Biol. Chem.*, **265**, 20727–30

Dahl, C. and Dahl, J. (1988). In Yeagle, P.L. (eds) *Biology of Cholesterol*, pp. 147–72. (CRC Press, Boca Raton)

Giraud, F. Claret, M., Bruckdorfer, K.R. and Chailley, B. (1981). *Biochim. Biophys. Acta*, **647**, 249–58

Straume, M. and Litman, B.J. (1988). *Biochemistry*, **27**, 7723–33

Yeagle, P.L. (1983). *Biochim. Biophys. Acta*, **727**, 39–44

Yeagle, P.L., Rice, D. and Young, J. (1988). *Biochemistry*, **27**, 6449–52

12
Hyporesponders and hyperresponders to changes in diet

Martijn B. Katan, PhD* and A.C. Beynen**

Department of Human Nutrition
Agricultural University
Wageningen, The Netherlands
**Department of Laboratory Animal Science*
State University
Utrecht, The Netherlands

Certain human subjects may have a consistently low or high response of serum cholesterol to dietary cholesterol. Responsiveness to dietary cholesterol appears to be associated with responsiveness to dietary saturated fatty acids. On the average, hyperresponders have a higher habitual cholesterol intake, higher levels of HDL cholesterol and a lower body weight than hyporesponders. The mechanisms underlying hypo- and hyperresponsiveness to either dietary cholesterol or saturated fatty acids have not yet been revealed. The phenomenon of hyporesponsiveness and hyperresponsiveness may have implications for the counselling of subjects who attempt to lower their serum cholesterol by diet. However, identification of true hyporesponders and hyperresponders is greatly hampered by within-person fluctuations of the level of serum cholesterol. No simple test is available to discriminate hyporesponders from hyperresponders. As yet, monitoring a person's response to diet should be based on relatively large numbers of serum cholesterol determinations.

13

Re-examination of the dietary fatty acid–plasma cholesterol issue: is palmitic acid (16:0) neutral?

K.C. Hayes

Professor of Biology (Nutrition)
Director, Foster Biomedical Research Laboratories
Brandeis University
Waltham, Massachusetts, USA

A series of studies in monkeys and hamsters, and re-evaluation of published human data, indicate that dietary saturated fatty acids exert a dissimilar metabolic impact on cholesterol metabolism. Myristic acid (14:0) appears to have a major cholesterol-raising effect by means of decreasing LDL receptor activity and by increasing the direct production of LDL (from sources other than VLDL-catabolism). Palmitic acid (16:0) appears neutral in most cases (plasma cholesterol < 200 mg/dl) or until the LDL receptor is down-regulated, as with high cholesterol intake or obesity. In such cases, the down-regulated LDL receptors coupled with an increased VLDL production (induced by 16:0 and 18:1) can divert VLDL remnants to LDL and expand the LDL pool. Furthermore, the cholesterolaemic impact of any saturated fatty acid can be countered up to a saturable 'threshold' level by dietary linoleic acid (18:2) which up-regulates the LDL receptor. Once above this 'threshold', the major fatty acids (16:0, 18:0, 18:1, 18:2, 18:3) appear to exert an equal impact on the circulating cholesterol concentration.

14
The potential health aspects of lipid oxidation products in food

Paul Bradley Addis

Professor
Department of Food Science and Nutrition
College of Agriculture and College of Human Ecology
University of Minnesota
St. Paul, Minnesota, USA

There are manifold ramifications of ongoing research on foods on the possible health aspects of lipid oxidation products in foods. Some of these aspects are briefly outlined in this section and a brief appraisal is given of the regulatory aspects of rancidity in foods and heated oils. The reader is referred to Addis and Park (1989) for suggestions for future research in this area.

There is, at the present time, little in the way of regulation of foods with regard to rancidity in the USA (Firestone and Summers, 1989). Certainly the presence of toxic xenobiotics will be a sufficient basis for FDA regulatory action against fats and oils, but the issue of process-induced deleterious substances, which would include lipid oxidation products, is not as clear cut and no federal regulation currently exists for control of rancidity. However, two municipalities, Chicago and San Francisco, do list rancidity as one factor which must be controlled in frying oils (Firestone, 1989).

In Europe, the laws are very explicit with regard to oxidation products in frying oils. Belgium, France, Germany, Spain and Switzerland restrict polar compounds to 25–27% as determined by IUPAC method 2.507 (Firestone, 1989).

Scandinavian countries do not have specific regulations but food inspectors employ a wide variety of tests to determine if oils should be discarded. These include 'food oil sensor', free fatty acids, smokepoint, taste, odour, foam and acid value. There is much current research concerning which method is the best for evaluating oils. Clearly, the area of heated-fats research is ripe for harvest in terms of research on toxicity, oil degradation, antioxidants, filtration, and methods of evaluation. These comments apply equally well to the many other ramifications of food lipid oxidation products. It is difficult to overestimate the potential importance, both from the scientific and health standpoints, of lipid oxidation products and it seems appropriate to attempt to discuss some of the broad significance of this exciting area of research. To begin with, it seems appropriate to consider some of the most fundamental ideas on CHD and challenge them based on the new findings on lipid oxidation products. It appears that dietary (pure) cholesterol is neither angiotoxic nor hypercholesterolaemic and, therefore, cannot initiate or promote CHD. It is tempting to speculate that lipid oxidation product consumption patterns may partially explain why some persons with low serum cholesterol are susceptible to CHD, while others with high serum cholesterol appear to escape the disease. The role of smoking, perhaps the single most important risk factor in CHD, may be linked to *in vivo* oxidation of blood and tissue lipids. Research is urgently needed on this point.

Lipid oxidation products in foods represent 'process-induced' toxicants and, therefore, are contrasted to the usual xenobiotic contaminant. Because such oxidation products are endogenously produced, as opposed to being derived from exogenous sources, the regulatory status is uncertain in the USA. Nevertheless, the FDA has established a program in 'process-induced' phenomena, indicating possible future regulatory interest. Heated oils would probably be targeted for early consideration of regulatory activity, based on activities in Europe. Interestingly, the recent popularity of a more polyunsaturated-type of frying oil will likely produce greater oxidation problems than use of tallow or shortening.

There may be a connection between dietary lipid oxidation products and mLDL and between both of these and the consumption of dietary antioxidants. The potential benefits of antioxidants would appear to be very great if the conversion of LDL to mLDL can be slowed by antioxidants.

15
Regulation of the concentration of cholesterol carried in low density lipoproteins in the plasma

John M. Dietschy, MD

The Jan and Henri Bromberg Professor
Chief, Gastroenterology
University of Texas
Southwestern Medical Center
Dallas, Texas, USA

The steady-state level of cholesterol can be calculated if, in a particular animal species, one has absolute values for the LDL-cholesterol production rate (J_t), whole animal receptor activity (J^m), the affinity of the LDL molecule for its receptor (K_m) and the proportionality constant for receptor-independent LDL-cholesterol transport (P). These studies outline the manner in which each of these four rate constants change in animals fed varying amounts of cholesterol and varying amounts of pure triacylglycerols containing only a single fatty acid. In addition, data are presented on the rates of net sterol balance and rates of cholesterol synthesis in the liver and other major organs under these same conditions. When small quantities of cholesterol are fed to animals receiving a lipid-free diet, there is a dose-dependent inhibition of hepatic cholesterol synthesis followed by an increase in the concentration of cholesteryl esters in the liver. This is subsequently followed by partial suppression of J^m and a small increase in J_t. As a consequence, there are modest increases in the circulating plasma LDL-cholesterol level. When triacylglycerol, containing a mixture of saturated fatty acids, is added to such diets, there is further suppression of LDL receptor activity and a more marked increase in the production rate: hence, there are marked increases in the level of LDL-cholesterol in the plasma. When triacylglycerols containing only a single fatty acid, varying in chain-length from 6:0 to 18:0, are fed to this same type of animal model, only the fatty acids 12:0, 14:0 and 16:0 cause these changes in production rate and receptor activity and significantly elevate the plasma LDL-cholesterol level. The 18:0 fatty acid does not alter any parameter of LDL-cholesterol metabolism even though feeding this fatty acid results in significant enrichment of the fatty acid pool in the liver cell membranes with the 18:0 compound. In similar experiments in which the animals were fed triacylglycerols containing a single species of unsaturated fatty acids, the 18:1 compound was the most potent in restoring receptor activity. There was no obvious correlation in these experiments between the concentration of total cholesterol in the liver and receptor activity. Thus, for example, the feeding of saturated fatty acids actually lowered the content of cholesterol in the liver cell while, at the same, suppressing receptor activity while unsaturated fatty acids tended to raise the content of cholesterol, particularly in the cholesteryl ester pool, while at the same time, increasing LDL receptor activity. Since the feeding of these various fatty acids did not appear to alter external sterol balance across the liver, these studies imply that fatty acids reaching the liver cell may alter that small pool of cholesterol in the cell which is unmeasurable, but which is actually the pool of sterol regulating the synthesis of LDL-receptor protein.

16

Plasma cholesterol responsiveness to saturated fatty acids

Gloria Lena Vega, PhD

Associate Professor
Department of Clinical Nutrition and
Center for Human Nutrition
University of Texas
Southwestern Medical Center
Dallas, Texas, USA

The variability in responsiveness to saturated fatty acids has not been studied systematically. For this reason data from three dietary studies carried out in our laboratory were pooled and used to evaluate how individuals vary in their responses in plasma concentrations of total cholesterol and low-density lipoprotein cholesterol to the substitution of saturated fatty acids for unsaturated fatty acids. The data showed a marked variability in response. Some patients demonstrated a striking rise in cholesterol levels whereas others had more modest increases. This finding points to the need for further investigation on this issue.

17

The role of n-3 fatty acids as modulators of n-6 fatty acid metabolism: health implications

Pierre Budowski, PhD

Professor (Emeritus)
Faculty of Agriculture
The Hebrew University of Jerusalem
Rehovot, Israel

Linoleic and α-linolenic acids are the parent fatty acids of the n-6 and n-3 series of polyunsaturated fatty acids (PUFA). In addition to their nutritional essentiality, these fatty acids also interact with each other at different metabolic levels. The formation of arachidonic acid (AA) from linoleic acid within the n-6 PUFA family, and the conversion of AA into eicosanoids, are effectively inhibited by n-3 PUFA. In addition, competition takes place between n-6 and long-chain n-3 PUFA moieties for incorporation into phospholipids of cell membranes and organelles. Conversely, linoleic acid is capable of interference with the biosynthesis of long-chain n-3 PUFA, provided it is present in large excess.

The relative dietary proportions and the metabolic interactions of the two PUFA families are of nutritional significance and have health implications, as they affect the properties of cell membranes and membrane-anchored proteins and receptors, as well as the production of AA-derived eicosanoids. *Unrestrained* AA metabolism, which results in excessive eicosanoid formation and side reactions leading to potentially damaging active oxygen species, is involved in various pathological processes ranging from immune-inflammatory reactions to thrombotic events.

Today, the PUFA intake in Western countries is heavily weighted in favour of linoleic acid which exceeds the intake of α-linoleic acid by roughly one order of magnitude. Under these conditions, the restraining action of α-linolenic acid on AA metabolism does not receive its full expression. Moreover, an excessive intake of linoleic acid interferes with the biosynthesis of docosahexaenoic acid, a n-3 PUFA which is of crucial importance for the normal development of brain and retina.

The present-day PUFA imbalance is a late consequence of the industrial revolution which has caused other changes in nutrient intakes and in life-style. Our enzymic equipment is ill adapted to cope with these changes.

18

The ratio of polyunsaturates to saturates and its role in the efficacy of n-3 fatty acids

K.S. Layne, E.A. Ryan, M.L. Garg, Y.K. Goh, J.A. Jumpsen and
M.T. Clandinin, PhD
Professor
Departments of Foods & Nutrition and Medicine
Nutrition and Metabolism Research Group
University of Alberta
Edmonton, Alberta, Canada

Dietary omega-3 fatty acids have been associated with a reduced incidence of coronary heart disease, probably due to altered eicosanoid metabolism and reduction in circulating serum lipoprotein fractions. Animal studies from our laboratory indicate that the efficacy of omega-3 fatty acids in lowering plasma cholesterol, triacylglycerol, and arachidonic acid depends on the dietary linoleic acid to saturated fatty acid (P/S) ratio.

Since omega-6 and omega-3 fatty acids compete at the level of the hepatic desaturases and for membrane incorporation, it is hypothesized that omega-3 fatty acids will reduce serum lipid and arachidonate levels more effectively when dietary linoleate levels are reduced. Currently we are investigating the effects of omega-3 fatty acid supplementation on serum lipoprotein profiles of normolipidaemic humans having a high or low dietary P/S ratio. Based on usual 7-day dietary records, 32 subjects were divided into high P/S (>0.8) or low P/S (<0.5) groups. All individuals were supplemented with olive oil for the first 3 months. The following 6 months involved a double blind, cross-over phase during which subjects were given modest intakes (35 mg omega-3 fatty acids/kg body weight) of either linseed oil ($18:3\omega3$) or fish oil ($20:5\omega3$, $22:6\omega3$) for 3 months in a randomized order, followed by the alternative oil for the final 3 months. Blood was sampled initially and after each treatment period for analysis of serum lipoprotein levels, fatty acid profiles, glucose, HbA$_1$c, glucagon, C-peptide, and insulin. The effects of these treatments and dietary P/S ratio on serum lipid levels will be discussed.

19
Lipoproteins, sex hormones and the gender difference in coronary heart disease

Ian F. Godsland, BA

Research Director
Wynn Institute for Metabolic Research
London, United Kingdom

In Western-industrialised societies coronary heart disease mortality is up to sixfold higher in men compared with women. Gender differences in lipoprotein risk factors for coronary heart disease may, in part, account for this difference: HDL cholesterol concentrations are lower and LDL cholesterol concentrations higher in men, in the age range when the gender difference in coronary heart disease is most apparent. Furthermore, when men and women are matched for HDL the difference in mortality rates is no longer apparent. Studies on the effects of exogenously administered gonadal steroids and sex hormones provide evidence for the hypothesis that the gender difference in lipoprotein concentrations is due to differing sex hormone concentrations in men and women. Androgenic activity is associated with low HDL and high LDL concentrations, and oestrogenic activity with the converse pattern. However, there are some exceptions, and these patterns are less clearly defined with the natural hormones. Associations between endogenous hormone levels and lipoprotein concentrations in men are the reverse of the pattern expected from the effects of exogenously administered steroids: HDL correlates positively with testosterone and negatively with oestradiol. Nevertheless, at puberty HDL concentrations fall in males, and in women at menopause HDL concentrations fall and LDL concentrations rise. These findings generally support the hypothesis that differences in sex hormone concentrations contribute to the gender difference in lipoprotein concentrations. However, these relationships are not seen in non-Western societies, indicating that some other factor, as yet unknown, is important for the gender difference in lipoprotein concentrations and coronary heart disease incidence to be manifest.

ABSTRACT

20
Children's health and the cholesterol/fat issue

Richard B. Goldbloom, OC, MD

Professor of Paediatrics
Dalhousie University
Director of Ambulatory Services
IWK Children's Hospital
Halifax, Nova Scotia, Canada

The methodological principles elaborated and adopted by the Canadian Task Force on the Periodic Health Examination and the US Preventive Services Task Force require that in making recommendations for preventive health care, scientific evidence take precedence over consensus and that the strength of that evidence be graded according to the quality of the studies on which it is based. When such methodology is used to formulate recommendations there is little place for concepts that say in effect: 'Well, it *probably* will do no harm and we think it *may* do some good'.

In discussing paediatric aspects of the fat and cholesterol issues, we must draw a clear distinction between the management of individual ostensibly healthy patients in clinical encounters, management of those already identified to be at high risk, recommendations for those with high risk, and recommendations directed at the entire population. Each situation has vastly different risk: benefit characteristics and cost implications.

In my view, in its 1986 statement on Dietary Fat and Cholesterol in Children, the American Academy of Pediatrics wisely suggested a range of intakes rather than a level which none should exceed. In doing so, they documented their respect for individuality and the glory of normal human variation – a respect that all of us should continue to emulate.

21
Coronary heart disease: prevention and treatment by nutritional change

William E. Connor, MD

Professor of Medicine
Head, Section of Clinical Nutrition and Lipid Metabolism
Oregon Health Sciences University
Portland, Oregon, USA

Diet greatly affects many of the risk factors which cause coronary heart disease. In fact, nutrition itself must be listed as one of the major risk factors because of its tremendous modifying effects on the disease process, atherosclerosis. The most important risk factor in which diet plays the major role, both in causation and in treatment, is hyperlipidaemia.

Hyperlipidaemia is important because it forms the basis for the excessive infiltration of lipid into the arterial intima with atherosclerosis an ultimate consequence. The cause of hyperlipidaemia for 99% of the population is a faulty life-style with excessive intakes of saturated fat, cholesterol and total calories in the diet.

The review of information on the vital role of plasma lipid and lipoprotein concentrations in the development of atherosclerosis raises a crucial question: Can dietary change lower elevated plasma lipid and lipoprotein concentrations in patients and in population subgroups of the Western world? The answer is an unequivocal yes.

The primary prevention of coronary heart disease is clearly the ultimate goal to deal most effectively with the current epidemic of coronary heart disease. Suggested dietary changes for the coronary patient are completely safe and are prudent measures to be followed by any population (i.e., Western) at serious risk for coronary disease. These nutritional changes should be instituted early in life when they will have the greatest impact. This is a familial disease and its control and treatment can best be approached on a family basis. The primary prevention of coronary heart disease is dependent upon the prevention of diet-induced hyperlipidaemia.

22

The relationship between serum cholesterol and the incidence of type-specific stroke in Honolulu Japanese men

Katsuhiko Yano, MD
Senior Investigator

and

Dwayne M. Reed, MD, PhD
Honolulu Heart Program
Honolulu, Hawaii, USA

During an average 20 years of follow-up of 7850 Japanese men in Hawaii aged 45 to 68 who were free of stroke at entry, 523 developed stroke, including 38 with subarachnoid haemorrhage (SAH), 78 with intracerebral haemorrhage (ICH), 355 with thrombo-embolic stroke (TE), and 52 with unspecified type. Age-adjusted incidence rates indicated that the baseline level of serum total cholesterol was associated inversely with SAH ($p=0.054$) and ICH ($p=0.015$), while it was directly associated with TE ($p=0.045$). Further adjustment for risk factors including hypertension, diabetes, body mass index, cigarette smoking, and alcohol consumption revealed that only the inverse association of serum cholesterol with ICH remained significant with the highest/lowest quintile relative risk of 0.46 (95% confidence interval: 0.24, 0.88). Separate analyses for hypertensive and normotensive men demonstrated that the inverse association with ICH and the direct association with TE were significant only in normotensive men. However, formal statistical tests for the interaction of serum cholesterol and blood pressure upon the risk of stroke were all negative. It was concluded that low serum cholesterol, especially below 4.14 mmol/l (160 mg/dl), significantly increased the risk of ICH even after adjusting for other risk factors.

ABSTRACT

23

Dyslipidaemias and the primary prevention of coronary heart disease: reflections on some unresolved policy issues

C. David Naylor, MD, DPhil, FRCP(C)

Director
Clinical Epidemiology Unit and Department of Medicine
Sunnybrook Health Science Centre
University of Toronto
Toronto, Ontario, Canada

Guidelines for prevention of CHD through detection of abnormal lipid profiles and manipulation of serum lipids have been promulgated in Europe and North America. Guidelines vary in several respects: e.g., target populations for case-finding; tests to be used; threshold values for further action; risk factors considered in treatment decisions; distinctions between primary and secondary prevention; and, role of a population strategy. The evidentiary base available to the various expert panels, consensus bodies, and task forces has been similar. Differing clinical and public policies clearly reflect divergent interpretation of evidence, perceived societal values and priorities, and – perhaps most important of all – the priorities and values of the experts and their sponsors.

The presentation will accordingly focus on several unresolved issues in clinical and public policy.

1. Predictive value and prognostic misclassification with current testing strategies
2. Matching treatment intensity to reversible risk in a multifactorial disease
3. The trial evidence: problems of generalizability in populations and design
4. All-cause mortality issues: clinical and public policy concerns
5. Role of patient preferences in decision-making and treatment dysutilities in broad policy determination
6. Discounting and time preference issues in treatment and policy decisions
7. Secondary versus primary prevention: the baby in the bathwater?

24

Canadian Consensus Conference on Cholesterol

Louis Horlick, MD, FRCP(C), FACP

Professor of Medicine (Emeritus)
Department of Medicine
University of Saskatchewan
Royal University Hospital
Saskatoon, Saskatchewan, Canada

Epidemiological studies carried out in Canada have revealed a very high burden of risk factors for coronary heart disease. The Nova Scotia Heart Health Study carried out in 1987 showed that 39% of males and 31% of females aged 35–64 had blood cholesterol levels above 220 mg/dl. It also showed that only 29% of the population aged 17–74, both sexes, was free of the three cardinal risk factors (hypercholesterolaemia, hypertension, smoking). It was this data that led us to opt for a population based strategy for control of hypercholesterolaemia. It would be based on health promotion strategies for the entire population, and would include action on all the risk factors rather than on cholesterol alone. It would require the collective involvement of health service personnel at all levels of government. We have therefore made important recommendations concerning dietary changes for the entire population, food products, and a new population goal for total cholesterol. In this respect, we differed from the American Consensus which initially opted for a high risk case finding strategy.

We did not ignore the problem of high risk individuals in our society. However, we gave it a lower priority than the population approach. The Panel made recommendations for screening which were aimed at individuals known to be at risk, but reserved universal screening for a time when resources would permit. It recommended the lipid parameters to be screened, and then made some basic recommendations for intervention. The emphasis in treatment was on the dietary intervention, and we gave only very general advice about drug treatment. Simplified cut-off points were used, stratified into two age classes, but not by sex. For men and women over age 30, a cholesterol level under 200 mg/dl was regarded as acceptable and should be rechecked in 5 years. Individuals in the range of 200–240 mg/dl should have dietary education provided, while those in this range but with LDL cholesterol levels above 130 or HDL cholesterol levels below 35 mg/dl required intensive dietary therapy. Cholesterol levels above 240 mg/dl, which were resistant to intensive dietary therapy might require pharmacological measures.

A vigorous high-risk approach will have important cost implications for the health care system, and will create major problems for physicians, dietitians, and laboratory services. Implementation of the public health/population model will greatly alleviate these problems.

Abstracts (French)

1
Nouveau profil de risque coronarien – énoncé pour les spécialistes de la santé

Keaven M. Anderson, PhD

Division de recherche-développement
Centocor, Inc.
Malvern, PA, États-Unis
(Ancien membre du National Heart, Lung, and Blood Institute, Framingham, MA)

Dans la plupart des pays du monde, les maladies cardiaques coronariennes sont encore la principale cause de décès et frappent souvent sans prévenir. Nous présentons une fiche qui stratifie à grande échelle les probabilités d'apparition des maladies cardiaques coronariennes chez des personnes sans antécédents pathologiques. Ces données reposent sur une équation qui permet de mettre à jour les publications découlant de l'étude de Framingham. Le rôle des profils de lipoprotéines dans la prédiction des risques en constitue l'axe principal. Les facteurs pris en compte sont le cholestérol total (C-T), le cholestérol porté par les lipoprotéines de haute densité (HDL-C), l'âge, le sexe, la tension artérielle systolique (TAS), le tabagisme, le diabète et l'hypertrophie ventriculaire gauche mesurée par électrocardiogramme (ECGHVG). L'équation est basée sur les cohortes originales de Framingham et sur leur descendance. Les premières évaluations ont été effectuées en 1968-1975 auprès de 5573 hommes et femmes âgés de 30 à 74 ans et l'incidence des maladies cardiaques coronariennes a été mesurée pendant les 12 années suivantes. Au départ, aucun des participants ne souffrait de maladie cardiaque coronarienne. Les risques liés à un profil lipidique donné varient considérablement selon l'existence ou l'absence d'autres facteurs de risques. Ainsi, un homme de 55 ans qui fume, dont le taux de cholestérol total est de 250 mg/dl, la tension artérielle systolique de 130 mmHg, l'HDL-C de 35 mg/dl, qui ne souffre pas de diabète et n'a pas d'hypertrophie ventriculaire gauche, selon les résultats de l'ECG, a 27 % de chance d'avoir une maladie cardiaque coronarienne sur dix ans. Une autre personne avec HDL-C de 60 mg/dl court 16 % de risques. Toutefois, si l'on supprime le tabagisme du profil et que le cholestérol total s'établit à 180 mg/dl, les risques sont de 6 %. Le choix des modèles et leurs répercussions font l'objet d'un débat. Ainsi, lorsque l'HDL-C est inclus au modèle, les effets du cholestérol total sont indépendants de l'âge et du sexe. La fiche insiste sur le fait qu'il existe plusieurs précurseurs des maladies cardiaques coronariennes et signale que tout profil des facteurs de risque des maladies cardiaques coronariennes doit être évalué et pris en compte dans son intégralité plutôt que de ne tenir compte que des facteurs de risque isolés.

2

Prévention des maladies cardio-vasculaires par le biais de changements alimentaires

Steven A. Grover, MD, MPA, FRCPCC
Directeur
Centre d'évaluation des risques cardio-vasculaires
Hôpital général de Montréal
Professeur adjoint
Département de médecine, d'épidémiologie et de biostatistique
Université McGill
Montréal (Québec)
Canada

Malgré les progrès opérés au niveau de leur diagnostic et de leur traitement, les maladies cardio-vasculaires restent la principale cause de décès chez des Canadiens. Il ne fait aucun doute que les maladies cardio-vasculaires peuvent être prévenues chez certaines personnes. Reste à savoir quelle sera l'ampleur des modifications nécessaires à leur prévention et quelle sera la portée de la prévention. Il faut déterminer ces « ordres de grandeur » pour comprendre l'efficacité potentielle des modifications alimentaires pour le Canadien moyen.

Pour répondre à ces questions, nous avons mis au point un modèle informatique capable d'anticiper les changements au titre de l'espérance de vie et de la morbidité en fonction de la modification des facteurs de risque. Le modèle de prévention primaire des maladies cardio-vasculaires permet de calculer la probabilité annuelle de décès par maladies cardio-vasculaires ou pour d'autres causes (n'ayant aucun rapport avec les maladies cardio-vasculaires) et le risque annuel de maladies cardio-vasculaires spécifiques pour une personne qui ne souffrait pas de maladie cardio-vasculaire lors de son inclusion dans le modèle.

Selon ce modèle informatique, les personnes qui peuvent tirer parti des modifications alimentaires sont celles à « haut risque » c'est-à-dire celles dont le taux de cholestérol sanguin est élevé et(ou) chez qui il existe d'autres facteurs de risque des maladies cardio-vasculaires. Par contre, les changements moyens au titre de l'espérance de vie pour de nombreux groupes de Canadiens risquent de ne pas dépasser un mois puisque ces personnes sont déjà dans la catégorie « à faible risque ».

Les risques, avantages et coûts inhérents à l'application de modifications alimentaires doivent être mieux compris avant que l'on procède à l'élaboration d'une stratégie nationale à ce chapitre. Ce n'est qu'alors qu'un programme scientifique et économiquement viable pourra être mis en oeuvre.

3

Les facteurs de risques coronariens aujourd'hui : perspective écossaise

Christopher G. Isles
Médecin consultant
Département de médecine
Dumfries and Galloway Royal Infirmary
Dumfries, Écosse

Objectif - Examiner les rapports entre les risques coronariens et les maladies coronariennes dans un échantillon de citadines de l'Ouest de l'Écosse.

Méthodologie - Étude longitudinale d'un échantillon général permettant d'établir un lien entre le cholestérol sanguin, le tabagisme, la tension artérielle diastolique, l'obésité et la classe sociale et la mortalité par maladies coronariennes après un suivi de 15 ans. Des comparaisons ont été effectuées avec des données comparables recueillies auprès d'un échantillon masculin.

Sujets- 15 399 adultes âgés de 45 à 64 ans dont 8262 femmes dépistées entre 1972 et 1976 à Renfrew et Paisley et suivis jusqu'à la fin de 1989.

Principale indice - L'analyse repose sur 490 décès féminins par maladies cardiaques coronariennes et 878 décès masculins.

Résultats - Les femmes de Renfrew et de Paisley sont plus susceptibles d'avoir un taux de cholestérol élevé, d'appartenir à la catégorie sociale 4 + 5 et moins susceptibles de fumer que les hommes. La répartition de la tension artérielle et de l'indice de masse corporelle est comparable pour les deux sexes. Le risque relatif (91 %) de décès par maladie coronarienne attribuable au cholestérol est comparable chez les femmes (1,56 [1,28, 1,90]) et chez les hommes (1,49 [1,26, 1,77]) mais le risque absolu est inférieur chez les femmes. Par conséquent, les femmes du quintile supérieur au titre du cholestérol affichent une mortalité par maladie coronarienne inférieure (6,1 décès par tranche de mille patientes par an) que les hommes du quintile inférieur (6,8 décès par tranche de mille patients par an). Les tendances qui révèlent un risque relatif comparable et une mortalité absolue inférieure chez les femmes valent également pour le tabagisme, la tension artérielle diastolique et la classe sociale. Il n'existe aucun lien entre l'obésité et les décès par maladies coronariennes une fois les données ajustées en fonction des autres risques. La mortalité par maladie cardiaque coronarienne spécifique à l'âge est toujours inférieure chez les femmes, même chez celles âgées de 60 à 64 ans au départ et pour lesquelles les taux ajustés de décès par maladie cardiaque coronarienne sont moitié moins importants que ceux correspondant aux hommes du même âge.

Conclusions - Ces résultats donnent à penser qu'un ou plusieurs autres facteurs diminuent les risques de maladie cardiaque coronarienne chez les femmes; il s'ensuit, par conséquent, que le potentiel des interventions comme l'interruption du tabagisme, l'abaissement de la tension artérielle et du taux de cholestérol à diminuer les décès par maladie cardiaque coronarienne est moindre chez les femmes que les hommes. Tant que les résultats des essais visant à abaisser le taux de cholestérol chez les femmes ne seront pas disponibles, les décisions à prendre au titre des traitements visant à abaisser les taux de lipides dans le sang devront reposer sur l'évaluation approximative des risques plutôt que sur des résultats vérifiés. Si l'on accepte que ces jugements soient déterminés par les risques absolus et non par les risques relatifs, alors l'étude de Renfrew et de Paisley donne à penser que le seuil des médicaments visant à abaisser le taux de cholestérol dans le cadre d'une prévention primaire des maladies coronariennes devra être de 1 à 2 mmol/l de plus chez les femmes que chez les hommes.

4

Effet d'un traitement visant à réduire le taux de cholestérol sur la morbidité et la mortalité par maladie cardiaque coronarienne : résultats de différents essais et autres

Martijn B. Katan, PhD
Professeur de nutrition humaine
Département de nutrition humaine
Université agricole Wageningen
Wageningen, Pays-Bas

Les résultats d'essais cliniques avec groupe témoin montrent avec éloquence que la réduction du taux de cholestérol sanguin par le biais d'un régime alimentaire ou d'un traitement médicamenteux réduit l'incidence des maladies cardiaques coronariennes. À l'échelle d'une population, la diminution du taux de cholestérol a pour principal effet de différer les premiers symptômes de la maladie plutôt que le décès car la plupart des décès par maladies cardiaques se produisent à un âge avancé. Aucune mortalité supérieure par cancer ne peut être décelée dans les populations dont les taux de cholestérol sanguin sont bas ou chez les patients qui, en raison d'une tare génétique, affichent un taux de cholestérol LDL nul. Il est donc peu vraisemblable que les traitements visant à abaisser le taux de cholestérol favorisent l'apparition de cancer. Cependant, les effets secondaires spécifiques et la toxicité des médicaments doivent faire l'objet d'un examen attentif; il reste que le régime alimentaire demeure le meilleur traitement contre l'hypercholestérolémie légère.

RÉSUMÉ

5

Tendances au titre de la consommation de cholestérol et de graisses, des taux de cholestérol sanguin et des maladies cardio-vasculaires au Japon

Hirotsugu Ueshima, MD

Directeur et professeur
Département des sciences de la santé
Université de médecine de Shiga
Shiga, Japon

Comparés à ceux d'Amérique et d'Europe, les taux de mortalité au Japon sont supérieurs au titre des accidents vasculaires cérébraux et inférieurs au titre des maladies cardiaques ischémiques. Les taux de mortalité relatifs aux accidents vasculaires cérébraux et aux maladies cardiaques ischémiques ont respectivement décliné depuis 1965 et 1970.

Les études de suivi épidémiologique entreprises au Japon montrent que l'hypertension est le principal facteur de risque des accidents vasculaires cérébraux. Une hypothèse veut qu'une consommation adéquate de graisses et de protéines animales prévienne les accidents vasculaires cérébraux. Par contre, plusieurs études épidémiologiques menées dans les pays industrialisés révèlent que l'hypertension, l'hypercholestérolémie et le tabagisme sont les principaux facteurs de risque des maladies coronariennes. Ces facteurs de risque pourraient fort bien s'appliquer aux Japonais, si l'on en croit les résultats d'études américano-japonaises et de certaines études de suivi japonaises.

Le taux de mortalité par accident vasculaire cérébral ajusté en fonction du sexe et de l'âge, a décliné de l'ordre de 64,9 % entre 1960 et 1985 et de 49,7 % entre 1975 et 1985 alors que la mortalité par maladie cardiaque ischémique a augmenté jusqu'en 1975 pour décroître par la suite. Entre 1975 et 1985, la mortalité par maladie cardiaque ischémique a baissé de 32,6 %. La consommation de graisses au Japon a plus que doublé au cours des 25 dernières années. Toutefois, elle reste deux fois inférieure à celle des Américains et des Européens. Par ailleurs, le rapport entre la consommation de graisse saturées et polyinsaturées reste supérieure à 1,0 et dépasse celle des Américains et des Européens qui s'établit à 0,5. La consommation de cholestérol a augmenté jusqu'en 1972 pour se stabiliser par la suite. Les Japonais mangent également plus de poisson, de coquillages, de mets frits dans l'huile végétale comme les « tempura » et moins de boeuf et de produits laitiers que les habitants des autres pays industrialisés.

Les tendances à l'augmentation de la consommation de graisses et le facteur lipidique au Japon viennent tout juste de ralentir. Les habitudes alimentaires des Japonais se reflètent dans leur taux de cholestérol sanguin. Il se peut qu'il existe encore une différence de 15-20 mg/dl dans le taux de cholestérol total des Japonais et des Américains, même si cette différence a tendance à décroître au fil des ans.

En conclusion, le régime alimentaire traditionnel des Japonais caractérisé par une faible consommation de graisses et un fort rapport P/S ainsi que des tendances favorables au titre de la consommation de protéines animales et de sel, ont peut-être contribué à la chute de la mortalité par accident vasculaire cérébral au cours des 25 dernières années et à la mortalité par accident cardiaque ischémique au cours des 15 dernières années.

6

La croisade contre les maladies cardiaques a-t-elle du bon?

Petr Skrabanek, PhD

Professeur
Département de santé communautaire
Trinity College
Université de Dublin
Dublin, Irlande

Les tentatives visant à manipuler le taux de « cholestérol national » en procédant à des changements au niveau du « régime alimentaire national », comme le recommandent différents comités de spécialistes, sont l'expression absurde du désir d'éliminer les maladies cardiaques coronariennes des rangs des causes de décès. Cette absurdité est double. Premièrement, les maladies cardiaques coronariennes sont caractéristiques d'un âge avancé, les décès par maladies cardiaques coronariennes se produisant en moyenne vers 75 ans. Ne pas mourir de maladie cardiaque coronarienne revient à mourir de cancer, d'accident vasculaire cérébral ou de démence de type Alzheimer. Deuxièmement, le rapport entre le cholestérol et les maladies cardiaques coronariennes n'est qu'hypothétique, ténu et non causatif.

L'hypothèse selon laquelle il existe un rapport entre le cholestérol et la maladie cardiaque coronarienne n'a pas été vérifiée ou ne l'a été que partiellement. Plusieurs études importantes dont celle de Framingham n'ont pas réussi à prouver qu'il existait un rapport entre le cholestérol alimentaire et le cholestérol sanguin. D'autres études ont par ailleurs démontré qu'il n'existait aucun rapport entre le cholestérol sanguin et l'importance des lésions athéromateuses coronariennes. Il n'existe en outre aucun rapport évident entre l'athérosclérose coronarienne et la maladie cardiaque coronarienne. Le cholestérol n'est ni une cause suffisante ni une cause nécessaire à l'apparition des maladies cardiaques coronariennes et il n'est par conséquent qu'un marqueur de risque par ailleurs très faible puisque le risque attribuable au cholestérol au titre des maladies cardiaques coronariennes n'est que de 10 % environ. Le consensus officiel voulant qu'il n'existe pas de seuil absolument sûr au titre du cholestérol est absurde et revient à prétendre qu'un taux de cholestérol nul est optimal.

Le test ultime pour vérifier l'hypothèse selon laquelle il existe un rapport entre le régime alimentaire et la maladie cardiaque est l'intervention à l'échelle de la population. Deux catégories de preuves sont disponibles : modification de l'hypercholestérolémie comme facteur de risque unique et intervention contre de multiples facteurs de risque. Dans les deux cas, les essais avec groupes témoins randomisés ne sont pas parvenus à en démontrer les avantages (McCormick et Skrabanek, 1988) et leur échec concerne à la fois les catégories à faible et à haut risque.

Si l'intervention au niveau des facteurs de risque multiples est inutile, il n'est par conséquent guère surprenant que l'intervention au niveau d'un seul facteur de risque (hypercholestérolémie) le soit également.

Les essais communautaires comme l'étude de Framingham et le projet de Northern Karelia attestent également de cet échec. À Framingham, en dépit d'une modification favorable des principaux facteurs de risque des maladies cardiaques coronariennes entre 1953 et 1983, l'incidence des maladies cardiaques coronariennes chez les hommes d'âge moyen pendant cette période a de fait *augmenté* (D'Agostino *et al*, 1989) au même titre que le taux de mortalité correspondant. À Northern Karelia, l'intervention communautaire n'a eu aucun effet sur la tendance sous-jacente au titre de la mortalité par maladies cardiaques coronariennes (McCormick et Skrabanek, 1988).

Quant aux vertus d'une intervention alimentaire, les nombreuses tentatives de cet ordre n'ont pas réussi à démontrer qu'elles étaient bénéfiques aux populations traitées. Dans le cadre du *Minnesota Coronary Survey* (Frantz *et al*, 1989), 4 500 hommes et 4 500 femmes d'établissements psychiatriques ont été affectés au hasard à un régime pauvre en graisses saturées et à un régime hospitalier normal. Même si le taux de cholestérol moyen du groupe suivant un régime pauvre en graisses a décru de 15 %, le suivi effectué cinq ans plus tard s'est soldé par 10 décès de plus par maladies cardiaques coronariennes et 21 décès de plus pour d'autres causes.

Malgré l'inutilité avérée des interventions à grande échelle pour prévenir les maladies cardiaques coronariennes, le fait que les spécialistes pertistent à formuler des recommandations qui ne sont finalement que l'expression de leurs voeux pieux et de leur dogmatisme constitue un phénomène sociologique fascinant. Ils font pourtant preuve d'un coupable manque d'éthique puisqu'ils imposent des interventions onéreuses et potentiellement dangereuses à des populations en bonne santé tout en leur cachant que la réduction du taux de cholestérol ne réduit pas le taux de mortalité (Oliver, 1988).

Bibliographie

D'Agostino, R., Kannel, W.B., Belanger, A.J. et Stytkowski, P.A. (1989). Trends in CHD and risk factors at age 55–64 in the Framingham study. *Int. J. Epidemiol.*, 3 (Suppl I), S67–S72

Frantz, I.D., Dawson, E.A., Ashman, P.L., Gatewood, L.C., Bartsch, G.E., Kuba, K. et Brewer, E.R. (1989). Test of effect of lipid lowering by diet on cardiovascular risk. *Arteriosclerosis*, 9, 129–35

McCormick, J. and Skrabanek, P. (1988). Coronary heart disease is not preventable by population interventions. *Lancet*, 2, 839–41

Oliver, M.F. (1988). Reducing cholesterol does not reduce mortality. *J. Am. Coll. Cardiol.*, 12, 814-17

7

Rôle du débit sanguin dans l'athérogenèse et hypothèse graisses-cholestérol alimentaires

William E. Stehbens, MD, DPhil

Professeur de pathologie
Wellington School of Medicine
Wellington Hospital
Newtown, Wellington
Nouvelle-Zélande

L'athérosclérose est une maladie dégénérative des vaisseaux sanguins qui touche tous les êtres humains et de nombreuses espèces inférieures. Sa gravité varie d'une personne à l'autre et d'un lit vasculaire à l'autre. Ses complications (déchirures de la tunique interne des vaisseaux, ulcères, thromboses murales, tortuosités, anévrismes) peuvent avoir pour origine une faiblesse murale acquise. Cette explication et la prédilection pour les fourches, jonctions et courbures artérielles ont abouti à l'hypothèse de la fatigue induite par hémodynamique qui fournit une explication plausible de ces complications. Or, l'hémodynamique a toujours été considérée comme un simple facteur de localisation de l'athérosclérose; sans manipulation alimentaire toutefois, l'athérosclérose accélérée peut être induite en modifiant chirurgicalement le débit sanguin des lapins et des moutons ainsi que de l'homme, dans les pontages coronaires par greffe veineuse et dans les veines des pontages artérioveineux thérapeutiques effectués dans le cadre des dialyses rénales. Ces observations contredisent radicalement l'hypothèse cholestérol/graisses alimentaires ou hypothèse des lipides qui n'est qu'une simple théorie sur l'accumulation de graisse dans les parois des vaisseaux sanguins et qui n'explique pas la pathogenèse ou les complications de l'athérogenèse.

L'hypothèse dite des lipides a dominé les recherches menées sur l'athérosclérose pendant plus de quarante ans, en dépit d'une représentation erronée de la pathologie vasculaire de l'animal soumis à un régime riche en cholestérol et de l'hypercholestérolémie familiale. La pathogenèse de l'ischémie myocardiale liée à un stockage lipidique dans ces conditions diffère de celle provoquée par l'athérosclérose, sans parler de multiples autres différences. L'absence de preuves pathologiques et expérimentales annule la valeur des études épidémiologiques sur l'athérosclérose. Parallèlement, les preuves épidémiologiques sur l'étiologie de l'athérosclérose sont assorties de nombreuses failles et incohérences dont 1) une mauvaise utilisation des causes et des facteurs de risque; 2) une mauvaise utilisation de la maladie cardiaque coronarienne à qui l'on a fait jouer le rôle de moniteur de substitution non pathognomonique et inadéquat de l'athérosclérose grave; 3) des extrapolations non valables des facteurs de risque des maladies cardiaques coronariennes à l'étiologie de l'athérosclérose; 4) un taux de mauvais diagnostic de l'ordre de ± 30 % au titre des maladies cardiaques coronariennes; 5) un manque d'objectivité au titre de la sélection des participants aux essais cliniques qui s'opère en fonction de l'âge et de l'hypercholestérolémie familiale; 6) l'utilisation de taux de mortalité incorrects et de mauvaises données alimentaires et 7) des erreurs écologiques. Pour l'heure, il n'existe aucune preuve scientifique qui permette d'affirmer que les graisses alimentaires/le cholestérol ou un taux de cholestérol sanguin élevé provoquent l'athérosclérose. Tant qu'il sera impossible d'évaluer avec précision la gravité de l'athérosclérose, les études épidémiologiques cliniques sur l'athérosclérose auront très peu d'intérêt.

8

Interactions cellulaires et lipoprotéiques dans l'athérogénèse précoce

<u>Mahamed Navab</u>, **PhD** et **Alan M. Folgelman**

Cardiologue résident adjoint
Division de cardiologie, École de médecine
Université de Californie à Los Angeles
Los Angeles, Californie, États-Unis

De plus en plus de preuves donnent à penser que les lipoprotéines oxydées jouent un rôle essentiel dans l'apparition de l'athérosclérose. Ces lipoprotéines ont été observées dans des plaques athérosclérotiques d'êtres humains et d'animaux de laboratoire. Par ailleurs, le développement des lésions chez des lapins Watanabe ou des lapins soumis à un régime riche en cholestérol peut être ralenti par le biais d'un traitement aux antioxydants. Les lipoprotéines de basse densité (LDL) subissent des modifications orchestrées par les cellules de la paroi artérielle et par les monocytes-macrophages de culture en l'*absence* de sérum. Les modifications que subissent les LDL dans la paroi artérielle n'interviennent néanmoins qu'en présence d'antioxydants plasmatiques comme α-tocophérol et β-carotène. Nous avons utilisé une coculture multicouches d'EC et de SMC aortiques humaines et étudié les modifications que subissaient les LDL originales en présence de sérum. Nous nous sommes aperçus que l'incubation des LDL dans les cellules de la paroi artérielle entraînaient une induction significative des protéines chimiotactiques 1 (MCP-1) ARNm des monocytes et des protéines et une augmentation marquée de la transmigration et de l'adhésion des monocytes sur les monocouches endothéliales des cocultures. Les lipoprotéines de haute densité (HDL) et les antioxydants préviennent les manifestations induites par les LDL. Sur la base des travaux récents effectués par notre laboratoire et par d'autres chercheurs, nous proposons un modèle de formation des cellules spumeuses dans la paroi artérielle. Dans les sites vulnérables aux lésions, les LDL plasmatiques pénètrent l'espace subendothélial largement acellulaire (SES) où elles sont maintenues dans des microenvironnements à l'abri des antioxydants plasmatiques. Les lipides LDL se modifient par oxydation, donnant naissance à des LDL légèrement oxydées, les MM-LDL. Une fois formées, les MM-LDL stimulent l'endothélium pour produire des molécules d'adhésion pour les monocytes sanguins, « M-ELAM », et secréter des MCP-1 et des M-CSF. Ces phénomènes moléculaires s'accompagnent des phénomènes cellulaires suivants : fixation des monocytes sur EC; migration des monocytes induite par les MCP-1 dans le SES de la paroi artérielle et

10

Obésité et anomalies apolipoprotéiques connexes: Rapport avec les maladies cardiaques coronariennes

Daniel A.K. Roncari, MD, PhD, FACP, FRCPC

Médecin en chef
Centre des sciences de la santé Sunnybrook
Professeur de médecine
Université de Toronto
Toronto (Ontario), Canada

L'obésité favorise et exacerbe tout à la fois les anomalies lipoprotéiques-apolipoprotéiques. Ce phénomène multiplie par conséquent les risques d'athérogénicité pour les personnes obèses. Cela est particulièrement vrai pour les sujets obèses avec prédisposition génétique spécifique à la dyslipoprotéinémie chez qui les anomalies de ce type sont alors beaucoup plus prononcées. La production hépatique de lipoprotéines de très basse densité (VLDL) est plus forte chez les obèses, surtout en cas d'augmentation du poids corporel ou de maintien de la corpulence. Les VLDL hétérogènes sont athérogéniques, notamment les particules qui sont plus denses du fait d'un rapport esters apoB/cholestérol supérieur. Les VLDL agissent à leur tour comme précurseurs de lipoprotéines plus athérogènes; les lipoprotéines de densité intermédiaire (IDL) et les lipoprotéines de basse densité (LDL). L'augmentation du débit des acides gras libres entre les tissus adipeux et le foie favorise la synthèse des VLDL. Les esters du cholestérol hépatique spécifique influencent par ailleurs de façon marquée la production d'apoB. L'apoB est essentiel au développement des particules VLDL qui finissent par être converties en LDL et dont l'apolipoprotéine exclusive est l'apoB. Parallèlement, la consommation alimentaire d'acides laurique, myristique et palmitique augmente le taux de cholestérol LDL sanguin; l'acide stéarique est neutre alors que les acides gras n-3, l'acide linoléique et l'acide oléique (qui sous certaines conditions est également neutre) font baisser les concentrations de cholestérol LDL. Chez les personnes obèses, et notamment chez celles avec expansion abdominale, les IDL contenant des isoformes E-2 et E-4 ont un rapport étroit avec les dyslipidémies, les isoformes E-2 favorisant l'augmentation des triglycérides VLDL dans le sang et la diminution du cholestérol HDL et les isoformes E-4 favorisant l'augmentation du cholestérol LDL, des LDL-apoB et des triglycérides dans le sang. Les IDL sont plus athérogènes que les VLDL. En supprimant la majorité des triglycérides restantes dans les IDL par lipoprotéine lipase (l'activité de la lipoprotéine lipase dont le principal activateur est l'apolipoprotéine C-II augmente dans le cas de l'obésité et favorise la progression de l'adiposité) et en transférant parallèlement les apoE et d'autres constituants avec différentes lipoprotéines, il se forme des lipoprotéines de basse densité. Ces particules hautement athérogènes contiennent de l'apoB-100 (apolipoprotéine exclusive) et sont enrichies d'esters de cholestérol. Dans le cas de l'obésité, le débit de VLDL, d'IDL et de LDL athérogènes augmente au même titre que leurs apolipoprotéines. Par conséquent, même en l'absence de concentrations sanguines élevées, leur vitesse excessive de remplacement crée un risque substantiel de maladies cardiaques coronariennes. Des concentrations VLDL plus denses engendrent, via les IDL, des lipoprotéines de basse densité dont le rapport esters de cholestérol/apoB est supérieur. Cette situation extrême se traduit par le syndrome de l'hyperapobetalipoprotéinémie décrite par A. Sniderman *et al.* Il s'agit d'un état athérogène important, même lorsque les concentrations de cholestérol et de triglycérides dans le sang sont normales. Des particules LDL et VLDL plus denses, comme c'est le cas dans l'hyperapobetalipoprotéinémie, se produisent fréquemment dans le cadre de l'hyperlipidémie combinée familiale dont l'expression varie d'un membre de la famille à l'autre. Alors que les anomalies lipoprotéiques-apolipoprotéiques se produisent généralement chez les personnes obèses, l'obésité abdominale est caractérisée par des concentrations élevées de VLDL-triglycérides et de LDL-apoB (l'influence des isoformes apoE ayant déjà été décrite) ainsi que par des anomalies HDL. Dans le cas de l'obésité abdominale et diffuse, les espèces HDL contenant des apoA-1 décroissent, partiellement en raison d'une élimination accrue dans les tissus adipeux; dans le cas de l'obésité abdominale, l'activité triglycéride lipase hépatique augmente. L'augmentation de la clairance est particulièrement évidente dans les dépôts abdominaux. Même si nos connaissances sur les lipoprotéines(a) sont encore très maigres, les concentrations de lipoprotéines diminuent relativement chez les sujets obèses et augmentent lorsqu'il y a perte de poids. En fait, chez les enfants comme chez les adultes, toutes ces anomalies s'estompent avec l'adoption d'un régime alimentaire efficace et la pratique d'exercices physiques, même si ce sont les facteurs génétiques qui déterminent le degré d'efficacité de ces interventions. Alors que le foie est le site d'élection principal de la production et du métabolisme des apolipoprotéines, des lipides et des lipoprotéines, les tissus adipeux modulent les fonctions hépatiques. Dans le cas de l'obésité, les tissus adipeux contribuent de façon marquée à la pathogenèse de lipoprotéines-apolipoprotéines anormales (tant au niveau de leur production que de leur clairance), en raison de leur influence sur le foie et de leur action sur les lipoprotéines (par le biais de la lipoprotéine lipase des cellules adipeuses). Les nombreuses anomalies moléculaires et cellulaires des cellules adipeuses qui favorisent le développement, la progression et la récurrence de l'obésité seront examinées dans le cadre de l'émergence d'un profil lipoprotéines-apolipoprotéines athérogène marqué et de son métabolisme.

RÉSUMÉ

11

Modulation de la fonction membranaire par le cholestérol

Philip L. Yeagle, PhD

Département de biochimie
University at Buffalo School of Medicine
State University of New York
Buffalo, New York, États-Unis

Le cholestérol est un constituant essentiel des membranes mammifères (et d'autres cellules). Les cellules mammifères ne peuvent croître, se reproduire ou se différencier sans l'intervention du cholestérol. Des comportements semblables s'observent dans d'autres organismes comme la levure où le stérol essentiel est l'ergostérol. Ces fonctions cellulaires ont besoin d'un certain niveau de stérol spécifique de structure; aucun autre stérol ne peut substituer ce stérol spécifique. Ainsi, l'ergostérol ne peut se substituer au cholestérol dans les cellules mammifères et le cholestérol ne peut se substituer à l'ergostérol dans les cellules de levure. Les effets structuraux du cholestérol sur les doubles couches lipidiques dans le cadre d'une concentration élevée de cholestérol sont aujourd'hui bien connus. Pourtant, le rôle que jouent les stérols spécifiques dans le fonctionnement normal de la cellule reste encore un mystère.

Des données récentes ont conduit à la formulation d'une hypothèse très poussée pour expliquer le rôle essentiel du cholestérol dans les cellules mammifères. Lorsque ses concentrations membranaires sont faibles, le cholestérol stimule l'activité des enzymes des membranes, qui sont essentiels aux fonctions cellulaires, par le biais d'une interaction protéine-stérol directe et spécifique de structure. Dans le cadre de concentrations membranaires élevées, le cholestérol module l'activité protéique des membranes en altérant l'ensemble des propriétés des doubles couches lipidiques de la membrane cellulaire. Ce phénomène correspond à un changement dans le « volume libre» au sein de la double couche qui affecte l'aptitude des protéines membranaires à subir les transitions conformationnelles nécessaires à leur fonction.

Les données disponibles seront examinées dans le cadre de cette hypo-thèse. Les données étudiées sont énumérés ci-dessous. Les expériences menées dans des conditions d'auxotrophie du stérol sur le mycoplasma et la levure révèlent un besoin en stérol spécifique de structure (Dahl & Dahl, 1988). Les études sur l'activité Na^+-K^+-ATPase dans les membranes plasmatiques de cellules mammifères montrent que le besoin en cholestérol spécifique de structure facilite l'activité de pompe, une enzyme de membrane essentielle à la fonction cellulaire (Yeagle *et al*, 1988). L'inhibition de Na^+-K^+-ATPase (Giraud *et al*, 1981; Yeagle, 1983) et du photorécepteur rhodopsine (Boesze-Battaglia & Albert, 1990; Straume & Litman, 1988) par le cholestérol à des concentrations membranaires élevées montre que l'altération des propriétés globales de la membrane par le cholestérol inhibe les fonctions membranaires.

Bibliographie

Boeze-Battaglia, K. et Albert, A. (1990). *J. Biol. Chem.*, **265**, 20727–30

Dahl, C. et Dahl, J. (1988). *Biology of Cholesterol* (Yeagle, P.L., eds), pp. 147-72. (CRC Press, Boca Raton)

Giraud, F., Claret, M., Bruckdorfer, K.R. et Chailley, B. (1981). *Biochim. Biophys. Acta*, **647**, 249–58

Straume, M. et Litman, B.J. (1988). *Biochemistry*, **27**, 7723–33

Yeagle, P.L. (1983). *Biochim. Biophys. Acta*, **727**, 39-44

Yeagle, P.L., Rice, D. et Young, J. (1988). *Biochemistry*, **27**, 6449–52

12
Hyporéactifs et hyperréactifs aux changements alimentaires

Martijn B. Katan*, PhD, A.C. Beynen**

*Département de nutrition humaine
Université agricole
Wageningen, Pays-Bas
**Département des sciences des animaux de laboratoire
Université d'État
Utrecht, Pays-Bas

La réponse du cholestérol sanguin de certains sujets humains au cholestérol alimentaire peut être légère ou prononcée. La réaction au cholestérol alimentaire semble dépendre de la réaction aux acides gras saturés alimentaires. En moyenne, les personnes qui ont tendance à hyperréagir consomment habituellement beaucoup plus de cholestérol, ont un taux de cholestérol HDL supérieur et un poids corporel inférieur aux personnes qui hyporéagissent. Les mécanismes sous-jacents à l'hypo- et à l'hyper-réactivité au cholestérol alimentaire ou aux acides gras saturés n'ont pas encore été caractérisés. Ces deux phénomènes d'hypo- et d'hyper-réactivité pourraient fort bien avoir des conséquences sur les conseils à prodiguer aux sujets qui essaient de faire baisser leur cholestérol sanguin en suivant un régime alimentaire spécifique. Toutefois, le dépistage d'une véritable hyporéactivité et d'une véritable hyperréactivité est difficile à cause des fluctuations intrapersonnelles du taux de cholestérol sanguin. Aucun test simple ne permet encore de différencier les hyperréactifs des hyporéactifs. Pour l'heure, la surveillance des réponses d'une personne au régime alimentaire doit s'opérer au moyen de nombreuses évaluations de son cholestérol sanguin.

13
Réexamen du rapport entre le cholestérol sanguin et les acides gras alimentaires : l'acide palmitique (16:0) est-il neutre?

K.C. Hayes

Professeur de biologie (nutrition)
Directeur
Foster Biomedical Research Laboratories
Université Brandeis
Waltham, Massachusetts, États-Unis

Une série d'études effectuées sur le singe et le hamster et la réévaluation des données humaines publiées, indiquent que les acides gras saturés alimentaires exercent une influence métabolique dissemblable sur le métabolisme du cholestérol. L'acide myristique (14:0) semble jouer un rôle important dans l'augmentation du taux de cholestérol en freinant l'activité des récepteurs LDL et en augmentant la production directe de LDL (à partir de sources autres que le catabolisme des VLDL). L'acide palmitique (16:0) semble neutre dans la plupart des cas (cholestérol sanguin < 200 mg/dL) ou tant que le récepteur LDL subit une régulation descendante, comme dans le cas d'une consommation abondante de cholestérol ou de l'obésité. Dans ces cas précis, les récepteurs LDL qui subissent une régulation descendante et l'augmentation simultanée de la production des VLDL (induite par 16:0 et 18:1) peuvent transformer les restes VLDL en LDL et augmenter le nombre de LDL. Par ailleurs, l'impact cholestérolémique de n'importe quel acide gras saturé peut être contrecarré par l'acide linoléique alimentaire (18:2) jusqu'à l'obtention d'un seuil « saturable » puisque l'acide linoléique fait subir une régulation ascendante aux récepteurs LDL. Lorsque ce « seuil » est dépassé, les principaux acides gras (16:0, 18:0, 18:1, 18:2, 18:3) semblent exercer une influence égale sur les concentrations de cholestérol en circulation.

RÉSUMÉ

14

Effets potentiels des produits d'oxydation des lipides alimentaires sur la santé

Paul Bradley Addis

Professeur
Département des sciences de l'alimentation et de la nutrition
Collège d'agriculture et d'écologie humaine
Université du Minnesota
St. Paul, Minnesota, États-Unis

Il existe plusieurs ramifications pour la santé des présentes recherches sur les aliments qui ont trait aux produits d'oxydation des lipides alimentaires. Certains de ces aspects sont décrits brièvement dans cet article qui donne également une brève évaluation des aspects régulatoires du rancissement des aliments et des huiles chauffées. Le lecteur est renvoyé à Addis et Park (1989) pour les suggestions de recherches dans ce domaine.

Il existe pour l'heure très peu de règlements sur le rancissement des aliments aux États-Unis (Firestone and Summers, 1989). Il va sans dire que la présence de xénobiotiques toxiques devrait suffir pour que la FDA prenne des mesures contre les graisses et les huiles. La question des substances délétères induites par transformation, qui concerne évidemment les produits d'oxydation des lipides, n'est pas clairement définie et aucun règlement fédéral n'existe à l'heure actuelle pour contrôler le rancissement. Deux municipalités, Chicago et San Francisco, ont toutefois inscrit le rancissement des huiles à friture au nombre des facteurs à surveiller (Firestone, 1989).

En Europe, les lois sur les produits d'oxydation des huiles à friture sont très explicites. La Belgique, la France, l'Allemagne et l'Espagne de même que la Suisse limitent les composés polaires à 25-27 %, conformément à la méthode IUPAC 2,507 (Firestone, 1989).

Les pays scandinaves n'ont adopté aucun règlement spécifique à ce chapitre mais leurs inspecteurs utilisent une vaste gamme de techniques pour déterminer à quel moment une huile est bonne à jeter. Parmi ces techniques figurent les sondes et les différents tests permettant de déterminer la teneur en acides gras libres et le point de fumée des huiles ainsi que leur goût, leur odeur, leur pouvoir moussant et leur acidité. Aucune recherche n'a encore été entreprise dans le but de déterminer quelle est la meilleure méthode d'évaluation de la qualité des huiles. Les recherches sur les huiles chauffées devraient de toute évidence fournir de précieux renseignements sur la toxicité, la dégradation des huiles, les antioxydants, la filtration et les méthodes d'évaluation. Ces commentaires s'appliquent également à tous les autres produits d'oxydation des lipides alimentaires. Il est difficile de surestimer l'importance potentielle, à la fois du point de vue scientifique et sanitaire, des produits d'oxydation des lipides et le moment est venu, semble-t-il, d'examiner de plus près certains des aspects importants de ce secteur de recherche.

Il est temps en effet de confronter les principales interprétations de l'étiologie des MCC aux résultats obtenus sur les produits d'oxydation des lipides. Il semble que le cholestérol (pur) alimentaire ne soit ni angiotoxique ni hypercholestérolémique et que par conséquent il ne peut ni favoriser ni déclencher les MCC. Il est tentant de supposer que ce sont les modes de consommation des produits d'oxydation des lipides qui expliquent partiellement pourquoi certaines personnes sont plus vulnérables que d'autres aux MCC. Le rôle du tabac, qui est peut-être le seul facteur de risque le plus important des MCC, joue peut-être un rôle dans l'oxydation du sang et des lipides tissulaires *in vivo*. Il faut impérativement mener des recherches sur ce sujet.

Les produits d'oxydation des lipides dans les aliments sont des toxiques « induits par transformation » et se distinguent, par conséquent, des contaminants xénobiotiques habituels. Puisque ces produits d'oxydation sont produits de façon endogène, plutôt que dérivés de sources exogènes, leur statut réglementaire aux États-Unis est très flou. Toutefois, la FDA a établi un programme d'études sur les phénomènes « induits par transformation », ce qui laisse présager d'une prochaine intervention à ce chapitre. Les huiles chauffées devraient faire l'objet de plusieurs règlements, comme c'est déjà le cas en Europe. La popularité que connaissent depuis peu les huiles très polyinsaturés risque d'entraîner des problèmes d'oxydation plus importants que le saindoux ou le shortening.

Il se peut qu'il y ait un rapport entre les produits d'oxydation des lipides alimentaires et les mLDL ainsi qu'un lien entre ces deux éléments et la consommation d'antioxydants alimentaires. Les avantages potentiels des antioxydants pourraient être considérables si ces derniers pouvaient ralentir la conversion des LDL en mLDL.

15
Régulation de la concentration de cholestérol porté par les lipoprotéines de basse densité

John M. Dietschy, MD
Professeur titulaire de la chaire Jan et Henri Bromberg
Chef, gastro-entérologie
Université du Texas
Southwestern Medical Center
Dallas, Texas, États-Unis

Il est possible de calculer les concentrations stables de cholestérol si, chez une espèce animale particulière, on dispose des valeurs absolues du taux de production de cholestérol LDL (J_t), de l'activité des récepteurs chez l'animal (J^m), de l'affinité de la molécule LDL pour son récepteur (K_m) et de la constante de proportionnalité pour le transport du cholestérol LDL indépendamment des récepteurs (P). Ces études illustrent les variations de ces quatre constantes chez les animaux soumis à des régimes dont la quantité de cholestérol est variable de même que la quantité de triacylglycérols purs ne contenant qu'un acide gras. L'article présente par ailleurs, des données sur les taux d'équilibre net en stérols et les taux de synthèse du cholestérol dans le foie et dans d'autres organes importants, dans les mêmes conditions. Lorsque de petites quantités de cholestérol sont administrées aux animaux soumis à un régime sans lipides, il se produit une inhibition de la synthèse du cholestérol hépatique dépendante de la dose administrée suivie d'une augmentation de la concentration en esters de cholestéryl dans le foie. Ce phénomène s'accompagne de la suppression partielle de J^m et d'une légère augmentation de J_t. Il en résulte de modestes augmentations du taux de cholestérol LDL dans le sang en circulation. Si l'on ajoute des triacylglycérols, contenant un mélange d'acides gras saturés, à ces régimes alimentaires, il se produit une autre suppression de l'activité des récepteurs LDL et une augmentation plus marquée du taux de production : d'où une augmentation marquée du taux de cholestérol LDL dans le sang. Lorsque des triacylglycérols contenant un seul acide gras, dont la longueur de chaîne varie entre 6:0 et 18:0, sont administrés au même modèle animal, seuls les acides gras 12:0, 14:0 et 16:0 provoquent des changements au niveau de la vitesse de production et de l'activité des récepteurs et augmentent significativement les concentrations de cholestérol LDL dans le sang. L'acide gras 18:0 ne modifie aucun paramètre du métabolisme du cholestérol LDL même si l'administration de cet acide gras enrichit de façon significative le pool d'acides gras dans les membranes cellulaires du foie. Dans le cadre d'expériences comparables, aux termes desquelles des triacylglycérols contenant une seule variété d'acide gras insaturé ont été administrés aux animaux, le composant 18:1 joue un rôle clé dans le rétablissement de l'activité des récepteurs. Il n'existe aucun rapport évident entre la concentration de cholestérol totale dans le foie et l'activité des récepteurs. Par conséquent, l'administration d'acides gras saturés fait chuter le contenu en cholestérol des cellules du foie tout en supprimant l'activité des récepteurs alors que les acides gras insaturés tendent à augmenter le contenu en cholestérol, particulièrement le pool d'esters de cholestéryl, tout en stimulant l'activité des récepteurs LDL. Puisque l'administration de ces différents acides gras ne semble pas modifier l'équilibre en stérols externe du foie, ces études donnent à penser que les acides gras qui parviennent aux cellules du foie peuvent altérer le petit pool de cholestérol dans les cellules qui, même s'il est impossible de l'évaluer, correspond en vérité au pool de stérols qui régule la synthèse des protéines des récepteurs LDL.

16
Réponse du cholestérol sanguin aux acides gras saturés

Gloria Lena Vega, PhD

Professeur adjoint
Département de nutrition clinique
et Centre de nutrition humaine
Université du Texas
Southwestern Medical Center
Dallas, Texas, États-Unis

La variabilité des réactions aux acides gras saturés n'a pas encore fait l'objet d'études systématiques. Pour cette raison, les données de trois études alimentaires entreprises par notre laboratoire ont été fusionnées et utilisées pour déterminer la variabilité des réactions de différentes personnes des concentrations plasmatiques de cholestérol total et de cholestérol à lipoprotéines de basse densité après substitution des acides gras saturés par des acides gras insaturés. Les données démontrent une variabilité marquée au titre des réactions. Certains patients réagissent par une augmentation spectaculaire de leur taux de cholestérol alors que d'autres n'enregistrent que de faibles augmentations. Ces résultats montent à quel point il convient de mener de plus amples recherches dans ce domaine.

17
Rôle des acides gras n-3 comme modulateurs du métabolisme des acides gras n-6 : conséquences pour la santé

Pierre Budowski, PhD

Professeur (émérite)
Faculté d'agriculture
Université hébraïque de Jérusalem
Rehovot, Israël

L'acide linoléique et l'acide alpha-linolénique font partie de la famille des acides gras polyinsaturés (AGP) n-6 et n-3. Outre leur valeur nutritive essentielle, ces acides gras interagissent également les uns les autres à différents niveaux métaboliques. La formation de l'acide arachidonique (AA) à partir de l'acide linoléique, au sein de la famille des AGP n-6, et la conversion de AA en éicosanoïdes sont inhibées par les AGP n-3. Par ailleurs, il se produit une véritable concurrence entre les fragments de molécules des AGP n-3 à chaîne longue et des AGP n-6, lors de l'incorporation dans les phospholipides des membranes et organelles cellulaires. Inversement, l'acide linoléique est capable d'interférer avec la biosynthèse des AGP n-3 à chaîne longue, à condition qu'il soit présent en quantité excédentaire.

Les proportions alimentaires relatives et les interactions métaboliques des deux familles d'acides gras polyinsaturés ont une importance nutritionnelle et sanitaire importante puisqu'elles affectent les propriétés des membranes cellulaires, des protéines ancrées sur les membranes et récepteurs ainsi que la production d'éicosanoïdes dérivés de AA. Le métabolisme *non limité* de AA, qui s'accompagne d'une formation excessive d'éicosanoïdes et de réactions secondaires aboutissant à la formation d'espèces oxygènes actives potentiellement nuisibles, intervient dans différents procédés pathologiques, allant des réactions inflammatoires immunologiques aux thromboses.

Aujourd'hui, la consommation en acides gras polyinsaturés dans les pays occidentaux privilégie très largement l'acide linoléique qui dépasse la consommation d'acide alpha-linolénique d'environ un ordre de grandeur. Dans ces conditions, l'action limitante de l'acide alpha-linolénique sur le métabolisme des AA ne s'exprime pas pleinement. Par ailleurs, une consommation excessive d'acide linoléique interfère avec la biosynthèse de l'acide docosahéxaénoïque, acide gras polyinsaturé n-3, qui est essentiel au développement normal du cerveau et de la rétine.

Le déséquilibre en acides gras polyinsaturés actuel est une conséquence tardive de la révolution industrielle qui a entraîné également d'autres changements au niveau de la consommation de nutriments et des modes de vie. Notre équipement enzymatique n'est pas adapté à ce type de changements.

18
Le rapport polyinsaturés–saturés et son rôle dans l'efficacité des acides gras omega-3

K.S. Layne, E.A. Ryan, M.L. Garg, J.A. Jumpsen et M.T. Clandinin, PhD

Professeur
Départements d'alimentation et de nutrition
et groupe de recherche sur le
métabolisme et la nutrition médicale
Université d'Alberta
Edmonton, Alberta, Canada

Il semble que les acides gras omega-3 alimentaires jouent un rôle dans la diminution de l'incidence des maladies cardiaques coronariennes en altérant vraisemblablement le métabolisme des éicosanoïdes et en réduisant les fractions de lipoprotéines dans le sang en circulation. Les études animales effectuées dans notre laboratoire indiquent que l'efficacité des acides gras omega-3 à faire baisser le cholestérol sanguin, les triacylglycérols et l'acide arachidonique dépend du rapport entre l'acide linoléique alimentaire et les acides gras saturés (P/S). Puisque les acides gras omega-3 et omega-6 se font concurrence au niveau des désaturases hépatiques et de l'incorporation dans les membranes, on suppose que les acides gras omega-3 sont capables de réduire les lipides sanguins et les taux d'arachidonates avec plus d'efficacité lorsque les concentrations de linoléate alimentaire sont réduites. Nous étudions pour l'heure l'effet qu'exerce un supplément d'acide gras omega-3 sur les profils lipoprotéiques sanguins de sujets humains normolipidémiques qui affichent un rapport P/S alimentaire élevé ou faible. Sur la base de rapports alimentaires de 7 jours, 32 sujets ont été divisés en groupes P/S élevés ($>0,8$) ou faibles ($<0,5$). Tous les sujets ont pris des suppléments sous forme d'huile d'olive pendant les trois premiers mois. Les six mois suivants correspondaient à un essai à double insu avec permutation pendant lequel les sujets devaient consommer en alternance de petites quantités (35 mg d'acide gras omega-3/kg de poids corporel) d'huile de lin ($18:3\omega$) ou d'huile de poisson ($20:5\omega3$, $22:6\omega3$). Des échantillons sanguins ont été prélevés au début et à la fin de chaque traitement puis analysés au titre des taux de lipoprotéines sanguines, des profils d'acides gras, du glucose, de HbA$_1$c, du glucagon, des C-peptides et de l'insuline. Les effets de ces traitements et le rapport P/S alimentaire sur les concentrations de lipides sanguines seront examinés.

19

Lipoprotéines, hormones sexuelles, sexe et maladies cardiaques coronariennes

Ian F. Godsland, BA

Directeur des recherches
Wynn Institute for Metabolic Research
Londres, Royaume-Uni

Dans les pays industrialisés occidentaux, la mortalité par maladies cardiaques coronariennes frappe six fois plus d'hommes que de femmes. Les différences hommes-femmes au titre des facteurs de risque lipoprotéiques liés aux maladies cardiaques coronariennes peuvent partiellement expliquer cette différence : les concentrations de cholestérol HDL sont inférieures et celles de cholestérol LDL supérieures chez les hommes, dans la tranche d'âge où la différence de sexe au titre des maladies cardiaques coronariennes est la plus apparente. Par contre, en appariant les concentrations de cholestérol HDL des hommes et des femmes, la différence au titre des taux de mortalité disparaît. Les études sur les effets de stéroïdes et d'hormones sexuelles administrés par voie exogène valident l'hypothèse selon laquelle les fluctuations au titre des concentrations de lipoprotéines chez les hommes et les femmes sont attribuables à différentes concentrations d'hormones sexuelles. L'activité androgène est liée à des concentrations LDL élevées et à des concentrations HDL faibles et inversement pour l'activité oestrogénique. Toutefois, il existe quelques exceptions et les hormones naturelles permettent de moins bien définir ces schémas. Les associations entre les concentrations d'hormones endogènes et les concentrations de lipoprotéines chez les hommes diffèrent radicalement du schéma attendu lorsque des stéroïdes leur sont administrés par voie exogène : un lien positif est établi entre les concentrations HDL et les testostérones et un lien négatif est établi avec les oestradiols. À la puberté, les concentrations de HDL baissent chez les hommes; à la ménopause, les concentrations de HDL baissent et les concentrations de LDL augmentent. Ces résultats valident l'hypothèse selon laquelle les différences au niveau des concentrations d'hormones sexuelles expliquent les différences hommes-femmes au titre des concentrations de lipoprotéines. Ce type de rapports ne s'observe pas dans les sociétés non occidentales, ce qui indique que certains autres facteurs, encore inconnus, jouent un rôle important dans la différence hommes-femmes au titre des concentrations de lipoprotéines et de l'incidence des maladies cardiaques coronariennes.

RÉSUMÉ

20

Santé infantile et le dilemme graisses/cholestérol

Richard Goldbloom, OC, MD

Professeur de pédiatrie
Université Dalhousie
Directeur des services ambulatoires
Hôpital IWK pour enfants
Halifax, Nouvelle-Écosse
Canada

Les principes méthodologiques énumérés et adoptés par le Groupe de travail canadien de l'Examen médical périodique et l'*U.S. Preventive Services Task Force* stipulent que la formulation de recommandations en médecine préventive privilégie les preuves scientifiques au consensus, et que ces preuves soient évaluées en fonction de la qualité des études dont elles découlent. Si ces principes président à la formulation de recommandations, plus rien alors ne justifie l'emploi du concept que « cela ne fera *probablement* pas de tort et nous croyons que cela fera *peut-être* du bien ».

En examinant les dimensions pédiatriques de la question des graisses et du cholestérol, il faut établir une distinction très claire entre le traitement de personnes visiblement saines vues en consultation et le traitement de celles identifiées comme étant à haut risque, d'une part et les recommandations qui s'appliquent aux personnes à haut risque et à l'ensemble de la population, d'autre part. Ces cas comportent des risques très différents : caractéristiques des avantages et coûts engagés.

Dans sa prise de position de 1986 sur les graisses alimentaires et le cholestérol chez les enfants, l'*American Academy of Paediatrics* proposait avec sagesse un écart de quantités à consommer plutôt qu'une limite à ne pas franchir. En agissant de la sorte, cet organisme témoigne du respect qu'il voue à l'individualisme et aux variations humaines normales - un respect qui devrait tous nous inspirer.

21

Maladies cardiaques coronariennes : prévention et traitement par intervention nutritionnelle

William E. Connor, MD

Professeur de médecine
Chef, section de nutrition clinique et de métabolisme des lipides
Université des sciences de la santé d'Oregon
Portland, Oregon, États-Unis

Le régime alimentaire modifie considérablement les nombreux facteurs de risque à l'origine des maladies cardiaques coronariennes. De fait, la nutrition à elle seule figure au rang des principaux facteurs de risque de cette maladie puisqu'elle peut modifier considérablement son évolution et la progression de l'athérosclérose. Le facteur de risque le plus important où le régime alimentaire joue un rôle essentiel, notamment dans la cause et le traitement, est l'hyperlipidémie.

L'hyperlipidémie est importante puisqu'elle facilite l'infiltration des lipides dans la paroi artérielle ce qui provoque ultérieurement l'athérosclérose. Pour 99 % de la population, l'hyperlipidémie est le résultat d'un régime de vie imprudent avec une consommation exagérée d'acides gras saturés, de cholestérol et de calories totales dans le régime alimentaire..

L'examen des données sur le rôle essentiel des concentrations de lipoprotéines et de lipides sanguins dans le développement de l'athérosclérose nous amène à nous demander si les modifications alimentaires peuvent baisser les concentrations de lipoprotéines et de lipides dans le sang des patients et sous-groupes de patients du monde occidental? La réponse est oui, sans équivoque.

La prévention primaire des maladies cardiaques coronariennes est de toute évidence l'objectif qu'il convient d'atteindre au plus vite pour endiguer la véritable épidémie de maladies cardiaques coronariennes à laquelle nous assistons à l'heure actuelle. Les changements alimentaires proposés aux patients coronariens sont sans danger et il serait prudent qu'ils soient suivis par tous ceux (dans les pays occidentaux) qui présentent des risques sérieux de maladies coronariennes. Ces changements nutritionnels doivent être apportés très tôt pour avoir le meilleur effet possible. La maladie cardiaque coronarienne est une maladie familiale et son contrôle de même que son traitement doivent être envisagés selon une perspective familiale. La prévention primaire des maladies cardiaques coronariennes dépend de la prévention de l'hyperlipidémie induite par le régime alimentaire.

22

Rapport entre le cholestérol sanguin et l'incidence des accidents vasculaires cérébraux spécifiques de type chez des Japonais d'Honolulu

Katsuhiko Yano, MD et Dwayne M. Reed, MD, PhD

Principal chercheur
Honolulu Heart Program
Honolulu, Hawaii, États-Unis

Dans le cadre d'un suivi moyen de 20 ans de 7 850 Japonais d'Hawaii âgés entre 45 et 68 ans qui, au début du suivi n'avaient jamais eu d'accident vasculaire cérébral, 523 ont fait un accident vasculaire cérébral dont 38 avec hémorragie sous-arachnoïdienne, 78 avec hémorragie intra-cérébrale, 350 avec thromboembolie et 52 avec complications non spécifiques. Les taux d'incidence ajustés en fonction de l'âge révèlent l'existence d'un rapport inverse entre le taux de cholestérol sanguin total au départ et les hémorragies sous-arachonidiennes ($p=0,054$) et intra-cérébrales ($p=0,015$) et d'un rapport direct avec les thromboembolies ($p=0,045$). D'autres ajustements en fonction des facteurs de risque comme l'hypertension, le diabète, l'indice de masse corporelle, le tabagisme et la consommation d'alcool révèlent que seul le rapport inverse entre le cholestérol sanguin et les hémorragies intracérébrales demeure significatif au titre du risque relatif de 0,46 du quintile inférieur/supérieur (intervalle de confiance de 95 % : 0,24, 0,88). Des analyses distinctes effectuées pour les hommes hypertendus et normotendus ont démontré que le rapport inverse avec les hémorragies intracérébrales et le rapport direct avec les thromboembolies n'était significatif que pour les hommes normotendus. Toutefois, les tests statistiques sur l'interaction entre le cholestérol sanguin, la pression artérielle et les risques d'accident vasculaire cérébral ont tous été négatifs. Par conséquent, il semble qu'un faible taux de cholestérol sanguin, notamment inférieur à 4,14 mmol/L (160 mg/dl), augmente significativement les risques d'hémorragie intracérébrale même après ajustement en fonction d'autres facteurs de risque.

23

Dyslipidémie et prévention primaire des maladies cardiaques coronariennes : réflexions sur quelques problèmes non résolus de politique

C. David Naylor, MD, DPhil, FRCP(C)

Directeur
Unité d'épidémiologie clinique
et département de médecine
Centre des sciences de la santé Sunnybrook
Université de Toronto
Toronto, Ontario, Canada

L'Europe et l'Amérique du Nord ont promulgué des directives pour la prévention des maladies cardiaques coronariennes, lesquelles consistent dans le dépistage des profils lipidiques anormaux et la manipulation des lipides sanguins. Ces directives diffèrent à plusieurs titres : populations cibles pour le dépistage des cas; tests à utiliser; seuils à partir desquels des interventions plus poussées doivent être menées; facteurs de risque pris en compte dans les décisions thérapeutiques; distinctions entre prévention primaire et secondaire et rôle d'une stratégie à l'échelle de la population. Les différents comités de spécialistes, organismes et groupes de travail avaient tous à leur disposition les mêmes preuves. Les divergences entre les politiques cliniques et publiques de chaque pays témoignent avec éloquence des différences d'interprétation, des priorités et valeurs sociales perçues et (par-dessous tout) des priorités et valeurs des spécialistes et des personnes qui les nomment.

Cette communication sera par conséquent axée sur plusieurs questions non résolues de politique publique et clinique.

1. Valeur prédictive et mauvaise classification des pronostics avec les stratégies de test actuelles.
2. Compatibilité entre l'intensité du traitement et les risques réversibles dans le cadre d'une maladie multifactorielle.
3. Preuves obtenues dans le cadre d'essais : problèmes inhérents à leur généralisation et conception.
4. Problèmes de la mortalité toutes causes confondues : préoccupations au titre des politiques publiques et cliniques.
5. Rôle des préférences des patients dans la prise de décisions et inutilité du traitement dans la détermination d'une politique globale.
6. Problèmes de décompte et de préférence temporelle dans les décisions politiques et le choix des traitements.
7. Prévention primaire - prévention secondaire : excès de zèle?

24
Congrès du consensus canadien sur le cholestérol

Louis Horlick, MD, FRCP(C), FACP
Professeur de médecine (émérite)
Département de médecine
Université de Saskatchewan
Hôpital universitaire Royal
Saskatoon, Saskatchewan, Canada

Les études épidémiologiques entreprises au Canada ont révélé l'existence de facteurs de risque importants des maladies cardiaques coronariennes. L'étude sur la santé cardiaque de Nouvelle-Écosse entreprise en 1987 démontre que 39 % des hommes et 31 % des femmes âgés de 35 à 64 ans ont des taux de cholestérol sanguin supérieurs à 220 mg/dl. Elle montre également que 29 % seulement des personnes âgées de 17 à 74 ans, tous sexes confondus, sont exemptes des trois principaux facteurs de risque (hypercholestérolémie, hypertension, tabagisme). Ce sont ces données qui ont conduit à l'adoption d'une stratégie globale de contrôle de l'hypercholestérolémie. Elle consiste dans l'adoption de stratégies de promotion de la santé à l'échelle de la population avec intervention sur tous les facteurs de risque plutôt que sur le cholestérol seulement. Pour ce faire, elle suppose la participation globale de tout le personnel des services de santé, à tous les paliers du gouvernement. Nous avons par conséquent formulé des recommandations importantes sur les changements alimentaires préconisés pour l'ensemble de la population, sur les produits alimentaires et sur l'objectif à atteindre en matière de cholestérol total. Nous nous éloignons à cet égard du consensus américain qui a opté pour une stratégie de dépistage des cas à haut risque.

Nous n'avons pas pour autant négligé le problème des personnes à haut risque dans notre société. Nous y donnons toutefois une moins grande priorité comparativement à l'approche globale. Le comité a recommandé le dépistage des personnes connues pour être à risque et réserve le dépistage universel à une époque où les ressources le permettront. Il énumère les paramètres lipidiques à dépister et formule ensuite des recommandations fondamentales en matière d'intervention. Le traitement consiste essentiellement dans une série d'interventions alimentaires et seuls des conseils d'ordre général sont formulés sur les traitements médicamenteux. Des points de coupure simplifiés ont été utilisés, divisés en deux catégories d'âge, indépendamment du sexe. Pour les femmes et les hommes de plus de 30 ans, un taux de cholestérol sanguin inférieur à 200 mg/dl est jugé acceptable et devrait être vérifié tous les cinq ans. Les personnes dont le taux de cholestérol se situe entre 200 et

240 mg/dl doivent pouvoir avoir accès à des conseils alimentaires et ceux dont le taux de cholestérol LDL est supérieur à 130 ou le cholestérol HDL inférieur à 35 mg/dl doivent suivre un régime alimentaire intensif. Les taux de cholestérol supérieurs à 240 mg/dl qui sont réfractaires à un régime alimentaire intensif devront par conséquent faire l'objet d'une intervention pharmacologique.

Il va sans dire qu'une approche rigoureuse orientée vers les personnes à haut risque est très coûteuse pour le système des soins de santé et risque de créer des problèmes importants aux médecins, aux diététistes et aux services de laboratoire. L'application d'un modèle de population/santé publique devrait considérablement minimiser les problèmes à ce chapitre.

Index